HOW THE Brain Learns to Read

David A. Sousa

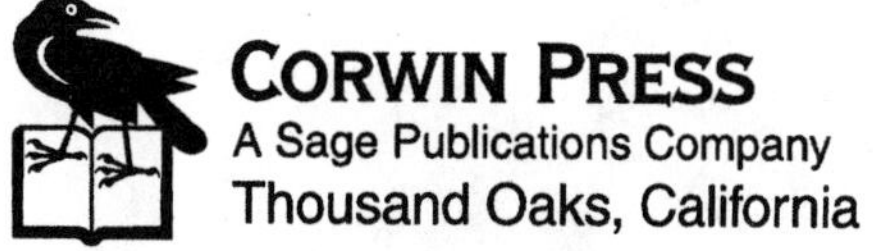

For information:

Corwin Press
A Sage Publications Company
2455 Teller Road
Thousand Oaks, California 91320
www.corwinpress.com

Sage Publications Ltd.
1 Oliver's Yard
55 City Road
London EC1Y 1SP
United Kingdom

Sage Publications India Pvt. Ltd.
B-42 Panchsheel Enclave
Post Box 4109
New Delhi 110 017 India

Printed in the United States of America

Library of Congress Cataloging-in-Publication Data

Sousa, David A.
How the brain learns to read / David A. Sousa.
p. cm.
Includes bibliographical references and index.
ISBN 1-4129-0600-8 (cloth) — ISBN 1-4129-0601-6 (pbk.)
1. Reading. 2. Reading disability—Physiological aspects.
3. Brain. I. Title.
LB1573.S7845 2005
418'.4'019—dc22 2004052713

This book is printed on acid-free paper.

05 06 10 9 8 7 6 5 4 3

Acquisitions Editor: Robert D. Clouse
Editorial Assistant: Jingle Vea
Production Editor: Diane S. Foster
Typesetter: C&M Digitals (P) Ltd.
Proofreader: Kristen Bergstad
Cover Designer: Tracy E. Miller
Graphic Designer: Anthony Paular

Contents

Acknowledgments

Corwin Press gratefully acknowledges the contributions of the following people:

Sandra Anderson
Educational Consultant
Exemplary Education, L.L.C.
Newcastle, VA

Lori Benton
Reading Specialist
Oakshire Elementary School
Orlando, FL

Diane Barone
Professor, Literacy Studies
Department of Educational Studies
University of Nevada, Reno
Reno, NV

Aileen Carew
Reading Specialist
Bel Aire School
Tiburon, CA

Robin Fogarty
Professional Development Consultant
Robin Fogarty & Associates, Ltd.
Chicago, IL

Jeanine Heil
Professional Development Coordinator
Office of Reading First
N. J. Department of Education
Trenton, NJ

Natalie McAvoy
Reading Specialist
Tibbets Elementary School
Elkhorn, WI

Harvey F. Silver & Richard Strong
Educational Consultants
Silver Strong Associates
Ho-Ho-Kus, NJ

Marilee Sprenger
Educational Consultant
Peoria, IL

Barbara Townsend
Reading Specialist
West Side Elementary School
Elkhorn, WI

Pat Wolfe
Educational Consultant
Napa, CA

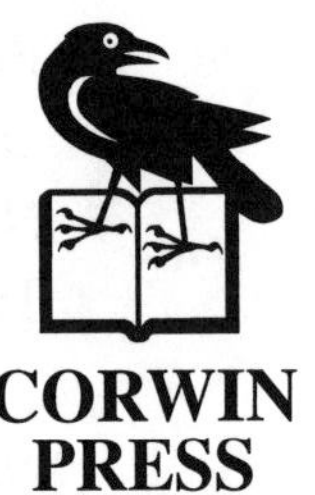

The Corwin Press logo—a raven striding across an open book—represents the union of courage and learning. Corwin Press is committed to improving education for all learners by publishing books and other professional development resources for those serving the field of K–12 education. By providing practical, hands-on materials, Corwin Press continues to carry out the promise of its motto: **"Helping Educators Do Their Work Better."**

About the Author

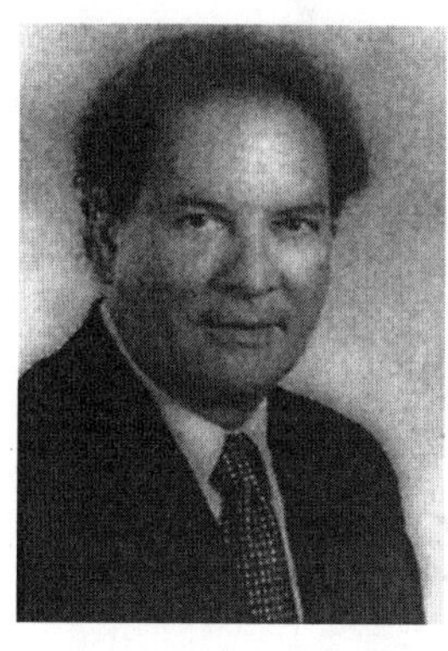

David A. Sousa, Ed.D., is an international educational consultant. He has made presentations at national conventions of educational organizations and has conducted workshops on brain research and science education in hundreds of school districts and at several colleges and universities across the United States, Canada, Europe, and Asia.

Dr. Sousa has a bachelor of science degree in chemistry from Massachusetts State College at Bridgewater, a master of arts in teaching degree in science from Harvard University, and a doctorate from Rutgers University. His teaching experience covers all levels. He has taught junior and senior high school science, served as a K–12 director of science, and was Supervisor of Instruction for the West Orange, New Jersey, schools. He then became superintendent of the New Providence, New Jersey, public schools. He has been an adjunct professor of education at Seton Hall University, and a visiting lecturer at Rutgers University. He was president of the National Staff Development Council in 1992.

Dr. Sousa has edited science books and published numerous articles in leading educational journals on staff development, science education, and brain research. He has received awards from professional associations and school districts for his commitment and contributions to research, staff development, and science education. He recently received the Distinguished Alumni Award and an honorary doctorate in education from Bridgewater (Mass.) State College.

He has appeared on the NBC *Today* show and on National Public Radio to discuss his work with schools using brain research. He makes his home in south Florida.

Reading is to the mind what exercise is to the body.

— Sir Richard Steele

Introduction

Most of us don't recall much about learning to talk. It just seemed to come naturally. We probably don't remember much about how we learned to read either. As adults, reading seems so effortless and automatic that we often assume it should be an easy skill for almost any child to acquire. But that is not the case. Learning to speak is an innate ability supported by specialized areas of the brain, and is automatic for almost all children raised in normal circumstances. But for many children, learning to read is a long, complicated task requiring years of conscious effort.

Have you ever thought about what your brain goes through when you read? First, your eyes have to scan those squiggly lines and curves called the alphabet and group them into the words as indicated on the page. Then, certain areas of the brain work to associate the written symbols with the sounds of language already stored in your head. As this association occurs, other neural networks decode the writing into a mental message that you understand. Incredibly, your brain can process and comprehend an entire sentence in a few seconds. It almost seems like magic. But it isn't magic. Reading is the result of an elaborate process that involves decoding abstract symbols into sounds, then into words that generate meaning. Can you remember the first time you encountered printed text and saw those letters? Just turn this page upside down and you get an idea of how alien those squiggles must have looked at first and what a struggle it was to make sense of them.

THE BAD NEWS AND THE GOOD NEWS

The Bad News

Educators have been well aware of the difficulties involved in learning to read and have long debated the best ways to teach beginning reading. No one method or program has triumphed, as evidenced by the lack of substantial progress in improving reading achievement scores. Despite all the time and resources devoted to reading programs, nearly two-thirds of low-income fourth graders cannot read at the proficient level. Grade 8 students have made no gains in reading achievement in the past decade, and the reading scores of grade 12 students have actually declined in that same time period (NAEP, 2003). The number of students identified with reading problems, including dyslexia, is growing rapidly. No one is sure if this is because more students are developing difficulties in reading or whether school districts are getting better at diagnosing previously unidentified students. One thing seems certain: Students who are poor readers in their early years remain poor readers in their later years.

A decades-long battle over the best way to help children learn to read has only polarized the educational community. Critics argue that reading instruction has been out of touch with research in that too many programs minimize the teaching of phoneme-grapheme relationships. The selection of reading programs has often been fueled by debates of philosophical stances and advocacies that have little to do with what research is uncovering about how children learn to read.

The Good News

Scientific methods are now available to study how the brain acquires reading skills. In the last two decades, brain researchers have developed new technologies for looking inside the living brain. These technologies fall into two major categories: those that look at brain *structure* and those that look at brain *function*. When aimed at the brain, computerized axial tomography (CAT) and magnetic resonance imaging (MRI) are very useful diagnostic tools that produce computer images of the brain's internal structure. For example, they can detect tumors, malformations, and the damage caused by cerebral hemorrhages.

Different technologies, however, are required to look at how the brain works. An alphabet soup describes the five most common procedures that can be used to isolate and identify the areas of the brain where distinct levels of activity are occurring. The technologies are the following:

- Electroencephalography (EEG)
- Magnetoencephalography (MEG)
- Positron Emission Tomography (PET)
- Functional Magnetic Resonance Imaging (fMRI)
- Functional Magnetic Resonance Spectroscopy (fMRS)

Here is a brief explanation of how each one works. A summary chart follows.

- ***Electroencephalography (EEG) and Magnetoencephalography (MEG).*** These two techniques are helpful in determining how quickly something occurs in the brain. To do that, they measure electrical and magnetic activity occurring in the brain during mental processing. In an EEG, anywhere from 19 to 128 electrodes are attached to various positions on the scalp with a conductive gel so electrical signals can be recorded in a computer. In a MEG, about 100 magnetic detectors are placed around the head to record magnetic activity. EEGs and MEGs can record changes in brain activity that occur as rapidly as one millisecond (one-thousandth of a second), typical times when the brain is processing language. When a group of neurons responds to a specific event (like a word), they activate and their electrical and magnetic activity can be detected above the noise of the nonactivated neurons. This response is called an *Event-Related Potential* or ERP. ERP evidence has provided information about the time needed for the brain to process reading, including times associated with recognizing the letters and hearing the sounds in one's head. EEG and MEG do not expose the subject to radiation and are not considered hazardous.

- ***Positron Emission Tomography (PET).*** The first technology to observe brain functions, it involves injecting the subject with a radioactive solution that circulates to the brain. Brain regions of higher activity accumulate more of the radiation, which is picked up by a ring of detectors around the subject's head. A computer displays the concentration of radiation as a picture of blood flow in a cross-sectional slice of the brain regions that are aligned with the detectors. The picture is in color, with the more active areas in reds and yellows, the quieter areas in blues and greens. Two major drawbacks to PET scans are the invasive nature of the injection and the use of radioactive materials. Consequently, this technique is not used with normal children because the radioactive risk is too high.
- ***Functional Magnetic Resonance Imaging (fMRI).*** This newer technology is rapidly replacing PET scans because it is painless, noninvasive, and does not use radiation. The technology helps to pinpoint the brain areas of greater and lesser activity. Its operation is based on the fact that when any part of the brain is used for thinking, the need for oxygen and nutrients increases. Oxygen is carried to the brain cells by hemoglobin. Hemoglobin contains iron, which is magnetic. The fMRI uses a large magnet to compare the amount of oxygenated hemoglobin entering brain cells with the amount of deoxygenated hemoglobin leaving the cells. The computer colors in the brain regions receiving more oxygenated blood and can locate the activated brain region to within one centimeter (less than a half-inch).
- ***Functional Magnetic Resonance Spectroscopy (fMRS).*** This technology involves the same equipment as fMRI but uses different computer software to record levels of various chemicals in the brain while the subject is thinking. Like the fMRI, fMRS can precisely pinpoint the area of activity, but it can also identify whether certain key chemicals are also present at the activation site. fMRS has been used to study language function in the brain by mapping the change in specific chemicals, such as lactate, that respond to brain activation during tasks involving language.

Techniques for Mapping Brain Functions		
Technique	**What It Measures**	**How It Works**
Electroencephalography (EEG) Magnetoencephalography (MEG)	The electrical and magnetic activity occurring in the brain during mental processing. The spikes of activity are called Event-Related Potentials (ERP).	In EEG, multiple electrodes are attached to the scalp to record electrical signals in a computer. In MEG, magnetic detectors are placed around the head to record magnetic activity. EEGs and MEGs record changes in brain activity that occur as rapidly as one millisecond. When a group of neurons responds to a specific event, they activate and their electrical and magnetic activity can be detected. This response is called an Event-Related Potential or ERP.
Positron Emission Tomography (PET)	Amount of radiation present in brain regions	The subject is injected with a radioactive solution that circulates to the brain. Brain regions of higher activity accumulate more radiation, which is picked up by a ring of detectors. A computer displays the concentration of radiation in a cross-sectional slice of the brain regions aligned with the detectors. The picture shows the more active areas in reds and yellows, the quieter areas in blues and greens.
Functional Magnetic Resonance Imaging (fMRI)	Levels of deoxygenated hemoglobin in brain cells	Any part of the brain that is thinking requires more oxygen, which is carried to the brain cells by hemoglobin. The fMRI uses a large magnet to compare the amount of oxygenated hemoglobin entering brain cells with the amount of deoxygenated hemoglobin leaving the cells. The computer colors in the brain regions receiving more oxygenated blood and locates the activated brain region to within one centimeter (half-inch).
Functional Magnetic Resonance Spectroscopy (fMRS)	Levels of specific chemicals present during brain activity	This technology involves the same equipment as fMRI but uses different computer software to record levels of various chemicals in the brain while the subject is thinking. fMRS can precisely pinpoint the area of activity, but it can also identify whether certain key chemicals are also present at the activation site.

Using these technologies, researchers have been able to explore how different brains function when carrying out certain tasks, including reading. Here are just a few of the fascinating things that have been uncovered:

- Novice readers use different cerebral pathways while reading than skilled readers
- People with reading difficulties use different brain regions to decode written text than do typical readers
- The brains of people with reading problems are working harder during reading than those of skilled readers
- Even though dyslexia is a brain disorder, it is treatable
- With proper instructional intervention, the brains of young struggling and dyslexic readers can actually be rewired to use cerebral areas that more closely resemble those used by typical readers

As a result of these discoveries, it is now possible to identify with a high degree of accuracy those children who are at greatest risk of reading problems, even before the problems develop, to diagnose the problems accurately, and to manage the problems with effective and proven treatment programs (Shaywitz, 2003). It is not exaggerating to say that reading is very likely the one area of school curriculum to date where neuroscience and cognitive psychology have made their greatest impact. The brain imaging studies have opened a new field in neuroscience that some call developmental cognitive neurology (Habib, 2003). Here one observes how the developing brain reacts to various kinds of environmental constraints. Future studies will enable scientists and educators to work together to better understand both the typical brain as well as the causes and possible treatments for learning deficiencies, including dyslexia.

> It is not exaggerating to say that reading is very likely the one area of school curriculum where neuroscience has made its greatest impact.

ABOUT THIS BOOK

I have been asked on many occasions to give specific examples of how the fruits of scientific research can have an impact on educational practice. That question is a lot easier to answer now than it was 15 years ago because recent discoveries in cognitive neuroscience have given us a deeper understanding of the brain. We now have more knowledge of our short-term and long-term memory systems, the impact of emotions on learning, and how we acquire language and motor skills. But the greatest contribution to date, in my opinion, is the growing body of research on how the brain learns to read.

Because reading is essential for success in our society, teaching all children to read is every school district's highest curriculum priority. Although many children learn to read well, too large a number encounter difficulties. Numerous reasons are cited for this unfortunate situation, such as poor home environment, physical and psychological deficits, and inadequate reading instruction. Regardless of the reasons, teachers of reading are still faced with the awesome responsibility of getting each child to learn the difficult task of reading. The more these teachers know about how the brain learns to read, the more likely they are to choose instructional strategies that will result in successful learning. The purpose of this book is to present what scientists currently believe about how young humans acquire spoken language and then use that capability when learning to read.

Questions This Book Will Answer

This book will answer questions such as these:

- *How do we learn spoken language?*
- *Does a family's socioeconomic status affect a child's vocabulary development?*
- *What must the brain be able to do in order to learn to read effectively?*
- *What has research found out about the effectiveness of the phonics and whole-language approaches to reading instruction?*
- *What are the implications of the current research in reading on everyday classroom practice?*
- *How important is spelling and invented spelling in learning to read?*
- *What strategies are effective in teaching students with limited English proficiency to read?*
- *Why is reading so difficult for so many children?*
- *What do we mean by reading problems?*
- *What have brain imaging scans revealed about the nature of dyslexia?*
- *How can elementary and secondary school classroom teachers successfully detect reading problems?*
- *What are the basic ingredients of successful early intervention programs?*
- *How have some intervention programs actually rewired the brains of struggling readers?*
- *What can secondary school content area teachers do to help their poor readers be more successful in comprehending the course material?*
- *What are the basics of a successful reading program?*
- *What do beginning readers need to learn and what do teachers need to know about teaching reading?*

Chapter Contents

Chapter 1. Learning Spoken Language. Children's competence in spoken language greatly influences how quickly and successfully they learn to read. This chapter examines how the young brain detects language sounds from the background noise and begins to recognize the words, pitch, and tempo of a native language. It looks at the specialized regions of the brain that work together and manipulate sounds to build words, phrases, and sentences, and at how the brain cleverly groups words and phrases to increase the speed of spoken language comprehension.

Chapter 2. Learning to Read. This chapter explores the various stages that the brain must go through while learning to read, including the process of building sounds into words, words into phrases, and phrases into sentences. The alphabetic principle is introduced here as well as the roles that short-term and long-term memories play in reading. Also discussed here are the fascinating discoveries that brain imaging scans have revealed about the cerebral mechanisms responsible for decoding written text and the different neural pathways used by novice and skilled readers.

Chapter 3. Teaching Reading. This chapter reviews the history of the debate over whether phonics or whole-language is the better method for beginning reading instruction. It cites the scientific studies that have gained a deeper understanding of how the brain learns to read. From these studies come valuable implications that educators can consider when deciding on the components of a reading program and on selecting instructional strategies in beginning reading that are likely to be more successful with more students.

Chapter 4. Recognizing Reading Problems. Because early detection of reading problems is essential for early intervention, this chapter focuses on the potential causes of reading difficulties, including what brain imaging scans have revealed about the nature of struggling readers and dyslexia. Also discussed here are the clues that teachers should look for at various grade levels to determine whether a student is having persistent difficulties with reading.

Chapter 5. Overcoming Reading Problems. Numerous suggestions are offered in this chapter for teachers and parents to help students overcome their reading problems. The components of early intervention programs are discussed in some detail as well as successful strategies for older students. Featured here is a discovery of great interest that came from imaging studies: certain reading interventions can actually rewire the brains of struggling readers so that they more closely resemble the neural mechanisms used for reading in the brains of skilled readers.

Chapter 6. Reading in the Content Areas. This chapter discusses the major differences between developmental reading (learning to read) and content area reading (reading to learn). It presents some tested strategies that secondary school content area teachers can use with students who are poor readers to help them understand vocabulary and gain a more accurate and deeper understanding of the content material they are reading. It highlights the value of graphic organizers and suggests some reading patterns that are unique to different subject areas.

Chapter 7. Putting It All Together. Finally, this chapter examines the essential pieces that are needed to develop, select, implement, and support an effective reading program, based on our current scientific understandings of how the brain learns to read. It suggests what beginning readers need to learn, what teachers need to know about teaching reading, and what kind of professional development needs to be implemented to support the reading program. Some suggestions for closing the reading achievement gap are proposed.

Most of the chapters contain suggestions for translating the research on reading into instructional practice. These suggestions are indicated with a checkmark (✓).

The information presented here was current at the time of publication. However, as scientists continue to explore the inner workings of the brain, they will likely discover more about the cerebral mechanisms involved in learning to read. These discoveries should help parents and educators understand more about reading, reading problems, and effective reading instruction.

ASSESSING YOUR CURRENT KNOWLEDGE OF READING

The value of this book can be measured in part by how much it enhances your knowledge about reading . This might be a good time for you to take the following true-false test and assess your current understanding of some concepts related to language, learning to read, reading difficulties, and reading instruction. Decide whether the statements are generally true or false and circle T or F. Explanations for the answers are identified throughout the book in special boxes.

1. **T** **F** The brain's ability to learn spoken language improves for most people during their early 20s.
2. **T** **F** Learning to read, like learning spoken language, is a natural ability.
3. **T** **F** There are about 200 ways to spell the sounds of the 44 phonemes in English.
4. **T** **F** Research studies have concluded that neither the phonological approach nor the whole-language approach is more effective in teaching most children how to read.
5. **T** **F** Non-English-speaking children can be taught to read English even if their spoken English vocabulary is weak.
6. **T** **F** Most children with attention-deficit hyperactivity disorder (ADHD) are also dyslexic.
7. **T** **F** Dyslexic students often have problems in other cognitive areas.
8. **T** **F** Many poor readers have attention problems that schools are not equipped to handle.
9. **T** **F** There is little that secondary school content area teachers can do to improve the comprehension skills of their students who are poor readers.

Children must learn to speak before they can learn to read. How we acquire spoken language is the subject of the first chapter.

CHAPTER 1
Learning Spoken Language

This chapter addresses several basic questions about how the human brain learns spoken language. They include:

- *Why does spoken language come so easily?*
- *How does a child's brain detect language sounds from background noise?*
- *Does a family's socioeconomic status really affect a child's vocabulary growth?*
- *How does a child learn the irregular forms of verbs?*
- *Can children tell the difference between explicit and inferred comprehension?*

How quickly and successfully the brain learns to read is greatly influenced by the spoken language competence the child has developed. How broad is the child's vocabulary? How many grammatical errors appear in speech? How sophisticated is the sentence structure? How well does the child comprehend variations in sentence structure? The answers to these questions help in determining the breadth and depth of the child's spoken language networks and become the starting points for assessing how well the child will learn to read. Therefore, it is important to understand what cognitive neuroscience has revealed about how the brain acquires and processes spoken words. Figure 1.1 presents a general timeline for spoken language development during the first three years of growth. The chart is a rough approximation. Obviously, some children will progress faster or slower than the chart indicates. Nonetheless, it is a useful guide to show the progression of skills acquired during the process of learning language.

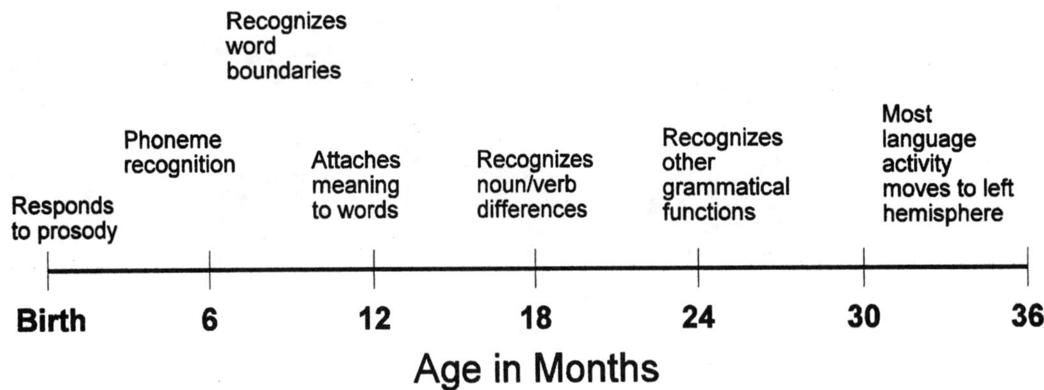

Figure 1.1 An average timeline of spoken language development during the child's first three years. There is considerable variation among individual children.

SPOKEN LANGUAGE COMES NATURALLY

One of the most extraordinary features of the human brain is its ability to acquire spoken language quickly and accurately. We are born with an innate capacity to distinguish the distinct sounds (phonemes) of all the languages on this planet. Eventually, we are able to associate those sounds with arbitrary written symbols to express our thoughts and emotions to others.

Other animals have developed ways to communicate with members of their species. Birds and apes bow and wave appendages; honeybees dance to map out the location of food; and even one-celled animals can signal neighbors by emitting an array of different chemicals. By contrast, human beings have developed an elaborate and complex means of spoken communication that many say is largely responsible for our place as the dominant species on this planet. Spoken language is truly a marvelous accomplishment for many reasons. At the very least, it gives form to our memories and words to express our thoughts. A single human voice can pronounce all the hundreds of vowel and consonant sounds that allow it to speak any of the estimated 6,500 languages that exist today. With practice, the voice becomes so fine-tuned that it makes only about one sound error per million sounds and one word error per million words (Pinker, 1994).

Before the advent of scanning technologies, we explained how the brain produced spoken language on the basis of evidence from injured brains. In 1861, French physician Paul Broca noticed that patients with brain damage to an area near the left temple understood

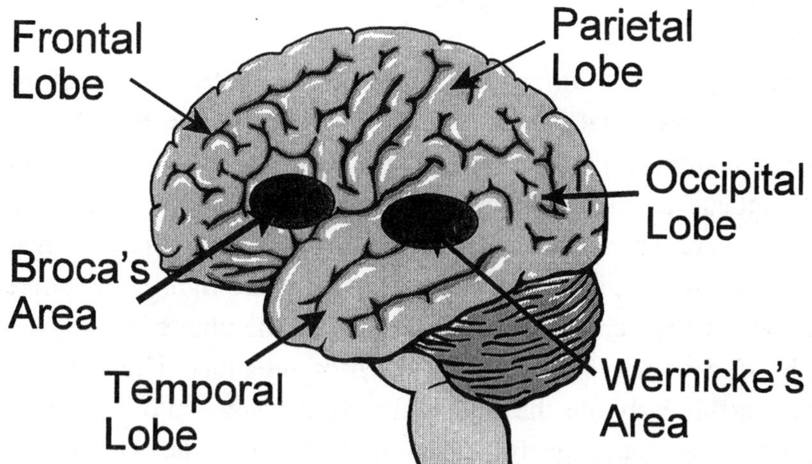

Figure 1.2 The language system in the left hemisphere is comprised mainly of Broca's area and Wernicke's area. The four lobes of the brain are also identified.

language but had difficulty speaking, a condition known as *aphasia.* About the size of a quarter, this region of the brain is commonly referred to as Broca's area (Figure 1.2).

In 1881, German neurologist Carl Wernicke described a different type of aphasia—one in which patients could not make sense out of words they spoke or heard. These patients had damage in the left temporal lobe. Now called Wernicke's area, it is located above the left ear and is about the size of a silver dollar. Those with damage to Wernicke's area could speak fluently, but what they said was quite meaningless. Ever since Broca discovered that the left hemisphere of the brain was specialized for language, researchers have attempted to understand the way in which normal human beings acquire and process their native language.

Processing Spoken Language

Recent research, using scanners, indicates that spoken language production is a far more complex process than previously thought. When preparing to produce a spoken sentence, the brain uses not only Broca's and Wernicke's areas, but also calls on several other neural networks scattered throughout the left hemisphere. Nouns are processed through one set of patterns; verbs are processed by separate neural networks. The more complex the sentence structure, the more areas that are activated, including the right hemisphere.

In most people, the left hemisphere is home to the major components of the language processing system. Broca's area is a region of the left frontal lobe that is believed to be responsible for processing vocabulary, syntax (how word order affects meaning), and rules of grammar. Wernicke's area is part of the left temporal lobe and is thought to process the sense and meaning of language. However, the emotional content of language is governed by areas in the right hemisphere.

Brain imaging studies of infants as young as four months of age confirm that the brain possesses neural networks that specialize in responding to the auditory components of language. Dehaene-Lambertz (2000) used EEG recordings to measure the brain activity of 16 four-month-old infants as they listened to language syllables and acoustic tones. After numerous trials, the data showed that syllables and tones were processed primarily in different areas of the left hemisphere, although there was also some right hemisphere activity. For language input, various features, such as the voice and the phonetic category of a syllable, were encoded by separate neural networks into sensory memory. These remarkable findings suggest that, even at this early age, the brain is already organized into functional networks that can distinguish between language fragments and other sounds. Another recent study of families with severe speech and language disorders has isolated a mutated gene believed to be responsible for their deficits. This discovery lends further credence to the notion that the ability to acquire spoken language is encoded in our genes (Lai, Fisher, Hurst, Vargha-Khadem, and Monaco, 2001).

The apparent genetic predisposition of the brain to the sounds of language explains why normal young children respond to and acquire spoken language quickly. After the first year in a language environment, the child becomes increasingly able to differentiate those sounds heard in the native language and begins to lose the ability to perceive other sounds. How long the brain retains this responsiveness to the sounds of language is still open to question. However, there does seem to be general agreement among researchers that the window of opportunity for acquiring language within the language-specific areas of the brain begins to diminish for most people around 10 to 12 years of age. Obviously, one can still acquire a new language after that age, but it takes more effort because the new language will be spatially separated in the brain from the native language areas (Gazzaniga, 1998). PET scans show that when children grow up learning two languages, all language activity is found in the same areas of the brain; those who learn a second language at a later age show that the two language areas are spatially separated (Kim, Relkin, Lee, and Hirsch, 1997).

> Most researchers agree that acquiring language within the language-specific areas of the brain diminishes for most people around 10 to 12 years of age.

Gender Differences in Language Processing

One of the earliest and most interesting discoveries neuroscientists made with functional imaging was that there were differences in the way male and female brains process language. Male brains tend to process language in the left hemisphere, while most female brains process language in both hemispheres. Figure 1.3 shows representational fMRIs with the solid white areas indicating areas of the brain that were activated during language processing. Of even greater interest was that these same cerebral areas in both genders were also activated during reading.

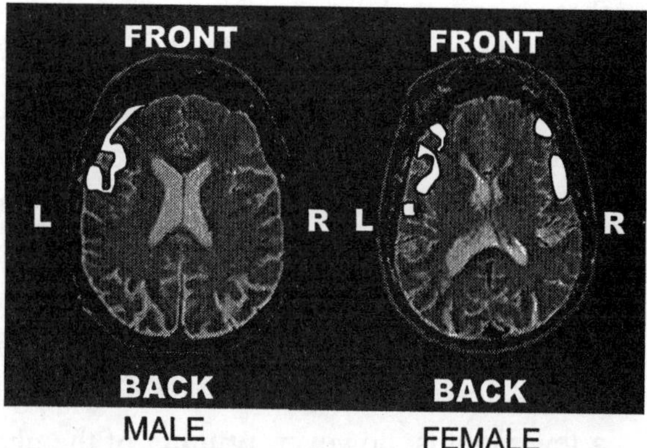

Figure 1.3 These are combined representational fMRIs showing the solid white areas of the male and female brains that were activated during language processing (Shaywitz et al., 1995).

Another interesting gender difference is the observation that the large bundle of neurons that connects the two hemispheres and allows them to communicate (called the *corpus callosum*) is proportionately larger and thicker in the female than in the male. Assuming function follows form, this difference implies that information travels between the two cerebral hemispheres more efficiently in females than in males. The combination of dual-hemisphere language processing and more efficient between-hemisphere communications may account for why young girls generally acquire spoken language easier and more quickly than young boys.

> **Answer to Test Question # 1**
>
> **Question:** The brain's ability to learn spoken language improves for most people during their early 20s.
>
> **Answer:** *False.* Numerous studies show that the brain's ability to acquire spoken language is best during the first 10 years. Of course, people can learn a new language any time during their lives. It will just take more effort.

STRUCTURE OF LANGUAGE

Learning Phonemes

Languages consist of distinct units of sound called *phonemes*. Although each language has its own unique set of phonemes, only about 150 phonemes comprise all the world's languages. These phonemes consist of all the speech sounds that can be made by the human voice apparatus. Phonemes combine to form syllables. For example, in English, the consonant sound "t" and the vowel sound "o" are both phonemes that combine to form the syllable *to-*, as in *tomato.* Although the infant's brain can perceive the entire range of phonemes, only those that are repeated get attention, as the neurons reacting to the unique sound patterns are continually stimulated and reinforced.

At birth (some say even before birth) babies respond first to the prosody—the rhythm, cadence, and pitch—of their mothers' voice, not the words. Around the age of six months or so, infants start babbling, an early sign of language acquisition. The production of phonemes by infants is the result of genetically determined neural programs; however, language exposure is environmental. These two components interact to produce an individual's language system and, assuming no abnormal conditions, sufficient competence to communicate clearly with others. Their babbling consists of all those phonemes, even ones they have never heard. Within a few months, however, pruning of the phonemes begins, and by about one year of age, the neural networks focus on the sounds of the language being spoken in the infant's environment (Beatty, 2001).

Learning Words and Morphemes

The next step for the brain is to detect words from the stream of sounds it is processing. This is not an easy task because people don't pause between words when speaking. Yet the brain has to recognize differences between, say, *green house* and *greenhouse*. Studies show that parents help this process along by slipping automatically into a different speech pattern when talking to their babies than when speaking to adults. Mothers tend to go into a teaching mode with the vowels elongated and emphasized. They speak to their babies in a higher pitch, with a special intonation, rhythm, and feeling. The researchers suggested that mothers are instinctively attempting to help their babies recognize the sounds of language. Researchers found this pattern in other languages as well, such as Russian, Swedish, and Japanese (Burnham, Kitamura, and Vollmer-Conna, 2002).

Remarkably, babies begin to distinguish word boundaries by the age of 8 months even though they don't know what the words mean (Van Petten and Bloom, 1999). They now begin to acquire new vocabulary words at the rate of about seven to 10 a day. By the age of 10 to 12 months, the toddler's brain has begun to distinguish and remember phonemes of the native language and to ignore foreign sounds. For example, one study showed that at the age of 6 months, American and Japanese babies are equally good at discriminating between the "l" and "r" sounds, even though Japanese has no "l" sound. However, by age 10 months, Japanese babies have a tougher time making the distinction, while American babies have become much better at it. During this and subsequent periods of growth, one's ability to distinguish native sounds improves, while the ability to distinguish nonnative speech sounds diminishes (Cheour et al., 1998). Soon, *morphemes,* such as *-s, -ed,* and *-ing,* are added to their speaking vocabulary. At the same time, working memory and Wernicke's areas are becoming fully functional so the child can now attach meaning to words. Of course, learning words is one skill; putting them together to make sense is another, more complex skill.

Verbal- and Image-Based Words

How quickly a child understands words may be closely related to whether the word can generate a clear mental image. A word like *elephant* generates a picture in the mind's eye and thus can be more easily understood than an abstract word like *justice*. Could it be that the brain maintains two distinct systems to process image-loaded words and abstract words?

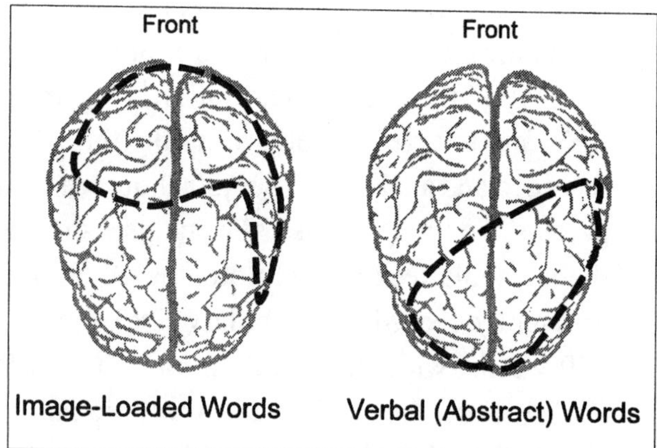

Figure 1.4 The dotted regions represent the areas of highest event-related potentials when subjects processed image-loaded words or verbal (abstract) words (Swaab, et al., 2002).

To further investigate this point, Swaab and her colleagues used numerous electroencephalographs (EEGs) to measure the brain's response to concrete and abstract words in a dozen young adults (Swaab, Baynes, and Knight, 2002). EEGs measure changes in brain wave activity, called *event-related potentials (ERPs),* when the brain experiences a stimulus. The researchers found that image-loaded words produced more ERPs in the front area (frontal lobe–the part thought to be associated with imagery) while abstract words produced more ERPs in the top central (the parietal lobe) and rear (the occipital lobe) areas. Furthermore, there was little interaction between these disparate areas when processing any of the words (Figure 1.4). The results support the idea that the brain may hold two separate stores for *semantics* (meaning), one for verbal-based information and the other for image-based information. This discovery has implications for language instruction. Teachers should use concrete images when presenting an abstract concept. For example, teaching the idea of justice could be accompanied by pictures of a judge in robes, the scales of justice, and a courtroom scene.

> Teachers should use concrete images when presenting an abstract concept.

Vocabulary Gaps in Toddlers

In the early years, toddlers acquire most of their vocabulary words from their parents. Consequently, children who experience frequent adult-to-toddler conversations that contain a wide variety of words will build much larger vocabularies than those who experience infrequent conversations that contain fewer words. The incremental effect of this vocabulary difference grows exponentially and can lead to an enormous word gap during the child's first three years.

A particularly significant two-part longitudinal study (Hart and Risley, 2003) documented the vocabulary growth of 42 toddlers from the age of 7 to 9 months until they turned 3 years old. Because parental vocabulary is closely associated with their socio-economic status (SES), part one of this study looked at toddlers in families from three different groups. On the basis of occupation, 13 of the families were upper SES, 23 were middle-lower SES, and 6 were on welfare. By the time the children were 3 years old, the researchers had recorded and analyzed over 1,300 hours of casual conversations between the children and their parents. To their surprise, the analysis showed a wide gap in the number of words present in the vocabularies of the children based on their SES. Children from the welfare families had an average recorded vocabulary size of just 525 words. Those from the middle-low SES had 749 words, while the children in the upper SES had average vocabularies of 1,116 words. Furthermore, the children from welfare families were adding words to their vocabulary more slowly than the other children throughout the length of the study.

Part two of the study was conducted six years later. The researchers were able to test the language skills of 29 of these children who were then in third grade. Test results showed that the rate of early vocabulary growth was a strong predictor of scores at ages 9 to 10 on tests of vocabulary, listening, speaking, syntax, and semantics. This study points out how important the early years are in developing a child's literacy and how difficult it is to equalize children's preschool experiences with language.

Early literacy problems can be addressed successfully through the publically-funded birth-to-school programs now available in just a few states. In these programs, school district personnel meet regularly with parents of infants in low SES households and provide them with inexpensive, age-appropriate resources to use with their children during the preschool years. The idea is to build the child's vocabulary and exposure to enriched language before entering school. Missouri began its Parents as Teachers (PAT) program in 1985, and has since provided preschool resources for more than 164,000 high-needs families. Independent evaluations have shown that PAT children were significantly more advanced in language development, problem solving, and social development at age 3 than comparison children. Furthermore, the program provides significant cost savings to local school districts by having fewer placements in special education, fewer grade retentions, and less remedial education (MDESE, 2003).

Syntax and Semantics

Language Hierarchy

With more exposure to speech, the brain begins to recognize the beginnings of a hierarchy of language (Figure 1.5). Phonemes, the basic sounds, can be combined into morphemes, which are the smallest units of language that have meaning. Morphemes can then be combined into words, and words can be put together according to the rules of syntax (word order) to form phrases and sentences with meaning. The difference in meaning (semantics) between the sentences "The woman chased the dog" and "The dog chased the woman" results from a different word order, or syntax. Toddlers show evidence of their progression through the syntactic and semantic levels when simple statements, such as "Candy," evolve to more complex ones, "Give me candy." They also begin to recognize that shifting the words in sentences can change their meaning.

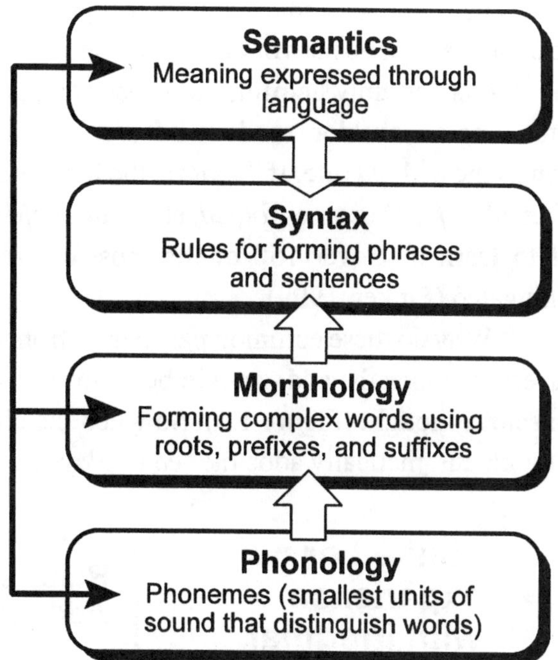

Figure 1.5 The diagram represents the levels of hierarchy in language and in language acquisition. Although the process usually flows from the bottom to the top, recycling from the top to lower levels can also occur, as indicated by the arrows to the left.

The Syntactic Network

The rules of syntax in English prohibit the random arrangement of words in a sentence. The simplest sentences follow a sequence common to many languages, that of subject-verb-object (or SVO) format, as in "He hit the ball." In more complex sentences, syntax imposes a stringent structure on word order to provide clarity and reduce ambiguity. Just look at what happens to meaning when writers neglect to follow the rules of syntax. The following examples are taken from actual headlines that appeared in the nation's newspapers (Cooper, 1987).

- "Defendant's speech ends in a long sentence"
- "Sisters reunited after 18 years in checkout line at supermarket"
- "Dr. Ruth talks about sex with newspaper editors"

Over time, the child hears more patterns of word combinations, phrase constructions, and variations in the pronunciation of words. Toddlers detect patterns of word order—person, action, object—so they can soon say, "I want cookie." They also note statistical regularities heard in the flow of the native tongue. They discern that some words describe objects while others describe actions. Other features of grammar emerge, such as tense. By the age of 3, over 90 percent of sentences uttered are grammatically correct because the child has constructed a syntactic network that stores perceived rules of grammar. For example, the child hears variations in the pronunciation of *walk* and *walked, play* and *played,* and *fold* and *folded.* The child isolates the *-ed* and eventually recognizes it as representing the past tense. At that point, the child's syntactic network is modified to include the rule: "add *-ed* to make the past tense." The rule is certainly helpful, but causes errors when the child applies it to some common verbs. Errors are seldom random, but usually result from following perceived rules of grammar such as the add *-ed* rule. If "I *batted* the ball" makes sense, why shouldn't "I *holded* the bat"? After all, if *fold* becomes *folded,* shouldn't *hold* become *holded*? Regrettably, the toddler has yet to learn that over 150 of the most commonly used verbs in English are irregularly conjugated (Pinker, 1999).

Why do these common past tense errors occur in a child's speech and how do they get corrected? Once the add *-ed* rule becomes part of the syntactic network, it operates without conscious thought (Figure 1.6). So when the child wants to use the past tense, the syntactic network automatically adds the *-ed* to *play* and *look* so that the child can say, "I *played* with

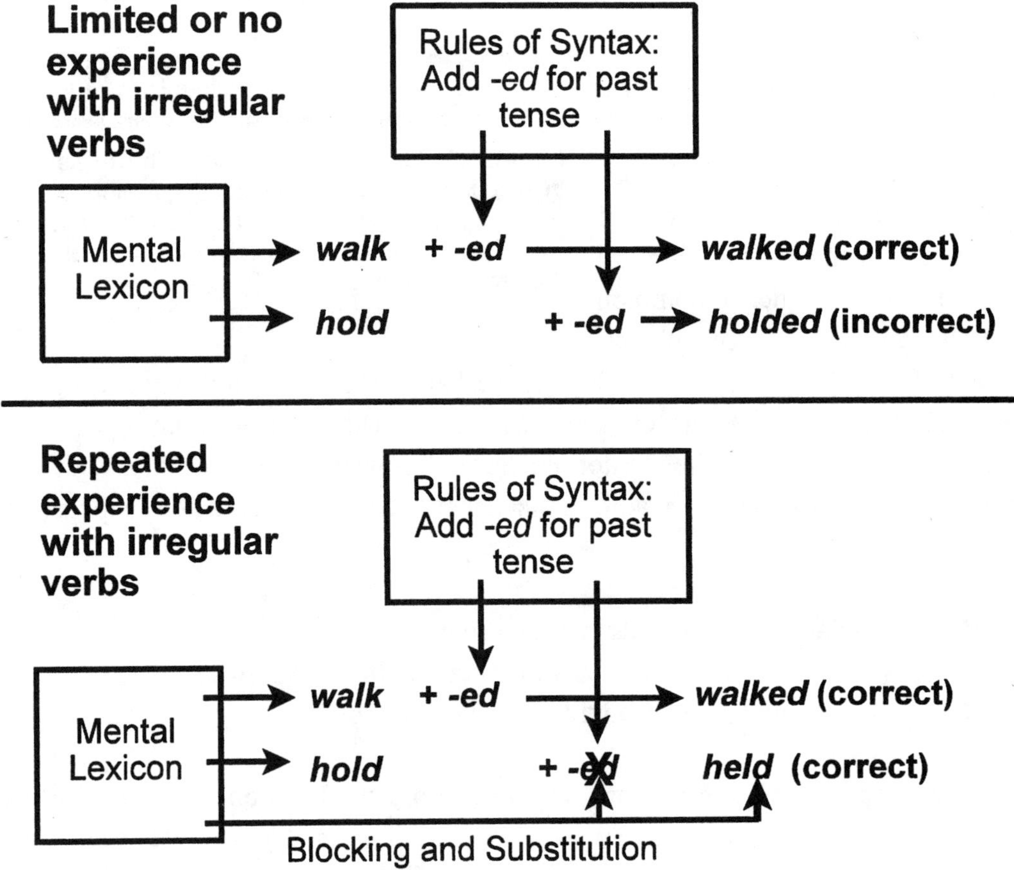

Figure 1.6 The diagrams illustrate how blocking becomes part of the syntactic network. Before a child encounters an irregular verb, the add *-ed* rule applies. Thus *walk* becomes *walked* and *hold* becomes *holded.* After several instances of adult correction and other environmental exposures (repetition is important to memory), the syntactic network is modified to block the rule for the past tense of *hold* and to substitute *held,* a word that now becomes part of the child's lexicon (Pinker, 1999).

Susan and we *looked* at some books." If, however, the child says "I *holded* the bat," repeated adult corrections, repetition, and other environmental encounters will inform the syntactic network that the add *-ed* rule is not appropriate in this case and should be blocked, and that a new word *held* should be substituted and added to the child's lexicon. This principle of *blocking* is an important component of accurate language fluency and, eventually, of reading fluency.

So how does the child eventually learn the irregular forms of common verbs? Long-term memory plays an important role in helping the child learn the correct past tense forms of irregular verbs. The more frequently the irregular verb is used, the more likely the child will remember it. Take a look at Table 1.1, which shows the ten most common verbs in English as computed by Brown University. The verbs are drawn from a million-word database of text used in magazines, newspapers, textbooks, popular books, and other sources (Francis and Kucera, 1982). Note all of these most common verbs are irregular. Interestingly enough, this tends to be true in many other languages. Pinker (1999) explains that irregular forms have to be repeatedly memorized to survive in a language from generation to generation, otherwise the verbs will be lost. He cites several infrequently used irregular verbs whose past tenses have slipped from common usage: *cleave–clove, stave–stove,* and *chide–chid.*

Most common verbs in English and many other languages are irregular.

Table 1.1 Frequency of Common Verbs in English in a Million Words of Text

Verb	Number of Occurrences
1. *be*	39,175
2. *have*	12,458
3. *do*	4,367
4. *say*	2,765
5. *make*	2,312
6. *go*	1,844
7. *take*	1,575
8. *come*	1,561
9. *see*	1,513
10. *get*	1,486

Source: Francis and Kucera, 1982

The ability of children to remember corrections to grammatical errors—including blocking—would be impossible without some innate mechanism that is genetically guided. No one knows how much grammar a child learns just by listening, or how much is pre-wired. What is certain is that the more children are exposed to spoken language in the early years, the more quickly they can discriminate between phonemes, recognize word boundaries, and detect the emerging rules of grammar that result in meaning.

Syntax and English Language Learners. Each language has its own rules of syntax. Consequently, children learning English as an additional language often have problems with English syntax. For example, unlike English, adjectives in Spanish, French, and other similar languages, are typically placed *after* the noun they modify. *Blue sky* is spoken in French as *ciel bleu.* German verbs usually are placed at the end of a clause and rarely follow the subject-verb-object (or SVO) sequence so common in English. For these beginning English language learners, special attention has to be paid to understanding how English rules of syntax differ from those of their native tongue.

> Beginning English language learners need to understand how English rules of syntax differ from those of their native tongue.

The Semantic Network

As phonemes combine into morphemes, and morphemes into words, and words into phrases, the mind needs to arrange and compose these pieces into sentences that express what the speaker wants to say. Meanwhile, the listener's language areas must recognize speech sounds from other background noise and interpret the speaker's meaning. This interaction between the components of language and the mind in search of meaning is referred to as *semantics.* Meaning occurs at three different levels of language: the morphology level, the vocabulary level, and the sentence level.

Morphology-Level Semantics. Meaning can come through word parts, or morphology. The word *biggest* has two morphemes, *big* and *-est.* When children can successfully examine the morphology of words, their mental lexicons are greatly enriched. They learn that words with common roots often have common meaning, such as *nation* and *national,* and that prefixes and suffixes alter the meaning of words in certain ways. Morphology also helps children learn and create new words, and can help them spell and pronounce words correctly.

Vocabulary-Level Semantics. A listener who does not understand many of the vocabulary words in a conversation will have trouble comprehending meaning. Of course, the listener may infer meaning based on context, but this is unreliable unless the listener understands most of the vocabulary. Children face this dilemma every day as adults around them use words they do not understand.

Sentence-Level Semantics. The sentence "Boiling cool dreams walk quickly to the goodness" illustrates that morphology and syntax can be preserved even in a sentence that lacks semantics. The words are all correct English words in the proper syntactic sequence, but the sentence does not make sense. Adults recognize this lack of sense immediately. But children often encounter spoken language that does not make sense to them. To understand language, the listener has to detect meaning at several different levels. Because adults do not normally speak sentences that have no meaning, a child's difficulty in finding meaning may result from a sentence having meaning for one person but not another. At this level, too, the listener's background knowledge or experience with the topic being discussed will influence meaning.

The cerebral processes involved in producing and interpreting meaning must occur at incredible speed during the flow of ordinary conversation. How it is that we can access words from our enormous storehouse (the mental lexicon) and interpret the meaning of conversation so quickly? What types of neural networks can allow for such speed and accuracy? Although linguistic researchers differ on the exact nature of these networks, most agree that the mental lexicon is organized according to meaningful relationships between words. Experimental evidence for this notion comes form numerous studies that involve word priming. In these studies, the subjects are presented with pairs of words. The first word is called the prime and the second word is the target. The target can be a real word or a nonword (like *spretz*). A real word target may or may not be related in meaning to the prime. After being shown the prime, the subject must decide as quickly as possible if the target is a word. The results invariably show that subjects are faster and more accurate in making decisions about target words that are related in meaning to the prime (e.g., *swan–goose*) than to an unrelated prime (e.g., *tulip–goose*). Researchers suspect that the reduced time for identifying related pairs results from these words being physically closer to each other among the neurons that make up the semantic network, and that related words may be stored together in specific cerebral regions (Gazzaniga, Ivry, and Mangun, 2002).

Additional evidence for this idea that the brain stores related words together has come from imaging studies using PET scans. Subjects in PET scanners were asked to name persons, animals, and tools. The results (Figure 1.7) showed that naming items in the same category activated the same area of the brain (Damasio, Grabowski, Tranel, Hichwa, and Damasio, 1996). It seems that the brain stores clusters of closely associated words in a tightly packed network so that words *within* the

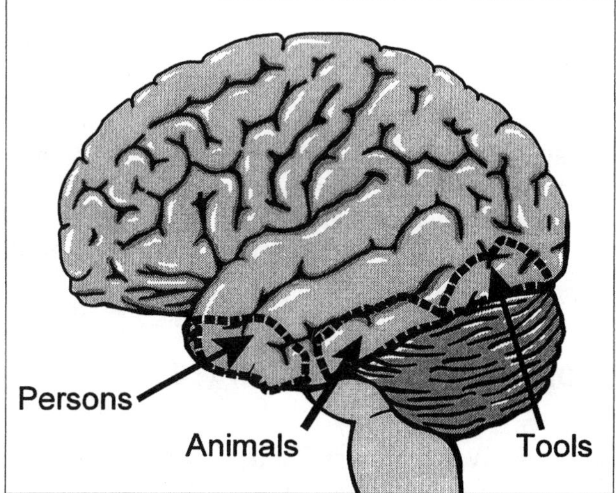

Figure 1.7 The diagram is a representation of the combined PET scan results showing that naming persons, animals, and tools mostly activated different parts of the brain's temporal lobe (Damasio et al., 1996).

network can activate each other in minimal time. Activating words *between* networks, however, takes longer.

How can we best represent these networks? Several different models have been proposed. One that seems to garner substantial support from contemporary neuroscientists is based on an earlier model first proposed by Collins and Loftus (1975) in the mid 1970s. In this model, words that are related are connected to each other. The distance between the connection is determined by the semantic relationship between the words. Figure 1.8 is an example of a semantic network. Note that the word *lemon* is close to—and would have a strong connection to—the word *grapefruit,* but is distant from the word *bird.* If we hear the word *lemon,* then the neural area that represents *lemon* will be activated in the semantic network. Other words in the network such as *lime* and *grapefruit,* would also be activated and, therefore, accessed very quickly. The word *bird* would not come to mind.

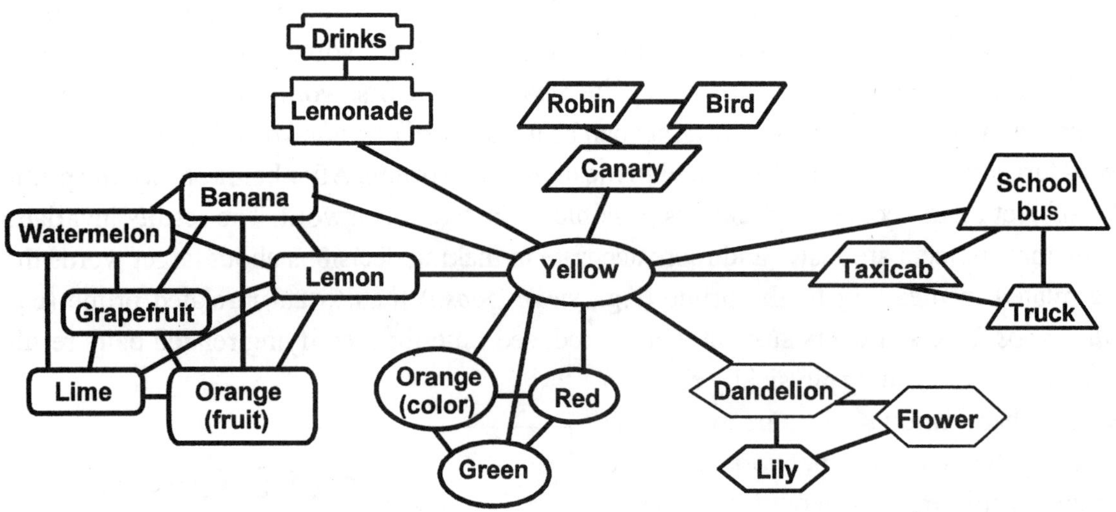

Figure 1.8 This is a representation of a semantic network. Words that are semantically related are closer together in the network, such as *lemon–yellow,* than words that have no close relationship, such as *lemon–bird.* Similar geometric figures identify semantically related words. The lines connect words from different networks that are associated, such as *lemon–yellow.*

From Words to Sentences

We have just discussed how the brain acquires, stores, and recognizes words. But to communicate effectively, the words must be arranged in a sequence that makes sense. Languages have developed certain rules—called grammar—that govern the order of words so that speakers of the language can understand each other. In some languages, such as English, different arrangements of words in a sentence can result in the same meaning. "The girl ate the candy" has the same meaning as "The candy was eaten by the girl." Of course, different word

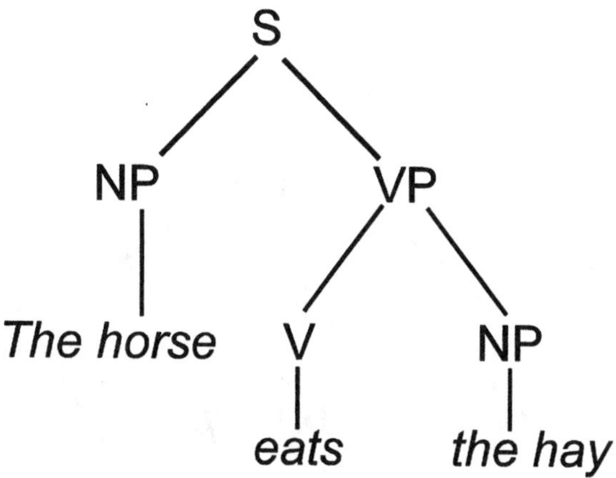

Figure 1.9 This model illustrates how the brain may process sentences to establish meaning. By grouping, or chunking, individual words into phrases, processing time is increased.

arrangements (syntax) can lead to different meanings, as in "The boat is in the water" and "The water is in the boat."

As a child's syntactic and semantic networks develop, context plays an important role in determining meaning. When hearing the sentence "The man bought a hot dog at the fair," the youngster is very likely to picture the man eating a frankfurter rather than a steaming, furry animal that barks. That's because the rest of the sentence establishes a context that is compatible with the first interpretation but not the second.

How does the young brain learn to process the structure of sentences? One prominent model suggests that words in a sentence are assigned syntactic roles and grouped into syntactic phrases (Pinker, 1999). For example, the sentence "The horse eats the hay" consists of a noun phrase (*the horse*), a verb (*eats*), and another noun phrase (*the hay*). A rule of grammar is that a verb (V) can be combined with its direct object to form a verb phrase (VP). In the preceding example, the verb phase would be *eats the hay.* The combination of the noun phrase (NP) and the verb phrase comprises the sentence (S), which can be represented by the syntactic model shown in Figure 1.9.

As sentences become more complicated, each module can contain another module within it. For example, the sentence "The parent told the principal her son is ill" contains a verb phrase that is also a sentence (*her son is ill).* To ensure rapid processing and accurate comprehension, the brain groups the phrases into the hierarchy as represented by the diagram shown in Figure 1.10.

How Can We Speak So Rapidly?

This module-within-a-module pattern (Figure 1.10) has two major advantages. First, by rearranging and including different phrase packets, the brain can generate and understand

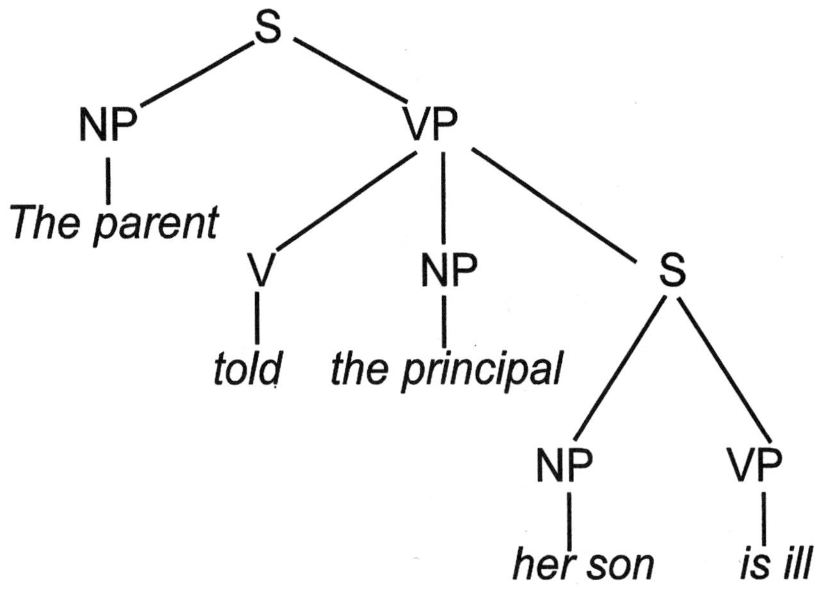

Figure 1.10 This illustrates how the brain proceeds to make additional chunks into phrases to ensure rapid processing and accurate interpretation.

an enormous number of sentences without having to memorize every imaginable sentence verbatim. Second, this pattern allows the brain to process syntactic information quickly so that it can meet the demanding comprehension time required for normal conversation. The efficiency of the system is amazing! The young adult brain can determine the meaning of a spoken word in about one-fifth of a second. The brain needs just one-fourth of a second to name an object and about the same amount of time to pronounce it. For readers, the meaning of a printed word is registered in an astounding one-eighth of a second (Pinker, 1999).

Recognizing Meaning

The brain's ability to recognize different meanings in sentence structure is possible because Broca's and Wernicke's areas establish linked networks that can understand the difference between "The dog chased the cat" and "The cat chased the dog." In an fMRI study, Dapretto and Bookheimer (1999) found that Broca's and Wernicke's areas work together to determine whether changes in syntax or semantics result in changes in meaning. For example, "The policeman arrested the thief" and "The thief was arrested by the policeman" have different syntax but the same meaning. The fMRI showed that Broca's area was highly activated when subjects were processing these two sentences. Wernicke's area, on the other hand, was more activated when processing sentences that were semantically—but not syntactically—different, such as "The car is in the garage" and "The automobile is in the garage."

How is it that Wernicke's area can so quickly and accurately decide that two semantically different sentences have the same meaning? The answer may lie in two other recently discovered characteristics of Wernicke's area. One is that the neurons in Wernicke's area are spaced about 20 percent farther apart and are cabled together with longer interconnecting axons than the corresponding area in the right hemisphere of the brain (Galuske, Schlote, Bratzke, and Singer, 2000). The implication is that the practice of language during early human development results in longer and more intricately connected neurons in the Wernicke region, allowing for greater sensitivity to meaning.

The second recent discovery regarding Wernicke's area is its ability to recognize predictable events. An MRI study found that Wernicke's area was activated when subjects were shown differently colored symbols in various patterns, whether the individuals were aware of the pattern sequence or not (Bischoff-Grethe, Proper, Mao, Daniels, and Berns, 2000). This capacity of Wernicke's area to detect predictability suggests that our ability to make sense of language is rooted in our ability to recognize syntax. The researchers noted that language itself is very predicable because it is constrained by the rules of grammar and syntax.

The Components of Speaking and Understanding Language

Any model for speaking and understanding language has to address the various stages of sound interpretation, beginning with the auditory input and ending with the formation of a mental concept represented by the word or words. Figure 1.11 shows the various neural components that linguistic researchers and neuroscientists believe are required for spoken language comprehension. It is a complex process, but the efficient organization of the linguistic networks that was built up through practice allows it to occur very quickly.

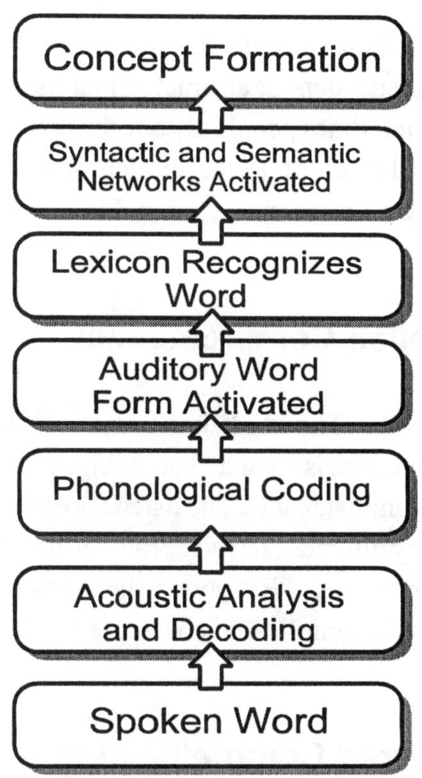

Figure 1.11 This schematic representation shows the major neural components required for spoken language processing. Feedback from higher to lower levels is possible. (Adapted from Gazzaniga et al., 2002).

To understand the different components, let's take the word *dog* through the model. After the spoken word *dog* enters the ear canal, the listener has to decode the sound pattern. In the word form area of the brain, acoustic analysis separates the relevant word sounds from background noise, decodes the phonemes of the word (*duh-awh-guh*), and translates them into a phonological code that can be recognized by the mental lexicon. The lexicon selects the best representation it has in store and then activates the syntactic and semantic networks, which work together to form the mental image of a furry animal that barks (concept formation). All this occurs in just a fraction of a second thanks to the extensive network of neural pathways that were established during the early years of speaking and listening.

Notice that the flow of information in this model is from the bottom up and, thus, appears linear. However, feedback from higher to lower levels is possible. For example, if the lexicon does not recognize the first set of signals, it could reactivate the phonological coding component to produce another set before they decay. It is important to understand how this spoken language processing works because, as we shall see in the next chapter, the process of reading words shares several steps with this model of spoken language processing.

LEVELS OF LANGUAGE COMPREHENSION

Parents speak differently to their children than to other adults. Elementary teachers use different language with their students than with their principal. Speech can be formal, as in the classroom, or informal, as around the dinner table. When young children use informal language, it is often context-dependent, that is, the conversation focuses on the immediate situation or activities at hand. On the other hand, formal speech may be more context independent or abstract in that the child may be relating different possible endings to a story. Sometimes people say one thing but really mean something else, and they hope that the listener will catch on to the subtler meaning. These different language forms are a recognition that there are several types and levels of spoken language and of language comprehension.

Explicit Comprehension

The most basic type of language comprehension is explicit comprehension—the sentence is clear and unambiguous. When someone says "I need a haircut," the interpretation is unmistakable. The listener knows exactly what the speaker means and does not need to draw any inferences or elaborate further. Adults tend to use explicit sentences with children to avoid ambiguity. "Eat your vegetables," and "Please be quiet" are clear statements. Whether the child complies, of course, is another story.

Inferred Comprehension

A more sophisticated form of language comprehension requires the listener to make inferences about meanings that go beyond what the speaker explicitly said. A principal who says to a tardy teacher, "Our school really gets off to a great start in the morning when all the staff is here by 8:15," is really saying, "Be on time." The teacher has to infer the statement's real intent by reading between the lines of what the principal explicitly said.

Young children have difficulty with inferred comprehension. If the parent says, "Vegetables are good for you," the child may not pick up on the underlying intent of this statement—eat your vegetables. Consequently, the child may not finish the vegetables and the parent may mistake this behavior as disobedience when it was really a lack of inferred comprehension.

Teachers sometimes use language requiring inferred comprehension when explicit comprehension would be much easier. A teacher who says, for example, "Do you think I should speak if someone else is talking?" may provoke a variety of responses in the minds of the children. One could think absolutely not, while another might hope she would just speak louder than everyone else so the lesson could move along. A few might get the real intent—oh, she wants us to be quiet.

Context Clues. We discussed earlier how context can be an important clue for determining the meaning of vocabulary words in a sentence. Context can also help with inferred comprehension. A first grade teacher who is telling her spouse over dinner how crowded her class is and that there are too many students who need special help may just be seeking sympathy. But in having the same conversation with her principal, she is really saying she needs an instructional aide. She never says that explicitly; the principal must infer the teacher's intent from her statement and the context.

Children need to develop an awareness that language comprehension exists on several levels. It involves different styles of speech that reflect the formality of the conversation, the context in which it occurs, and the explicit as well as underlying intent of the speaker. When children gain a good understanding of these patterns in speech, they will be better able to comprehend what they read.

What's Coming?

The child's brain has now acquired the fundamentals of spoken language. Neural networks are developing rapidly in Broca's and Wernicke's areas, and every day brings new vocabulary and understanding to the expanding mental lexicon. How will these newly-acquired language skills and knowledge help the child accomplish the next major cognitive task: learning to read? All the steps the brain must go through to progress from spoken to written language are unveiled in the next chapter.

CHAPTER 2
Learning to Read

This chapter addresses several basic questions about how the human brain learns to read. They include:

- *What must a child be able to do in order to read effectively?*
- *What role does working memory play in learning to read?*
- *What happens in the brain when a child goes from a non-reader to a novice reader, and finally to a skilled reader?*

One of the first things to recognize is that intelligence generally does not play a critical role in learning to read. Three sources of evidence indicate this. First, studies of children who learn to read before entering school indicate that there is not a strong relationship between IQ and early reading. Second, studies have shown that IQ is only weakly related to reading achievement in grades 1 and 2. Finally, children who have difficulty learning to read often have above-average IQs (Rawson, 1995; Shaywitz, 2003). It appears then that, to a large degree, learning to read is independent of intelligence.

READING IS NOT A NATURAL ABILITY

Humans have been speaking for tens of thousands of years. During this time, genetic changes have favored the brain's ability to acquire and process spoken language, even setting aside specialized areas of the brain to accomplish these tasks. Consequently, the brain's proficiency at hearing and quickly remembering words is natural, though no less remarkable. Children begin to learn words before their first birthday and during their second year are acquiring them at the rate of 8

> To a large degree, learning to read is independent of intelligence.

to 10 per day. By the time they enter school, they have a well-developed language system consisting of an active vocabulary of about 3,000 words and a total mental lexicon of over 5,000 words. At some point, the child's brain encounters the written word and wonders, "What are those symbols? What do they mean?"

Speaking is a normal, genetically-hardwired capability; reading is not. No areas of the brain are specialized for reading. In fact, reading is probably the most difficult task we ask the young brain to undertake. Reading is a relatively new phenomenon in the development of humans. As far as we know, the genes have not incorporated reading into their coded structure, probably because reading, unlike spoken language, has not emerged over time as a survival skill. If reading were a natural ability, everyone would be doing it. But in fact, there are nearly 40 million adults in the USA alone who are functionally illiterate.

> Speaking is a normal, innate ability; reading is not.

Renewed emphasis in recent years on improving the basic cognitive skills of students has increased pressure to start reading instruction sooner than ever before. In many schools, reading instruction starts in kindergarten. Some neuropsychologists are now debating whether kindergartners are developmentally ready for this challenging task. Are we creating problems for these children by trying to get them to read before their brains are ready? Because boys' brains are physiologically one or two years less mature than girls' brains at this age, are boys at greater risk of failure? To answer these questions, let's examine what researchers have discovered about how the brain learns to read, and the problems that can develop.

Some children—perhaps 50 percent—make the transition from spoken language to reading with relative ease, once exposed to formal instruction. It appears, however, that for the other 50 percent, reading is a much more formidable task, and for about 20 to 30 percent, it definitely becomes the most difficult cognitive task they will ever undertake in their lives.

Answer to Test Question # 2

Question: Learning to read, like learning spoken language, is a natural ability.

Answer: *False.* Unlike spoken language, the brain has no areas specialized for reading. The skills needed to link the sounds of language to the letters of the alphabet must be learned through direct instruction.

EARLY STAGES OF READING

Before children learn to read, they acquire vocabulary by listening to others and by practicing the pronunciation and usage of new words in conversation. Adult correction and other sources help to fine-tune this basic vocabulary. Because the ability to read is strongly dependent on the word forms learned during this period, a child's beginning reading will be more successful if most of the reading material contains words the child is already using. The phoneme-grapheme connection can be made more easily. Reading, of course, also adds new words to the child's mental lexicon. Consequently, there must be some neural connections between the systems that allow the brain to recognize spoken words and the system that recognizes written words.

Learning to read starts with the awareness that speech is composed of individual sounds (phonemes) and a recognition that written spellings represent those sounds (*the alphabetic principle*). Of course, to be successful in acquiring the alphabetic principle, the child has to be aware of how the phonemes of spoken language can be manipulated to form new words and rhymes. The neural systems that perceive the phonemes in our language are more efficient in some children than in others. Just because some children have difficulty understanding that spoken words are composed of discrete sounds doesn't mean that they have brain damage or dysfunction. The individual differences that underlie the efficiency with which one learns to read can be seen in the acquisition of other skills, such as learning to play a musical instrument, playing a sport, or building a model. To some extent, neural efficiency is related to genetic composition, but these genetic factors can be modified by the environment. Nonetheless, being aware of sound differences in spoken language is crucial to learning to read written language.

Phonological and Phonemic Awareness

Phonological awareness is the recognition that oral language can be divided into smaller components, such as sentences into words, words into syllables and, ultimately, into individual phonemes. This recognition includes identifying and manipulating onsets and rimes as well as having an awareness of alliteration, rhyming, syllabication, and intonation. Being phonologically aware means having an understanding of all these levels. In children, phonological awareness usually starts with initial sounds and rhyming, and a recognition that sentences can be segmented into words. Next comes segmenting words into syllables and blending syllables into words.

Phonemic awareness is a subdivision of phonological awareness and refers to the understanding that words are made up of individual sounds (phonemes) and that these sounds can be manipulated to create new words. It includes the ability to isolate a phoneme (first, middle, or last) from the rest of the word, to segment words into their component phonemes, and to delete a specific phoneme from a word. Children with phonemic awareness know that the word *cat* is made up of three phonemes, and that the words *dog* and *mad* both contain the phoneme */d/*. Recognition of rhyming and alliteration are usual indications that a child has phonological awareness, which develops when children are read to from books based on rhyme or alliteration. But this awareness does not easily develop into the more sophisticated phonemic awareness, which is so closely related to a child's success in learning to read (Chard and Dickson, 1999). Nonetheless, reading programs that emphasize phonological and phonemic awareness have proved to be successful in schools (Wise, Ring, and Olson, 1999).

Phonemic awareness is different from *phonics*. Phonemic awareness involves the auditory and *oral* manipulation of sounds. A child demonstrates phonemic awareness by knowing all the sounds that make up the word *cat*. Phonics is an instructional approach that builds on the alphabetic principle and associates letters and sounds with *written* symbols. To demonstrate phonics knowledge, a child tells the teacher which *letter* is needed to change *cat* to *can*. Although phonemic awareness and phonics are closely related, they are not the same. It is possible for a child to have phonemic awareness in speech without having much experience with written letters or names. Conversely, a child may provide examples of letter-sound relationships without ever developing phonemic awareness. In fact, simply learning these letter-sound relationships during phonics instruction does not necessarily lead to phonemic awareness (SEDL, 2001).

> Simply learning letter-sound relationships during phonics instruction does not necessarily lead to phonemic awareness.

The terms phonological awareness, phonemic awareness, and phonics have different meanings, but they can be easily confused. Table 2.1 defines these terms. In this book, I will refer mainly to phonemic awareness because many of the research studies on learning to read focus specifically on phonemes.

Phonemic Awareness and Learning to Read

New readers must learn the alphabetic principle and recognize that words can be separated into individual phonemes, which can be reordered and blended into words. This enables learners to associate the letters with sounds in order to read and build words. Thus, phonemic awareness in kindergarten is a strong predictor of reading success that persists throughout school. Early instruction in reading, especially in letter-sound association, strengthens phonological awareness and helps in the development of the more sophisticated phonemic awareness (Snow, Burns, and Griffin, 1998).

Numerous research studies over the past two decades have established a strong positive link between phonemic awareness and success in early reading. About 70 to 80 percent of children are able to learn the alphabetic principle after one year of instruction. For the rest, additional study is needed (Shaywitz, 2003).

Table 2.1 Definitions of Terms Related to Speech and Reading

Term	Definition	Example
Phonological awareness	The awareness of any size unit of sound, including the ability to separate words into syllables, to count syllables, to identify phonemes in words, and to generate and recognize rhyming words	The word *carpet* has two syllables, each one composed of three phonemes
Phonemic awareness	The awareness that spoken language is made up of individual units of sound	The word dog has three phonemes, */d/-/ô/-/g/*
Phonics	An instructional approach for teaching reading and spelling that emphasizes sound-symbol relationships	The symbol *p* is used to represent the italicized sounds in the words *p*ot, jum*p*, and co*p*y

Source: Yopp and Yopp, 2000

Sounds to Letters (Phonemes to Graphemes)

To be able to read, the brain must memorize a set of arbitrary squiggles (the alphabet) and identify which symbols, called *graphemes,* correspond to the phonemes already stored in the mental lexicon. Many European languages use abstract letters (i.e., an alphabetic system) to represent their sounds so that the words can be spelled out in writing. The rules of spelling that govern a language are called its *orthography.* How closely a language's orthography actually represents the pronunciation of the phoneme can determine how quickly one learns to read that language correctly. Some languages, like Spanish, Italian, and Finnish, have a very close correspondence between letters and the sounds they represent. This is known as a *shallow* orthography. Once the rules of orthography in these languages are learned, a person can usually spell a new word correctly the first time because there are so few exceptions.

English, on the other hand, often has a poor correspondence between how a word is pronounced and how it is spelled. This is called a *deep* orthography. It exists because English does not have an alphabet that permits an ideal one-to-one correspondence between its phonemes and its graphemes. Consider that just when the brain thinks it knows what letter represents a phoneme sound, it discovers that the same symbol can have different sounds, such as the *a*'s in *cat* and in *father.* Consider, too, how the pronunciation of the following English words differs, even though they all have the same last four letters, and in the same sequence: *bough, cough, dough* and *rough.* This lack of sound-to-letter correspondence makes it difficult for the brain to recognize patterns and affects the child's ability to spell with accuracy and to read with meaning. Eventually, the brain must connect the 26 letters of the alphabet to the 44-plus sounds of spoken English (phonemes) that the child has been using successfully for years. Table 2.2 illustrates the complexity of English orthography, compared to some other related languages. There are more than 1,100 ways to spell the sounds of the 44 phonemes in English.

Table 2.2 Language Sounds and Their Spellings

Language	Number of Sounds (Phonemes)	Number of Ways to Spell Sounds
Italian	33	25
Spanish	35+	38
French	32	250+
English	44	1,100+

Alphabetic Principle

The alphabetic principle describes the understanding that spoken words are made up of phonemes and that the phonemes are represented in written text as letters. This system of using letters to represent phonemes is very efficient in that a small number of letters can be used to write a very large number of words. Matching just a few letters on a page to their sounds in speech enables the reader to recognize many printed words: for example, connecting just four letters and their phonemes /a/, /l/, /p/, and /s/ to read *lap, pal, slap, laps,* and *pals.*

Despite the efficiency of an alphabetic system, learning the alphabetic principle is not easy because of two drawbacks. First, the letters of the alphabet are abstract and thus unfamiliar to the new reader, and the sounds they represent are not natural segments of speech.

Answer to Test Question # 3

Question: There are about 200 ways to spell the sounds of the 44 phonemes in English.

Answer: *False.* Actually, there are more than 1,100 ways to represent the sounds of the 44 English phonemes. This condition, known as deep orthography, is one major reason that English is a difficult language to learn, especially for those whose native language has a more reliable letter-to-sound correspondences, such as Spanish.

Second, because there are about 44 English phonemes but only 26 letters, each phoneme is not coded with a unique letter. There are over a dozen vowel sounds but only five letters, *a, e, i, o,* and *u,* to represent them. Further, the child needs to recognize that how a letter is pronounced depends on the letters that surround it. The letter *e,* for example is pronounced differently in *dead, deed,* and *dike.* And then there are the consonant digraphs, which are combinations of two consonants, such as *ch, sh,* and *ph,* that represent a single speech sound. There are also three-letter combinations, called trigraphs, such as *tch* and *thr.* With more practice at word recognition, the reader must work toward fast and accurate word recognition in order to increase reading fluency.

Unfortunately, the human brain is not born with the insight to make sound-to-letter connections, nor does it develop naturally without instruction. Children of literate homes may encounter this instruction before coming to school. Others, however, do not have this opportunity during their preschool years. For them, classroom instruction needs to focus on making the phoneme-phonics connections before reading can be successful. If children cannot hear the *-at* sound in *bat* and *hat* and perceive that the difference lies in the first sound, then they will have difficulty decoding and sounding out words quickly and correctly.

> The human brain is not born with the insight to make sound-to-letter connections, nor does it develop naturally without instruction.

Whether children learn the alphabetic principle by direct or implicit instruction, the problems of inconsistent orthography are resolved the same way other learning challenges are—through practice. With sufficient, effective practice, children develop a context-sensitive understanding of letter-to-sound correspondence. Eventually, they learn that *-ough* in the context of *c*_ _ _ _ is pronounced differently from the context *thr*_ _ _ _.

Letters to Words

Decoding

Phonological awareness helps the beginning reader decipher printed words by linking them to the spoken words that the child already knows. This process is called *decoding.* It involves realizing that a printed word represents the spoken word through a written sequence of letters (graphemes) that stand for phonemes, and then blending the phonemes to pronounce the word. Research studies indicate that a child must be able to decode with accuracy and fluency in order to read proficiently (Moats, Furry, and Brownell, 1998).

Decoding starts with learning the letters of the alphabet and the basic sounds they represent. There has been some discussion among researchers over whether beginning readers should learn the letters of the alphabet by their *names* (that is, *ay, bee, cee, dee,* etc.) or whether they should learn the letters by how the generally *sound* (that is, *ah, beh, cuh, duh,* etc.). Some linguists believe that learning how the letter sounds will accelerate the child's ability to link sounds to letters. At the time of this writing, the research literature was mixed as to whether either method is more effective.

Early decoding most likely starts when children match symbols in their environment to concrete objects in contextual situations. For example, many children recognize the golden arches and the McDonald's sign as a place they like to eat, yet they might not be able to read the word *McDonald's* out of context. Children might also recognize the word *corn* on a cereal box, but might not recognize it in a story. This situation is called *environmental print reading.*

Exactly how the human brain developmentally makes the connections between sounds and words needed for successful decoding is still unclear. But research studies, including some that used brain scans, have helped neurolinguists gain a better understanding of how written word knowledge develops in the beginning reader. One model was developed by Ehri (1998), who proposed four phases of word recognition during early reading (Figure 2.1). The phases are described as follows (Morris, Bloodgood, Lomax, and Perney, 2003):

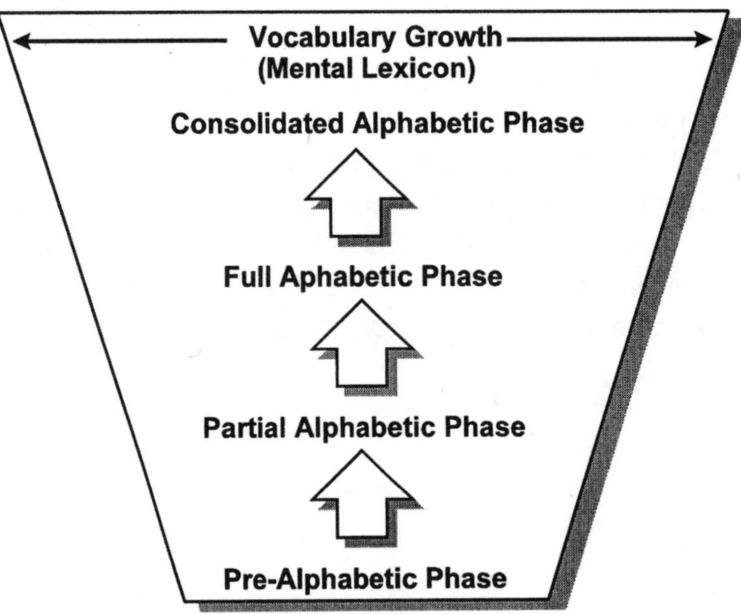

Figure 2.1 As word recognition develops over time from the pre-alphabetic phase to the consolidated alphabetic phase, the reader's vocabulary (the mental lexicon) grows dramatically (Ehri, 1998).

1. ***Pre-alphabetic phase.*** In this phase, children remember words by connecting visual cues in the word (such as the two *l*s in *bell* or the curve at the end of *dog*) with the word's meaning and pronunciation. There is no systematic letter-sound connection. Consequently, the child's ability to commit new words to memory or

retain old words is overwhelmed when visually similar words (such as *bell, ball, will,* or *dog, bug, dig*) are encountered in the text.

2. ***Partial alphabetic phase.*** In this phase, the child commits printed words to memory by connecting one or more printed letters with the corresponding sound(s) heard during pronunciation. For instance, a child might remember the word *talk* by joining the beginning and ending letters (*t* and *k*) with their corresponding spoken sounds *tuh* and *kuh.* New readers enter this phase when they know some letter-sound correspondences and can separate the beginning or ending sounds from the word. Words now become easier to remember because they can be processed through a more reliable letter-sound system rather than the unreliable visual cues used in the pre-alphabetic phase. This phase is sometimes called *sight-word reading* and the readers develop the ability to recognize certain familiar and high-frequency words. However, because these readers still have a limited memory, the ability to remember new words diminishes. They will confuse letters, misreading *take* or *tack* for *talk,* and usually cannot read text that has words outside their mental lexicon.
3. ***Full alphabetic phase.*** As reading progresses, phonemic awareness improves and the reader moves into this phase. Here, the child remembers how to read a specific word by making accurate connections between the letters seen in the word and the phonemes that are used in the word's pronunciation. For example, when reading the word *trap*, the child recognizes the initial consonant blend, */tr/,* then the medial vowel, */u/,* and then to the final consonant, */p/.* This complete phoneme-grapheme connection will facilitate committing this word to long-term memory, thus leading to more accurate reading.
4. ***Consolidated alphabetic phase.*** In this phase, the beginning reader begins to notice multi-letter sequences that are common to words stored in memory (such as the ending *-ake* in *cake, make,* and *take,* or the *-ent* in *bent, cent,* and *tent*). By forming a chunk for each common sequence, word reading becomes faster and more efficient. When encountering a new word containing the chunk (such as *dent*), the child just processes the beginning consonant and the chunk, instead of processing each letter separately. Chunking is particularly helpful when reading longer, multisyllable words like *practice, measurement,* and *traditional.*

As children master each phase, their mental lexicons grow dramatically. Ehri's model is consistent with others (Gough and Juel, 1991), all of which describe an increasing degree of phoneme awareness that occurs in stages. Beginning readers focus on the initial sound of a word *(bug = /b/ /-/ /-/).* Then they progress to processing the beginning and ending sounds *(bug = /b/ /-/ /g/),* and finally to each sound in the word *(bug = /b/ /u/ /g/).*

It should be noted that not all researchers believe that children acquire word recognition skills in a series of stages identified by different decoding strategies. Another theory suggests that children develop these skills gradually on the basis of many experiences with language and reading (Munakata, McClelland, Johnson, and Siegler, 1997). The idea is that children's decoding skills improve based on exposure to many examples and increased sensitivity to the internal structure of words, their components, and their corresponding pronunciations. In other words, progress in decoding is incremental and based on repeated word exposure rather than separated into stages that are based on the manipulation of letter cues. Regardless of whether decoding skills are acquired in stages or incrementally, no one doubts that a firm understanding of the alphabetic principle is essential for early success in learning to read.

Morphemes

What Are Morphemes and Morphology? As reading practice continues, the neural systems are no longer decoding words letter by letter, but are becoming better at recognizing *morphemes.* Morphemes are the smallest word elements that can change a word's meaning, such as the *-ing* that changes *signal* to *signaling*. They can stand on their own as a complete word (free morphemes) or exist as prefixes and suffixes (bound morphemes) that must be added to a root word. When readers understand morphemes, they can separate unfamiliar words into comprehensible parts. If the reader understands what *hate* means and also what *-ful* means, then the reader is likely to comprehend the meaning of *hateful.* This component of grammar that builds words out of pieces (morphemes) is called *morphology.*

There are two types of bound morphemes:

1. *Inflectional morphemes.* These are suffixes that provide information such as case (*Tommy's dog*), number (*dog/dogs*), tense (*he called*), and person (*she calls*).
2. *Derivational morphemes.* These are affixes (prefixes and suffixes) that create new words by changing the meaning of the root words. Some derivational morphemes change the root word's part of speech (*attend* is a verb, add *-ance* and *attendance* becomes a noun). Others, like *un-* and *re-*, change the root word's meaning but not the part of speech.

Morphology is an important component of our language, even to young brains. Research studies confirm that before they learn to read, children are more cognizant of morphology than phonology (Mann, 2000). This means they comprehend more easily that the inflectional morpheme *-s* in *dogs* represents the plural of *dog* than that the *-s* in *yes* represents a phoneme. They also understand more easily that the *-er* in *bigger* is a comparison to something that is already big than that the *-er* represents the second syllable in a word like *power.*

Morphological and Phonemic Awareness. Of course, when students first learn to read, phonemic awareness becomes all important as the young brain tries to match letters to sounds. But by grade 3, morphological awareness begins to surpass phonemic awareness in the development of decoding skills (Singson, Mahony, and Mann, 2000). Morphological awareness helps these students when they encounter multisyllabic words. A word like *indisputable* will be separated into its affixes and root word: *in-, dispute, -able.* Because such words do not appear frequently in their texts, the ability to understand these words will depend far more heavily on the reader's morphological awareness than on word recognition skills (Mahony, Singson, and Mann, 2000).

Other than helping to decode unfamiliar words, morphemes can also help the reader decide whether a word is an adjective (*singing*), noun (*singer*), or verb (*sing*), and thus assist in determining the word's meaning. The syntactic position of the word also helps determine its grammatical aspects, and this redundant information makes the sentence easier to understand and increases reading speed. At this point, word recognition is largely automatic and the reader can understand familiar words without consciously analyzing and decoding their phonemic characteristics. When a student can recognize enough words, the next step is to read sentences and paragraphs fluently.

Is Spelling Crucial to Reading?

Spelling becomes important almost as soon as the child has mastered phonemic awareness and begins to make the letter-sound correspondences. Now the new reader must match the variety of spellings to their sounds. Research studies have found that preschool children are sensitive to patterns in the way words are spelled and the pieces (morphemes) that can be attached to them (Treiman and Cassar, 1997). By grade 1, children note that *ck* never comes at the beginning of a word, and it is always preceded by a short vowel. Older children are not likely to spell *dirty* as *dirdy* because they recognize the morpheme *dirt* and a suffix.

As children progress in mapping letters and sounds, they discover an important reality about spelling: Usually, the mapping from spelling to pronunciation is more reliable than from pronunciation to spelling—the same sound can be spelled in different ways. This fact apparently causes some hesitation in word identification during reading. Recent research has shown that the more ways a sequence of phonemes can be spelled, the longer it takes to read a sentence containing that sequence. For example, *shelf* is read more quickly than *sneer* because the rime unit */ɛlf/* is always spelled *elf* whereas the rime unit */ir/* can be spelled as *ere, eer, ier,* or *ear* (Stone, Vanhoy, and Van Order, 1997; Peereman, Content, and Bonin, 1998). The researchers suspect that the hesitation is caused by a feedback mechanism in the reader's brain that verifies whether past experience supports the pronunciation of *eer* as */ir/.* This notion demonstrates at least one way in which reading and spelling may be closely related.

> Success in reading does not automatically result in success in spelling.

Success in reading does not automatically result in success in spelling. Reading requires recognition whereas spelling requires production—a more complex skill that utilizes additional mental processes. Indeed, many skilled readers consider themselves to be terrible spellers. This is because so many English words do not adhere to strict phonetic rules. Almost every spelling-to-sound convention has exceptions. Nonetheless, good spelling is crucial for recognizing and decoding the meaning of words. To become an expert decoder, the reader will need to learn how to correctly identify and spell the exceptions. Studies show that the accuracy of a student's spelling in kindergarten and grade 1 is a predictor of later reading ability (Moats et al., 1998).

As students develop their spelling skills, they also increase their word recognition speed during reading. Word recognition becomes automatic, and skilled readers are now able to recognize new words based on their morphemes. For example, a student who recognizes the spelling of *react* in *reaction*, will realize that the words are related and make connections between their meanings. This is the primary way in which students expand their lexicon in grade 3 and beyond (Anglin, 1993). In sum, good spelling skills often lead to rapid word recognition and comprehension.

READING COMPREHENSION

Words to Sentences

Comprehension of reading material occurs when readers are able to place the meaning of individual words into the structure and context of the entire sentence. Furthermore, the reader's ability to remember the sentence's structure (syntax) relies on working memory. Let's examine first the role of syntax in sentence comprehension; working memory is discussed later in this chapter.

Syntax and Comprehension

When children read simple sentences, they grasp meaning mainly through simple associations that are already stored in the brain's word form area and the mental lexicon. The syntax is easy and there is little risk of ambiguity of meaning. In the sentence "The cat is white," only one interpretation is possible. But as sentences get more complex, syntax plays an important role in comprehension. Readers are more likely to encounter ambiguity in reading than in speech because written texts tend to use complex grammatical structures more often than casual conversation.

Before beginning to read, children already have a good sense of syntax as a result of speaking and listening. They learn that "I want cookie" sounds better (and may get more results) than "Cookie, I want" or "I cookie want." Their brains soon recognize a speech pattern: Who's acting? (subject), What's the action? (predicate), What's being acted upon? (object). Interestingly enough, this syntax pattern is common to many Indo-European languages. Sentence structure gets more complicated in reading, however. There are three types of syntactic structure for sentences, as follows (SLC, 2000):

- *Simple:* A simple sentence contains just one main clause, for example, "The boy rowed the boat."
- *Compound:* A compound sentence has two or more main clauses joined by connecting words, for example, "The boy rowed the boat while his mother watched."
- *Complex:* A complex sentence contains a main clause and one or more dependent or relative clauses. An example would be: "The boy who rowed the boat waved to his mother."

Many syntactic changes can occur within these three categories that change the meaning of these sentences. Some clauses can include negation ("The boy didn't row the boat.") or contain prepositional phrases ("to his mother"), or conjunctions ("The boy and his mother rowed the boat."). Using the passive voice will reverse the relative position of the subject and the object ("The boat was rowed by the boy."). Relative clauses can further complicate the matter, by being relative to the subject ("The boy who rows the boat is lost.") or relative to the object ("The boy rows the boat that is leaking.").

So how is a beginning reader going to deal with differences in meaning that result from variations in syntax? The following six syntactic variations can be particularly troublesome and require some basic strategies that, by the way, do not always work (SLC, 2000).

- Word order
- Minimum-distance principle
- Analysis of conjoined clauses
- Passive voice
- Negation
- Embedding

Word Order. As mentioned earlier, prereading children are accustomed to the subject-verb-object (SVO) sequence and rely heavily on it to decode early reading. This reliance is fine as long as the sentences are in the active voice, such as "He chased the dog." Difficulties arise, however, when sentences are in the passive voice, such as "He was chased by the dog." In the latter case, order of the words, *He, chased,* and *dog* was preserved, so the reader might misinterpret the sentence to mean "He chased the dog."

Minimum-Distance Principle. Beginning readers assume that words in a sentence refer to their closest related words, verbs referring to their closest preceding nouns, and pronouns to their closest noun of the same gender. The minimum-distance principle is easily applicable to the sentence "He rowed the boat all by himself," but not to "He rowed the boat that belonged to the fisherman all by himself." Readers are apt to rely more on the minimum-distance principle when the number of words they have to remember in the sentence exceeds the capacity of their working memory.

Analysis of Conjoined Clauses. While attempting to comprehend a sentence with two clauses, the young reader may assume that the two clauses are conjoined by a conjunction such as "and." Consequently, the reader may misinterpret the sentence "The man chased the dog that ate the steak" to mean "The man chased the dog, and the man ate the steak."

Passive Voice. For the young reader, the passive voice is particularly difficult to understand and learn. They violate the SVO sequence, and they can be particularly troublesome if they are reversible, such as "She was called by him," which could be mistakenly read as "She called him." Sometimes, common sense helps the reader to comprehend passive voice sentences correctly. For example, in the sentence "The window was broken by the baseball," it is clear that the window couldn't break the baseball, so only one interpretation makes sense.

Negation. Sentences written in the negative are usually more difficult for the young brain to comprehend. That is because the brain tends to interpret the sentence in the positive sense, and then moves to the second phase to process the negative sense. Consequently, the young reader will find the sentence, "Circle the picture that shows cows and sheep" easier to understand than "Circle the picture that has cows but not sheep." Substantial practice with negation can improve a reader's comprehension and fluency with these types of sentences.

Embedding. Embedded clauses can lead to ambiguity or misinterpretation. In grades 2 and 3, readers encounter the following three types of embedded clauses:

1. *The subject of the main clause is the same as the subject of the embedded clause.* Example: "The boy rowed the boat and waved to his mother." These are usually easy for young readers to understand.
2. *The object of the main clause is the subject of the embedded clause.* Example: "The man chased the dog that ate the steak." These are more difficult to comprehend accurately. The reader may incorrectly apply the conjoined-clause strategy here and read the sentence as "The man chased the dog, and the man ate the steak."
3. *The subject of the main clause is the object of the embedded clause.* Example: "The boat that the boy rowed belongs to the fisherman." Ambiguity arises because these types of sentences violate both the SVO sequence as well as the minimum-distance principle.

As students read more and as their working memory becomes more efficient, they gradually switch from using these rudimentary strategies to paying closer heed to the actual syntax of sentences.

Morphology and Comprehension

Morphology, you will recall, studies how words are put together from pieces (e.g., prefixes and suffixes), and how these pieces can change the meaning of words or create new ones. Morphological awareness contributes to reading comprehension in the following ways (Mahony et al., 2000):

- *Meaning.* The reader is able to distinguish the difference between nouns formed by adding *-tion* and nouns formed by adding *-ive.* Thus, *operation* and *operative* are formed from the same root word but have different meanings.
- *Syntactic properties.* The reader understands that a particular suffix indicates a part of speech. For example, *-y* indicates an adjective (*noisy*) and *-ly* indicates an adverb (*noisily*).
- *Phonological properties.* The reader understands that derivational suffixes can alter the pronunciation of the root word. For example, adding *-ic* to *hero* involves a shift in emphasis from the first syllable of *heroic* to the second, and adding *-al* to *hymn* involves pronouncing the previously silent consonant *-n* in *hymnal.*
- *Relational properties.* The reader understands the relationship between words formed by adding different prefixes and suffixes to the same root word, as in *import* and *export* or in *operation* and *operative.* When readers use relational properties effectively, their reading fluency, pronunciation, and comprehension improve. Furthermore, they get better at distinguishing between true morphological relationships, such as *sail-sailor,* and false ones, such as *may-mayor.*

Decoding Ability, Intelligence, and Comprehension

Research studies have shown that phonemic awareness is a stronger predicator of success with reading comprehension than intelligence during the stages of early reading (Torgesen, 1999). As children progress, however, the research evidence suggests that decoding speed as well as intelligence (as measured by standard IQ tests) are closely related to reading comprehension. One recent study involving 124 children found that decoding ability was the best single predictor of how well the child comprehended the reading. The child's IQ was also a significant predictor, although not as strong as decoding ability (Tiu, Thompson, and Lewis, 2003).

> Research studies show that during early reading phonemic awareness is a stronger predictor of success in reading comprehension than intelligence.

Reading Comprehension and Language Comprehension

Research studies have demonstrated that reading comprehension is very closely related to spoken language comprehension. If that is the case, how do we explain those children who can read words but whose comprehension in reading is not as good as their spoken language comprehension? One possible explanation is that children learn spoken language in settings that are different from where they learn to read. Written language generally adheres to stricter grammatical structures and uses more formal vocabulary than spoken language. Consequently, how well a child comprehends a written text is determined by how well that child comprehends the same text when it is spoken.

How well a child comprehends a written text is determined by how well that child comprehends the same text when it is spoken.

HOW MEMORY AFFECTS LEARNING TO READ

To understand how memory affects reading, we need a brief review of the brain's memory components. As researchers gain greater insight into the brain's memory processes, they have had to devise and revise terms that describe the various stages of memory. If you took a psychology course more than a decade ago, you learned that we had two memories, short-term (temporary) memory and long-term (permanent) memory. Neuroscientists now believe that we have two temporary memories that perform different tasks. It is a way of explaining how the brain deals briefly with some data, but can continue to process other data for extended periods of time. For now, short-term memory is used by cognitive neuroscientists to include the two stages of temporary memory: immediate memory and working memory (Squire and Kandel, 1999). Figure 2.2 illustrates the stages of temporary and permanent memory.

Immediate Memory

Immediate memory is one of the two temporary memories and is represented in Figure 2.2 by a clipboard, a place where we put information briefly until we make a decision on how to dispose of it. Immediate memory operates subconsciously or consciously and holds data for up to about 30 seconds. (Note: The numbers used in this chapter are averages over time. There are always exceptions to these values as a result of human variations or pathologies.) The individual's experiences determine its importance. If the information is of little or no

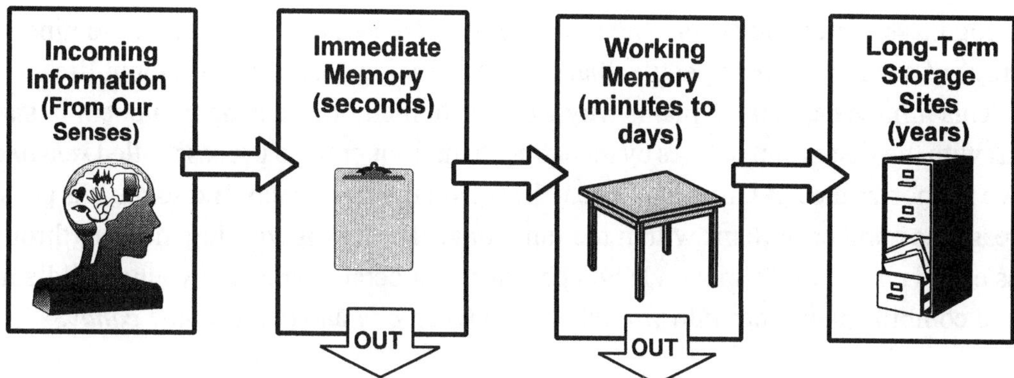

Figure 2.2 The diagram illustrates the theory of temporary and permanent memories. Information gathered from our senses lasts only a few seconds in immediate memory. Information in working memory usually endures for minutes or hours, but can be retained for days if necessary. The long-term storage sites (also called permanent memory) store information for years.

importance within this time frame, it drops out of the memory system. For example, when you look up the telephone number of the local pizza parlor, you usually can remember it just long enough to make the call. After that, the number is of no further importance and drops out of immediate memory. The next time you call, you will have to look up the number again.

Working Memory

Suppose, on the other hand, you can't decide whether to call the pizza parlor or the Chinese take-out place, and you discuss these options with someone else in the room. This situation requires more of your attention and is shifted into working memory for conscious processing. Working memory is the second temporary memory and the place where conscious, rather than subconscious, processing occurs. In Figure 2.2, working memory is shown as a work table, a place of limited capacity where we can build, take apart, or rework ideas for eventual storage somewhere else. When something is in working memory, it generally captures our focus and demands our attention. Scanning experiments show that most of working memory's activity occurs in the frontal lobes, although other parts of the brain are often called into action (Goldberg, 2001; Sousa, 2001a).

Capacity of Working Memory

Working memory can handle only a few items at one time. This functional capacity changes with age. Preschool infants can deal with about two items of information at once. Preadolescents can handle three to seven items, with an average of five. Through adolescence, further cognitive expansion occurs and the capacity increases to a range of five to nine, with an average of seven. For most people, that number remains constant throughout life.

This limited capacity explains why we have to memorize a song or a poem in stages. We start with the first group of lines by repeating them frequently (a process called *rehearsal*). Then we memorize the next lines and repeat them with the first group, and so on. It is possible to increase the number of items within the functional capacity of working memory through a process called *chunking*. In spoken language, chunking occurs when the young child's mind begins to combine phonemes into words, such as when *can* and *dee* become *candy.*

Time Limits of Working Memory

Working memory is temporary and can deal with items for only a limited time. For preadolescents, it is more likely to be 5 to 10 minutes, and for adolescents and adults, 10 to 20 minutes. These are average times, and it is important to understand what the numbers mean. An adolescent (or adult) normally can process an item in working memory intently for 10 to 20 minutes before fatigue or boredom with that item occurs and the individual's focus drifts. For focus to continue, there must be some change in the way the individual is dealing with the item. As an example, the person may switch from thinking about it to physically using it, or making different connections to other learnings. If something else is not done with the item, it is likely to drop from working memory.

This is not to say that some items cannot remain in working memory for hours, or perhaps days. Sometimes, we have an item that remains unresolved—a question whose answer we seek or a troublesome family or work decision that must be made. These items can remain in working memory, continually commanding some attention and, if of sufficient importance, interfere with our accurate processing of other information. Eventually, we solve the problem and it clears out of working memory.

Reading Comprehension and Working Memory

Spoken language uses memory systems for meaning. Memory helps students remember a set of oral directions: "Take out you math book and do the even-numbered problems on pages 18 and 19, and then check your answers on page 237." But reading is a far more complicated skill involving a number of brain systems. When reading a word, the decoding process breaks the word into its segments and, while being retained in working memory, the phonemes are blended to form words that the reader can recognize. The ability to retain verbal bits of information is referred to as *phonologic memory.*

When reading sentences, the visual and memory systems of the brain must decode and then retain the words at the beginning of a sentence for a period of time while the reader's eyes move to the end of the sentence. In a short sentence like "See the dog run," that is no problem because the memory time-span requirement is minimal. However, when reading complex sentences, such as "The boy ran down the street to tell his friend that the ice cream truck was just around the corner and would be here soon," requires much more memory time. Furthermore, the brain must pay attention to syntax and context in order for the sentence to be accurately understood. Because of working memory's limited capacity, beginning readers will have difficulty understanding long sentences or sentences with complex structure or syntax. They may be able to read the sentence aloud, but may not comprehend its meaning.

A child's ability to store words temporarily in working memory depends on several factors, such as age, experience, and language proficiency. But the code that readers of any age use to store written words and phrases is a phonological code. Consequently, phonological coding skills are crucial for using and developing the ability of working memory to store representations of written words. A reader with efficient phonological decoding skills will be able to quickly generate and retain phonetic representations of written words as well as preserve the words themselves and their sequence in the sentence. By developing these working memory skills, the reader with appropriate background knowledge can comprehend not only the sentence, but also the paragraph and the chapter (SLC, 2000).

> Because of working memory's limited capacity, beginning readers will have difficulty understanding long sentences.

During reading, working memory helps comprehension in the following two ways.

- *Understanding complex structure.* In complex sentences, such as "The woman who is getting into the blue car dropped her key," working memory holds the decoded results of the first part of a sentence while the visual cortex processes the words and phrases in the rest of the sentence. Working memory then puts all the pieces together to establish the sentence's meaning.
- *Preserving syntax (word order).* Take the sentence "The driver of the blue car, not the red car, honked his horn." Here, working memory preserves the word order so that the reader can process the sequence, recognize negation, and correctly identify who honked the horn.

As reading progresses, the meaning of each sentence in a paragraph must be held in memory so that they can be associated with each other to determine the intent of the paragraph and whether certain details need to be remembered. Working memory must then link paragraphs to each other so that, by the end of the chapter, the reader has an understanding of the main ideas encountered. With extensive practice the working memory becomes more efficient at recognizing words and at chunking words into common phrases. As a result, the child reads faster and comprehends more.

Forming Gists

Because working memory has a limited capacity, it cannot hold all the words of a long sentence. To deal with this limitation, working memory merges words within a clause to form a *gist* (the memory device known as *chunking*) that is then temporarily stored in place of the words. As reading continues, the brain adds new gists of clauses until the sentence is completed. Then a gist of the sentence is generated. Gists from other sentences in the paragraph are chunked to form a higher level gist of the paragraph. Then, gists of paragraphs are chunked to form an even higher level gist of the chapter, and eventually for the entire text. Table 2.3 shows how gists at one level combine to form gists of the next level.

Table 2.3 Levels of Reading Comprehension Gists in Working Memory

4th Level:	Chapter #1 gist ✚ Chapter #2 gist ✚ Chapter #3 gist ➔ **Text gist**
3rd Level:	Paragraph #1 gist ✚ Paragraph #2 gist ✚ Paragraph #3 gist ➔ **Chapter #1 gist**
2nd Level:	Sentence #1 gist ✚ Sentence #2 gist ✚ Sentence #3 gist ➔ **Paragraph #1 gist**
1st Level:	Clause #1 gist ✚ Clause #2 gist ✚ Clause #3 gist ➔ **Sentence #1 gist**

Source: SLC, 2000

Early reading makes heavy demands on both the processing and storage functions of a young working memory. Chunking the representations of word forms into gists is an efficient way of managing the competition for space and time in working memory. Gists take up less space and are retained while individual word forms are deleted. Sentence gists are then deleted when paragraph gists are formed, and so on. Clause gists endure for about 30 seconds; chapter gists can last for 15 minutes or more (SLC, 2000).

Other factors affect the ability of working memory to retain or lose information during reading (Figure 2.3). New reading that the child finds interesting is likely to make it past immediate memory to working memory for conscious processing. And if the new reading activates material recently learned, long-term storage retrieves that information and moves it into working memory where it enhances the acquisition of the new learning. This process is called *transfer* and represents one of the most powerful principles of learning (Sousa, 2001a).

Reading information can also leave working memory. This can occur if

- Too many minutes have elapsed since the information was last activated. For instance, just after reading the first sentence of a lengthy paragraph, the reader gets involved in a brief conversation with another child. When the reader returns to the text, the previously-read material has faded and the child must start again from the beginning.

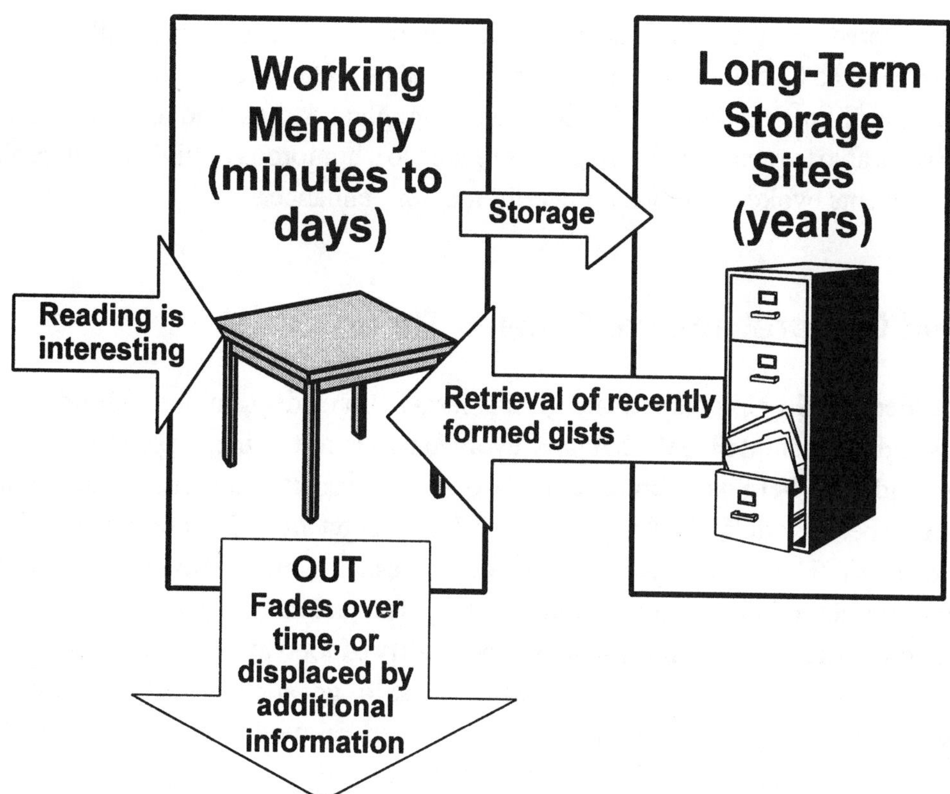

Figure 2.3 Reading and memory interact in several ways. Reading that is interesting to the reader will pass through immediate memory into working memory for conscious processing. New reading may activate long-term storage to retrieve related gists already learned. Reading information can fall out of working memory by fading or by being displaced by additional information.

- The information is displaced when additional information is placed in working memory and its capacity is exceeded. This can happen if the child is reading faster than he can comprehend, thus giving the brain insufficient time to form the necessary gists and then clear out the individual words. In this case, the words are removed from memory before the gist is generated, and comprehension suffers.

As more demands are placed on working memory during reading, other difficulties may arise. A young child who is just learning to read using a book with advanced vocabulary words will have trouble with comprehension because so much memory capacity is being used trying to decode unfamiliar words. Research studies on the pace at which people read have offered further insights into how memory affects comprehension. For example, the studies found that readers spent more time reading the topic sentence of a paragraph. This may indicate that working memory is exerting more effort to generate and ensure the retaining of this gist because it is most useful in understanding the rest of the passage, and for creating the gist of the entire paragraph. The research studies also demonstrated, to no one's surprise, that readers remembered best those ideas and concepts that were referenced repeatedly, as well as those that were linked through cause and effect (SLC, 2000). On the other hand, readers spent the least amount of time reading the details of a paragraph and, thus, had difficulty recalling them. They were able to recall, however, details related to a humorous or vivid event, probably because such events evoke emotion, a powerful memory enhancer.

Memory and Comprehension: Schema Theory

A reader's ability to comprehend gists is largely dependent on that individual's past experiences and the mental models that have evolved as a result of those experiences. We all use mental models to help us interpret the world and to predict situations occurring in our environment. These models, first suggested by Jean Piaget in 1926, are called *schemata* (singular, *schema*). They develop over time and represent frameworks or scripts that use general concepts stored in long-term memory to help us make meaning out of situations. For example, if some friends are telling you about the quality of food at a new restaurant, there is no need for them to also tell you that they sat at a table, got menus, and left a tip. These incidentals are filled in because they are part of your general model, or schema, about your past experiences at restaurants, and are implicitly understood.

Schemata are important in helping to comprehend text. Readers use their schemata to interpret cause and effect, to compare and contrast, and to make inferences about the author's meaning. Information that does not fit into these schemata may not be understood or may be understood incorrectly. This is one reason why readers may have problems comprehending text on a subject in which they have no experiences even though they understand the meaning of every word in the text (Driscoll, 1994). Schemata are greatly influenced by an individual's culture. Thus, young readers who were not brought up in the United States may have a difficult time reading and answering questions about George Washington.

Modifying Schemata

Schemata are created through repeated experiences with events, people, and objects that we encounter in our world. When we encounter a new experience, our schemata can be modified in any of the following three ways (Figure 2.4):

- *Accretion:* The learner incorporates the new information into an existing schema without altering that schema. For example, suppose I visited a public library and all that I experienced there fit into my long-held schema of a library as a place with just print material and a card catalog. As a result, I did not alter my library schema in any appreciable way.

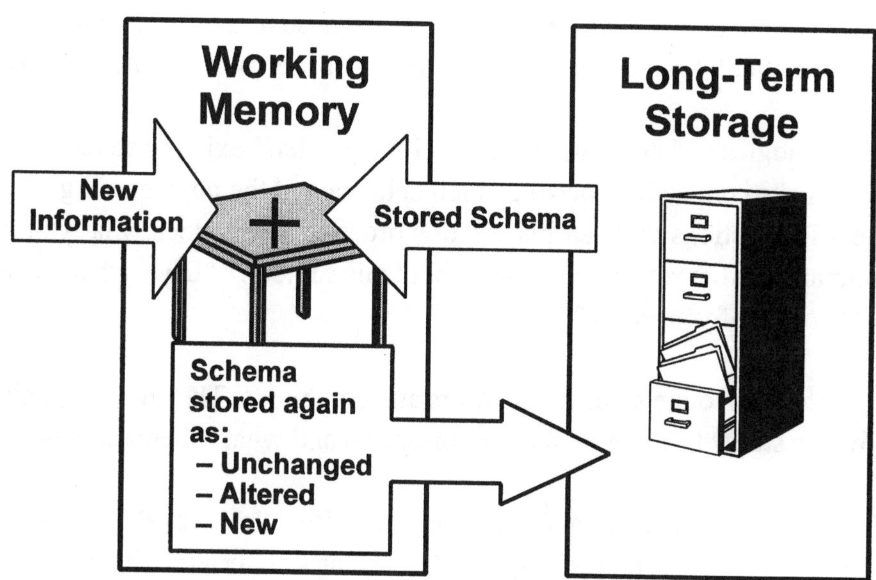

Figure 2.4 This illustration shows how a stored schema helps us to interpret new information. As the new information is processes, the schema can be returned to long-term memory unchanged or altered to accommodate the new experience. In some cases, the new information cannot be accommodated by the current schema, so a new one is created.

- *Tuning:* The learner realizes that the existing schema is inadequate to accommodate the new information, and alters the existing schema to be more consistent with the experience. For example, when I visited a modern public library and realized that the card catalog was replaced by a computer database, I had to modify my library schema to accommodate this experience.
- *Restructuring:* The learner realizes that the new information is so inconsistent with the existing schema that a new schema has to be created. For example, now my ability to access the print information at the local public library directly from my computer at home any time of the day or night has forced me to create a new schema.

Using Schema Theory in Teaching and Learning

Schema theory reaffirms the importance of the role of prior knowledge in learning. Teachers of reading should consider using strategies that activate the reader's prior knowledge, thus enabling them to better understand the text. Effective strategies include the following (Armbruster, 1996):

✓ Read the heading and title. Have the readers examine visuals in the text, and make predictions based on the title and visuals.

✓ Provide content that has unifying themes, because information that lacks a theme can be difficult to understand, especially for readers with limited experiences.

✓ Use analogies and comparisons to elicit the readers' existing schema and to help them make connections between their schema and the new learning. Ask readers specific questions that can help in this process: "How does what you have read compare to what you already know about this subject?" "Does what you have read change any of your ideas?"

✓ Pay attention to the students' answers and comments. They may give clues about how the students are organizing information and what schemata they are using.

✓ Keep in mind how cultural differences may affect the reader's ability to interpret text, and avoid text that is so culture-biased as to interfere with a reader's ability to correctly comprehension the passage.

WHAT DO BRAIN SCANS REVEAL ABOUT READING?

Reading Pathways

Using functional imaging scans, neuroscientists have discovered the neural mechanisms involved in reading. As would be expected, the scans have shown that all readers use neural circuitry dedicated to visual processing, because the curves and lines of the alphabet need to be visually analyzed to distinguish one letter from another. In addition to the visual processing area, Shaywitz (2003) and other researchers (Indefrey et al., 1997; McCandliss, Cohen, and Dehaene, 2003) noted that three other areas of the brain were involved in reading. However, which of these three areas the brain used was dependent on how skilled the person was at reading. Apparently, beginning readers use different neural pathways than skilled readers, most likely because their needs are different. Here is what the researchers found.

> Beginning readers use different neural pathways than skilled readers.

Pathway for Novice Readers

The brain of a beginning reader needs to analyze each new word it encounters. It must pull it apart and associate the letters with their sounds. A region of the brain that overlaps portions of the parietal and temporal lobes—called the parieto-temporal area—is shown in Figure 2.5 and is the area where this important word analysis occurs. In this area, located

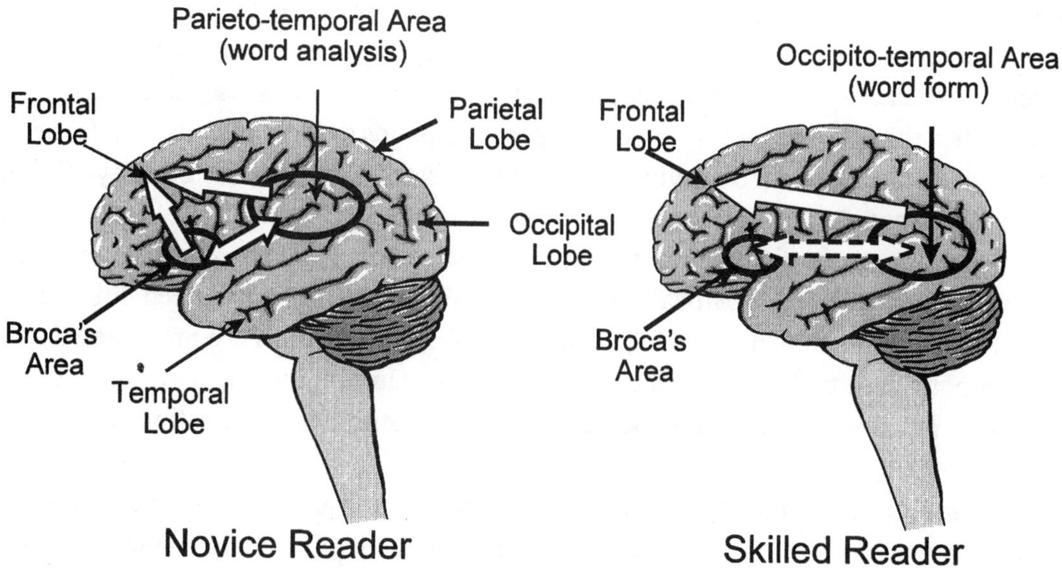

Figure 2.5 These diagrams show the brain systems used for reading. The novice reader uses the parieto-temporal area to slowly analyze new words with considerable help from Broca's area. However, the skilled reader uses the occipito-temporal area to quickly identify previously learned word forms, with just a little help from Broca's area, as indicated by the dotted arrow. Both types of readers activate the frontal lobe to generate meaning (McCandliss et al., 2003; Shaywitz, 2003).

above and slightly behind the ear, the brain begins to recognize certain relationships between the sounds of spoken language and the letters of the alphabet that represent them. Broca's area, specialized region for language located behind the left temple, is also significantly involved in this word analysis.

When, for example, the child's brain first sees the word *dog* in print, the word analysis area (parieto-temporal area) records the three alphabetic symbols and matches the *duh-awh-guh* sounds to their appropriate letters, *duh=d, awh=o,* and *guh=g.* We know this developing sound-to-letter relationship as the alphabetic principle. Eventually, a mental image of a furry animal is conceptualized in the mind's eye, adding meaning to the symbolic representation, *d-o-g.*

Pathway for Skilled Readers

With repeated encounters of the same word, the child's brain makes a neural model—called a word form—that encompasses the spelling, pronunciation, and meaning of that word. Current interpretation of the functional imaging scans supports the notion that word forms are stored in a region that overlaps the occipital and temporal lobes—called the occipito-temporal area—located toward the lower rear part of the brain. Here, all the important information about a word is stored, including its spelling, pronunciation, and meaning. Thus, when the word form is produced, the child can read this word far more quickly. Just seeing it activates all the components at once without any conscious thought on the part of the reader. As more word forms collect in this cerebral region, reading becomes more fluent and reading skill levels rise dramatically. Broca's area now plays only a minor role in assisting this region. The more skilled the reader, the more quickly this area responds to seeing a word—in less than 150 thousandths of a second (150 milliseconds), much faster than the blink of an eye (Price, Moore, and Frackowiak, 1996).

It is important to note that the occipito-temporal region is not an area specialized for reading in the same way that Broca's and Wernicke's areas are specialized for spoken language. Studies have shown that other types of sensory information are processed by the occipito-temporal area that are not related to word forms (Joseph, Noble, and Eden, 2001). However, with practice, this area can become exceptionally efficient at generating visual word forms during reading.

To summarize: Beginning readers use both Broca's area and the word analysis region to slowly analyze each word. Skilled readers, on the other hand, rely mainly on the word form area to rapidly produce meaning from words, with only marginal help from Broca's area when needed. As we shall see later on, children and adults with reading difficulties, including dyslexia, show distinctly different patterns of brain activation when reading from those described here.

MODELS OF READING PATHWAYS

Now that functional imaging scans have given us a clearer picture of the neural areas involved in reading, we can develop models that represent how the novice and skilled brains read.

The Novice Reader

Figure 2.6 shows the pathway and the components for the novice reader, one who usually sounds out new words while reading. The visual cortex records the word *dog* and sends the visual information to the word analysis region (parieto-temporal area). Working with Broca's area, these two networks analyze the word for its component phonemes and pronunciation. The pathway is indicated in the diagram by the white arrows labeled "N" (Shaywitz, 1996).

A visual word form is then produced and the mental lexicon is activated to identify the visual form. If the visual form for dog is retrieved, a conceptual representation is generated of a furry, barking animal. This is a relatively slow process because each step—spelling, pronunciation, and meaning—is treated separately. In the event that the lexicon cannot identify the visual form, a feedback loop may reactivate the visual cortex as well as the decoding and

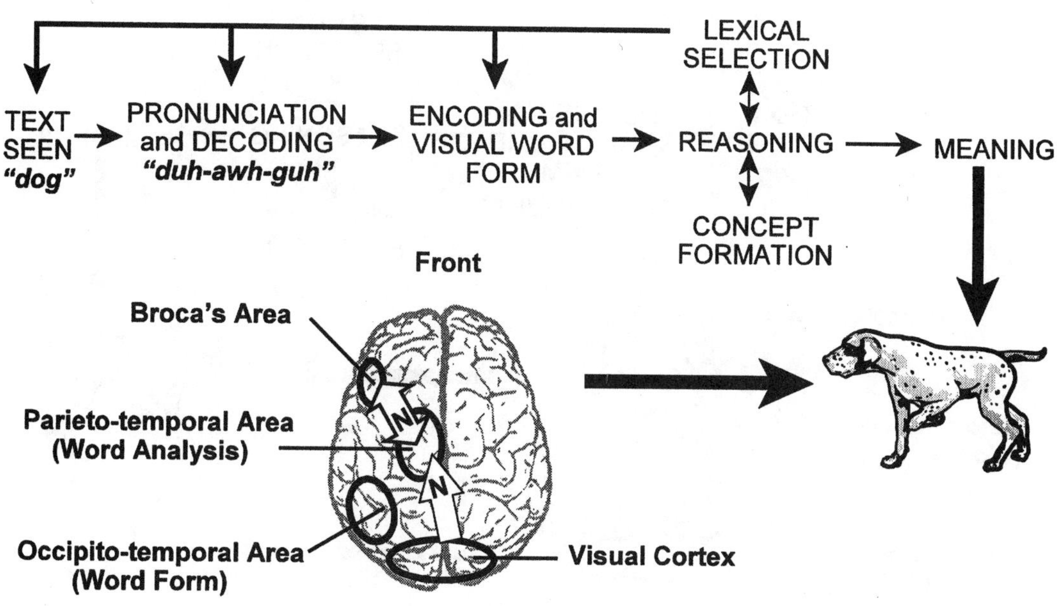

Figure 2.6 The diagram represents the neural pathways and linguistic components of the novice reader. The printed word stimulates the visual cortex, which passes the visual input information to the word analysis region (parieto-temporal area). Working with Broca's area, these two networks slowly analyze the word for its constituent phonemes and pronunciation (pathway indicated by the white arrows marked "N"). A visual word form is produced and the mental lexicon is activated to identify the word form and generate the concept of a furry animal that barks. If the lexicon cannot retrieve the word form, the visual cortex and coding areas may be reactivated to provide more input, thus slowing down the process.

encoding areas to provide more information, adding further delay. Although this feedback process takes more time, it can still be completed correctly.

The Skilled Reader

Following repeated encounters with the same word, the child's brain forms a composite neural model of the word that includes its spelling, pronunciation, and meaning. This word form model gets stored in the occipito-temporal area. As the number of words in the word form area grows, the child becomes a more skillful reader.

Figure 2.7 shows the neural pathway and components for the skilled reader. Note that the visual information about *dog* is sent to the word form region (occipito-temporal area) where all the relevant linguistic information is stored (indicated in the diagram by the white arrow labeled "S"). The mental image can be generated quickly, and the reader moves on to the next word. Imaging scans show that the word form area is in full activation when highly-

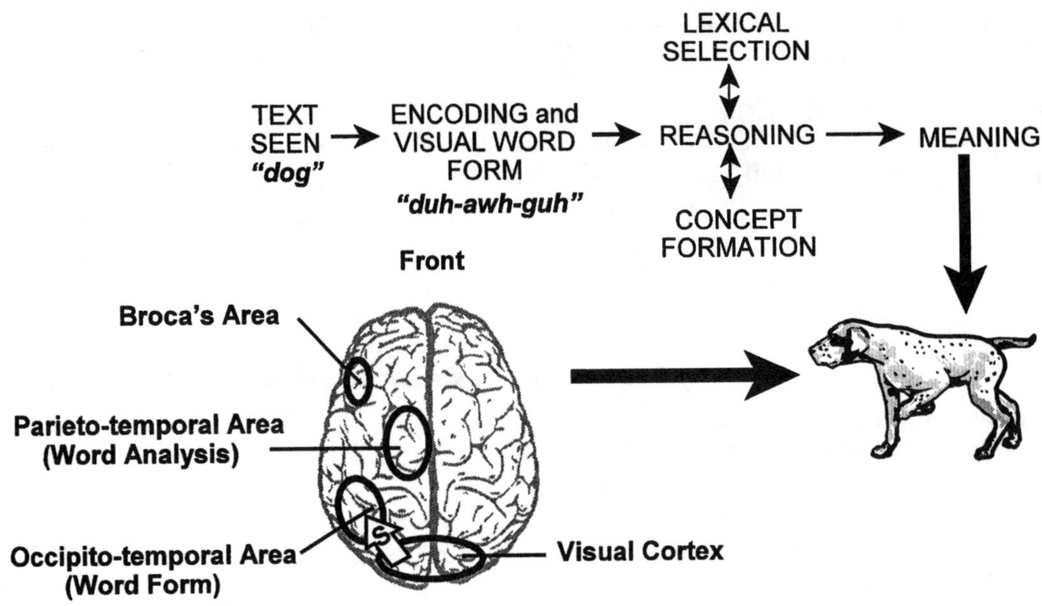

Figure 2.7 This diagram shows the pathway for the skilled reader. Visual information about the word *dog* is passed along to the word form region (occipito-temporal area) where all the linguistic and visual information about a dog is generated, indicated by the white arrow labeled "S." The lexical representation is quickly activated and a mental concept is formed.

skilled readers are moving through text. This indicates that reading skill relies heavily on the word form area (McCandliss, et al., 2003; Shaywitz, 2003). Keep in mind that although the processes outlined in Figures 2.6 and 2.7 appear linear and singular, they are really bidirectional and parallel, with many phonemes being processed at the same time.

Eye Movements During Reading

When we read, our eyes make rapid movements across the page, stopping for certain periods of time, called *fixations.* It is during these fixations of about 200 to 250 milliseconds that the eyes actually acquire information from the text. Then the eyes take about 20 to 40 milliseconds to move to the next fixation point, a distance of about nine letter spaces. During this time, vision is suppressed and no new information enters the processing system. Skilled readers also move their eyes backwards about 10 to 15 percent of the time in order to reread material. These *regressions* are needed when the reader has difficulty comprehending the text (Rayner, Foorman, Perfetti, Pesetsky, and Seidenberg, 2001).

Research studies on eye movements during reading lend further support to the notion that novice and skilled readers are processing written information differently. Novice readers fixate on every word in a text and they often fixate on the same word several times. Their fixation points are only about three letter spaces apart and their fixation periods run longer, from 300 to 400 milliseconds. Furthermore, up to 50 percent of their eye movements are regressions. These eye movements most likely indicate the difficulty the novice reader is having encoding the text. The longer fixation time may also result from the slower process of word analysis that occurs in the brain's parieto-temporal area. Table 2.4 shows a comparison of the eye movements of novice and skilled readers.

Table 2.4 Comparison of Eye Movements of Novice and Skilled Readers

Reading Skill Level	Fixation Time (in milliseconds)	Fixation Span (in letter spaces)	Percentage in Regression
Novice	300 to 400	3	Up to 50
Skilled	200 to 250	9	10 to 15

Source: Rayner et al., 2001

Combining Written and Spoken Words

You will recall in the previous chapter we discussed a schematic representation of how the brain processes and recognizes spoken language (Figure 1.11). We mentioned then that written language must share some of the steps with the spoken language model. Figure 2.8 is a schematic representation of how the spoken and written language processing systems might interact. Words can enter the system through either pathway. However, words entering through the spoken word pathway are more likely to be learned easier because that process is facilitated by genetic influences and by Broca's and Wernicke's areas that specialize in spoken language processing.

The processing of written words, however, is not facilitated at the lower levels by any brain areas specialized for reading. Remember that to the occipito-temporal area, reading is just another collection of sensory stimuli that must be decoded and encoded in order to derive meaning. Several fMRI studies have shown that both Broca's and Wernicke's areas (sites of phonologic processing) were activated when participants were asked to generate written words (Joseph et al., 2001). Apparently, as you can see from the model, the formation of visual word forms (orthographic coding) relies strongly on the ability to generate auditory word forms (phonologic coding). How well and how quickly a child learns to read even common words depends a great deal on how well that child has acquired and practiced spoken language.

How well and how quickly a child learns to read even common words depends a great deal on how well that child has acquired and practiced spoken language.

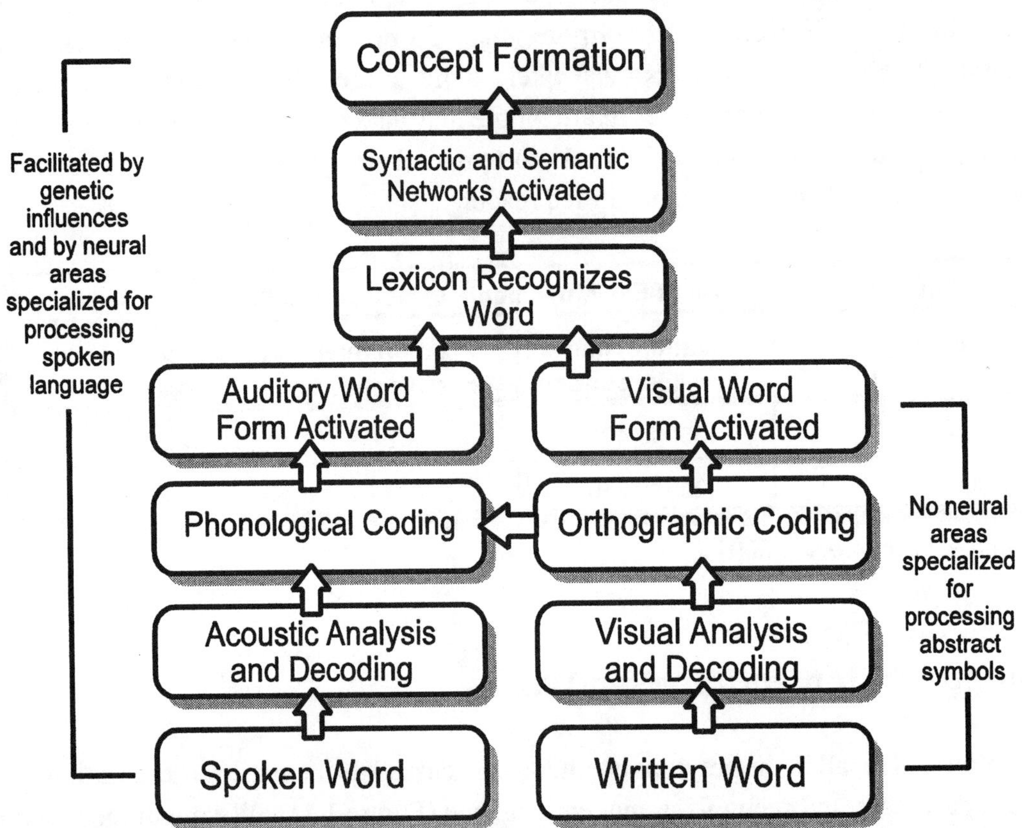

Figure 2.8 This is a schematic representation of the components involved in spoken and written language processing. Words can enter the system through either pathway. Words entering through the spoken word pathway are learned quicker because that process is facilitated by genetic influences and by brain areas specialized for spoken language. Note the horizontal arrow at the third step, which indicates that the ability to encode visual word forms (orthographic coding) relies strongly on the brain's ability to generate auditory word forms (phonological coding) (Gazzaniga et al., 2002).

THE IMPORTANCE OF PRACTICE

For most children, reading improves with practice. Experience in reading improves several components of the decoding and comprehension processes (Rayner et al., 2001). For example, practice

- Allows the mental lexicon and word form areas of the brain to acquire increasingly accurate representations of a word's spelling, thereby strengthening the connection between how the word sounds (the phonological form) and its spelling (the orthographic representation). This is called the *phonological-orthographic connection.* The stronger this connection, the faster one reads.

- Results in an increasing facility with words because it increases the quality of the words' representation in the lexicon, thereby enhancing comprehension.
- Turns low-frequency words into high-frequency words, improving the fluency of reading. Fluency involves developing rapid and automatic word-identification processes as well as bridging the gap between word recognition and comprehension.
- Increases familiarity with the patterns of letters that form printed words, thereby improving spelling. This is referred to as the *lexical-orthographic connection.* It is not the same as the phonological-orthographic connection. Both contribute in their own way to support the brain's ability to read words.
- Improves comprehension because the reader is exposed to both familiar and new words used in many different contexts. This helps the reader recognize that two words can have the same spelling, but have different meanings, grammatical functions, and pronunciation, such as: "I *lead* a team that tests our drinking water for *lead* and other metals."

Less able readers are likely to get less practice than more able readers. Consequently, the gap between more and less able readers increases over time. It was not surprising, then, that Cunningham and Stanovich (1997) found that reading ability in grade 1 was a strong predictor of reading ability in grade 11. This evidence contradicts a common belief that initial differences in reading ability wash out over time.

> Reading ability in grade 1 is a strong predictor of reading ability in grade 11.

Being a Skilled Reader

Skilled readers do not read each word individually, nor do their eyes move from word to word until they reach the end. Rather, they scan the text searching for patterns that will make the task of reading easier. To illustrate this, look at the following block of text and note any irregularities:

Q Q Q Q Q Q Q Q
Q Q Q Q Q Q Q Q
Q Q Q Q Q P Q Q
Q Q Q Q Q Q Q Q
Q O Q Q Q Q Q Q
Q Q Q Q Q Q Q Q

What did you notice? Most people will spot the letter "P" almost immediately, but miss the letter "O" in the fifth line. This illustrates the selectivity of vision. We notice something that violates the pattern but skim over something that very closely resembles it. These expectations of conformity guide our reading and allow us to increase our reading speed. This activity also shows the faster we read, the more detail we miss.

Another interesting characteristic of skilled reading is that the phonologic module becomes so adept at recognizing common words that it can do so even if the word is significantly misspelled. Can you understand the following text?

> Aoccdrnig to rseerach at an Elingsh uinervtisy, it deosn't mttaer in waht order the ltteers in a wrod are, the olny iprmoetnt tihnh is taht the frist and lsat ltteer is in the rghit pclae. The rset can be a total mses and you can sitll raed it outhit a porbelm. Tihs is bcuseae we do not raed ervey letetr by itslef, but the wrod as a wlohe.

Most skilled readers can read this paragraph despite the misspellings. Apparently, the beginning and ending letters as well as the context supply enough clues for the phonologic module to recognize the words and determine meaning.

What's Coming?

That the brain learns to read at all attests to its remarkable ability to sift through seemingly confusing input and establish patterns and systems. For a few children with exceptional language skills, this process comes naturally; most, however, have to be taught. In the next chapter, we discuss some considerations that parents and teachers should keep in mind when teaching children to read.

CHAPTER 3
Teaching Reading

This chapter addresses several basic questions about teaching reading. They include:

- *What are the basic characteristics of the various approaches to reading instruction?*
- *What strategies are effective for teaching phonemic awareness, phonics, spelling, fluency, vocabulary, and comprehension?*
- *What strategies are effective for teaching reading to students who have limited English proficiency?*

BRIEF HISTORY OF TEACHING READING

Reading instruction in the United States over the past 130 years has involved two general methods: an analytical method called the *phonics* approach and a global method called the *whole-word* (now, *whole-language*) approach (Figure 3.1). Phonics instructioı was the earliest method for teaching reading. Children were taught the letter names and simple syllables from which they then constructed words. Emphasis was on phonics drill. In this analytical approach, bits of words were used to build syllables, then words and meaningful phrases.

At the beginning of the twentieth century, the emphasis shifted to a more global approach and choral reading emerged. Students would spell the syllable aloud together and then pronounce it. A few decades later, the pendulum swung back and phonics drill returned. But dissatisfaction with this method arose again in the 1940s, and the emphasis shifted back to a global approach known as whole-word instruction. The whole-word method placed little emphasis on phonics drill and more on recognizing entire words as the meaningful units of reading. The teacher showed the students a flash card with a word on it. After the teacher

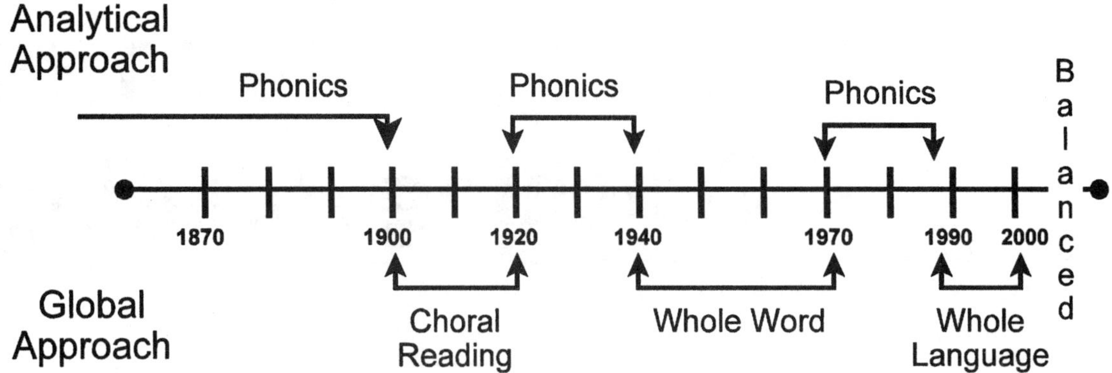

Figure 3.1 The timeline from 1870 to the present shows how the predominant method of reading instruction has alternated between analytical and global approaches. Today, the emphasis has shifted toward a balanced approach that seeks to combine phonics instruction with enriched reading text.

pronounced the word, the children would say it aloud. The small set of beginning vocabulary words was gradually expanded.

One major reason for advocating the whole-word approach was that the irregularities in the pronunciation of common words, such as *pint* (violates the pattern of *hint, mint, tint,* etc.) and *have* (violates the pattern of *gave, pave, save*, etc.) meant that the letter-to-phoneme correspondence was not very reliable. Therefore, emphasis should be on learning to memorize the pronunciation of whole words, not parts of words. Another argument for whole-word instruction was that it promoted comprehension early in the learning of reading: words have meaning, speech sounds do not (Rayner et al., 2001).

In the early 1970s, concerns over the poor results on standardized reading tests prompted a shift in emphasis back to phonics drill. At the same time, a psycholinguistic approach to reading was emerging, based on the work of Smith and Goodman (1971). Psycholinguistic advocates suggested that reading was like a guessing game in which readers determined meaning through a variety of redundant cuing systems present in rich literature. This approach, which became known as the whole-language method, also suggested that phonics not be taught separately because they were boring and failed to show the child that learning to read could be enjoyable. The proponents of phonics, however, were not convinced that the whole-language method (sometimes called the literature-based method) was effective. Thus, the so-called "reading wars" began in earnest and continued through the 1990s.

> For over a century, reading instruction in the United States has shifted between the phonics and whole-language approaches.

Basic Rationale for Phonics Instruction

Phonics instruction is based on the following concepts:

- Learning to read is not a natural ability for the human brain.
- Spoken language and written language are very different, and thus require the mastery of different skills.
- The alphabetic principle must be taught because it is not learned merely by exposure to print.
- The most important skill at the beginning stages of reading is the ability to read single words accurately, completely, and fluently.
- Context is not the primary factor in beginning word recognition.

Basic Rationale for Whole-Language Instruction

Whole-language instruction is based on the following concepts:

- Reading knowledge can be developed in the same natural way as spoken language.
- Children can often determine the meaning of an unfamiliar word by searching for semantic, syntactic, and phonetic cues in the text.
- Experiencing words in context leads to greater improvement in word reading than experiencing words out of context.
- Phonics knowledge is important but should not be explicitly taught.
- Reading should be a pleasurable experience for the child.

Figure 3.2 shows a comparison between the phonics and whole-language approaches to teaching reading. Obviously, the methods used to teach reading will dramatically affect the young brain's ability to decode abstract symbols into sounds and words that will result in obtaining meaning from print. Despite the passion of the supporters for both the phonics and whole-language approaches, experience has taught us that no one mix of instructional strategies and curriculum materials will work for every child. As a result of the reports of the National Research Council (Snow et al., 1998) and the National Reading Panel (NRP, 2000), many educators now suggest that the teaching of reading should use a balanced approach that includes a phonics component as well as enriched text. Figure 3.3 shows one way to look at the balanced approach to teaching reading.

> Experience has taught us that no one mix of instructional strategies and curriculum materials on teaching reading will work for every child.

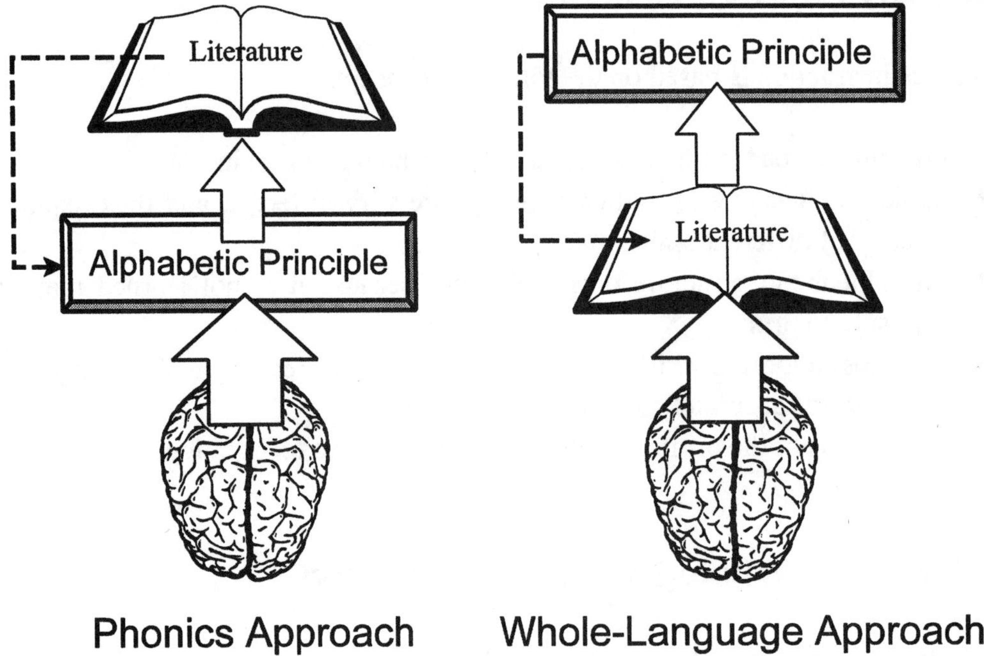

Figure 3 .2 A comparison of the phonics and whole-language approaches to teaching reading. The phonics approach focuses on developing the alphabetic principle through decoding text before moving on to enriched literature. As reading progresses, letter-to-sound correspondences are strengthened and new ones learned (dotted arrow). The whole-language method focuses on reading literature early so that letter-to-sound correspondences develop naturally. As the alphabetic principle strengthens, more unfamiliar words can be read (dotted arrow).

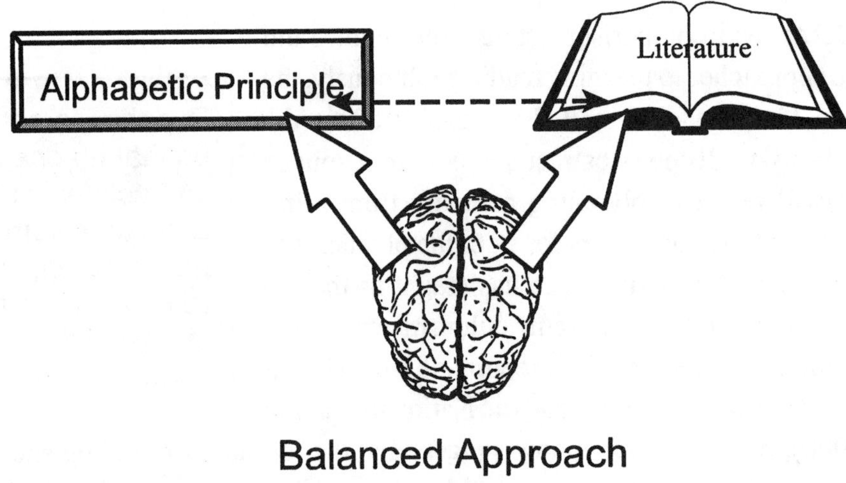

Figure 3.3 In the balanced approach to teaching reading, students learn the alphabetic principle and use enriched literature together.

Basic Rationale for the Balanced Approach

The balanced approach is based on the following considerations:

- No one reading program is the best program for all children.
- Children need to develop phonemic awareness in order to learn to read successfully.
- Children need to master the alphabetic principle.
- Phonics are important but should not be taught as a separate unit through drill and rote memorization.
- Phonics should be taught to develop spelling strategies and word analysis skills.
- An important component is learning to read for meaning.
- Enriched literature helps students develop a positive dispositions toward reading and develops their ability to think imaginatively and critically.

There is still some persistent debate about what constitutes a balanced reading program. The question now is whether reading programs built around a balanced approach are based sufficiently on scientific research to meet the requirements of the No Child Left Behind Act. Regardless of their biases and perspectives, educators, parents, and policymakers must now recognize that reading is a *learned* skill, and the curriculum programs selected to teach reading must reflect what science continues to learn about how we acquire skills.

BRAIN RESEARCH AND LEARNING A SKILL

Research in cognitive neuroscience indicates that learning any skill, including reading, requires some basic elements if such learning is to be successful. These elements include the following (SLC, 2000):

- *Practice.* For the brain to build and strengthen the neural pathways required to learn a new skill, the learner must be repeatedly exposed to, and process, the material being learned. But the practice cannot be haphazard. Practice leads to permanency, so it is important that the activities associated with practice be carefully planned to ensure that the learning being stored is correct. As for reading, practice brings about true accomplishment. Studies show that the more a person reads, the better that person will be at reading at any age and at any level of proficiency.
- *Intensity.* Learning a new skill requires focus and concentration. Intense focus on a new skill allows the learner's brain to build more neural support for that skill in a short period of time. If you are planning on running a marathon, occasional

jogging will not have sufficient intensity to prepare and train your body. To become a skilled reader, the learner must first focus intently on the basic skills needed to learn the correct letter-to-sound relationships.

- *Cross-training.* Learning any skill is easier if it can be supported by other skills the student already knows or is learning at the same time. Cross-training involves bringing together a wide range of skills that reinforce overall comprehension of the material. Accomplished reading requires that the learner be simultaneously proficient in many different skills, such as spoken language fluency and comprehension.
- *Adaptivity.* When teaching a new skill, the teacher needs to assess the student's current skill level and adapt the new instruction accordingly. If the instructional skill level is too low, the learner may get bored and lose interest. If the skill level is too high, the learner may get frustrated and lose motivation. Reading instruction should include constant monitoring of the learner's progress so that the teacher can adapt the instructional strategies as needed.
- *Motivation and attention.* Motivation is the key to successfully learning a skill because it keeps students interested in paying attention and in practicing the skill. Reading instruction needs to include motivational strategies and texts that keep students interested and thus sustain attention.

None of the elements mentioned above will come as a surprise to any person who has taught. Nonetheless, they are worth reviewing. With so many reading programs available, these elements become important measures that teachers can use to assess the effectiveness of materials designed to support the teaching of reading.

MODERN METHODS OF TEACHING READING

With the growing support in the late 1990s for the balanced approach to teaching reading, the reading wars abated. But now a new war seems to have taken its place. The reports of the National Research Council (Snow et al., 1998) and the National Reading Panel (NRP, 2000) concluded that, based on scientific evidence, reading programs that included a strong phonics component were more likely to be successful with more beginning readers than programs lacking this component. At the same time, the research using fMRI technology described in Chapter 2 offered new insights into how the brains of novice, skilled, and struggling readers differed. Furthermore, intensive interventions with struggling readers (described later in Chapter 5) changed their fMRI images to resemble those of typical readers.

It did not take long for some researchers to question the findings of the National Reading Panel (Camilli and Wolfe, 2004; Krashen, 2001, 2002; Yatvin, 2003). Their criticisms included (1) concerns over whether the Panel's methodology was truly scientific, (2) suggestions that the results were crafted to fulfill a political agenda, and (3) cautions that the Panel's conclusions would promote one philosophical view of reading (i.e., phonics) over others. Even the results of the fMRI studies were challenged (Coles, 2004) as being of questionable value and deliberately misinterpreted to support the prescriptive approaches mandated by the No Child Left Behind legislation. Not surprisingly, other researchers responded in defense of the Panel's two years of work (Ehri, Shanahan, and Nunes, 2002; Shaywitz, 2003). Consequently, a new debate is in progress, this one over what constitutes good research in reading. School districts, meanwhile, are caught in the middle. The No Child Left Behind legislation requires districts to use scientifically-based reading programs just as researchers and politicians debate the meaning and intent of scientific evidence.

Where Do We Go From Here?

So, where do we go from here? Educators should become familiar with all positions so that they can understand the major issues involved in the debate. Ultimately, however, they need to make important recommendations regarding the type of reading program that is most likely to help young children learn to read successfully. Accordingly, let's consider what the major research studies have revealed about how the brain learns to read. The evidence presented here comes from the following sources:

- *The National Research Council (NRC) (Snow et al., 1998).* This 1998 report from the research arm of the National Academy of Sciences focused on how to reduce children's reading difficulties. It looked at how parental influences, family literacy, and preschool environments affect reading development. Although it did not make specific suggestions for reading curriculum, the report did make recommendations about teacher preparation, both in preservice and inservice training programs. However, the NRC report did not specifically address how critical reading skills are most effectively taught.
- *The National Reading Panel (NRP, 2000).* The report the NRP issued in 2000 was the result of two years of effort that included reviewing thousands of research studies on reading, interviewing parents and teachers, and recommending the most effective and scientifically proven methods for teaching reading. The NRP report took into account the report of the National Research Council and focused on the specific topics of alphabetics (phonemic awareness and phonics), fluency, vocabulary and text comprehension, teacher preparation, and the use of computer technology in reading instruction. Many of the recommendations of the NRP were translated into teaching strategies in a publication developed by the Center for the Improvement of Early Reading Achievement and funded by the National Institute for Literacy (NIFL, 2001).

- *Laboratory Studies.* Experimental studies conducted in laboratories are also providing new information about the reading process. Using brain imaging and mapping technologies, scientists are learning more about the brain regions associated with the different stages of learning to read. These studies include looking at the brains of people with reading problems.
- *Best Practices Research.* Best practices research on reading conducted in schools involved case studies that assessed whether certain instructional practices were more effective than others. These studies examined the practices of exemplary teachers to sort out what they were doing differently from others that resulted in greater student achievement. Several of these reports have been published recently, and they offer valuable insights into the effectiveness of various strategies for teaching reading. Although some of the studies involved a small sample of students, their results cannot be dismissed.
- *Evidence-based Practices.* Other research studies have looked at the effectiveness of practices in longitudinal and multi-level designs rather than just at exemplary teachers. Results from these types of studies are particularly valuable because they generally involve a large sample of students whose achievement is monitored for a year or more.

In this chapter, we will discuss the findings of these research studies and reports as they apply to the teaching of reading to children without any reading difficulties. Diagnosing children with reading problems, and how to address those problems, will be discussed in subsequent chapters. Figure 3.3 reminds us that reading involves the two major processes of decoding and comprehension. Successful decoding includes phonemic awareness, phonics, and fluency. Comprehension requires a developed vocabulary, interaction with the text, and a teacher whose training provides strategies for advancing the learner's ability to understand what is read.

RESEARCH FINDINGS ON READING INSTRUCTION — DECODING

Phonemic Awareness Instruction

Phonemic awareness, you will recall, is the ability to manipulate individual sounds in *spoken* language. Children have phonemic awareness when they can (1) recognize words beginning with the same sound, (2) isolate and say the first and last sounds in a word, (3) combine and blend sounds in a word, and (4) break a word into its separate sounds. Phonemic awareness and letter knowledge are the two best predictors of how well children will learn to read during their first two years of instruction. Even for middle and high school students, phonemic

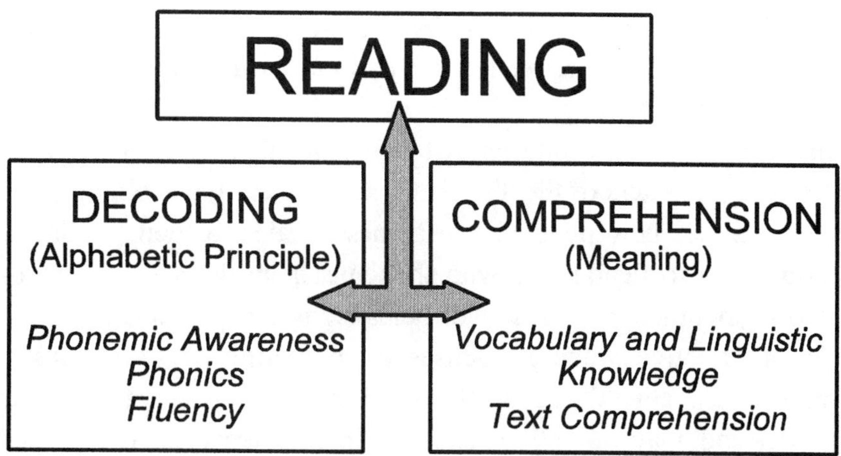

Figure 3.3 Successful reading is the result of the interaction between the decoding and comprehension processes. Decoding includes phonemic awareness, phonics, and fluency. Comprehension requires adequate vocabulary and linguistic knowledge, and interaction with text to capture meaning.

awareness is a good predictor of their ability to read accurately and quickly (Shaywitz, 2003). Phonemic awareness can be taught and learned.

The findings in the research examined by the NRC were (Snow et al., 1998):

- Learning to read depends critically on mapping the letters and the spellings of words onto the sounds of speech and speech units they represent.
- Explicit instruction in the phonological structure of speech and of phonemes and their spellings helps children acquire the alphabetic principle and use it appropriately when they encounter unfamiliar words in text.

> Even for middle and high school students, phonemic awareness is a good predictor of their ability to read accurately and quickly.

The findings in the research examined by the NRP showed that phonemic awareness instruction (NIFL, 2001):

- Helps children learn to read. Phonemic awareness is the first step in mastering the alphabetic principle, the ability to map letters onto the spoken sounds of language. As their mapping skills get better, they can read faster and with greater comprehension.

- Helps children learn to spell. Children who have phonemic awareness understand that letters and sound are related in a particular way, and that these relationships are important in spelling.
- Is most effective when children are taught to manipulate phonemes while handling cutouts of the letters of the alphabet that represent those phonemes. This allows children to see how phonemic awareness relates to their reading and writing. Learning how to blend letters with phonemes helps them to *read* words, and learning to segment letters with sounds helps them to *spell* words.
- Is most effective when it focuses on only one or two types of phoneme manipulation, rather than several types. Teaching too many types at once confuses children and may not allow enough time to teach each type well. Another possibility is that it may inadvertently result in teaching more difficult types before the children have learned the simpler ones.
- Is effective under a variety of teaching conditions with a variety of learners across a range of grade and age levels. Furthermore, the improvements in reading lasted well beyond the end of the phonemic awareness training, indicating mastery in most children.

After children are introduced to new letter-sound relationships, practice ensures that the learning is committed to long-term memory.

Recent brain imaging studies have shown

- How effective practice can build new neural circuits. After children are introduced to new letter-sound relationships, additional practice is necessary to ensure that the learning is committed to long-term memory.

How Do I Teach Phonemic Awareness?

✓ Assess each child's phonemic awareness capabilities before beginning instruction. This will help identify which students should start with simple manipulation and which can move on to more advanced manipulation activities.

✓ A complete phonemic awareness program provides activities that include matching, isolating, substituting, blending, segmenting, and deleting sounds in words (Yopp and Yopp, 2000).

✓ Teach one or two types of phoneme manipulation to produce a greater benefit rather than teaching several types at once.

✓ Teach students to manipulate phonemes along with letters to enhance their mental lexicon. Have them say the whole word aloud and then the individual phonemes. Then write each letter on the board as they sound out its phoneme. This helps the students acquire the alphabetic principle.

✓ Remember that phonemic awareness instruction can benefit **all** children, including preschoolers, kindergartners, first graders, and even less able readers.

✓ Avoid spending too much time on phonemic awareness activities. The whole program should average out to about 10 minutes per day. Obviously, some students will need more time than others, perhaps up to 30 minutes per day (Brady and Moats, 1998).

✓ Small groups are usually more productive for phonemic awareness instruction. Children can benefit from hearing their classmates and receiving feedback from the teacher.

✓ Preschool (and parental) instruction should focus on

- developing an awareness of rhyme
- separating words into syllables and syllables into phonemes

✓ Kindergarten instruction should focus on

- practicing the sound structure of words
- the recognition and production of letters
- knowledge of print concepts.

✓ Grade 1 instruction should provide

- explicit instruction and practice with sound structures that lead to phonemic awareness
- familiarity with sound-spelling correspondences and common spelling conventions and their use in identifying written words
- sight recognition of frequent words
- independent reading, including reading aloud

✓ Remember that phonemic awareness instruction is only one important part of a reading program. How well students learn to read and comprehend will depend not just on phonemic awareness but also on the effectiveness of the other components in the literacy curriculum.

Phonemic awareness is only one important part of a literacy curriculum.

✓ Keep in mind the importance of practice. When children learn new letter-sound correspondences, they should practice them in isolation and then in reading aloud simple sentences and books. With every bit of practice and corrective feedback, the word form that will be stored in the brain's memory is likely to be accurate in pronunciation, spelling, and meaning. Through additional practice in spelling-sound patterns, a precise replica of the word form will be established in the neural circuits, and recognition of that word again in the future becomes easier.

Phonics Instruction

Phonics instruction teaches the relationship between phonemes of spoken language and the graphemes of *written* language, and how to use these relationships to read and write words. It includes helping children use the alphabetic principle to recognize familiar words automatically and accurately, and to decode unfamiliar words. Critics of phonics say that English spellings are too irregular for phonics instruction to be of any value. Nonetheless, phonics instruction teaches children a system for remembering how to read words. For example, when children learn that *ghost* is spelled this way and not *goast,* their memory helps them to remember the spelling and to recognize the word instantly. Although many words are spelled irregularly, most of them contain some regular letter-sound relationships that help children learn to read them. Moreover, students at risk for reading failure, such as those in special education and Title I programs, benefited the most from phonics-based programs (Foorman, Francis, Fletcher, Schatschneider, and Mehta, 1998). The NRP report summarizes the research on phonics instruction as follows (NIFL, 2001).

Phonics instruction that is systematic and explicit

- Makes a bigger contribution to a child's growth in reading than little or no phonics instruction.
- Significantly improves kindergarten and grade 1 children's word recognition and spelling when compared to children who do not receive systematic instruction. It should be noted that the effects of phonics instruction on students in grades 2 through 6 are limited to improving their oral text and word reading skills. Explicit phonics instruction beyond grade 6 is not generally productive for most students.
- Significantly improves children's reading comprehension. This is because their increased ability for automatic word recognition allows them more time to focus on and process the meaning of text. Contrary to what some believe, research studies indicate that phonics instruction contributes to comprehension skills rather than inhibiting them.
- Is effective for children from various economic and social levels.

- Particularly helps children who are having difficulty learning to read and who are at risk for developing future reading problems.
- Is most effective when introduced in kindergarten or grade 1.

How Do I Teach Phonics?

✓ Systematic instruction is characterized by the direct teaching of the letter-sound relationships of both consonants and vowels in a clearly defined sequence. Such programs give children substantial practice in applying these relationships as they read and write, as well as opportunities to spell words and write their own stories. Several approaches to teaching phonics exist, depending on the unit of analysis or how letter-sound combinations are presented to the student. They include

- *Analogy-based phonics* - using parts of word families to identify unknown words that have similar parts
- *Analytic phonics* - analyzing letter-sound relationships in previously learned words
- *Embedded phonics* - learning letter-sound relationships during the reading of connected text
- *Onset-rime phonics* - identifying the sound of the letter or letters before the first vowel (onset) in a one-syllable word and the sound of the remaining part of the word (the rime)
- *Phonics through spelling* - learning to segment words into phonemes and to make words by writing letters for phonemes
- *Synthetic phonics* - learning how to convert letters or letter combinations into sounds, and then how to blend the sounds together to form recognizable words.

✓ Effective programs for phonics instruction

- Include knowledge of the alphabet, phonemic awareness, vocabulary development, the reading of text, and systematic instruction in phonics.
- Help teachers systematically and explicitly instruct students in how to relate sounds and letters, how to break words into sounds, and how to blend sounds to form words.
- Help children understand why they are learning relationships between sounds and letters.
- Help children apply their knowledge of phonics as they read text.
- Help children apply what they learn about sounds and letters to their own writing.
- Can be adapted to the needs of individual students.

✓ Systematic programs in phonics introduce the child to different letter-sound pairings, starting with the simplest and most frequent combinations and then progressing to more complex and unusual ones. One approach (Carnine, Silbert, and Kame'enui, 1997) suggests

- *Start with one-to-one letter-sound relationships.* Introduce consonants that are predictable in their relationships between the letter and their sounds. A possible sequence could begin with : *m, t, s, f, d,* and *r,* and ending with *k, v, w, j, p, y.*
- *Continue with vowel sounds.* Vowels are needed to help make up words, but they can be more difficult for young children to pronounce than consonants. Identify long vowels that say their name, as the */a/* in *made,* the */e/* in *be,* the */i/* in *mine,* the */o/* in *row,* and the */u/* in *used.* Short vowels do not say their name, such as in *dad, tell, kid, top,* and *run.*
- *Phonic units.* These usually contain six to eight consonants and two vowels. As the children master more phonic units, they should be able to pronounce a larger number of words.
- *Complex letter-sound combinations.* Introduce common digraphs, such as *sh-* in *should, ch-* in *chip, th-* in *thing,* and the *wh-* in *what.* Later, the children will recognize larger phonetic combinations, such as *-tch* (*witch*), *-dge* (*fudge*),and *-ough* (*cough, rough*).

✓ Practice materials should include stories that contain words using the specific letter-sound correspondences the children are learning (often called decodable texts). They should also have practice writing letter combinations and using them to write their own stories.

✓ Phonics instruction can be taught effectively to individual students, small groups, or the whole class, depending on the needs of the students and the number of adults working with them.

✓ Phonics lessons should last typically from 15 to 20 minutes a day, but should also be reinforced during the remainder of the day with other activities in the child's reading program, including opportunities to read and write.

✓ Phonics instruction should be taught for about two years for most students, usually kindergarten and grade 1. If begun in grade 1, it should be completed by grade 2.

✓ Phonics instruction is but one of the necessary components of a comprehensive reading program, including phonemic awareness, fluency, and text reading and comprehension skills.

✓ Role reversal can be an effective strategy for helping children acquire the alphabetic principle. Ask the students to make up vocabulary words for you to write down. They should be nonsense words that the children create. Ask them to clearly enunciate each sound so that you can write the word down accurately (SEDL, 2001).

✓ Pay close attention to how children write. To assess their understanding of the alphabetic principle, it is not necessary for them to write accurately. It is important, however, that they write one symbol per sound; that is, a word with three phonemes should be represented in writing by three symbols.

Spelling and Invented Spelling

Spelling is closely linked to reading because it involves breaking apart a spoken word into its sounds and encoding them into the letters representing each sound. While learning to read words, children also learn how to spell those words. As children try to represent words with the alphabet, they often encode words by their initial consonants, followed by their ending sounds. Middle sounds, usually vowels, are omitted at first. Thus, *horse* might be written as *hrs,* and *monster* as *mstr.* The pronunciation of this *invented spelling* is very close to that of the intended word. Invented spelling allows children to practice applying the alphabetic principle and gain in phonemic awareness. It serves as a transitional step and assists in the development of reading and writing.

Invented spelling allows children to practice applying the alphabetic principle and gain in phonemic awareness.

Studies on early literacy development have shown that invented spelling is a reliable measure of early reading achievement. One study found that preschool and kindergarten children who were inventive spellers performed significantly better on word reading and on storybook readings. In a literacy study of four grade 1 classrooms, two teachers encouraged invented spelling while the other two teachers encouraged traditional spelling. The inventive spellers scored significantly better than the traditional spellers on several measures of word reading that were administered during the second semester in grade 1 (Ahmed and Lombardino, 2000). Uhry (1999) found that invented spelling was the best predictor of how well kindergartners could match, through finger-point reading, spoken words to printed words in reading a sentence—a skill known as *concept of a word in text.*

When their invented spelling is accepted, children feel empowered to write more and with purpose, communicating their messages from the very beginning of school. Writing slows down the process of dealing with text, allowing children more time to recognize and learn about sound-letter relationships. For some children, writing may be an easier way to literacy than reading. In reading, the process involves changing letter sequences to sounds, whereas in writing the process is reversed—going from sounds to letters. Accordingly, writing may be a simpler task because it involves going from sounds in the child's head that are already known and automatic, to letters, rather than from the unknown letters in reading to what is known (Chomsky, 1979).

Some researchers in the past have raised concerns about whether the persistent use of invented spelling leads to confusion and the formation of bad spelling habits. But research studies indicate that, with appropriate teacher intervention, the invented spellings gradually come closer to conventional forms. Consequently, spelling errors should not be seen as an impediment to writing but as an indication of the child's thought processes while making sense of letter-sound relationships. From that perspective, the errors could yield important information about a child's internal reading patterns (Sipe, 2001). On the other hand, remember that practice eventually makes permanent. The consistent repetition of incorrect spellings will, in time, lead to their storage in long-term memory. Therefore, teachers should use strategies that will help children transform invented spelling into conventional spelling.

How Do I Teach Spelling?

✓ Effective spelling instruction focuses on helping children go from sound to letter, which strongly reinforces their reading—going from letter to sound. Spelling instruction is more than memorizing word lists. It should follow a logical sequence that starts with phonemic awareness, demonstrates which letters represent which sounds, and introduces the notion that the same sound can have different spellings (Shaywitz, 2003).

✓ *Moving away from invented spelling.* Techniques, such as using sound boxes (also known as Elkonion boxes) drawn on paper, can help the child enunciate the word slowly and recognize other sounds that need to be represented by letters. For example, if the child spells *dog* as *dg,* you draw a box for the first sound */d/ = duh* and the child enters the letter *d* and puts a marker or coin on it. By stretching out the pronunciation of the word, the child hears the */ô/ = auh* sound. Now draw another box, enter the letter *o* and ask the child to push a marker into it. This continues until the last phoneme, */g/ = guh* is represented by the letter *g.* The process can be repeated until the child is confident in hearing the middle vowel sound (Figure 3.4).

✓ Another technique for correcting spelling is the Have-a-Go chart (Bolton and Snowball, 1993). Students use this chart (Figure 3.5) when they need your assistance with words they have misspelled. The student writes the misspelled word in the first column. Use the sound box (Figure 3.4) to stretch the word and

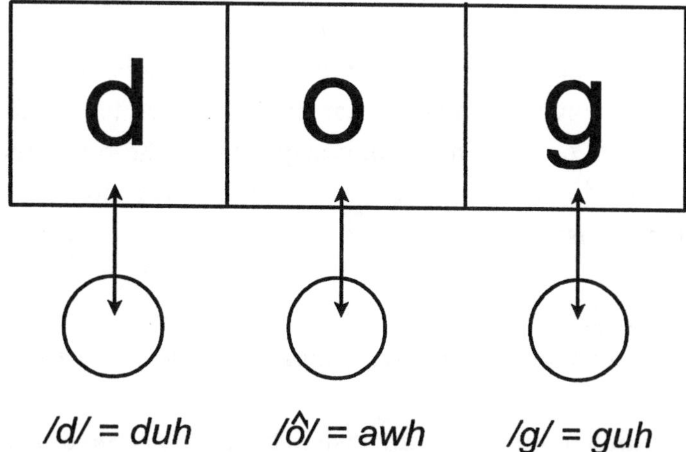

Figure 3.4 This sound (Elkonion) box technique requires the student to move a marker (or coin) into the box several times while pronouncing the letter's sound. It helps the child detect the middle vowel sounds and thus represent them in spelling (Sipe, 2001).

ask the student to listen for phonemes. After sounding out the word several times, the student writes the word again in the Have-a-Go column. If incorrect, you can write the word correctly. The student then writes the correct word in the third column. Now encourage the student to recall the correct spelling mentally and to write it again in the fourth column to enhance retention of the correct spelling in long-term memory.

Have-a-Go Chart

Misspelled Word	Have-a-Go	Correct Spelling	Copied Spelling
Bots	*Boats*		*Boats*
Clen	*Cleen*	*Clean*	*Clean*

Figure 3.5 Students write the misspelled word in the first column. The teacher might use the sound box (Figure 3.4) to stretch the word and ask the student to listen for phonemes. The student writes the word again in the Have-a-Go column. If incorrect, the teacher either writes the word or refers the student to a dictionary. The student then writes the correct word in the third column and copies it again in the fourth column to enhance retention in long-term memory (Bolton and Snowball, 1993).

✓ As spelling progresses, introduce children to spelling strategies they can use to help spell new words. Later, tell them about words, like *colonel* and *could,* that do not match the spelling rules they were taught.

✓ A study conducted by Ahmed and Lombardino (2000) analyzed the spelling of 100 kindergarten children for letter omission, letter substitution, as well as letter voicing and devoicing. Based on their spelling scores, the children were identified as low, middle, or high in spelling acquisition. The researchers suggested that teachers consider the following strategies, based on the students' spelling acquisition levels:

Low-level spellers:

✓ Teach that a monosyllabic word must be spelled with a vowel (Example: *cat,* not *ct*).

✓ Show children how to distinguish between the name of a vowel letter and its sound in closed monosyllabic words (Example: the letter *a* has a different sound from its name in the word *cat.*

✓ Help children master spelling consonants that have only one letter form and a corresponding letter name (Examples: *b, d, m, p, t*).

✓ Have children practice closed monosyllables consisting of the five vowel sounds (*a, e, i, o, u*) and the consonants that have one corresponding letter (Examples: *bat, met, sit, not,* and *put*).

Mid-level spellers:

✓ Teach the vowel lengthening rule by adding the silent letter *e* after a consonant (Examples: in *lake* and in *time*).

✓ Help children learn to spell consonants that do not have a corresponding letter name (Examples: *ch-* as in *child,* and *sh-* as in *shop*).

✓ Teach how to spell consonant blends (Examples: *dr-* as in *drink, tr-* as in *trap, -mp* as in *damp, -ng* as in *wing,* and *-nk* as in *think*).

High-level spellers:

✓ Have children practice the spelling of frequently occurring vowel digraphs (Examples: *-ai* as in *sail, -ee* as in *bee, -oa* as in *coat*).

✓ Then practice the floss rule—double a word's final *-f, -l,* or *-s* if it follows a short vowel (Examples: *buff, fill,* and *toss*).

✓ Help children understand the meaning of the suffixes *-ed* and *-ing,* and practice their spellings.

In the past, writing was often delayed until children could spell every word correctly. Such an approach inhibited the flow of thoughts necessary for children to attain literacy. Accepting invented spelling allowed children to engage in meaningful writing more than they ever expected. Furthermore, the processes used by teachers to correct spelling develops phonemic awareness and reading. The key to corrective spelling lies with the interventions that teachers *purposefully* use to guide children's writing from invented to conventional spellings. If left alone to grapple with the bizarre nature of English orthography, children will grow frustrated with spelling. But with appropriate teacher interventions, children can overcome the orthography maze and eventually learn the rules, patterns, and exceptions that control spelling in English.

How Teaching Writing Can Affect Spelling and Reading

Few research studies have examined the links between beginning writing and its influence on spelling accuracy and reading. Nonetheless, there is growing evidence that these skills are interrelated. Handwriting is not just a motor skills process or exercise in penmanship. It draws on letter knowledge because to write a letter, the child must attach a verbal label (the letter's name) to the letter symbol, have a precise image of the letter in memory, and be able to retrieve that letter from memory when needed. Some researchers suggest that this direct link between letter knowledge and writing letter forms may indicate that poor handwriting is the result of weak letter knowledge rather than the result of motor difficulties (Berninger et al.,1997).

> Studies have found that explicit instruction in spelling for kindergarten children improved both their spelling and reading abilities.

Studies by O'Connor and Jenkins (1995) and Vandervelden and Siegel (1997) found that explicit instruction in spelling for kindergarten children not only improved the children's spelling ability but also improved their reading ability. The explicit instruction in these studies included using magnetic letters to spell words, speech-print matching of words, Elkonion boxes (Figure 3.4) for spelling, and onset deletion and substitution activities.

What should be the nature of writing instruction in kindergarten classes? Despite the limited research, some suggestions do emerge from these studies (Berninger et al., 1997; Graham, Harris, and Fink, 2000; Vandervelden and Siegel, 1997).

- ✓ Writing instruction is equally effective whether it is distributed throughout the kindergarten day or taught as a single daily activity.
- ✓ The instruction should include components related to handwriting, letter writing accuracy and fluency, spelling, and, if appropriate, simple compositions.
- ✓ Kindergarten children, even those with reading and writing difficulties, can be taught how to form and write letters. This can be accomplished by modeling newly introduced letters, practicing letter names while writing letters, tracing letters with numbered arrow cues, practicing letters from memory, and asking children to circle letters that represent their best work.

- ✓ Kindergarten children can learn to spell consonant-vowel-consonant (CVC) words as they learn beginning reading skills related to letter-sound correspondences, blending, and segmenting.

- ✓ At the beginning of the year, writing lessons in kindergarten that feature specific instruction in letter formation and spelling could be extended to include short compositions later in the year; for example, write a sentence describing a picture, or write a short story explaining what is happening in the wordless picture book.

Fluency Instruction

Fluency is the ability to read a text orally with speed, accuracy, and proper expression. Case studies report that fluency is one component that is often neglected in the classroom. Children who lack fluency read slowly and laboriously, often making it difficult for them to remember what has been read (recall the limited capacity of working memory) and to relate the ideas expressed in the text to their own experiences. Frequent practice in reading is one of the main contributors to developing fluency.

Fluency bridges the gap between word recognition and comprehension. Because fluent readers do not need to spend much time decoding words, they can focus their attention on the meaning of the text. With practice, word recognition and comprehension occur almost simultaneously. Of course, a student will usually not read all text with the same ease. Fluency depends on the reader's familiarity with the words, and with the amount of practice reading the text. The fluency of even skilled readers will slow down when encountering unfamiliar vocabulary or topics. To read with expression, readers must be able to divide sentences into meaningful chunks that include phrases and clauses. As comprehension speed increases, readers develop a sense of knowing when to pause appropriately at the ends of sentences, and when to change tone and emphasis.

> Frequent practice in reading is one of the main contributors to developing fluency.

Fluency and Automaticity. Although the terms are often used interchangeably, it should be noted that fluency is not the same as automaticity. Automaticity is the fast and effortless word recognition that comes after a great deal of reading practice. It does not refer to reading with expression. Thus, automaticity is necessary, but not sufficient, for fluency. Two approaches, each of which has several variations, have been used to teach fluency.

- *Guided repeated oral reading.* This approach encourages students to read passages aloud several times and receive systematic and explicit guidance and feedback from the teacher.
- *Independent silent reading.* This approach encourages students to read silently on their own, inside and outside the classroom, with minimal guidance and feedback.

Researchers have investigated these two main approaches and have found the following (NIFL, 2001):

- *Repeated oral reading.* Monitored repeated oral reading improves reading fluency and overall reading achievement. Students who read passages aloud and receive guidance from their teachers become better readers because this process improves word recognition, speed, accuracy, and fluency. It also improves reading comprehension, but to a lesser extent. This approach even helps struggling readers at the higher elementary grade levels.
    - Round-robin reading—where students take turns reading parts of a text aloud, but not repeatedly—in itself does not increase fluency. This may be because students usually read a small amount of text and only once. Furthermore, the children are likely to pay attention only when it is their turn to read.
    - Children become good readers when they gain an increased sensitivity for how the printed word relates to how it is pronounced. This ability requires the child to pay attention to letter strings and the phoneme sequences in those strings. Children who have attained this ability can read pronounceable nonwords, and the pronunciation errors that they make in reading are plausible. When this occurs, the child's brain is apparently doing some form of phonological recoding, that is, recoding the spellings so they can be pronounced. Opportunities for this recoding occur when children read aloud to a parent or teacher. Feedback from these attempts build up the child's recognition of the written (orthographic) form of unfamiliar words. Several research studies conclude that reading aloud promotes the acquisition of printed word representations in the child's mental lexicon (Share and Stanovich, 1995).
    - Many studies indicate that good readers read the most and poor readers read the least. The suggestion here is that the more children read, the better their fluency, vocabulary, and comprehension. However, these findings do not indicate cause and effect. It is possible that the more children read, the better their fluency. But it may just be that better readers simply choose to read more.
    - The popular belief that fluency was a direct result of proficiency in word recognition is not supported by recent research. Although word recognition is a necessary skill, fluency is now seen as a separate component that can be developed through instruction. Informal Reading Inventories (IRIs), running

records, and miscue analysis are appropriate measures for identifying problems that students are having with word recognition, but are not suitable measures of fluency. Simpler measures, such as calculating words read correctly per minute, are more appropriate for monitoring fluency.

- *Independent silent reading.* No research evidence is currently available to confirm that instructional time spent on silent, independent reading with minimal guidance and feedback improves fluency and overall reading achievement in young readers. Given that instructional time is limited, there may be better ways to spend reading time in the classroom than silent reading. Nonetheless, you should encourage students to read more outside of school rather than devote instruction time to independent reading. Students could also read on their own in class during independent work time when, for example, they have finished one activity and are waiting for another one to begin. Independent reading does build a reader's vocabulary. Some researchers estimate that young readers who engage in independent reading for just 10 minutes a day read over 600,000 more words each year than students who do no independent reading. Increasing the reading time to 20 minutes a day raises the words read to over two million a year (Cunningham and Stanovich, 1998; Hart and Risley, 2003).

How Do I Teach Fluency?

✓ Have students read aloud and provide effective guidance and feedback to improve their fluency. Students need instruction in fluency when

- Their word recognition errors exceed 10 percent when reading a text they have not practiced.
- They cannot read orally with expression.
- Their comprehension is poor after reading a text orally.

✓ *Literature Circles.* Combine reading instruction with opportunities for them to read books at their independent level of reading ability. One technique is to use literature circles where small groups of students discuss a piece of literature in depth. The group is formed by the choice of the book rather than by ability. Literature circles allow students to discuss, on their own, events, characters, and their own personal experiences related to the story. This process helps students engage in reflection and critical thinking as well as construct meaning in their interactions with other students. For more information on literature circles, see the **Resources** section.

✓ Read aloud daily to your students. By your being a good model of fluent reading, students learn how a reader's voice can help text make sense. Then have the students reread the text, perhaps up to four times to improve fluency. Students can practice reading aloud in several ways. The methods are listed in Figure 3.6 in the order of increasing student independence and of decreasing teacher involvement (Carbo, 2003).

- *Shared reading.* This is an interactive reading activity in which students join in the reading of a large book as guided by the teacher. After placing the book on an easel so it can be easily seen, the teacher uses a pointer to guide the reading, pointing to the words as they are read. The teacher may wish to read the text first, asking students to predict a word or phrase or summarize what is happening. Later, the teacher and students take turns reading, and choral reading may also occur. The goal is to work toward phrase fluency rather than reading the text word by word.
- *Student-adult reading or neurological impress.* In this one-on-one method, the adult provides a model of fluent reading by reading the text first. The student then reads the text and the adult provides encouragement and assistance as needed. The student rereads the passage three or four times until fluency is attained. In a variation of this method, called neurological impress, the teacher reads a passage softly into the student's dominant ear as they both use their fingers to follow along in the text.

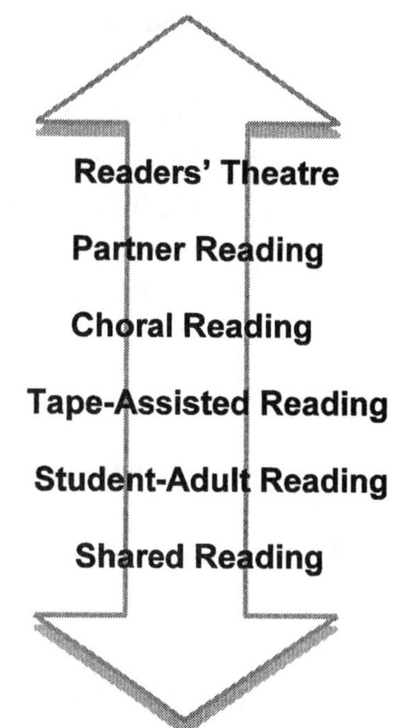

Figure 3.6 The diagram illustrates the range of teacher and student involvement for various models of teaching reading (Adapted from Carbo, 2003).

- *Tape-assisted reading.* An audiotape of a fluent reader is used for this strategy. The reader should read at a speed of about 80 to 100 words per minute to ensure that the students can follow the words and gain meaning. At first, the students read the passage to themselves. Then they listen to the tape and follow along, pointing to the words in their books as the reader says them. Next, the students read aloud along with the tape several times until they can read the text independently.

- *Choral (unison) reading.* Students read along as a group with an adult reader, either from a big book or from their own copy. Choose a text that is short and aimed at the independent reading ability of most students. Begin reading and invite students to join in as they recognize the words you are reading. After three or four readings, the children should be able to read the text independently.
- *Partner or paired reading.* This technique pairs a more fluent reader with a less fluent reader. The more fluent student reads first, providing a model of fluency. Then the less fluent student reads aloud while the stronger partner provides assistance with word recognition and feedback. Another format is to pair readers of similar fluency to reread parts of a story to each other.
- *Readers' theatre.* In this activity, students rehearse (but not memorize) and then perform a play in front of their classmates. They read from scripts that have been taken from books rich in dialogue. A narrator may be used to give any necessary background information, and the students read lines as characters in the play. This novel approach provides an enjoyable opportunity for rereading text, practicing fluency, and promoting cooperation among the students in the class. In one study, students participating in this activity for a period of ten weeks made an entire year's gain in improving their reading rates (Martinez, Roser, and Strecker, 1999). Readers' theatre is appropriate for students in second grade through high school.

✓ Consider having other adults, such as parents and other family members, read to the class and to their children at home. The more models of fluent reading the children hear, the better. Such an approach increases the children's vocabulary, their familiarity with written language, and their knowledge of the world.

✓ In primary grades, read aloud from a big book while pointing to each word as you read it. The children will notice when you are raising or lowering your voice, and you may need to explain to them why you are reading a sentence in a certain tone.

✓ Fluency develops when students can read a text repeatedly with a high degree of success; that is, they can decode and understand about 95 percent of the words. If the text is more difficult, students will spend so much effort and time on decoding that they will not develop fluency. Restrict text to 50 to 200 words, depending on the age of the reader, and include a variety of nonfiction, poetry, and stories to maintain interest.

✓ Because they contain rhyme, rhythm, and meaning, poems are an easy and enjoyable way for children to practice reading.

✓ One measure of fluency is the average number of words the student can read correctly in a minute. Graphing words correct per minute (WCPM) throughout the year can show a student's reading growth. These values can be compared to published norms to determine whether students are making suitable progress in their reading fluency. Table 3.1 explains how to calculate words correct per minute. After making the calculation, compare the result to average oral reading frequency norms. Some local school districts have set their own norms to help teachers assess their students' progress in fluency. Table 3.2 lists oral reading frequency norms compiled from Hasbrouck and Tindal (1992), Mather and Goldstein (2001), NAEP (2003), and NIFL (2001). Figure 3.7 suggests a sample graph for grade 2 that you could use to show a student's progress in WCPM throughout the school year.

Decoding and the Balanced Approach

In response to the renewed interest in phonemic awareness, some schools adopted a modified form of whole-language that includes teaching modules for explicit phonics instruction in addition to the literature-based instruction. A few studies have shown that reading achievement for students in these "balanced" programs improved more than those in the pure whole-language programs, provided certain conditions were met (Fitzgerald and Noblit, 2000; Pressley, 1998). The programs that showed improvement were those where the instruction in phonological awareness followed a scope and sequence with texts based on developing letter-sound correspondences. Further, the phonological and literature-based components represented an integrated balance of skills and meaningful applications of the research on reading and reading instruction.

It seems, then, that a balanced approach involving adequate, purposeful instruction in phonological awareness (including phonemic awareness) and supplemented later by literature is a workable framework for teaching young children to read. Children bring a knowledge of spoken language when they encounter the printed page. They need to learn the written symbols that represent speech, and to use them accurately and fluently. Reading instruction should begin with phonics, using decodable text, and then move to contextual and enriched reading as the student gains competency and confidence. Thus, some of the principles of whole language can be incorporated later as part of reading development.

> Reading instruction should begin with phonics, using decodable text, and then move to enriched texts as the student gains competency and confidence.

Table 3.1 Calculating Words Correct Per Minute (WCPM) and Reading Accuracy

Steps	Example
Select three brief passages from a grade-level basal text. Have the student read each passage aloud for exactly one minute. Count the total number of words the student read for each passage.	Words read per minute: Passage 1: 88 Passage 2: 83 Passage 3: 85
Compute the average number of words read per minute.	Average is: 88 + 83 + 85 = 256 / 3 = 85.3
Count the number of errors the student made on each passage.	Errors made per minute: Passage 1: 10 Passage 2: 7 Passage 3: 8
Compute the average number of errors per minute.	Average is: 10 + 7 + 8 = 25 / 3 = 8.3
Subtract the average number of errors read per minute from the average number of words read per minute. The result is the average number of words correct per minute (WCPM).	Average words less average errors: 85.3 – 8.3 = **77.0 WCPM**
The WCPM can also be used to calculate a student's average percentage of accuracy when reading. Simply divide the WCPM figure by the average number of words read per minute and multiply by 100.	Percent accuracy: 77.0 / 85.3 x 100 = **90.3%**

Table 3.2 Average Reading Rates for Students in Grades 1 to 12	
Grade Level	Words Correct per Minute by End of Year (50th Percentile and Above)
1	50 – 75
2	90 – 120
3	110 – 135
4	115 – 145
5	125 – 165
6	177
7	191
8	205
9	219
10	233
11	247
12	261

Sources: Hasbrouck and Tindal (1992), Mather and Goldstein (2001), NAEP (2003), and NIFL (2001).

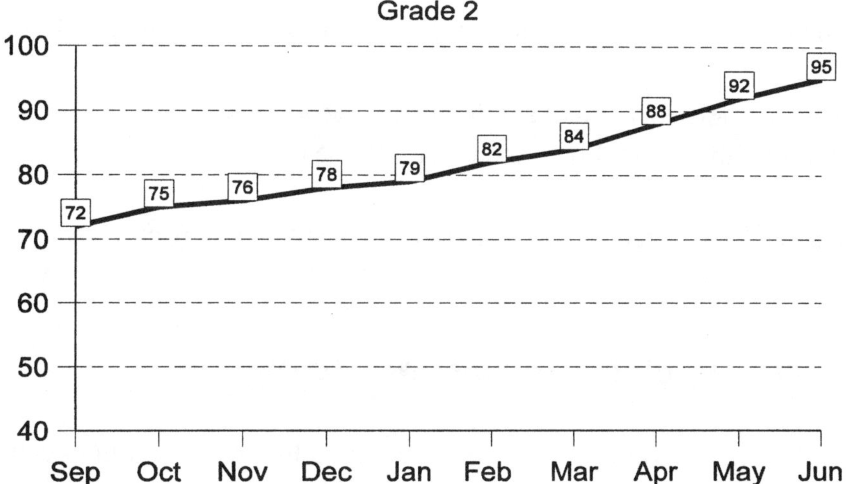

Figure 3.7 This is a sample graph of a student's words correct per minute scores throughout the school year. It is an easy way to show progress in developing reading fluency. In this example, the student's progress was monitored monthly, but less frequent assessments are also appropriate.

Answer to Test Question # 4

Question: Research studies have concluded that neither the phonological approach nor the whole-language approach is more effective in teaching most children how to read.

Answer: *False.* Numerous research studies have found that mastering the alphabetic principle does not come naturally to most children, and that instructional techniques that explicitly teach this principle through phonological awareness are more effective with most children than those that do not.

RESEARCH FINDINGS ON READING INSTRUCTION — COMPREHENSION

The ultimate goal of reading is for children to become sufficiently fluent to understand what they read. This understanding includes literal comprehension as well as more sophisticated reflective understandings, such as "Why am I reading this?" and "What is the author's point?" Reading comprehension depends heavily on spoken language comprehension. As children master the skill of word identification, their reading comprehension improves dramatically. Reading comprehension is a complex cognitive process that relies on several components to be successful. To develop reading comprehension skills, children need to

- Develop their vocabulary and linguistic knowledge
- Thoughtfully interact with the text to derive meaning

Let's take a look at each of these areas and review the relevant research.

Vocabulary and Linguistic Knowledge Instruction

Vocabulary refers to the words we know that allow us to communicate effectively. Words that we use in our speech or that we recognize when listening comprise our oral vocabulary. Words we recognize or use in print comprise our reading vocabulary. Oral vocabulary becomes the basis for comprehension in reading. A child with a good grasp of the alphabetic principle can encounter an unfamiliar printed word and decode the word into

What Are Decodable Texts?

Some confusion exists about what constitutes a decodable text. Two reasons may explain the confusion. First, the word "decodable" is used differently by researchers and by educators and policymakers. In research studies, "decodability" is a measure of the regularity of word pronunciation as decoded by the reader's phonological module. It does not refer specifically to phonics instruction. To educators and policymakers, however, decodable text contains a certain number of words that could be expected to be pronounced (i.e., decoded) as a result of phonics lessons already taught.

Second, the documents issued by educators and policymakers offer many different definitions of a decodable text. In general, the documents state that a decodable text should be composed of words that use the letter-to-sound correspondences that have already been taught, but there is no agreement on what the percentage of such words should be. There is no research available at this time to support any specific recommendation of a particular proportion of decodable words in beginning reading texts (Allington and Woodside-Jiron, 1998).

speech. If the word is in the mental lexicon, the child will be able to understand it. However, if the word is not in the lexicon, the child will have to determine its meaning by other means. Consequently, the larger the child's oral vocabulary, the more easily the child will comprehend text. As children learn, pronounce, and use more words in their speech and reading, their linguistic knowledge develops. They get more confident in their understanding of letter-sound combinations, more adept at recognizing semantic differences, and more aware of the various classes of words (e.g., adjectives, nouns, and verbs) used in a sentence.

The scientific research on vocabulary instruction reveals that some vocabulary must be taught directly but that most vocabulary is learned indirectly. The research also has shown the following:

- Children learn the meanings of most words indirectly, through everyday experiences with oral and written language. These experiences include conversations with other people, listening to adults read to them, and reading on their own. They learn vocabulary words directly when they are explicitly taught individual words and word-learning strategies.
- Some vocabulary should be taught directly. Direct instruction is particularly effective for teaching difficult words representing complex concepts that are not part of the children's everyday experiences.

- Repeated exposure to vocabulary in many contexts aids word learning and linguistic knowledge. The more children see, hear, and read specific words, the better they learn them and their various meanings.
- Vocabulary acquisition can be affected by several factors. In a broad review of the research literature on vocabulary, Swanborn and de Glopper (1999) found that factors such as ability, age, and text density had an impact on the chances that students will learn new words in context. Table 3.3 shows the factors and their influence on vocabulary acquisition. Low-ability students have only an 8 percent chance of learning new words in context, but that number climbs to 19 percent for high-ability students. Not surprisingly, older students in grade 11 have a 33 percent chance of learning new words while fourth-graders have only an 8 percent chance. Text density measures the number of new words per given number of words. The lower the text density (1 new word in 150), the greater the chances of learning a new word (30 percent). The chances drop to only 7 percent when the text density reaches to 1 new word in 10.

Table 3.3 Factors Influencing Chances of Learning New Words in Context

Factor	Chances of Learning New Word
Ability: Low	8 percent
Medium	12 percent
High	19 percent
Age: Grade 4	8 percent
Grade 11	33 percent
Text Density:	
1 new word in 10 words	7 percent
1 new word in 74 words	14 percent
1 new word in 150 words	30 percent

Source: Swanborn and de Glopper, 1999

- Linguistic knowledge includes one's ability to (1) hear, distinguish, and categorize the sounds of speech (phonology), (2) understand the rules that constrain how words are put together in phrases and sentences (syntax), and (3) understand the meaning of individual words and sentences and the relationships between them (semantics).

How Do I Teach Vocabulary?

Selecting Vocabulary. Selecting which vocabulary words to teach separately is an important instructional decision. To help in this selection process, consider the following:

✓ Be sure to teach those terms that are central to the unit of study. These should be terms that are so important that students who do not understand them will have difficulty comprehending the text. Avoid selecting words that will have little value to students after they complete the unit test.

✓ Remember the capacity limits of working memory and keep the number of new words per lesson to no more than five for elementary students and up to seven for secondary school students. This will give you more time to teach each word in depth, resulting in greater student comprehension.

✓ Choose other new words with care. Although a chapter may have 10 to15 new words, only 3 or 4 may address critical components of the chapter. Avoid selecting words in the text just because they are italicized or in boldface print, or words that the student will never encounter again.

✓ Include words that will be used continually throughout the text or unit of study. Having a deep understanding of these words will allow students to build on them as they develop new information over the long term.

Other Guidelines. Here are some other guidelines for teaching vocabulary.

✓ You can promote indirect learning of vocabulary by

- Reading aloud to your students, regardless of the grade level or subject that you teach. Students of all ages will learn vocabulary better if you read text containing difficult words. Discuss the text before, during, and after you read to help students attach meaning to unfamiliar words by connecting them to past knowledge and experiences. Then ask the students to use the newly-learned words in their own sentences.
- Encouraging students to read extensively on their own.

✓ You will not have time to teach directly all the words that students might not know in a text. In fact, it is better not to try to teach all the unknown words so that students can develop their own word-learning strategies. Word-learning strategies include using

- *Dictionaries and other reference aids.* Students need to learn how to use dictionaries, thesauruses, and glossaries to deepen and broaden their knowledge of words. You can show them how to find an unknown word in the classroom dictionary and note that there may be several different definitions for the word. Read the definitions one at a time and have the class discuss which one is more likely to fit the context of the story. For example, in the sentence "The workers went into the mine," the children may confuse *mine* with the possessive word form. After you finish reading the various definitions from the dictionary, the students can eliminate the inappropriate definitions and settle on "a hole made in the earth to find coal or minerals."
- *Information about word parts to figure out the meanings of words in text.* Word parts include affixes (prefixes and suffixes), base words, and word roots. Students learn that certain affixes change the meaning of words in a specific way. For example, the prefix *dis-* usually means the negative or reverse of the root word's meaning (*disrespect* means showing no respect). Base words are words from which many other words can be formed. The base word *complete* can form the words *completely, incomplete, incompleteness, completion, completing.* Word roots are the words from other languages (mainly Latin and Greek) that are the origin of many English words.
- *Context clues to determine the meaning of words.* Context clues are hints about the meaning of an unknown word that are provided by the words, phrases, and sentences that surround the word. The clues may be descriptions, examples, definitions, or restatements. However, not all context clues are helpful, because they give little information about a word's meaning. Descriptive words that are used in a literary or obscure way are particularly difficult to comprehend through context clues. For example, in the sentence "She gave a strained response," *strained* could have a number of meanings in this context, such as *squeaky, hoarse, noisy, difficult, tense,* and so on.
- *Associating an image with a word.* Imagery is a powerful memory device. Whenever students can associate an image (or other symbolic representation) with a new word, they are more likely to remember the word and its meaning.

✓ With early readers you will probably be able to teach about 10 new words per week. Focus your teaching time on the following types of words:

- *Important words.* Directly teach those new words that are important for comprehending a concept or the text. Give the students some word-learning strategies to figure out the meanings of other words in the text.
- *Useful words.* Teach directly words that students are likely to encounter and use repeatedly. For example, it is more useful for students to learn the word *biology* than *bionic,* and the word *journey* is more useful than *excursion.*

- *Difficult words.* Provide instruction for words that are particularly difficult for the students. Especially challenging are words that are spelled or pronounced the same but have different meanings, depending on the context. Here are but a few examples of words that are spelled the same but have different meanings in a sentence:

  The bandage was *wound* around the *wound.*
  When shot at, the *dove dove* into the bushes.
  She did not *object* to the *object.*
  They were too *close* to the door to *close* it.

  Problems also arise with words that are spelled and pronounced the same, but have different meanings, such as *store* (place to buy things) and *store* (to put away), *land* (piece of ground) and *land* (bring down an airplane), and *arms* (limbs) and *arms* (weaponry).

With early readers you will probably be able to teach about 10 new words per week.

✓ When selecting reading texts, it is important to know the level of word knowledge that students will have for those texts. Students know the vocabulary words in their mental lexicon in varying degrees that researchers divide into the following three levels:

- *Unknown.* A word that is completely unfamiliar and its meaning is unknown.
- *Acquainted.* A word that is somewhat familiar and the student has some idea of its basic meaning.
- *Established.* A word that is very familiar and the student can immediately recognize its meaning and use the word correctly.

Assess the child's level of familiarity with the words in a specific text according to these three categories. If the assessment indicates few or no unknown words, consider selecting a more difficult text to challenge the child and to build vocabulary.

How Do I Teach Linguistic Knowledge?

✓ Linguistic knowledge (SEDL, 2001).

- *Phonology.* To assess phonological skill, play the "same or different" game by generating pairs of words that are either identical or differ in some subtle way. Say them aloud and ask if they are the same or different. Most children should not miss hearing the different ones. Sometimes children can hear the differences between similar sounding words, as *glow* and *grow,* but have difficulty articulating that difference in their own speech. Difficulty with articulation does not mean difficulty with perception. When a child mispronounces a word, say the mispronounced word back to the child as a question. The child with normal phonologic skills will repeat the statement, trying to make you understand the meanings.

- *Syntax.* The rules of English prohibit the haphazard arrangement of words in a sentence. Poor syntax can make meaning ambiguous (see Chapter 2). One way to assess syntactic skill is to give the children sentences with a key word missing. Ask them to supply the word that would correctly fill the blank. Remember that a child's answer may not make sense, yet still be syntactically correct. Develop syntactic skills by helping children build more complex sentences. For example, after showing a short video, ask students to describe something they saw or heard ("I saw a tree" or "I heard a bird."). Then ask them to build their sentences ("I saw a tree and heard the bird singing.").
- *Semantics.* Semantics describes meaning. One way to assess semantics is to create sentences and stories that have logical inconsistencies and see if the children can detect them ("Mary went to the store because she enjoys staying home."). Instructional activities that develop semantics include asking children to substitute words (synonyms) that would have the same meaning in context, and suggesting that they use context to guess the meaning of unknown words.

Text Comprehension

Just because readers are able to sound out words does not guarantee that they will comprehend what they read. Many reading teachers have witnessed group reading sessions where students could sound out a story with great effort but really had little understanding of what had been read. Children who are first learning to sound out words are using substantial mental effort, so fewer cerebral resources remain for the cognitive operations needed to comprehend the words being read aloud. It is critical for children to develop fluency in word recognition. When they are fluent, word recognition requires far less mental effort, freeing up the child's cognitive capacity for understanding what is read. Thus, explicit instruction in word recognition to the point of fluency is a vital component for text comprehension.

Tan and Nicholson (1997) conducted a study that showed the importance of word-recognition instruction to the point of fluency. Struggling primary-level readers who were taught new words with instruction that emphasized word recognition to the point of fluency (i.e., they practiced reading the individual words until they could recognize them automatically) answered more comprehension questions correctly than did students who experienced instruction emphasizing individual word meanings (i.e., instruction involving mostly student-teacher discussions about word meanings).

Text comprehension occurs when readers derive meaning as a result of intentionally interacting with the text. Such comprehension is enhanced when readers actively relate the ideas represented in print to their own knowledge and experiences and can construct mental representations in their memory. Hence, good readers are both purposeful and active. Purposeful means they may read to find out how to use a computer, read a magazine for entertainment, read a classic novel for enjoyment, read a guidebook to gather information about a tourist spot, or read a text book needed for a course. Good readers are active in that they get the most out of their reading by using their experiences and knowledge about the world, their understanding of vocabulary and language structure, and their knowledge of reading strategies. When problems with reading occur, they know how to solve them.

The scientific research on text comprehension reveals the following:

✓ Comprehension is a complex interactive process that begins with identifying words by using knowledge outside the text, accessing word meaning in context, recognizing grammatical structures, drawing inferences, and self-monitoring to ensure that the text is making sense. When confronted with several meanings for a word in a sentence, the brain needs to select the one that makes sense in context. How this happens is the subject of much research. One possible mechanism, called the *structure-building framework* (Gernsbacher, 1990), suggests that readers construct meaning by activating mental representations of concepts that are relevant to the text and blocking those that are irrelevant. Figure 3.8 illustrates the cognitive mechanism, using the example of a reader encountering the sentence "The man planted a tree on the bank." *Bank* has two common meanings, but only one fits the context of this sentence. The mental lexicon may activate both at first, but skilled readers quickly suppress the irrelevant meaning. Less skilled readers, however, spend more time considering alternative meanings and may not make the correct selection in the end. Many English words have dozens of meanings, depending on their context. Thus, developing the ability to quickly block irrelevant meanings becomes a necessity for reading fluency and comprehension. (This process is similar to the syntactic blocking described in Chapter 2, whereby syntactic rules are blocked for the formation of irregular verbs.)

✓ Text comprehension is improved by direct, explicit instruction that helps readers use specific strategies to make sense of the passage. These strategies represent the purposeful steps that enable readers to reason strategically whenever they encounter barriers to understanding what they are reading. Comprehension strategies include self monitoring, graphic and semantic organizers, answering questions, generating questions, recognizing story structure, and summarizing.

✓ Teaching comprehension strategies in the context of specific academic areas can be effective at all grade levels. Cooperative learning is a particularly useful technique for helping students to understand content-area texts (see Chapter 6).

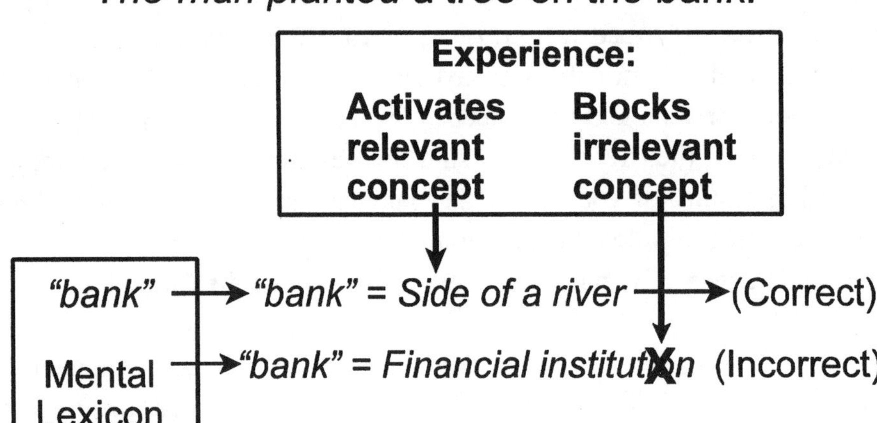

Figure 3.8 The diagram illustrates how the brain deals with multiple meanings of a word. Spoken language experience activates the relevant meaning while blocking the irrelevant meaning.

How Do I Teach for Text Comprehension?

Text comprehension occurs when the brain's frontal lobe is able to derive meaning by processing the visual and auditory input that resulted from reading with the reader's prior knowledge. Teachers should emphasize text comprehension as early as the primary grades, rather than waiting until children have mastered reading basics. The basics of decoding can be learned in a few years, but reading to learn subject matter does not occur automatically and requires constructing meaning at all grade levels.

Start Teaching Comprehension Strategies Early. At what grade level can teachers begin to include instruction in comprehension strategies? Tradition curricula have favored honing word-recognition skills in the primary grades while developing comprehension skills in the later grades. Recent research (NRP, 2000; Snow et al., 1998) studies suggest, however, that instruction aimed at improving comprehension (i.e., instruction beyond word-recognition) does make a significant impact on literacy during the primary years. Student reading achievement in the primary grades improved when decoding and word recognition were taught systematically with comprehension strategies. This approach was particularly effective in raising reading achievement for children in high-poverty schools (Taylor, Pearson, Clark, and Walpole, 2000).

The instructional approaches that have received the strongest support from scientific research are the following (NIFL, 2001):

✓ *Comprehension monitoring.* This is a self-monitoring strategy to help students recognize when they understand what they are reading and when they do not. They also learn appropriate strategies for resolving problems in comprehension. Metacognition (thinking about our own thinking) is an effective means of monitoring comprehension. Before reading, simply ask them to clarify their purpose for reading this text and preview the text with them. As part of the preview, ask the students what they already know about the content of the selection. During reading, they should monitor their understanding and adjust their reading speed to match the difficulty of the text. Students can use several different forms of monitoring, such as

- Identifying where the difficulty occurs ("I don't understand the third paragraph on page 10.").
- Identifying what the difficulty is ("I don't know what the author means when he says...").
- Restating the difficult passage in their own words ("Oh, so the author means...").
- Looking back through the text ("The author talked about . . . in the previous chapter. Maybe I should reread that chapter to find out what he is talking about now.").
- Looking ahead in the text for information that might help resolve the difficulty ("Oh, the next section seems to have some information that may help me here.").

After reading, they should summarize in their own words what they understood from the passage. Their summaries can be addressed to the teacher or shared with other students in cooperative learning groups.

✓ *Using graphic and semantic organizers.* Graphic organizers are effective visual tools for illustrating the interrelationships among concepts in a text. Known by many different names (e.g., frames, clusters, webs, text maps, visual organizers), they provide cues about connections between and among ideas that can help students better understand difficult concepts. Semantic organizers look a little like a spider web. They have lines connecting a main idea to a variety of related ideas and events. Both of these types of organizers help students read to learn subject matter in all content areas because they capitalize on the brain's innate aptitude for remembering patterns. Figure 3.9 illustrates examples of a spider map and a semantic map that can be used to enhance reading comprehension. Chapter 6 contains more on different types of graphic organizers.

> Graphic organizers are effective visual tools for illustrating how concepts in a text are related.

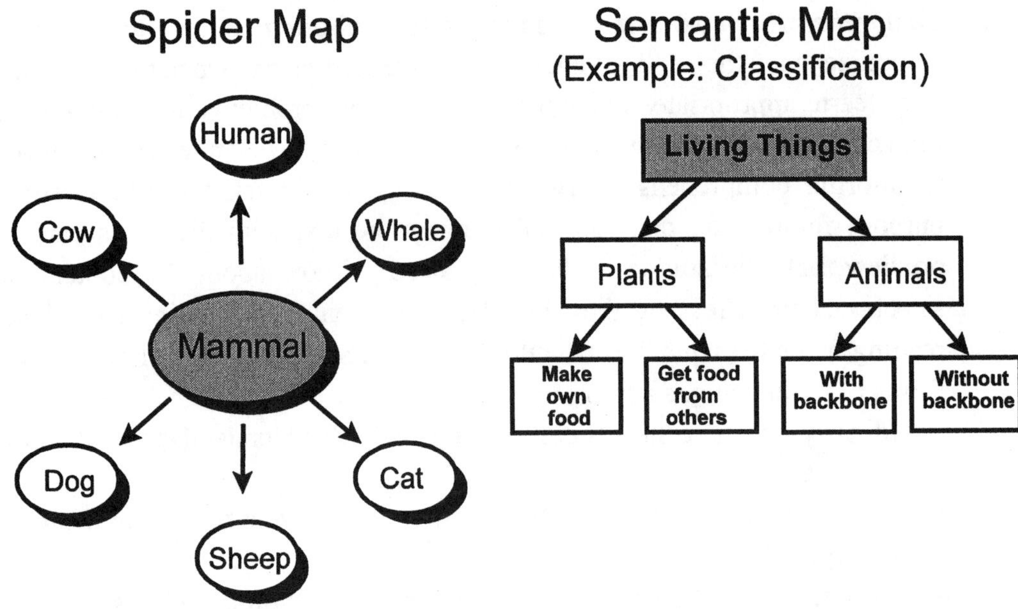

Figure 3.9 Visual organizers come in many forms. Here are examples of a spider map of types of mammals (left) and a semantic map for a simple classification of living things.

✓ *Answering questions.* Research studies show that teachers' questions strongly support and advance how much students learn from reading. The questions are effective because they

- Give students a purpose for reading
- Focus the students' attention on what they are to learn
- Help students to interact with what they read
- Encourage students to monitor their comprehension
- Help students relate what they are learning to what they already know. The instruction helps readers learn to answer questions that require an understanding that is

  Text explicit – stated explicitly in a single sentence
  Text implicit – implied by information presented in two or more sentences
  Scriptal – not found at all in the text, but part of the reader's prior knowledge or experience.

✓ *Generating questions.* Teaching students to ask their own questions helps them become aware of whether they understand what they are reading. By generating their own questions, students focus on the purpose of the reading, improve their active mental processing, and learn to integrate information from different segments of the text.

- ✓ *Recognizing story structure.* Story structure describes how the events and content of a story are organized into a plot. Teaching about story structure helps student learn to identify categories of content, such as initiating events, goals, setting, internal reactions, and outcomes. How this content is organized into a plot can often be revealed through story maps. Story maps are a type of graphic organizer that illustrates the sequence of events in a simple story. They can be powerful aids for understanding and remembering stories (see Figure 5.2).

- ✓ *Summarizing.* When summarizing, students synthesize and integrate the most important information and concepts in the text. To do this successfully, students must identify the main ideas, connect them to each other, eliminate unnecessary information, and remember what they read.

- ✓ *Mental imagery.* Readers (especially young readers) who form mental pictures, or images, during reading understand and remember what they read better than readers who do not visualize. Urge readers to form visual images of what they are reading, such as picturing a character, event, or setting described in the text. This will not be easy because children today are exposed to technology that provides many images for them. Consequently, they have little practice at imaging and need to be given clear directions on how to do it.

- ✓ *Paraphrasing.* This strategy aids in comprehension by having students first hear the text read aloud, then reading it quietly themselves and taking notes, rewriting it in their own words, and discussing their paraphrased text with their classmates. Paraphrasing is effective because it involves reading, writing, speaking, and listening, all of which lead to a deeper understanding and greater memory of the text (Fisk and Hurst, 2003).

Another particularly effective strategy for developing comprehension focuses on reading and other activities related to a central theme. Because the varied classroom activities center around this theme, students can more easily comprehend their related readings (NIFL, 2001).

- ✓ *Concept-oriented reading instruction (CORI).* The teaching framework for CORI includes four phases: (1) observe and personalize, (2) search and retrieve, (3) comprehend and integrate, and (4) communicate to others. Here is an example of how CORI was implemented in one school. First, the teachers identified a conceptual theme for instructional units to be taught for 16-18 weeks in the fall and spring. The themes selected by third-grade teachers were the adaptations and habitats of birds and insects for the fall. In the spring, the third-grade units were weather, seasons, and climate. Fifth-grade units in the fall were life cycles of plants and animals, and the spring units emphasized earth science, including the solar system and geological cycles.

At the beginning of each unit, students performed observation and hands-on activities both outside and inside the classroom. Third and fifth graders participated in such activities as collecting and observing crickets, constructing spider webs, dissecting owl pellets, and building weather stations. Within each activity, students personalized their learning by composing their own questions as the basis for observing, reading, and writing. Student questions included a structural focus, such as, "How many types of feathers does a bird have?" Then conceptual questions, such as, "Why does that bird have such a long beak?" evolved as students attempted to explain the phenomena they had observed. These questions generated opportunities for self-directed learning. Students chose their own subtopics, found particular books, selected peers for interest-based activities, and constructed their goals for communicating to others.

The second phase of the CORI framework consisted of searching and retrieving information related to the students' questions. Students were taught how to use the library, find books, locate information within expository texts, and use a diversity of community resources. In addition, direct strategy instruction was provided to help students integrate information across sources including texts, illustrations, references, and human experts. Along with informational texts, woven through the instruction were stories, folklore, novels, and poetry. Most of the teachers began the units with a narrative related to the theme that students read at the same time they were conducting science observations. Following observation and the formation of conceptual questions, teachers moved to the informational texts. As students concluded their indepth study of multiple informational texts, teachers introduced novels, novelettes, and poetry related to the conceptual theme of the unit.

The last phase of the CORI framework is communicating to others. Having gained expertise in a particular topic, students were motivated to speak, write, discuss, and display their understanding to other students and adults. In both third- and fifth-grade classrooms, students made posters, wrote classroom books, and composed extended displays of their knowledge. One class made a videotape of its weather unit, providing a lesson on weather prediction and an explanation for the rest of the school.

✓ *Transactional strategies.* Transactional strategies combine some of the preceding strategies with whole-language instruction to improve reading comprehension. They begin with the teacher explaining to students how they can

- Make predictions about upcoming contents

- Relate the text to prior knowledge
- Ask questions about the information
- Seek clarification when the meaning is not clear
- Visualize the meaning
- Summarize along the way.

Students learn to use these strategies, especially in small reading groups that focus on high-quality literature. As students have trouble decoding a word, the teacher helps them use fix-up strategies they have learned, such as sounding out the word, rereading it, looking it up, and even skipping the word. Skipping the word is acceptable because main ideas are often expressed in several different ways in the text. This approach empowers students to read more challenging material by suggesting that they should not avoid reading texts that contain some unfamiliar words. For transactional strategies to be successful, teachers need to thoroughly understand the components of skilled reading and how to teach the related strategies (Pressley and Afflerbach, 1995).

✓ *The SAIL program.* Transactional strategies can even be used in the primary grades. One comprehensive program for reading comprehension instruction is known as SAIL (Students Achieving Independent Learning). In this program, the teachers

- Use explicit instruction, modeling, and discussion as a means of teaching comprehension strategies, focusing particularly on visualizing, questioning, predicting, clarifying, and making associations between the text and the students' experiences
- Emphasize not only the nature of the strategy but also when and how to apply it in actual reading
- Model the use of the strategies by thinking aloud in the presences of students about their own use of comprehension strategies
- Encourage students to discuss their comprehension of texts as well as the strategies they are using to achieve that comprehension
- Teach students to attend to their own reading processes, to the context in which they are reading, and to the text.

SAIL suggests a menu of strategies that can be used to enhance comprehension. Teachers and students select from this menu the strategies that are best suited to promoting understanding of the text being read. The menu includes (Pearson and Duke, 2002)

- Thinking aloud (talking about character development, identifying with a character, imaging how a character might feel)
- Constructing images (using visualization to create themes)
- Summarizing (especially reading for multiple meanings)

- Predicting (activating prior knowledge)
- Questioning (looking for different points of view)
- Clarifying (including relating text to personal experience)
- Story grammar analysis (relating one text to another)
- Text structure analysis (looking for specific text features, such as point of view, tone, or mood)

A study of SAIL with low-achieving students in second-grade classrooms (Brown, Pressley, Van Meter, and Schuder, 1996) found that the SAIL students performed considerably better on standardized measures of reading comprehension and word attack than the students of teachers who were not using the SAIL methods. Furthermore, the SAIL students made richer interpretations of text and acted like more strategic readers. (For more information on SAIL, see the **Resources** section.) SAIL is only one member of a family of approaches that use transactional strategy instruction. There is no indication that primary-grade students are unable to handle this approach to text comprehension instruction.

Developing Critical Reading Strategies in Older Students

Students read thousands of pages of text as they progress through secondary school. They often need to make judgments about what they are reading. These judgments are based largely on the prior knowledge, beliefs, and values that students bring to the reading process.

Critical readers assess the reliability and validity of the text, and ask questions about themselves, the writer, and the writing.

The brain's frontal lobe is thought to be the place where critical thinking occurs. Here, past experiences are mingled with the reading to construct meaning and to acquire new knowledge. Critical readers assess the reliability and validity of the text, and ask questions about themselves, the writer, and the writing. They read beyond the obvious meanings to the assumptions, strategies, and arguments behind them. How does the writer reason with readers and manipulate them? Reading critically helps learners separate nonfiction from fiction, creativity from fantasy, fact from opinion, and is thus a valuable lifelong skill. Regrettably, not enough time is devoted to teaching students how to become critical readers.

If teachers want students to develop critical reading strategies, they should create a classroom climate that fosters inquiry by encouraging students to question, to make predictions, and to support their value judgments. Students employ higher-order thinking skills to evaluate evidence, draw conclusions, make inferences, and defend their line of thinking. This process is made somewhat easier if, when reading text critically, the students (Paterno, 2001)

- Underline key words, phrases, and sentences
- Write comments or questions in the margin
- Number related points in sequence
- Bracket important sections of the text
- Connect ideas with lines or arrows
- Make note of anything important, questionable, or interesting

Critical reading strategies include the following:

Previewing. This strategy allows students to get an overview of the content and organization of the reading by skimming the headnotes, captions, summaries, and other introductory material.

Contextualizing. As students read, what they comprehend is colored by their own experiences and by living in a particular time and place. But some of the texts they read were written in a radically different place and time. To read critically, they need to put the text in its biographical, cultural, and historical contexts to recognize the differences between their own contemporary values and those represented in the text.

Questioning to Understand and Remember. Students write down questions that come to mind as they read the material for the first time. The questions should focus on main ideas, not details, and should be expressed in their own words. This activity also helps in retention of new learning.

Challenges to the Students' Beliefs and Values. Students put a mark next to sections that challenge their attitudes, beliefs, and values. They make notes in the margin about how they feel or about what particularly challenged them. Then they review their notes and look for any patterns.

Evaluating an Argument. Writers make assertions that they want the reader to accept as true. Critical readers do not accept anything at face value but evaluate the claim and support for each argument. Students assess the reasoning process as well as its truthfulness. The support should be appropriate to the claim, and the statements should be consistent with each other.

Outlining and Summarizing. Students use an outline to reveal the basic structure of the text, its main ideas, subtopics, and supporting details. This requires a close analysis of each paragraph and a listing of the main ideas. In summarizing, however, the students write a synopsis in their own words of what they have read. Thus, students experience creative synthesis by putting ideas together in a condensed and new form.

Comparing and Contrasting Related Readings. Different authors discuss the same issues in different ways. Comparing and contrasting the arguments of various authors on a particular issue helps to better understand the approach each author used.

Questions That Promote Critical Reading

Critical reading can be prompted by specific questions that relate to the reader, the author, and the writing. Students can use the following questions to sharpen their critical reading skills (Paterno, 2001):

About the reader

- What do I know about this topic?
- What are my beliefs and values about this topic?
- Why am I reading this material?

About the writer

- What is the writer's background?
- How might that background affect the writer's approach to the topic as well as the selection and interpretation of the evidence presented?
- What are the writer's value assumptions about this topic?

Writer's arguments, evidence, and conclusions

- What is the basis for the writer's argument?
- What evidence does the writer present to support the argument?
- What is the writer's conclusion?

Writer's use of evidence to support the conclusion

- Are there any logical fallacies?
- What evidence does the writer use to support the conclusion(s)?
- Are the writer's sources credible?
- If the writer uses research studies:
  - Is the research timely?
  - Is the sample group representative of the target population?
  - Who conducted the research and what was its purpose?
  - Has the research been replicated?
  - Do the graphic illustrations represent the data in a truthful manner?
  - What is the source of the data in the illustration?
  - Do the physical dimensions of the graphic illustration accurately portray numerical relationships?

- Are the statistical findings and the writer's conclusion focused on the same topic?

Reader's reaction to the reading

- Do I accept the writer's evidence as reliable and as a valid support of the conclusion?
- How does the conclusion relate to what I already know about this topic?
- How has the writer's argument changed my views on this topic?

Teaching students to read, write, and think critically takes time and may represent a shift from what happens in many secondary school language arts classes. Teachers feel pressed for time and face the ever-increasing demands of high-stakes testing. Nonetheless, critical reading strategies can make reading much more productive and satisfying and thus help the students handle difficult material well and with confidence.

Students Who Are English Language Learners (ELL)

Children for whom English is a new language have been entering schools across the country in ever-increasing numbers, posing unique challenges to teachers of reading. These challenges have been intensified by recent state and federal policy initiatives mandating that all students demonstrate adequate yearly progress. Thus, schools with large English language learner populations are under pressure to help these students succeed. One of the more vexing problems is whether it is better to promote literacy in these children's native or second language. The research evidence, though small, suggests that initial reading instruction in a child's home language (e.g., Spanish) contributes positively to that child's ability to attain literacy in both languages, and also to the prevention of reading difficulties. It is generally counterproductive to hasten young non-English-speaking children into reading in English without adequate preparation. Reading in any language requires a solid mental lexicon of spoken vocabulary. Thus, learning to *speak* English becomes the child's first priority, because it provides the foundation for hearing and reflecting on the structure of spoken words and then to learning the alphabetic principle as it applies to the sounds of English. Likewise, learning to read for meaning depends on comprehending the language of the text being read.

> It is generally counterproductive to hasten young non-English-speaking children into reading in English without adequate preparation in speaking English.

The report of the National Research Council (Snow et al., 1998) suggested that if children come to school with no proficiency in English but speaking a language for which there are instructional guides, materials, and locally proficient teachers, then these children should be taught how to read in their native language while acquiring oral, and eventually, reading, proficiency in the English language. Those non-English speaking children with a native language for which there are no materials, should focus on developing their oral proficiency in English. Formal reading instruction should be postponed until the child can speak English with an adequate level of proficiency.

One format for providing this type of instruction is paired bilingual instruction whereby ELL students are taught to read in their native language and in English at different times of the day. This can be expanded to two-way bilingual instruction in which ELL and native English speakers both learn to read in both languages (Calderón and Minaya-Rowe, 2003). In an analysis of 17 research studies, Slavin and Cheung (2003) found that most studies showed significant positive effects of the bilingual approach, especially the two-way format, on the students' reading performance. Most of these studies evaluated the Success for All program, which is a comprehensive reading program emphasizing systematic phonics, cooperative learning, tutoring for struggling students, and family support programs. Evaluations of both the English and Spanish versions of the Success for All program have consistently found them to improve English and Spanish reading performance in beginning readers. Two other programs that have been successful with helping ELL students learn to read in their native language and then in English are the Spanish version of Reading Recovery (Escamilla, 1994) and the small-group version of Direct Instruction (Gunn, Biglan, Smolkowski, and Ary, 2000).

Cooperative Learning Strategies With ELL Students

As children with limited English proficiency begin to acquire English, cooperative learning seems particularly appropriate and effective for bilingual education. First of all, cooperative learning should improve the reading performance of students in their native language. In an analysis of nearly 100 studies, Slavin (1995) showed that student achievement in a variety of settings using cooperative learning methods increased significantly those of the control groups.

Answer to Test Question # 5

Question: Non-English-speaking children can be taught to read English even if their spoken English vocabulary is weak.

Answer: *False.* During reading, the brain relies heavily on a person's spoken vocabulary to decode words. With only a small number of English words in the mental lexicon, learning to read in English becomes very frustrating. Bilingual programs that build a child's native reading skills while also enhancing English language skills have shown success in helping the child learn to read English.

Research on second-language learning has found that students need to engage in a great deal of oral interaction, jointly solving problems and determining meaning, if they are to achieve a high level of proficiency in the new language. Because cooperative learning provides many opportunities for students to work together to share understandings, it is likely to be an especially beneficial strategy for students making the transition to reading in English.

One form of cooperative learning has been particularly successful with bilingual students. Known as Bilingual Cooperative Integrated Reading and Composition (BCIRC), this method assigns students to four-member heterogeneous learning teams. After their lesson, the students work in teams on cooperative learning activities including identification of main story elements, vocabulary, summarization, reading comprehension strategies, partner reading, and creative writing using a process writing approach. In a major study (Calderón, Hertz-Lazarowitz, and Slavin, 1998) of 222 students with limited English proficiency in grades 2 and 3, teachers used the BCIRC model, working first with students in their native language and then helping them to make the transition to English. As part of BCIRC, the teachers used a total of 15 different strategies before, during, and after reading. Most of the activities were completed in a five-day cycle. They were the following:

1. *Building background and vocabulary.* Teachers select vocabulary that might be particularly difficult, strange, or important. They write the words on chart paper and develop semantic maps with the students. The maps are displayed on a wall and are used later during reading, discussion, and writing activities.
2. *Making predictions.* Teachers model how to make and confirm predictions. Students then work in their teams with the title and illustrations of a story and predict the elements of that story.
3. *Reading a selection.* Students track as the teacher reads aloud the first part of a story. During the second part, the students are encouraged to read in a whisper with the teacher.
4. *Partner reading and silent reading.* For partner reading, the students sit in pairs and take turns reading alternate paragraphs aloud. They assist each other in pronouncing and decoding the meaning of words. Then each student reads the assigned text silently.
5. *Treasure hunting: Story comprehension.* After partner reading, pairs discuss the answers to questions about key elements of a narrative, such as characters, setting, problems, and problem solutions. Working together, students help each other to understand the questions, to look up the answers, to look for clues to support their answers, to make inferences, and to reach consensus.
6. *Mapping the story.* After the treasure hunts are done, each team reviews a variety of graphic organizers and chooses one to map the story. This visual aid helps to organize the story elements. After discussing story elements, such as character names, the setting, the main idea, major events of the story, and problems the

characters encountered, the team members represent these creatively in the story map. They can use the maps later to provide visual clues for retelling the story and for story-related writing later in the cycle.

7. *Retelling the story.* Students use the maps to retell the stories to the partners within their teams and evaluate their partners' verbal summaries. Afterward, the students discuss with their partners what they liked about the story.
8. *Story-related writing.* In this part of the lesson cycle, students engage in a variety of writing activities that are related to the selection they have been reading all week. For the students who are acquiring English, the teacher models the writing process extensively each time. Then, with a partner or in teams of four, students write in various genres. During this time, the students help each other to develop story lines and characters, to sequence events, and to give each other feedback. They are also learning to engage in a process of drafting, revising, rewriting, editing, and publishing.
9. *Saying words aloud and spelling.* Words from the story become the word bank to be used throughout the week. Students say the words aloud to ultimately master their meaning, pronunciation, and spelling. This activity includes 10 to 12 words from the story that students must be able to read fluently, spell, and use correctly in meaningful sentences.
10. *Checking the partner.* When students complete the activities listed above, their partners initial a student assessment form indicating that they have completed and achieved the task. The teacher gives the student teams the daily expectations about the number of activities to be completed. However, the teams can proceed at their own rate and complete the activities earlier if they wish, creating additional time for writing and for independent reading of other books on the same theme. Because the scores of individual students also become the team's score, the partners have a vested interest in making sure all students correctly finish their work.
11. *Making meaningful sentences.* The students carefully select five or more words from the story. They discuss their meanings and use these words to write meaningful sentences that denote the definitions and give a clear picture of the word's meaning.
12. *Taking tests.* After three class periods, the teacher gives the students a comprehension test on the story. It includes asking them to write meaningful sentences for each vocabulary word and to read the word list aloud to the teacher. Students are not permitted to help one another on these tests because the test scores and evaluations of the story-related writing are the major components of students' weekly team scores. These weekly tests provide teachers a progressive view of the students' listening, speaking, reading, and writing performance.

13. *Direct instruction in reading comprehension.* Throughout the lesson cycle, the teacher provides direct instruction in reading comprehension skills such as identifying main ideas, drawing conclusions, and comparing and contrasting. The students practice these skills in their teams and take quizzes on them individually (without the help of their teammates) to contribute to their team scores.
14. *Writing workshops.* These workshops consist of a series of mini-lessons on the writing process. First, the teacher gives step-by-step explanations and ideas for completing a writing assignment. Then the students work closely with their peers and with the teacher through the phases of pre-writing, writing, revising and editing.
15. *Independent reading.* The teacher asks students to read a book of their choice for at least 20 minutes each evening. Parents are encouraged to discuss the reading with their children and to initial forms indicating that the children have read for the minimum time. The students earn points for their team if they submit a completed form each week. Additional points can be earned by completing a book report every two weeks.

The students who were part of the BCIRC program in the second and third grades performed significantly better on tests of Spanish and English reading than comparison students. Second graders taught primarily in Spanish scored significantly higher on a Spanish writing scale and somewhat higher on the reading scale than comparison students. Third-grade students who had been in the program for two years were more likely than the comparison group to meet the criteria necessary for exiting the bilingual program in language and reading.

My purpose in this chapter was to present the latest research on the effectiveness of models that educators use for teaching reading. In the past few decades, methods for teaching reading have become highly politicized. The proponents of literature-based and skills-based programs have attacked each other's research and practices, leaving the classroom teacher confused about which program to use. Given the wide variation in the cognitive abilities of children and their environments as well as the complexities involved in learning to read, it is clear that no one approach will be successful for all children. Some preschool children will have had such rich exposure to spoken language and print that they are already mastering the alphabetic principle and are prepared for enriched reading experiences as early as kindergarten. Others can be so language deprived that instruction will need to focus mainly on developing phonemic awareness. And, of course, there are all the possible variations in between.

Faced with this heterogeneous mix, teachers of reading still need sound guidance, not rhetoric, regarding research-based methods for teaching beginning reading. Despite the controversy, the latest review of scientific research on reading leads us to the following three conclusions. For *most* children,

- Mastering the alphabetic principle is essential to learning how to read successfully.
- Instructional techniques that explicitly teach this principle are more effective than those that do not.
- The reading teacher remains the most critical component of any reading program.

These conclusions are even more important when applied to children who are at risk for having difficulty learning to read. This is not to deny that literature-based activities that supplement phonics instruction can help to ensure the application of the alphabetic principle to enriched readings. Such activities can make reading meaningful and enjoyable.

When children receive instruction in phonemic awareness and the alphabetic principle and learn to apply that knowledge to decoding words, they are likely to succeed at learning to read. But once they fall behind, they almost never catch up. As noted earlier, a child's reading level in first grade is an astonishingly reliable predictor of reading achievement in high school (Cunningham and Stanovich, 1997). Consequently, the sooner that parents and teachers can recognize children with reading problems, the better.

What's Coming?

We now know that many reading difficulties can be overcome with early diagnosis and systematic intervention. Just how to go about determining whether a child has a reading problem is the topic of the next chapter.

CHAPTER 4
Recognizing Reading Problems

This chapter addresses several basic questions about how to recognize reading problems. They include:

- *What are the most common causes of reading problems?*
- *What have brain imaging scans revealed about struggling and dyslexic readers?*
- *What are some methods for detecting reading problems?*

THE READING GAP

Recent NAEP Assessments

About one student in three has reading problems. The 2003 report from the National Assessment of Educational Progress on reading described the reading achievement of students in the fourth, eighth, and twelfth grades (NAEP, 2003). It included comparisons between NAEP reading performance of students in 2002 and 2003 to the performance of their counterparts in previous assessments. Reading performance is reported in two ways: (1) average scale scores, and (2) achievement levels. The average scale score reflects the overall reading performance of a particular group, using a scale of 0 to 500 to provide information about student performance for all three grades. Achievement levels describe what students should know and be able to do at each of three levels, *Basic*, *Proficient*, and *Advanced*.

The Basic achievement level represents partial mastery of prerequisite knowledge and skills that are fundamental for efficient work at each grade. The Proficient achievement level indicates that students have demonstrated competency over challenging subject matter, including subject-matter knowledge, the application of such knowledge to real-world situations, and analytical skills appropriate to the subject matter. The Advanced achievement level represents superior performance in all these areas (NAEP, 2003).

National Scale Scores

Figure 4.1 shows the average reading scale scores for the three grades tested during 1992 through 2002 as well as the 2003 results for grades 4 and 8. In 1998, NAEP began testing the use of accommodations in reading, such as assessing these students in small groups or allowing them extra time as a way to increase participation. However, the NAEP does not allow having the reading assessment read aloud or translated because that would alter the skills being assessed.

In 2002, about 19 percent of grade 4 students selected for the NAEP were identified as special needs students. This is almost double the size of the special needs population tested in 1992. About 68 percent of these students participated in the 2002 testing, and 31 percent of them required accommodations.

Regrettably, little progress has been made in improving the average reading scale scores over the decade. The fourth-grade average score increased from 2000 to 2003, but it is not significantly higher than in 1992. NAEP explained these results by noting that more Hispanic and special needs students are now being assessed. When the scores of these students are removed from the totals, the average score is somewhat higher for the remaining fourth-grade population. The 2003 eighth-grade average score is the same as in 1998, but is an improvement over the1992 score.

The twelfth-grade average score in 2002, however, is significantly lower than the 1998 score and represents a continuing decline since 1992. NAEP noted that fewer students in twelfth grade are participating in these assessments, and it has established a commission to examine the issues involving twelfth grade participation in future assessments (NAEP, 2003).

Achievement Levels for Fourth Grade

NAEP (2003) gives the following specific definitions of the Basic, Proficient, and Advanced achievement levels in reading for grade 4:

- *Basic:* Fourth-grade students at the Basic level should demonstrate an understanding of the overall meaning of what they read. When reading text appropriate for fourth-graders, they should be able to make obvious connections between the text and their own experiences and extend the ideas in the text by making simple inferences.

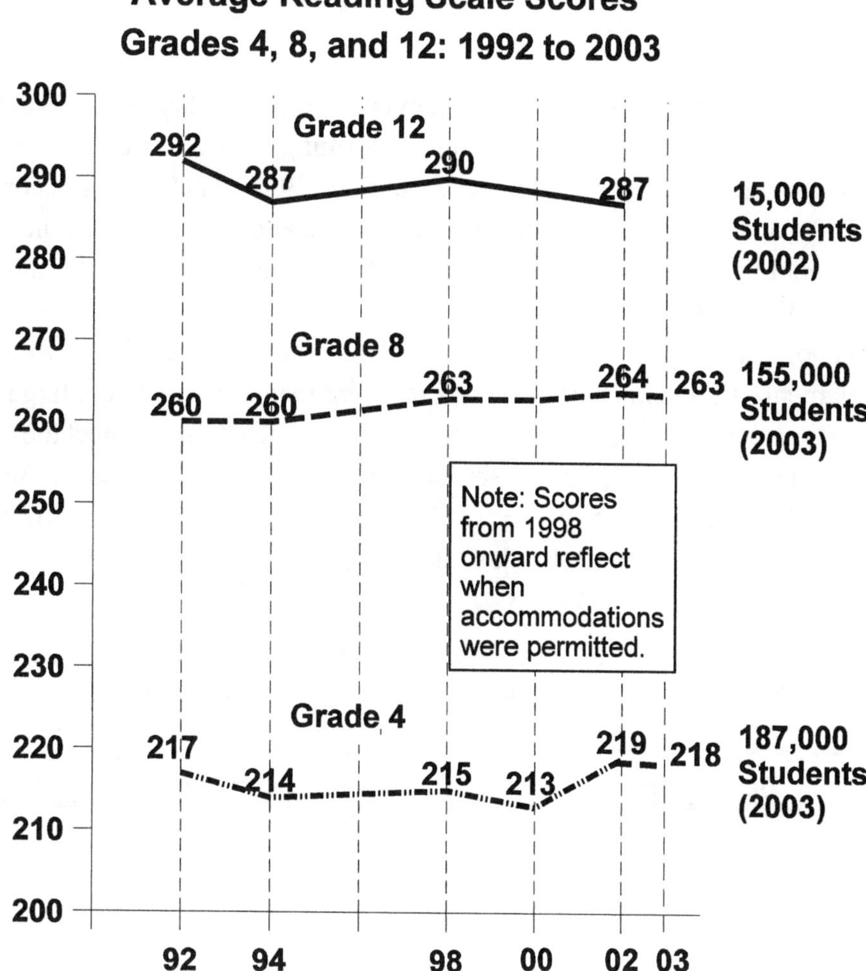

Figure 4.1 The chart shows the average NAEP reading scale scores for grades 4 and 8 for 1992 to 2003, and the grade 12 scores for 1992 to 2002. The tests were not administered in 1996. Grades 8 and 12 were not assessed in 2000. Scores from 1998 through 2003 reflect when testing accommodations were permitted (NAEP, 2003).

- *Proficient:* Fourth-grade students at the Proficient level should be able to demonstrate an overall understanding of the text, providing inferential as well as literal information. When reading text appropriate to fourth grade, they should be able to extend the ideas in the text by making inferences, drawing conclusions, and making connections to their own experiences. The connection between the text and what the student infers should be clear.
- *Advanced:* Fourth-grade students at the Advanced level should be able to generalize about topics in the reading selection and demonstrate an awareness of how authors compose and use literary devices. When reading text appropriate to fourth grade, they

should be able to judge text critically and, in general, to give thorough answers that indicate careful thought.

The fourth-grade results by reading achievement level are displayed in Table 4.1. They show that over one-third of these students are performing below Basic achievement levels, although that is an improvement over the percentages in 1998 and 2000 when accommodations are included. Thus, there are more fourth-grade students at or above Proficient in 2003 than in 1992. The report also noted that there were no differences between males and females in these results (NAEP, 2003).

Indications are that little progress is being made toward significantly increasing the number of elementary students who become Proficient readers, despite the large amounts of resources and time devoted to teaching reading. If school districts are to meet the expectations and deadlines regarding reading that are set forth in the No Child Left Behind Act, educators must reexamine how and when they are identifying students with reading problems, and what steps they are taking to help these at-risk students.

Table 4.1 Percentage of Fourth Grade Students by Reading Achievement Level NAEP 1992 to 2003 (*Accommodations Permitted)

Year	Below Basic	At Basic	At Proficient	At Advanced
1992	36	34	22	6
1994	40	31	22	7
1998*	40	30	22	7
2000*	41	30	23	7
2002*	36	32	24	7
2003*	37	32	23	8

Source: NAEP, 2003

Achievement for Black and Hispanic Students

Of continuing concern is the consistently low achievement levels for Black (Figure 4.2) and Hispanic (Figure 4.3) students over the last decade when compared to White students. There were no significant changes in fourth-grade and eighth-grade average scores for Black and Hispanic students from 2002 to 2003, although the 2003 scores were slightly higher for both grade levels than in 1992. In 2003, Hispanic students scored higher on average than Black students. This persistent poor performance of minority students in reading can be explained only in part by specific cognizant impairments, such as dyslexia. After all, the White student

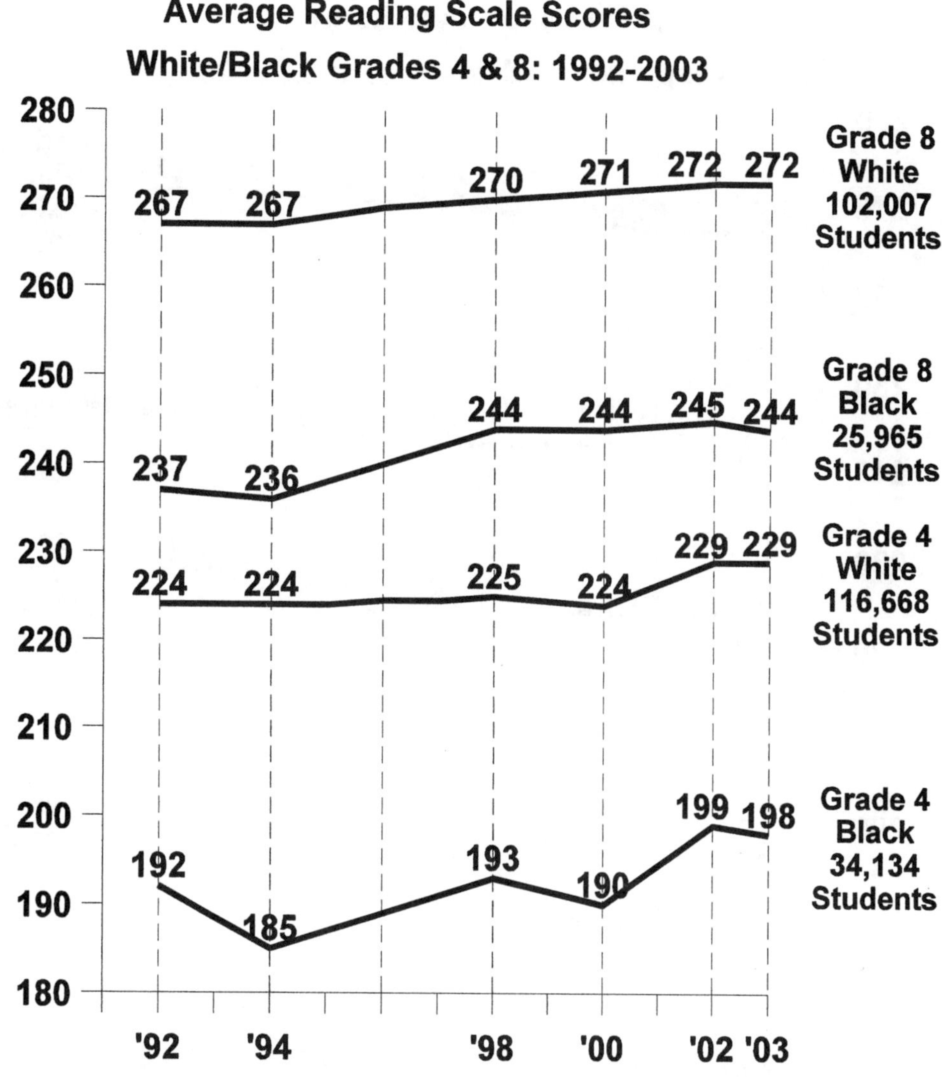

Figure 4.2 Since 1992, grade 4 and 8 Black students consistently scored below White students. Grade 4 Black students have made some gains in the last three years but the scores of grade 8 Black students have changed little in recent years (NAEP, 2003).

population also includes children with reading problems, yet their average scores remain higher. Furthermore, there is little scientific evidence that Black and Hispanic children are at a substantially greater risk for developmental dyslexia than these testing results would suggest. The size of the reading gap and the number of students involved suggests that this problem has roots in at least three separate but related areas: inadequate reading instruction, social and cultural conditions, and physical causes.

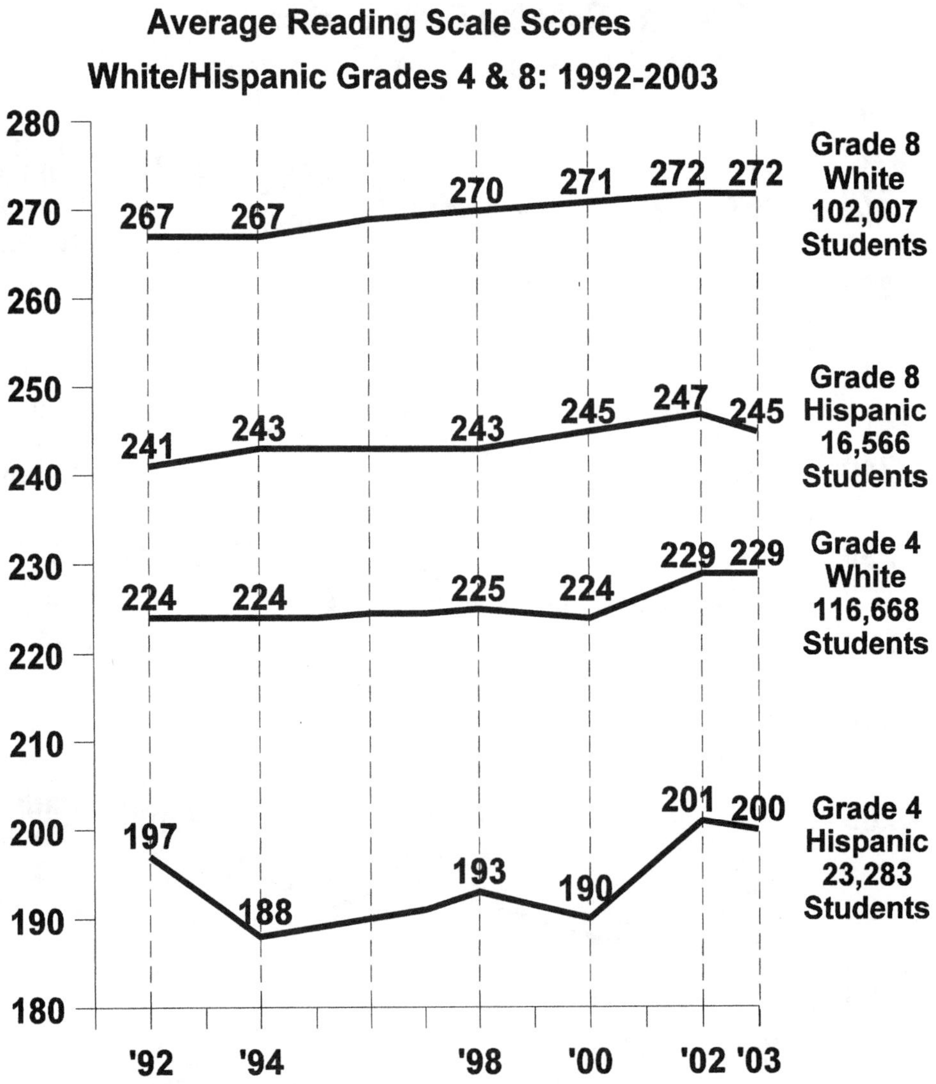

Average Reading Scale Scores
White/Hispanic Grades 4 & 8: 1992-2003

Grade 8 White 102,007 Students: '92 267, '94 267, '98 270, '00 271, '02 272, '03 272

Grade 8 Hispanic 16,566 Students: '92 241, '94 243, '98 243, '00 245, '02 247, '03 245

Grade 4 White 116,668 Students: '92 224, '94 224, '98 225, '00 224, '02 229, '03 229

Grade 4 Hispanic 23,283 Students: '92 197, '94 188, '98 193, '00 190, '02 201, '03 200

Figure 4.3 Since 1992, grade 4 and 8 Hispanic students consistently scored below White students. The scores of grade 4 Hispanic students have shown some improvement in the last four years but those of grade 8 Hispanic students have changed little (NAEP, 2003).

INADEQUATE READING INSTRUCTION

Some children have reading problems because they did not get adequate instruction in the skills needed for decoding, such as concepts about the nature of print, recognizing letters, and the alphabetic principle. They may not have had ample opportunities for systematic and focused practice in decoding real words. As a result, they failed to develop a rich mental lexicon, which is essential for promoting fluency and comprehension. To successfully understand a language, children need to develop a rich vocabulary and an appreciation for semantics, and combine that understanding with what they know about the real world. They also need to have a good understanding of the mechanics of language (syntax) and they need to be attuned to the phonology of the language so that they do not confuse similar sounding words, such as *chair* and *cheer*.

None of these areas can be described as social, cultural, or physical problems that lead to reading difficulties. These deficits are not intrinsic to the child, but to the classroom and to the school system that has not provided the appropriate instructional environment. Schools situated in high-poverty areas are often competing for limited materials and resources. Conscientious but inadequately trained teachers may be using outdated programs and methodologies. This unfortunate combination can be the cause of some children's reading difficulties. Children in this situation are not dyslexic. Their problem is that they were simply never taught the skills needed to learn how to read. To be successful in teaching all children, teachers need to become extremely knowledgeable about effective strategies as well as diagnostic in their approach to reading instruction.

SOCIAL AND CULTURAL CAUSES OF READING PROBLEMS

A large number of Black and Hispanic children performing below White children in reading display no signs of specific learning impairments. Clearly other factors are at work. Multiple studies have identified social conditions that have an impact on the achievement of children in inner-city schools. Limited teacher training, large class sizes, the absence of literature in the home, and poor parental support for schools have all been cited as causes for lack of student progress. Although these conditions cannot be ignored, schools need to focus more on the direct connections between what we are learning about how the brain learns to read and the *linguistic* barriers interfering with that learning.

Some researchers believe that these children are performing poorly on reading tests because their home language differs substantially from the language used in reading instruction (Labov, 2003). Bailey (1993) suggested a decade ago that Black children were being immersed in a language dialect that has become known as African-American Vernacular English (AAVE). Residential desegregation has increased the impact of AAVE. Meanwhile, as Spanish-speaking populations increase, children are faced with learning to read English in school while speaking Spanish at home.

> Teachers of reading should be trained to recognize when a child's reading problems are the result of linguistic clashes and not a pathology.

Consequently, some of the causes of poor performance by Black and Hispanic children can be attributed to impediments resulting from linguistic differences. That is, their native dialect or language is different in significant ways from what is being taught in school. They come to school with a mental lexicon whose word representations often do not match what they are trying to decode on the printed page. Learning to read involves determining which words *are* present in their mental lexicon, what they represent, and whether they can be comprehended in context. This is not a physiological deficit; it is a social and cultural problem. For these children, we should not be looking at what is wrong with them but how we can alter instruction to make them more successful in learning to read. Such alterations can be made when teachers of reading are properly trained to recognize w hen a child's reading problems are the result of linguistic clashes and not a pathology. Furthermore, that training should also help teachers understand how they can use some of the linguistic attributes of AAVE and Spanish to help children pronounce, decode, and understand standard English.

PHYSICAL CAUSES OF READING PROBLEMS

As noted earlier, nature long ago crafted sophisticated neural networks in the brain to process spoken language. But decoding written text is a wholly artificial creation that calls upon neural regions designed for other tasks. Because there is no single neural region for reading, numerous brain areas must be recruited to perform the task of decoding artificial symbols into sound. Reading is so complex that any small problem along the way can slow or interrupt the process. It is small wonder that children have more problems with reading than with any other skill we ask them to learn. Difficulties result essentially from either environmental or physical factors, or some combination of both. Environmental factors include limited exposure to language in the preschool years, resulting in little phoneme sensitivity, letter knowledge, print awareness, vocabulary, and reading comprehension. Physical factors include speech, hearing, and visual impairments and substandard intellectual capabilities. Any combination of environmental and physical factors makes the diagnosis and treatment more difficult.

Successful decoding and comprehending of written text involves the coordination and integration of three separate neural systems.

Recent research into the causes and nature of reading problems has revealed more about the neural processes involved in reading. Recall that successful reading involves two basic processes—decoding and comprehension—that are generated by three neural systems. Figure 4.4 illustrates how these three systems interact. Decoding written text into sounds that represent words results when the visual and auditory processing systems see and sound out the words in the reader's head. The frontal lobe interprets the meaning conveyed by those word representations.

Problems with any one or more of these systems can cause reading difficulties. In some children, the problems occur during early brain development and affect their ability to process

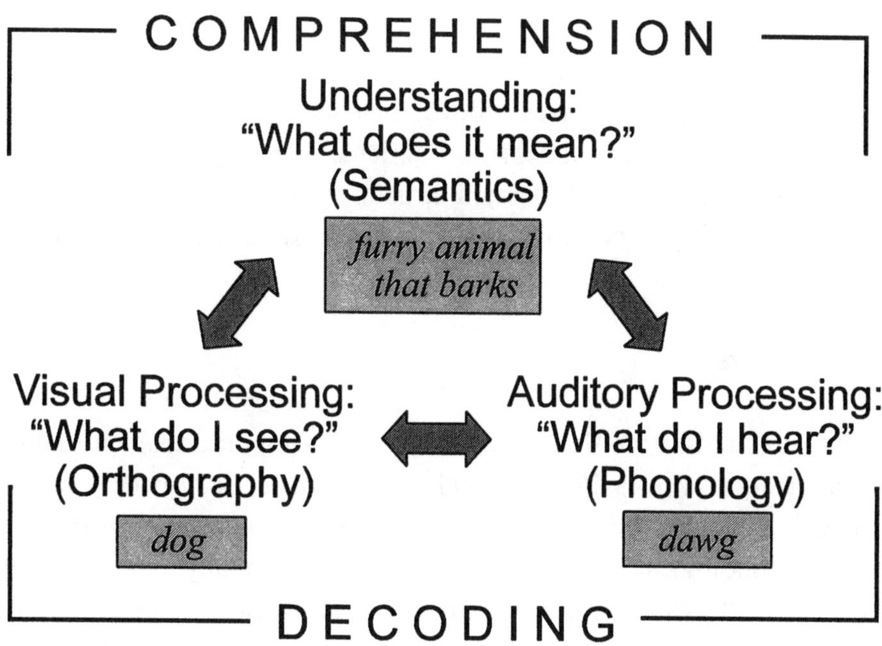

Figure 4.4 Successful reading requires the coordination of three systems: visual and auditory processing to decode the words, and frontal lobe processing to determine meaning.

the sounds of language and, eventually, to decode written text. This developmental deficit appears to be the most common cause of reading difficulties, and usually results in a life-long struggle with reading. Less common are problems with reading caused by impairments in hearing and vision that can occur at any time in a person's life.

Most research studies on reading have focused primarily on developmental reading problems that scientists refer to as *developmental dyslexia.* In developmental dyslexia, the child experiences unexpected difficulty in learning to read despite adequate intelligence, environment, and normal senses. It is a spectrum disorder, varying from mild to severe. Neuroimaging studies have established that there are significant differences in the way normal and dyslexic brains respond to specific spoken and written language tasks. Furthermore, there is evidence that these differences may weaken with appropriate instructional interventions.

Scientists have long been searching for the causes of reading problems. This has not been an easy task because of the large number of sensory, motor, and cognitive systems that are involved in reading. Struggling readers may have impairments in any one or more of these systems, but not all struggling readers have dyslexia. Specifically, dyslexia seems to be caused by deficits in the neural regions responsible for language and phonological processing or by problems in nonlinguistic areas of the brain.

Linguistic Causes

Several potential linguistic causes of developmental dyslexia that have emerged from recent research studies, including phonological deficits, differences in auditory and visual processing speeds, the varying sizes of brain structures, memory deficits, genetics, brain lesions, and word-blindness. It is possible that several of these causes are related to each other and can coexist in the same individual.

Phonological Deficits

The ability to sound out words in one's head plays an important role in reading familiar words and sounding out new ones. Phonological information is used by the working memory to integrate and comprehend words in phrases and sentences. Extensive evidence has existed for decades that phonological operations are impaired in many dyslexics (Harm and Seidenberg, 1999). But the causes of the impairment were not clear. Because many dyslexics have normal or above normal intelligence, researchers suspected that the phonological processing deficits appeared only when the brain was trying to decode writing. Exactly why that happens is not fully known. However, studies of the differences in auditory and visual processing speeds as well as fMRI scans of the brain during reading are shedding new light on the possible causes of the phonological impairments.

Differences in Auditory and Visual Processing Speeds

One of the more intriguing explanations of some reading difficulties, including dyslexia, has come from research studies using magnetoencephalography (MEG), a technique for measuring the electric signals emitted during brain activation as a result of mental processing. These studies noted abnormal auditory activation but normal visual activation during reading (Helenius, Salmelin, Richardson, Leinonen, and Lyytinen, 2002; Renvall and Hari, 2002; Tallal et al.,1996; Temple et al., 2003). Sometimes referred to as *temporal processing impairment,* the differences in the processing speeds could explain some of the symptoms common to dyslexia.

The explanation goes like this: When reading silently, our eyes scan the words on the page (visual processing) and we sound out those words in our head. This sounding out represents the auditory processing necessary for us to decode and interpret what we are reading. To read successfully, the visual and auditory processing systems have to work together, that is, be in synchrony.

When a child begins to learn to read, it is essential that the letter (grapheme) the child sees corresponds to what the child hears (phoneme) internally. In Figure 4.5, the child with normal auditory processing (left) is looking at the letter *d* and the auditory processing system is simultaneously sounding out */d/* or *duh.* As the eye moves to *o,* the phoneme */ô/* or *awh*

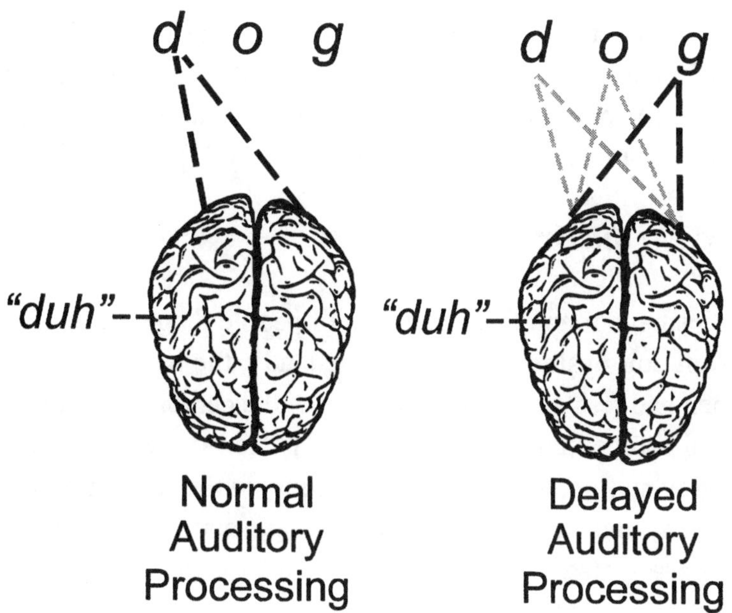

Figure 4.5 In normal auditory processing (left), the phoneme that the child hears correctly matches the letter that the eyes see—in this case, the sound "duh" corresponds to the letter "d." If the auditory processing system is delayed, however, the child's eyes are already on the letter "g" while the "duh" phoneme is still sounding in the child's head. The brain errs in matching "duh" with "g."

will sound out and then *g* produces the phoneme */g/* or *guh.* Later, when this child is asked to write *dog,* the */d/* phoneme will recall the letter *d,* and so on.

However, if the auditory processing system is impaired and lags behind the visual processing system, then the child's eye is already scanning to the letter *g* while the phoneme */d/* or *duh* is still being processed in the auditory system. As a result, the child's brain incorrectly associates the letter *g* with the phoneme sound of */d/* or *duh.* Now, when we ask the child to write the word *dog,* the child hears the first phoneme */d/* or *duh* but incorrectly recalls the letter *g,* perhaps eventually writing the word *god.*

If this notion is correct, then finding a way to bring the auditory and visual processing systems in closer synchrony should help to remedy the problem. That is exactly what several researchers tried. They developed a computer program, known as Fast ForWord, designed to help poor readers slow down visual processing to allow the auditory processing sufficient time to recognize the sound of the initial phoneme. Using this program with children who had reading problems produced surprisingly successful results. The program and process are discussed in greater detail in Chapter 5.

Some scientists are even suggesting that this time delay problem could lead to a simple test for early diagnosis of dyslexia. Researchers at Wake Forest University asked dyslexic and non-dyslexic people to tell which of two lights appeared first. Both groups performed much better when they heard sounds through headphones. For non-dyslexic participants, the sound needed to occur within 150 milliseconds of the light for them to perform better. Longer intervals did not improve their performance. However, dyslexic participants performed better with longer delays up to 350 milliseconds. Because the test did not involve reading, this time difference could help identify young children with potential reading problems before they reach school age (Burdette, Hairston, Flowers, and Wallace, 2003).

Structural Differences in the Brain

Some MRI studies have found that the brains of people diagnosed with dyslexia are structurally different from non-dyslexic brains. In one study, the researchers noted that the dyslexic brains of 16 men had less gray matter (surface of the cerebrum) in the left temporal lobe, the frontal lobe, and cerebellum than the brains of 14 non-dyslexic subjects (Brown et al., 2001). Having less gray matter (and thus fewer neurons) in the left temporal lobe (where Wernicke's area is located) and in the frontal lobe (where comprehension occurs) could contribute to the deficits associated with dyslexia.

Phonologic Memory Deficits

Skilled reading requires an ability to retain verbal bits of information (phonemes) in working memory. Recent studies have shown distinct deficits in this phonologic memory among poor readers. The deficits more commonly involve serial tasks, such as holding a string of phonemes to make a word and a sequence of words to generate a sentence (Howes, Bigler, Burlingame, and Lawson, 2003).

Genetics and Gender

Studies of genetic composition have shown strong associations between dyslexia and genetic mutations in twins and families (Pennington, 1990), and recent investigations may have actually identified some of the specific genes involved (Kaminen et al., 2003). Thus, dyslexia is a life-long condition and not just a "phase." The genetic mutations could impede the development of systems that the typical brain utilizes to decode written text, forcing the brain to construct alternate and less efficient pathways.

> Boys tend to be over-identified with reading problems; girls, on the other hand, tend to be under-identified.

Nationwide, there are three to four times more boys identified with reading problems than girls. Although this was once thought to be the result of genetic deficits, the true reason may be because boys are over-identified (often due to their rambunctious behavior) and girls are under-identified (sit quietly in class and obey the rules). Recent studies indicate that many girls are affected as well but are not getting help (Shaywitz, 2003).

Lesions in the Word Form Area

Researchers using PET scans have noticed that some developmentally dyslexic people have lesions in the left occipito-temporal area of the brain. You may recall from Chapter 2 that this area is identified as the word form area most used by skilled readers to decode written text. Another discovery in these studies was that the amount of blood flowing to this brain region predicted the severity of the dyslexia (Rumsey et al., 1999). Regardless of the cause, a lesion and reduced blood flow would likely hamper the ability of this patch of neurons to decode written text.

Word-Blindness

Word-blindness is the inability to read words even though the person's eyes are optically normal. Two forms exist: *Congenital word-blindness* involves a glitch in the wiring of neurons during embryonic development and is usually confined to those neural systems associated with reading. This disorder may go unnoticed for years, affecting reading and occasionally spoken language. *Acquired word-blindness* results from some traumatic insult to the brain, such as a stroke or a tumor, occurring during a person's lifetime and interfering with already established systems. The damaged area is usually on the left side of the brain, causing weakness in the right side of the body and difficulty pronouncing words or naming objects (Shaywitz, 2003).

Nonlinguistic Causes

Some people, who are otherwise unimpaired, have extreme difficulties in reading because of deficits in auditory and visual perception not related to linguistic systems. This revelation was somewhat of a surprise because conventional wisdom held that impairments in reading (and also in oral language) were restricted to problems with linguistic processing. The following are some possible nonlinguistic causes found in the research literature.

Perception of Sequential Sounds

The inability to detect and discriminate sounds presented in rapid succession seems to be a common impairment in individuals with reading and language disorders. These individuals also have difficulty in indicating the order of two sounds presented in rapid succession. This particular deficit is related to auditory processing of sound waves in general and is not related directly to distinguishing phonemes as part of phonological processing. Hearing words accurately when reading or from a stream of rapid conversation is critical to comprehension (Wright, Bowen, and Zecker, 2000).

Sound-Frequency Discrimination

Some individuals with reading disorders are impaired in their ability to hear differences in sound frequency. This auditory defect can affect the ability to discriminate tone and pitch in speech. At first glance, this may seem like only an oral language-related impairment. However, it also affects reading proficiency because reading involves sounding out words in the auditory processing system (Wright et al., 2000).

Detection of Target Sounds in Noise

The inability to detect tones within noise is another recently discovered nonlinguistic impairment. When added to the findings in the two deficits mentioned above, this evidence suggests that auditory functions may play a much greater role in reading disorders than previously thought (Wright et al., 2000).

Visual Magnocellular-Deficit Hypothesis

The interpretation of some research studies has lead to a hypothesis about the functions of the visual processing system. This proposes that certain forms of reading disorders are caused by a deficit in the visual processing system, which leads to poor detection of coherent visual motion and poor discrimination of the speed of visual motion. This part of the visual system involves large neurons and so is referred to as the magnocellular system. Impairment in this system may cause letters on a page to bundle and overlap, or appear to move—common complaints from some struggling readers and dyslexics (Demb, Boynton, and Heeger, 1998). Other scientists, however, question this interpretation of the research mainly because it is not known how the visual impairments relate to the phonological impairments (Amitay, Ben-Yehudah, Banai, and Ahissar, 2002). Current evidence suggests that visual impairments by themselves are a very small part of dyslexia (Rayner et al., 2001).

Motor Coordination and the Cerebellum

Several imaging studies show that many dyslexic readers have processing deficits in the cerebellum of the brain (Nicolson, Fawcett, and Dean, 2001). Another study determined that nearly 75 percent of the dyslexic subjects had smaller lobes on the right side of the cerebellum compared to non-dyslexic participants (Eckert et al., 2003). The cerebellum is located at the rear of the brain just below the occipital lobe (Figure 4.6). It is mainly responsible for coordinating learned motor skills. Deficiencies in this part of the brain could result, according to researchers, in problems with reading, writing, and spelling. Problems in reading may result if cerebellar deficits delay the time when an infant sits up and walks, and begins babbling and talking. Less motor skill coordination can mean less articulation and fluency in speech. This, in turn, leads to less sensitivity to onset, rime, and the phonemic structure of language.

Handwriting, of course, is a motor skill that requires the precise coordination and timing of different muscle groups. Lack of coordination of these muscles due to a cerebellar deficit would create difficulties in writing, a characteristic that many dyslexics display. Problems with spelling would arise from poor phonological awareness, trouble with word recognition, and difficulties in automating spelling rule skills.

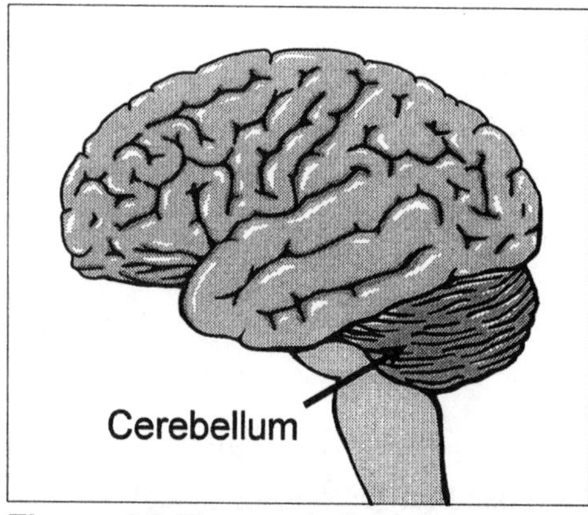

Figure 4.6 The cerebellum is located at the rear of the brain and is responsible for coordinating learned motor skills.

The possibility of deficits in visual and auditory perception and memory as well as in motor coordination on various reading tasks accounts for the wide range of individual differences observed among those with reading disorders. Analyzing these differences leads to a better understanding of the multidimensional nature of reading disorders and possible treatment.

Attention-Deficit Hyperactivity Disorder

Attention-deficit hyperactivity disorder (ADHD) is a developmental disorder characterized by difficulty in focusing and sustaining attention. Children with ADHD are often assumed to also have developmental reading problems. But that is not usually the case. ADHD and developmental dyslexia are separate disorders, and less than 25 percent of ADHD children also have dyslexia.

Answer to Test Question # 6

Question: Most children with attention-deficit hyperactivity disorder (ADHD) are also dyslexic.

Answer: *False.* ADHD and developmental dyslexia are separate disorders. Only about 25 percent of ADHD children also have dyslexia.

Is Dyslexia Present in Readers of Other Languages?

Dyslexia appears in all languages, including those that are read from right to left, as Hebrew and Arabic. People with dyslexia who speak highly phonetic languages, such as Spanish and Finnish, are identified with the disorder later than those who speak deep morphological languages such as English, where the linguistic demands of the language are more challenging. English speakers experience the complex phonetic structure early on in their schooling. Readers can also experience difficulties in logographic languages, such as Chinese, due to visual confusion or problems with memory recall.

BRAIN IMAGING STUDIES

You will recall from the Introduction that brain imaging technologies are of two kinds: those that look at the structure of the brain (e.g., MRI and CAT scans) and those that look at how the brain functions (e.g., PET and fMRI scans). In recent years, these scans have revealed differences in both the structure and function of dyslexic brains compared to non-dyslexic brains. Eventually, these types of investigations may lead to more accurate diagnosis and treatment.

Studies of Brain Structure

MRI studies that have compared the brain structure of dyslexic individuals to normal readers have found some interesting differences. These differences were more evident in dyslexics who had early spoken language problems than in dyslexics whose speech progressed normally. The regions of the brain that showed structural variations were consistent across multiple MRI studies and were closely associated with those neural areas involved in spoken language processing (Beaton, 1997; Leonard, 2001). The implication here is that an individual with atypical brain structures that hamper speech is likely to have difficulties in learning to read as well.

Studies of Brain Function

Newer research in brain function is shedding more light on dyslexia. Because dyslexics often confused *b* and *d,* psychologists thought for many years that dyslexia was merely a vision problem. Researchers now believe that the letters can also be confused because they sound alike. This is the brain's inability to process what it hears, not what it sees. Other imaging studies show an imperfectly functioning system for dividing words into their phonological units—a critical step for accurate reading. Letter reversals can be the result of phonological missteps in the decoding of print to sound and back to print. It is likely that the learner has problems in assigning what he says or hears in his head (the phoneme) to the letters he sees on paper (the grapheme). Thus, remedial strategies should focus on reestablishing correct phonemic connections with intense practice.

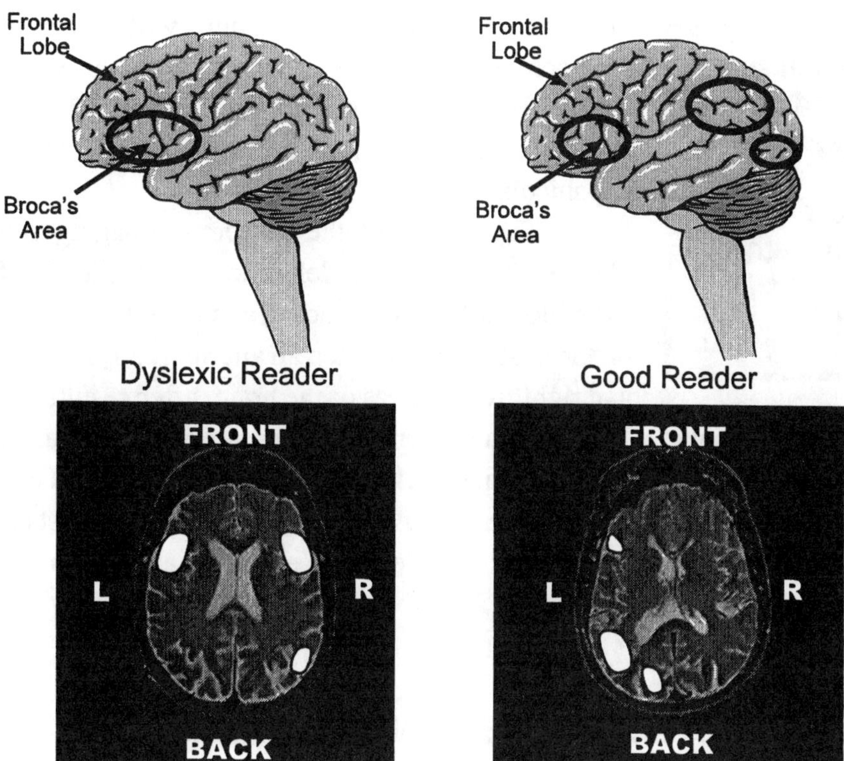

Figure 4.7 The brain regions that are activated during reading are shown as black ovals in the upper diagrams and as white areas in the lower representative fMRI scans. Dyslexic readers (left) use different brain regions during reading than do good readers (right). Note that dyslexic readers show little activation in the back of the brain but strong activation in the front regions, especially in Broca's area. Good readers, on the other hand, show strong activation in the back of the brain with lesser activation in the front (Richards, 2001; Shaywitz, 2003; Simos et al., 2000).

Numerous functional imaging studies clearly indicate that poor readers use different brain pathways than good readers. As discussed in Chapter 2, good readers of all ages rely more on the occipito-temporal areas in the back of the brain to decode word forms, and require only a little input from Broca's area (Figure 4.7). By using just these three left-side areas, their ability to recognize word forms, with practice, is automatic and their reading becomes fluent.

The studies further show that dyslexic readers at an early age do not use the word processing regions in the left rear part of the brain. Rather, they rely more on Broca's area for decoding text. This reliance increases with age so that, as adolescents, they are overactivating Broca's area and recruiting other frontal regions as they try to read. Apparently, the increased use of frontal brain areas is an attempt to compensate for the disruptions in the rear of the brain. In the cross-sectional picture in Figure 4.7, note how during reading a dyslexic reader's brain activates an area in the right frontal lobe—used primarily for visual memory—in addition to Broca's area. But rote-based learning of words can get a reader only so far before the memory systems begin to fail. This overreliance on memory results in slow and laborious reading because the disruption in the rear brain areas prohibit automatic word recognition.

The different brain scan patterns between good and dyslexic readers are so consistent that they may one day allow for early diagnosis, perhaps even before a child begins to read.

Functional imaging studies of adults with dyslexia, including high-achieving university students, reveal this same pattern of strong frontal area use during reading (Richards, 2001; Shaywitz, 2003; Simos, Breier, Fletcher, Mergman, and Papanicolaou, 2000).

The results of the numerous imaging studies seem clear: Good readers use left-side posterior areas of the brain for rapid, automatic decoding and reading. Dyslexic readers, on the other hand, develop an alternative system that uses left and right frontal areas of the brain, often resulting in accurate but slow reading. Moreover, dyslexic brains during reading are working harder—that is, employing more neurons—than the brains of good readers (Brun et al., 2003). These different patterns between good and dyslexic readers are so consistent that neuroscientists believe that functional imaging may one day allow for early detection of dyslexia, perhaps even before a child begins to learn to read (Nandy et al., 2003).

DETECTING READING PROBLEMS

In recent years, researchers have made significant progress using fMRI scans to understand how novice, skilled, and dyslexic brains read. Yet, despite these advancements, fMRI scans are not a practical tool at present for diagnosing dyslexia in a single individual. That is because the results of fMRI studies are usually reported for groups rather than for individuals. Researchers have found some variations in the activated areas of the brain among individuals within both the dyslexic and control groups. More research is needed to clarify these differences before fMRI or any other imaging techniques can be used for diagnostic purposes (Richards, 2001). Until that time, however, researchers can use the information gained from imaging studies to develop other kinds of diagnostic tests that more closely align with our new understanding of dyslexia.

For the moment, critical observation of a child's progress in learning to speak, and eventually in learning to read, remains our most effective tool for spotting potential problems. Most difficulties associated with reading do not go away with time. Therefore, the earlier that parents and teachers can detect reading problems in children, the better. The problems often begin to reveal themselves first in spoken language and later while learning to read.

Spoken Language Difficulties

I discussed in previous chapters that learning to read is closely connected to fluency in spoken language. Both speaking and reading rely on the proper functioning of the phonologic module, that brain region where sounds are combined to form words and words are broken down into their basic sounds. Consequently, difficulties that children have with spoken language are often clues to potential reading problems. Parents and teachers should remember that it is normal for all children to make occasional language errors while speaking. But frequent language errors, stemming from any one or a combination of the following conditions, could indicate that a child may run into trouble when beginning to learn to read.

Some of the spoken language difficulties may involve any one or more of the following (IDA, 2003; NAEYC, 1998; Shaywitz, 2003):

- *Delay in speaking.* Children generally say their first words at about 12 months of age and follow with phrases when between 18 and 24 months old. Because learning to read is closely linked to a child's phonologic skills in spoken language, delays in speaking may be an early indication of potential reading problems, espe-cially in a family that has a history of dyslexia.
- *Difficulties with pronunciation.* Children should have little difficulty pronouncing words correctly by 5 or 6 years of age. Difficulties in pronouncing words (sometimes referred to as "baby talk") may be an indication of future reading problems. Such trouble pronouncing long or complicated words could signal a snag in the parts of the brain that generate spoken language, causing a mix-up in the processing of the phonemes. Mispronunciations often involve mixing syllables within words (*aminal* for animal) and leaving off the beginning syllables (*luminum* for aluminum).
- *Difficulty in learning the letters of the alphabet.* Learning the names of the letters of the alphabet is an important, though not essential, step in learning to read. Marked difficulties in learning the letters could indicate a potential reading problem.
- *Recalling incorrect phonemes.* A child looks at a picture of a donkey and recalls the word *doggie,* a word similar in sound but not in meaning. This recall of incorrect phonemes may cause a child to talk about a word without actually recalling it. The child may get frustrated because of the inability to say the word. As these children get older, they may resort more to vague words in order to mask their difficulties in retrieving specific words. They use general words like *things* and *stuff,* making their conversations hard to follow. It is important to remember that the problem here is not with their thinking, but with their ability to use expressive language, that is, to recall a word on command.
- *Insensitivity to rhyme.* Part of a young child's enjoyment of spoken language is playing with rhyme. Hearing and repeating rhyming sounds demonstrates how words can be separated into smaller segments of sound, and that different words may share the same sound. Children with good rhyming skills are showing their readiness for learning to read. Those with little sensitivity to rhyme, on the other

hand, may have reading problems because they are unable to detect the consonant sound that changes the meaning of closely rhyming words.

- *Genetics.* Looking at the family tree for signs of dyslexia in close relatives is a clue because about 25 to 50 percent of the children born to a dyslexic parent will also be dyslexic (Kaminen et al., 2003; Londin et al., 2003; Shaywitz, 2003). Whether the child actually displays dyslexia depends somewhat on that child's environment. This revelation came from studies of identical twins. Because they share the same genes, if one twin has dyslexia, so should the other. But in reality, in 30 to 35 percent of the cases, one twin is dyslexic while the other is not (Fisher and DeFries, 2002). Apparently, even though these children had a genetic predisposition for dyslexia, differences in the home and school environments played important roles in determining how successful these children would be at reading.

Looking for Early Indicators of Reading Problems

Until the time that brain imaging becomes a standard diagnostic tool, researchers will continue to look for ways to accurately identify students with reading problems as early as possible. Multiple research studies have sought to find indicators of reading problems that are more valid than solely the professional judgment of the evaluating team. The obvious problem here is that the application of professional judgment is only as good as the training and competence of the team members. This approach can often lead to considerable variability in identification from district to district and even from state to state. Using more objective measures would reduce this variability. Research studies have found that letter fluency is a useful measure in kindergarten, while response to instruction can be a valuable measure in second grade.

Letter Fluency Tasks as Kindergarten Indicators

The earlier that children who are at risk for reading problems can be identified, the better. Trying to carry out such identification procedures in kindergarten is difficult because of the broad range of background experience these children bring to the classroom. Nonetheless, studies involving kindergarten children do seem to indicate that letter-name fluency and nonsense word fluency can be valid indicators of early reading skills, such as oral reading fluency (ORF).

One study (Speece and Mills, 2003) tested 39 kindergartners in the Spring in several language skill areas, including receptive vocabulary, phonological awareness, letter-name knowledge, letter-sound knowledge, letter-name fluency, and nonsense word fluency. These same children were again tested one year later in first grade in similar skills, plus oral reading fluency. Nonsense word fluency and letter-word fluency, respectively, were the highest predictors of oral reading fluency. In fact, the fluency measures were more accurate at predicting ORF than national normed measures of reading and phonological awareness, which identified only 33 percent of the poor readers in this study.

Using Response to Instruction as an Indicator in Second Grade

Another technique for avoiding the misidentification or nonidentification of students with reading problems is to place increased emphasis on measures of school performance. The response-to-treatment model identifies students based on low achievement, application of certain criteria for exclusion, and then response to interventions. Those who would be identified as having reading problems are children who did not respond to treatment and still display low achievement in reading, especially where the primary cause is not considered to be social and economic disadvantages, mental deficiency, or linguistic and cultural diversity.

Studies that tested this approach (Torgesen, 2001; Vellutino et al., 1996) provided children in primary grades with incremental periods of instruction and moved them out when they made adequate progress. One study (Vaughn, Linan-Thompson, and Hickman, 2003) of 45 second-grade, largely Hispanic students at risk for reading difficulties, sought to identify students by providing increments of supplemental instruction (10 weeks in length, 5 sessions per week, and about 35 minutes per session). The instruction included fast-paced lessons that focused on phonemic awareness, phonics, fluency, comprehension, and spelling, with correction and feedback and many opportunities for reading practice. Students were tested after each 10 weeks of supplemental instruction to determine if they met the exit criteria. Those who met the criteria were exited from the program and those who did not received another 10 weeks of supplemental instruction.

The exit tests included tests of oral reading fluency (ORF), word attack, passage comprehension, phonological processing, and general language proficiency. Ten students exited after the first 10 weeks of intervention, 14 after 20 weeks, and another 10 after 30 weeks. Even after 30 weeks of supplemental instruction, 11 students still did not meet the exit criteria, although most showed small improvements in reading fluency. The study showed that using a set of exit criteria linked to 30 weeks of supplemental instruction led to the identification of a distinct group of students who required substantial support and more explicit and intensive instruction, perhaps in special education. The researchers suggested that using response to treatment (1) provides supplemental instruction to a large number of at-risk students, (2) requires consistent monitoring of student progress, and (3) reduces the many biases inherent in the traditional referral systems that rely heavily on the interpretations and perceptions of classroom teachers.

Remember that all children make errors in spoken language and while reading. But the number of errors should decrease with time, and there should be clear evidence of growth in vocabulary and reading comprehension. Determining whether a child has consistent problems with reading requires careful and long-term observation of the child's fluency in speaking and reading. Most children display obvious improvements in their speaking and reading skills over time. Researchers, clinicians, and educators who study dyslexia and who work with poor readers look for certain clues that will show whether a child's reading ability is progressing normally.

The checklists that follow contain indications of reading problems commonly found in struggling readers, including people diagnosed with dyslexia. The indications have been gathered from several sources (Brady and Moats, 1997; IDA, 2003; NAEYC, 1998; Shaywitz, 2003; Stinson, 2003) and are separated into grade-level groupings. **The lists are not intended to be used for final diagnosis. Diagnosis of dyslexia or any other learning disorder can be made only by experienced clinicians.** However, the lists will help you to assess the degree of difficulty a child may be having in learning to read and to determine whether additional testing and consultations are required.

Use the following checklist to determine whether a child may be displaying problems. Circle the appropriate response to the right of each indicator. Those indicators marked "often" should be discussed among parents, teachers, and specialists in speech and language pathologies.

Preschool

Indicator (Inconsistent with the child's age or cognitive abilities) After the skills have been taught, the child . . .	**Rating**		
has difficulty pronouncing words	Rarely	Sometimes	Often
has difficulty with rhymes	Rarely	Sometimes	Often
is unable to recall the correct word	Rarely	Sometimes	Often
has difficulty in learning/remembering the names of letters	Rarely	Sometimes	Often
has difficulty following multi-step directions or routines	Rarely	Sometimes	Often
has difficulty telling/retelling a story in correct sequence	Rarely	Sometimes	Often
has trouble learning common nursery rhymes	Rarely	Sometimes	Often
has difficulty separating sounds in words	Rarely	Sometimes	Often

has difficulty blending sounds to make words	Rarely	Sometimes	Often
has difficulty listening to and discussing storybooks	Rarely	Sometimes	Often

Kindergarten and First Grade

Indicator (Inconsistent with the child's age or cognitive abilities) After the skills have been taught, the child . . .	**Rating**		
has difficulty recognizing that words can be separated into their basic sounds, such as *shoe* can be broken down into */sh/* and */oo/*	Rarely	Sometimes	Often
has difficulty recognizing that words can be separated, such as *horseshoe* into *horse* and *shoe*	Rarely	Sometimes	Often
has trouble sounding out individual words in isolation	Rarely	Sometimes	Often
has difficulty using descriptive language	Rarely	Sometimes	Often
says that reading is difficult	Rarely	Sometimes	Often
has difficulty connecting letters to their sounds	Rarely	Sometimes	Often
says a word that is very different from its text, such as saying *house* when reading *giant*	Rarely	Sometimes	Often
has difficulty pronouncing the beginning sounds in words	Rarely	Sometimes	Often
has difficulty spelling high frequency short words	Rarely	Sometimes	Often
has difficulty reading orally with fluency	Rarely	Sometimes	Often
has difficulty using context to identify new words	Rarely	Sometimes	Often
has difficulty learning new vocabulary	Rarely	Sometimes	Often
has difficulty following simple directions, such as "Take out your notebook."	Rarely	Sometimes	Often
has difficulty retelling a story	Rarely	Sometimes	Often
has difficulty comprehending what was read	Rarely	Sometimes	Often

Second to Fourth Grade

Indicator (Inconsistent with the child's age or cognitive abilities) After the skills have been taught, the child . . .	Rating		
makes letter reversals, as *b* for *d* and *q* for *p*	Rarely	Sometimes	Often
makes letter inversions, as *n* for *u* and *w* for *m*	Rarely	Sometimes	Often
makes word reversals, as *pot* for *top*	Rarely	Sometimes	Often
confuses small words, as *and* for *said* and *goes* for *does*	Rarely	Sometimes	Often
has difficulty pronouncing long, unfamiliar words	Rarely	Sometimes	Often
confuses words that sound alike, as *left* for *felt* or *ocean* for *motion*	Rarely	Sometimes	Often
relies on guessing and context to decode new words rather than sounding them out	Rarely	Sometimes	Often
omits parts of words when sounding them out, as *enjble* for *enjoyable*	Rarely	Sometimes	Often
has difficulty breaking multisyllabic words into their component syllables	Rarely	Sometimes	Often
avoids reading aloud	Rarely	Sometimes	Often
pauses and hesitates during speech, lots of *ums*	Rarely	Sometimes	Often
has difficulty responding orally when questioned	Rarely	Sometimes	Often
relies heavily on memorizing instead of comprehending	Rarely	Sometimes	Often
has difficulty remembering facts	Rarely	Sometimes	Often
transposes number sequences	Rarely	Sometimes	Often
confuses arithmetic signs	Rarely	Sometimes	Often
has difficulty finishing written tests on time	Rarely	Sometimes	Often
has difficulty planning and organizing time and tasks	Rarely	Sometimes	Often
has difficulty representing the complete sound of a word when spelling	Rarely	Sometimes	Often

Fifth to Eighth Grade

Indicator **(Inconsistent with the child's age or cognitive abilities)** **After the skills have been taught, the child . . .**	**Rating**		
reverses letter sequences, as *soiled* for *solid*	Rarely	Sometimes	Often
has difficulty identifying and learning prefixes, suffixes, and root words	Rarely	Sometimes	Often
spells the same word differently on the same page	Rarely	Sometimes	Often
reads aloud slowly, laboriously, and without inflection	Rarely	Sometimes	Often
performs disproportionately poorly on multiple choice tests	Rarely	Sometimes	Often
avoids reading aloud	Rarely	Sometimes	Often
relies on guessing and context to decode new words rather than sounding them out individually	Rarely	Sometimes	Often
avoids writing	Rarely	Sometimes	Often
has difficulty with word problems in mathematics	Rarely	Sometimes	Often
has difficulty with comprehension when reading	Rarely	Sometimes	Often
has difficulty remembering facts (rote memory)	Rarely	Sometimes	Often
has difficulty responding orally when questioned	Rarely	Sometimes	Often
has difficulty with non-literal language, such as idioms, jokes, slang, and proverbs	Rarely	Sometimes	Often
avoids reading for pleasure	Rarely	Sometimes	Often
has difficulty planning and organizing time, materials, and tasks	Rarely	Sometimes	Often
has difficulty learning a foreign language	Rarely	Sometimes	Often
writes with difficulty with illegible handwriting	Rarely	Sometimes	Often

These lists can be useful tools in assessing whether a child (or adult) displays the symptoms common to those diagnosed with reading problems, including dyslexia. The symptoms must be persistent and not the occasional error. Persistence over a prolonged period of time is the key to determining the likelihood of dyslexia or any other physical condition that is interfering with the child's ability to read.

It is not unusual for struggling readers and dyslexic students to be depressed by their reading failures and self-conscious about their difficulties in the classroom. They often find the classroom a very stressful environment and are likely to exhibit behavior problems if they do not receive the special consideration that they need. Because dyslexia is a spectrum disorder ranging from mild to severe, children who are only mildly affected may exhibit one or a few of the problems mentioned in the checklists.

Remember the Strengths of Struggling Readers

Remember that struggling readers frequently have strengths in other areas, such as higher-order cognitive thinking that can help them manage or overcome their difficulties with reading. Many students with dyslexia are able to go on to higher education and be successful. But their phonologic deficits do not go away. Wilson and Lesaux (2001) studied the phonological processing skills of university students with dyslexia. Not surprisingly, the dyslexic students performed less well than the control group on measures of word recognition, word attack, reading vocabulary and comprehension, and spelling. However, the scores of the students with dyslexia in reading comprehension were not as low as expected. The researchers explained this finding by noting that there was no time limit for interpreting their reading, and that there were indications that the dyslexic students were using strategies different from typical university students in order to derive meaning from text. Apparently, these students were able to compensate for their persistent difficulties with phonological processing and become sufficiently competent readers to survive successfully in a university.

Growing scientific evidence continues to support the notion that most dyslexia is caused by deficits in phonological processing. It is important to recognize that dyslexia does not reflect an overall impairment in language, intelligence, or thinking skills. Many smart people are dyslexic. Rather, for most people it reflects an overall problem with the ability of a specific brain system, referred to earlier as the *phonologic module,* to put together the sounds of language to form words and to break words down into their basic sounds. This focus allows research to more closely examine the nature of these deficits and to explore methods for remediation. Other research evidence suggests that dyslexia may have multiple causes that require different forms of intervention. No doubt,

Famous dyslexics include:
- Hans Christian Andersen
- Winston Churchill
- Tom Cruise
- Leonardo da Vinci
- Walt Disney
- Albert Einstein
- Jay Leno
- Auguste Rodin
- Steven Spielberg
- W. B. Yeats

some individuals display dyslexic symptoms because of visual and auditory problems not directly associated with phonological processing, but their numbers are small.

Because reading does not come naturally to the human brain, children learning to read have to put much effort into associating their spoken language with the alphabet and with word recognition. To do this successfully, phonemic awareness is essential. In light of recent research, educators should have second thoughts about reading programs that delay phonemic awareness or that treat it as an ancillary skill to be learned in context with general reading.

In light of recent research, educators should have second thoughts about reading programs that delay the teaching of phonemic awareness or treat it as an ancillary skill.

Educators should also become more aware of the scientific research into dyslexia and be able to recognize when students are having persistent reading problems. Early identification of struggling readers leads to early intervention. Researchers agree that a systematic, intensive, and comprehensive approach to early intervention can significantly reduce the number of students reading below the Basic level of proficiency.

A Note About "Cures" for Dyslexia

From time to time we read about a newly-discovered scientific "cure" for dyslexia. One recent claim from Britain was that dyslexia was caused by an underdeveloped cerebellum—the part of the brain responsible for motor coordination. Treatment involves stimulating the cerebellum by repeated physical activities and balancing exercises. According to the proponents, dyslexic students using this intervention showed improvement in reading and writing.

Another claim is that dyslexia is caused by a deficiency in the Omega-3 fatty acids that are essential for proper brain function. The "cure" involves administering very large doses of Omega-3 in capsule form. Here, too, proponents claim that dyslexic children have improved their reading skills.

Neither of the above claims is supported nor explained by current scientific knowledge or research. The scientific community is generally skeptical of any claims of curing developmental dyslexia. It is a life-long spectral disorder that can be overcome best through early and appropriate interventions that are systematic, sequential, and focused on developing phonological awareness.

Answer to Test Question # 7

Question: Dyslexic students often have problems in other cognitive areas.

Answer: *False.* Dyslexic students have had to construct extensive neural pathways and enhance specific neural regions when struggling to read. As a result, they often have strong capabilities in problem solving, reasoning, critical thinking, and concept formation.

What's Coming?

After recognizing that certain students are having reading problems, the next step is to select interventions that have been shown to be successful in helping struggling readers. All teachers are teachers of reading, and thus should have the training to strengthen the reading skills of students at every grade level. How to teach students with difficulties in reading is the focus of the next chapter.

CHAPTER 5
Overcoming Reading Problems

This chapter addresses several basic questions about overcoming reading problems. They include:

- *What are the basic ingredients of early intervention programs?*
- *What types of intervention programs are more successful with older students?*
- *How have some interventions actually rewired the dyslexic brain?*
- *What advice should be given to struggling readers and students with dyslexia and their parents?*

Many teachers work hard every day trying to help students with reading problems overcome their difficulties. Just how successful are these teachers? One study of fourth and fifth graders in special education classes showed virtually no change in their rate of reading growth when compared to their rate of growth in their regular education classes (Hanushuk, Kain, and Rivkin, 1998). Other studies have found that the reading programs being used in resource rooms lacked the effective interventions needed for learning the alphabetic principle and for developing skills in word recognition and text decoding (Vaughn, Moody, and Schumm, 1998). Even children taught in inclusion classrooms—where they receive special reading assistance within their regular classrooms—showed little change in their reading ability compared to their classmates (Zigmond and Jenkins, 1995). Conversely, the students receiving instruction in *scientifically-based programs* demonstrated rapid growth in reading achievement (Temple et al., 2003; Torgesen et al., 2001).

The secret to helping children overcome reading problems is early diagnosis. Chapter 4 dealt with the various clues that can alert parents and teachers to potential difficulties in learning to read. When there is sufficient evidence that a child is at risk for developing reading problems, quick intervention is essential. There are now several reading programs that are based on the more recent research and that have proven successful with struggling readers. The programs adhere to the notion that for children to become literate, they must break the reading code. Children with dyslexia may use different neural pathways and may have to work harder, but they still must master the skills of decoding printed text into recognizable sounds.

SOME CONSIDERATIONS FOR TEACHING STUDENTS WITH READING PROBLEMS

It is usually the regular classroom teacher who works the most with struggling readers and who helps them learn to read. The following thoughts may make the instructional process somewhat easier and more successful for all students (DITT, 2001).

General Considerations

✓ Make your classroom expectations clear.

✓ Ensure that classroom procedures are orderly, structured, and predictable.

✓ Remember that many struggling readers *can* learn to read. They just need different kinds of instructional strategies.

✓ Be constructive and positive. Labeling can often be disabling when you label the child rather than the behavior. Avoid labels and sarcasm that undermine the instructional environment and adversely affect the child's self-concept and performance.

✓ Recognize that struggling readers will take up to three times longer to complete work and will tire quickly.

✓ Avoid appeals to "try harder." The brains of struggling readers are already expending extra effort while decoding print, and these appeals will not improve performance. What is needed is slower speed with clearer comprehension.

✓ Determine and then complement these children's abilities, and teach through their strengths. Plan lessons so the students experience a sense of accomplishment rather than failure.

In the Elementary Classroom

- ✓ Get a complete explanation of the child's history of problems encountered when learning to read.
- ✓ Select scientifically-researched reading strategies and use a multi-sensory approach.
- ✓ Recognize the frustration that these students feel as they struggle to read.
- ✓ Show concern and understanding.
- ✓ Recognize that performance may be well below the child's potential.
- ✓ Remember that this child learns in different ways, but can learn.
- ✓ Realize that the child may have behavioral and self-esteem problems.
- ✓ Develop good student-teacher rapport.
- ✓ Maintain contact with the child's parents and give them periodic progress reports. Make suggestions of what they can do with the child at home to complement your classroom strategies.
- ✓ Ensure that other classmates understand the nature of dyslexia so that the child is not bullied or mocked.
- ✓ Assign a buddy to help the struggling reader in the class and school.
- ✓ Encourage the child to point out talents and strengths.

In the Secondary Classroom

- ✓ Get a complete explanation of the student's history of reading problems.
- ✓ Use a multi-sensory approach in classroom instruction.
- ✓ Recognize the compounded frustrations of a dyslexic teenager.

✓ Remember that dyslexic students learn in different ways, but they *can* learn.

✓ Realize that these teenagers may have problems with their self-esteem.

✓ Recognize that these students may have behavior or truancy problems.

✓ Realize that these students often have a significant gap between their performance and their potential.

✓ Show concern and understanding.

✓ Use diagrams and graphic organizers when teaching. Advanced organizers that contain important notes about the lesson are also very helpful and can help prevent failure.

✓ Develop good student-teacher rapport.

✓ Maintain contact with the student's parents and give them periodic progress reports. Make suggestions of what they can do with the student at home to complement your classroom strategies.

✓ Ensure that these students' legal rights are adhered to when taking tests.

✓ Mild dyslexics often develop coping strategies in elementary school. Be aware that these strategies may be inadequate for the complex and multi-faceted secondary curriculum.

✓ Ensure that any remedial materials are relevant to the maturity and not the academic level of the student.

✓ Be aware that struggling readers can have great difficulty reading an unseen text aloud in class. Asking them to do this can adversely affect their self-esteem.

BASIC INGREDIENTS OF EARLY INTERVENTION PROGRAMS

The National Reading Panel (NRP, 2000) has strongly recommended that beginning reading programs focus on systematic and explicit instruction in helping children master the alphabetic principle, especially for children at risk for reading difficulties. Dozens of reading programs flood the market every year. Deciding which program can best meet the needs of struggling readers is now easier thanks to our greater understanding of how the brain learns to read. Based on this understanding, a reading program is likely to be successful in helping children with reading difficulties if it includes explicit instruction in phonological awareness as well as word identification skills that lead to accurate, fluent reading and comprehension. Multiple research studies demonstrate the success of this approach (Chard and Dickson, 1999; Coyne, Kame'enui, and Simmons, 2001; Torgesen, 2002, 2004).

How Do I Develop Phonemic Awareness in Struggling Readers?

Training in phonemic awareness needs to be more intense for children with reading disabilities. Reading programs are filled with activities for separating words into phonemes, synthesizing phonemes into words, and deleting and substituting phonemes. Research suggests that the development of phonemic awareness is more likely to be successful if it follows these general principles (Chard and Osborn, 1998):

- ✓ *Continuous sounds before stop sounds.* Start with continuous sounds such as */s/, /m/,* and */f/* that are easier to pronounce than the stop sounds of */b/, /k/,* and */p/.*
- ✓ *Modeling.* Be sure to model carefully and accurately each activity when it is first introduced.
- ✓ *Easy to complex tasks.* Move from easier tasks, such as rhyming, to more complex tasks, such as blending and segmenting.
- ✓ *Larger to smaller units.* Move from the larger units of words and onset-rimes to the smaller units of individual phonemes.
- ✓ *Additional strategies.* Use additional strategies to help struggling readers, such as concrete objects (e.g., bingo chips or blocks) to represent sounds.

We have already discussed how early awareness of phonemes is a strong indicator of later reading success. Further, the research on interventions clearly demonstrates the benefits of explicitly teaching phonemic awareness skills. No students benefit more from this instruction than those already burdened with reading problems. The development of phonemic awareness occurs over several years. It is the last step in a developmental continuum that begins with the brain's earliest awareness of rhyme. Figure 5.1 illustrates the continuum from rhyming to full phoneme manipulation (Chard and Dickson, 1999).

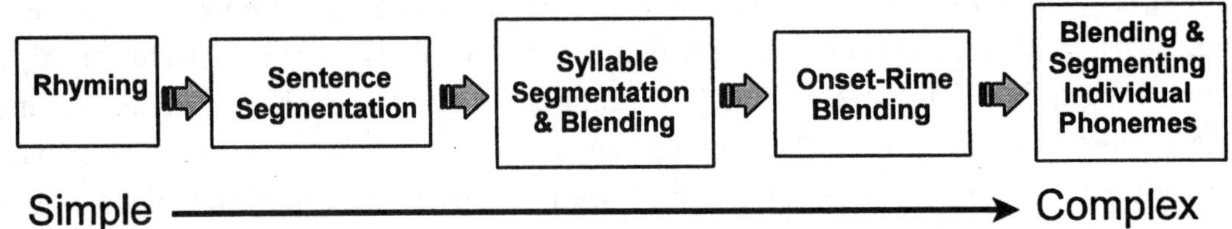

Figure 5.1 The development of phonemic awareness is a continuum that begins with simple rhyming and ends with the manipulation of individual phonemes.

General Guidelines

The first four steps in Figure 5.1, from rhyming to onset-rime blending, can occur during the preschool years in the appropriate environment. If the parent sings rhyming songs and reads to the child from rhyming books, the child's brain begins to recognize the sounds that comprise beginning language. However, many children begin school with a very weak phonological base. Teachers must then assess where students lie on the phonological continuum and select appropriate strategies to move them toward phonemic awareness. Edelen-Smith (1998) offers teachers the following guidelines to consider when selecting strategies to help students recognize and successfully manipulate phonemes.

✓ *Be specific.* Identify the specific phonemic awareness task and select the activities that are developmentally appropriate and that keep the students engaged in the task. Select words, phrases, and sentences from curricular materials to make this meaningful. Look for ways to make activities enjoyable so students see them as fun and not as monotonous drills.

✓ *Avoid letter names.* Use the phoneme sounds of the alphabet when doing activities, and avoid letter names. Letters sounded as they are named only confuse the learner. Keep in mind that one sound may be represented by two or more letters. Target specific sounds and practice beforehand so students can hear them clearly.

✓ *Treat continuant and stop sounds differently.* Continuant sounds are easier to manipulate and hear than the stop sounds. When introducing each type, treat them differently so students become aware of their differences. Exaggerate continuant sounds by holding on to them: *sssssing* and *rrrrrun.* Use rapid repetition with the stop consonants: */K/-/K/-/K/-/K/-/K/-/K/-athy.*

✓ *Emphasize how sounds vary with their position in a word.* Generally, the initial position in the word is the easiest sound. The final position is the next easiest and the middle position is the most difficult. Use lots of examples to make this clear, such as *mop, pin,* and *better.*

✓ *Be aware of the sequence for introducing combined sounds.* When introducing the combined sounds, a consonant-vowel pattern should come first, then a vowel-consonant pattern, and finally, the consonant-vowel-consonant pattern. For example: first *tie*, next *add,* and then *bed.*

Simple Phonemic Awareness

Young students are usually unaware that words are made of sounds that can be produced in isolation. This leaves it up to the teacher to find ways to emphasize the concept of speech sounds through *systematic* and *direct* instruction. An effective reading program should include activities that help children manipulate phonemes. Here are some ways to do this (Edelen-Smith, 1998):

✓ *Recognizing isolated sounds.* Associate certain speech sounds with an animal or action that is familiar to the students. For example, the buzzing sound of a bee or snoring in sleep is *zzzzzzzz–*, the hissing of a snake, *ssssssss–*, the sound of asking for quiet, *shhhhhhhh–,* or the sound of a motor scooter or motor boat, *pppppppp–*. Alliteration also helps with this task. Talking about Peter Piper picking a peck of peppers affords the valuable combination of sound recognition, story telling, and literary context. It also provides self-correcting cues for initial-sound isolation and for sound-to-word matching.

✓ *Counting words, syllables, and phonemes.* It is easier for a child's brain to perceive words and syllables than individual phonemes. Thus word and syllable counting is a valuable exercise for sound recognition that can lead later to more accurate identification of phonemes. Start with a sentence from the curriculum and say it aloud. Do not write it out because the students should focus on listening. Ask the students to count the number of words they think are in the sentence. They can use markers or tokens to indicate the word number. Then show or write the sentence and have the students compare the number of words to their own count. Syllable counting can be done in many ways. Students can count syllables in the same way they identified the word count. Also, they can march around the room while saying the syllables, they can clap hands, tap pencils, or do any other overt activity that indicates counting.

✓ *Synthesizing sounds.* Sound synthesis is an essential yet easily performed skill for phonemic awareness. Start with using the initial sound and then saying the remainder of the word. For example, the teacher says, "It starts with *b* and ends with *-and,* put it together and it says *band.*" The students take turns using the same phrasing to make up their own words. Variations include limiting the context to objects in the classroom or in the school, or to a particular story that the class has recently read.

Guessing games can also be productive and fun activities for playing with sounds. One game involves hiding an object in a bag or some other place and then giving clues to its name sound-by-sound or syllable-by-syllable. When a student guesses the word correctly, you reveal the object. Songs can also be used. Blending the music with the sounds of words increases the chances that the phonemes will be remembered.

✓ *Matching sounds to words.* This activity asks the learner to identify the initial sound of a word, an important skill for sound segmentation. Show the student a picture of a kite and ask, "Is this a *dddd-ite,* or a *llll-ite,* or a *kkkk-ite?*" You could also ask, "Is there a *k* in *kite?,*" or "Which sound does *kite* start with?" This allows the students to try three onsets with three rimes and to mix and match until they get it correct. Consonants make a good beginning because they are easier to emphasize and prolong during pronunciation. Have students try other words in threes. Be sure to use the phoneme sound when referring to a letter, not the letter name.

✓ *Identifying the position of sounds.* Segmenting whole words into their components is an important part of phonemic awareness. This ability is enhanced when learners recognize that sounds occur in different positions in words: initial, medial, and final. Edelen-Smith (1998) suggests explaining that words have beginning, middle, and end sounds just like a train has a beginning (engine), middle (passenger car), and end (caboose). Slowly articulate a consonant-vowel-consonant (CVC) word at this time, such as *c-a-t,* and point to the appropriate train part as you sound out each phoneme. Then have the students sound out other CVC words from a list or recent story, pointing to each train part as they say the parts of the word.

One of the more difficult phonemic tasks for children is to separately pronounce each sound of a spoken word in order.

✓ *Segmenting sounds.* One of the more difficult phonemic tasks for children is to separately pronounce each sound of a spoken word in order. This process is called sound segmentation. Developing this skill should start with isolating the initial phonemes. The previous activities—matching sounds to words and identifying the position of sounds—help the learner identify and recognize initial phonemes. Visual cues can also play an important part in segmenting sounds. Select words that are familiar to the students (or have the students select the words) so that they can use contextual clues for meaning. After sufficient practice, eliminate the cards so that students can perform the sound segmenting task without visual cues.

✓ *Associating sounds with letters.* For the reading process to be successful, the brain must associate the sounds that it has heard during the pre-reading years of spoken language with the written letters that represent them. This is particularly difficult for students with disabilities that hamper the learning of reading. Consequently, extensive practice is essential. Nearly all of the activities mentioned above —especially those involving visual cues—can be modified to include associations between sounds and letters. As the students master individual sounds, their corresponding letter names can then be introduced. A type of bingo game can also be used to practice sound-with-letter association. Each student gets a card with letters placed into a bingo grid. Draw a letter from a container and call out the phoneme. Students place tokens on the letter that corresponds to the phoneme. The student who first gets "phoneme bingo" names the letters aloud. Teachers can devise all types of variations to this bingo game to maintain the practice while keeping the task interesting and fun.

Compound Phonemic Awareness

In compound phonemic awareness, the learner must hold one sound in memory while matching it to a second sound. For example, "Do *dog* and *deer* begin with the same sound?" The two activities that develop compound phonemic awareness involve matching one word to a second word and the deleting of sounds in a word.

✓ *Matching one word to another word.* Byrne (1991) has suggested three games to develop phonemic word matching skills. The words and pictures used in each of these games should relate to themes and readings done in the classroom. One involves making a set of dominoes that have two objects pictured on each tile. The students have to join the tiles that share the same beginning or ending sounds.

A second game uses picture cards that are placed face down in a pile. Each student draws a card from the pile and places it face up. Students continue to draw cards and place them in the face-up pile. The first student to match the beginning or ending sound of a drawn card with the top card on the face-up pile says the match aloud and collects the pile.

The third game is a variation of bingo. Each bingo card contains pictures, which the students mark when their picture has the same beginning or ending sounds as the word said by the caller (student or teacher).

✓ *Deleting sounds.* Deleting sounds from words and manipulating phonemes within words are more difficult tasks for the young brain to accomplish. Studies show that most children must attain the mental age of seven years before this task can be accomplished adequately (Cole and Mengler, 1994). Furthermore, segmentation skills and letter names must be mastered before sound deletion tasks can be successfully learned.

Three tasks seem to be particularly important to mastering this skill: deleting parts of a compound word, identifying a missing sound, and deleting a single sound from a word.

1. *Deleting parts of a compound word.* To illustrate deleting parts of a compound word, point to a picture or an object that is a compound word and demonstrate how each word can be said with one part missing. For example, "This is a classroom. I can say *class* without the *room.* And this is a farmhouse (or greenhouse). I can say *farm* (*green*) without *house.* Now you try it. This is a playground." Use other common examples, such as *lighthouse, airplane, grandmother, seashore, sandbox, toothpaste,* and *nightlight.*
2. *Identifying the missing sound.* In this task, focus on deleting the initial and final sounds instead of the medial sounds, which is the first step to master for the young brain. Take word pairs, such as *ate-late,* and ask "What's missing in *ate* that you hear in *late*?" Other examples are *ask-mask, able-table,* and *right-bright.* After a few trials, have the students make up their own word pairs, preferably from lesson material.
3. *Deleting a single sound from a word.* This task should begin with segmentation practice. First, separate the sound for deletion. For example, separate *g* from *glove.* "Glove. It starts with *g* and ends with *love.* Take the first sound away and it says *love.*" Use words for which a sound deletion results in another real word. Other examples are *spot-pot, train-rain, scare-care,* and *snap-nap.* After practicing this skill, say a word aloud and ask students to say the word with the initial sound missing: "Say *mother* without the *m.*" Visual clues can help those who have difficulty saying a word with the deleted sound.

Onset and Rime

The young brain's awareness of onsets, rimes, and syllables develops before an awareness of phonemes. Onsets are the initial consonants that change the meaning of a word; rimes are the vowel-consonant combinations that stay constant in a series. For example, in *bend, lend,* and *send,* the onsets are *b, l,* and *s;* the rime is *-end.* Using literature, word families, and direct instruction are strategies that focus on word play designed to enhance onset and rime recognition (Edelen-Smith, 1998).

> The young brain's awareness of onsets, rimes, and syllables develops before an awareness of phonemes.

✓ *Literature.* Books with rhyming patterns (like many books by Dr. Seuss) are easily recalled through repeated exposure. Almost any literary source that plays with word sounds is valuable. Books that particularly develop awareness of sound patterns associated with onset and rime are those using alliteration (the repetition of an initial consonant across several words, e.g., *Peter Piper picked a peck of peppers*) and assonance (the repetition of vowel sounds within words, e.g., *The rain in Spain stays mainly on the plain*).

✓ *Word families charts.* Using words from a story or book, construct a chart that places a different beginning letter in front of a rime. For example, start with the rime *-at* and add *f, h, b,* and *s* to form *fat, hat, bat,* and *sat.* Have the students make up a story line whenever the word changes (e.g., *The fat cat chased a hat*). Encourage the students to make their own charts with different rimes and to keep them for future reference.

✓ *Direct instruction.* Students who have difficulties distinguishing the sounds among rhyming words need more direct instruction. Model rhyming pairs (e.g., *sun-fun* and *hand-band*) using flash cards so students match what they see with what they hear. Be sure they repeat each rhyming pair several times to reinforce auditory input. Another activity includes three cards, only two of which have rhyming words. Ask students to pick out and say the two that rhyme, or the one that doesn't. Later, change the rhyming words to two rhyming pictures out of three (e.g., a nose, a rose, and a horse).

Successful Early Intervention Programs

Several early intervention programs have been consistently successful for years and deserve to be mentioned here. Two notable ones are Reading Recover and Success for All.

Reading Recovery

Started in 1984, Reading Recovery has served more than one million children. This program is designed for the lowest-achieving readers in first grade. Specially trained teachers meet with the children individually for 30 minutes daily for 12 to 20 weeks. Instruction focuses on developing phonemic awareness, practice learning letter-sound relationships through phonics, strategies to enhance text comprehension, and teaching for fluency and phrasing. The children are tested before entering the program, at the end of the Reading Recovery instruction, and at the end of first grade. Their scores are compared with a random sample of their peers. A Spanish version is available.

Numerous studies and research reports over the last 15 years document the effectiveness of Reading Recovery for the lowest-performing first graders. Cumulative 17-year results show that 81 percent of children who have the full series of lessons can read at the class average. Furthermore, most of these children maintain and improve their gains in later grades (Reading Recovery Council, 2002).

Success for All — Reading First

Based on the widely-used Success for All comprehensive reform model introduced in 1987, this adaptation is a core reading program for grades K to 3 designed to strengthen the students' phonemic awareness, phonics, vocabulary, fluency, and comprehension. Students have a 90-minute reading period daily with specially trained teachers. The program uses proven instructional strategies, such as cooperative learning, partner reading, a rapid pace of instruction, frequent standards-based assessments, and effective classroom management techniques to engage each student. Also included are activities that build around existing textbooks to emphasize comprehension of narrative and expository texts, metacognitive comprehension strategies, writing, study skills, and home reading. Children are assessed every eight weeks in decoding, reading comprehension, and fluency. Based on these assessments, teachers regroup the children across grade lines so that each teacher can work with children at one reading level. This program is also available in Spanish.

Since the inception of the basic program, Success for All has been evaluated in grades K to 3 through several major experimental studies. The studies found that, in comparison to matched control schools, students in Success for All schools read significantly better, are promoted regularly from grade to grade, are less often referred to special education, and attend school more regularly (Weiler, 1998).

PROGRAMS FOR OLDER STUDENTS

How Do I Develop Fluency and Comprehension in Older Struggling Readers?

Older struggling readers are able to develop strong reading capabilities when provided with effective instructional conditions (Lyon, 2002). To be effective, reading programs must include activities that promote reading fluency. Shaywitz (2003) strongly supports the notion of short, intense daily practice sessions in reading in order to develop fluency. The children's practice continues over weeks and months as they reread passages until they attain high accuracy. Intense practice helps children build fluency because decoding becomes automatic, the same way that practice assists athletes and musicians perform motor skills almost without thinking (Shaywitz calls this *overlearning*, the ability to perform something without attention or conscious thought).

Fluency comes through repetition of words and sentences. Such repetition increases the chances that words and common phrases will be stored in long-term memory, allowing for faster word recognition during subsequent encounters. The National Reading Panel (NRP, 2000) recommended reading programs that emphasize repeated oral reading accompanied by teacher feedback and guidance, a strategy referred to as *guided repeated oral reading*. The feedback is necessary because it gives children the opportunities to modify their pronunciation so that the stored representation of the word in their mental lexicon continues to approach its correct pronunciation and spelling. Whenever readers mispronounce words, it means that they do not have accurate mental representations of those words in their brains and will thus have difficulty storing or retrieving information related to that word. Guided repeated oral reading is an especially effective technique for helping readers practice aloud unfamiliar vocabulary. Such practice builds accurate neural representations of the vocabulary and enhances comprehension.

What Strategies Teach Fluency and Comprehension to Struggling Readers?

Studies have shown that children with reading problems are able to master the learning strategies that improve reading comprehension skills. For students with learning problems, learning to use questioning strategies is especially important because these students do not often spontaneously self-question or monitor their own reading comprehension.

Here are three strategies that researchers and teachers have found particularly effective. Some of the strategies have been around for over 20 years, but their fundamental premises have been reaffirmed by recent research.

Questioning and Paraphrasing: Reciprocal Teaching

Reciprocal teaching is a strategic approach that fosters student interaction with the text being read (Palincsar and Brown, 1984). In reciprocal teaching, students interact deeply with the text through the strategies of questioning, summarizing, clarifying, and predicting.

Reciprocal teaching involves
- Questioning
- Summarizing
- Clarifying
- Predicting

Organized in the form of a discussion, the approach involves one leader (students and teacher take turns being the leader) who, after a portion of the text is read, first frames a question to which the group responds. Second, participants share their own questions. Third, the leader then summarizes the gist of the text, and participants comment or elaborate upon that summary. At any point in the discussion, either the leader or participants may identify aspects of the text or discussion that need to be clarified, and the group joins together to clarify the confusion. Finally, the leader indicates that it is time to move on and solicits predictions about what might come up next in the text.

The value of paraphrasing, self-questioning, and finding the main idea are well researched strategies. Students divide reading passages into smaller parts, such as sections, subsections, or paragraphs. After reading a segment, students are cued to use a self-questioning strategy to identify main ideas and details. The strategy requires a high level of attention to reading tasks because students must alternate their use of questioning and paraphrasing after reading each section, subsection, or paragraph.

Reciprocal teaching is an effective strategy because it requires the brain to integrate prior knowledge with new learning, to make inferences, to maintain focus, and to use auditory rehearsal to enhance retention of learning. Research studies support the value of reciprocal teaching. One study of 50 at-risk post-secondary students enrolled in a community college showed that the reciprocal teaching group performed significantly better than the comparison group on reading comprehension and strategy acquisition. There were no differences on perception of study skills. Poorer readers in the reciprocal teaching group outperformed poorer readers in the comparison group on both reading comprehension and strategy acquisition measures (Hart and Speece, 1998). See more about reciprocal teaching in Chapter 6.

Questioning to Find the Main Idea

This self-questioning strategy focuses primarily on identifying and questioning the main idea or summary of a paragraph. Here's how it works. Students are first taught the concept of a main idea and how to do self-questioning. Students then practice, asking themselves questions aloud about each paragraph's main idea. They can use a cue card for assistance. Following the practice, the teacher provides immediate feedback. Eventually, following successful comprehension of these short paragraphs, students are presented with more lengthy passages, and the cue cards are removed. Continuing to give corrective feedback, the teacher finishes each lesson with a discussion of students' progress and of the strategy's usefulness. Studies show that students with learning disabilities who were trained in a self-questioning strategy performed significantly higher (i.e., demonstrated greater comprehension of what was read) than untrained students (Idol, 1987; Sousa, 2001b).

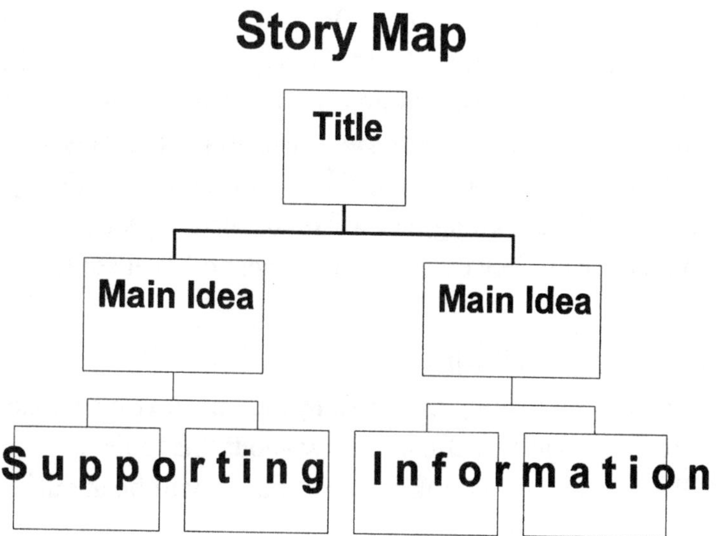

Figure 5.2 This is just one example of a story map. It helps students discover the author's main ideas and to search out information to support them (Sousa, 2001a).

Story-Mapping

In this strategy, students read a story, generate a map of its events and ideas, and then answer questions. (Figure 5.2 is one example of a story map.) In order to fill in the map, students have to identify the setting, characters, time, and place of the story; the problem, the goal, and the action that took place; and the outcome. The teacher models for students how to fill in the map, then gives them many opportunities to practice the mapping technique for themselves and receive corrective feedback. The map is an effective visual tool that provides a framework for understanding, conceptualizing, and remembering important story events. The reading comprehension of students can improve significantly when the teacher gives direct instruction on the use of the strategy, expects frequent use of the strategy, and encourages students to use the strategy independently.

Focusing on Comprehension: The PASS Process

Students with reading disorders often have difficulty deriving meaning from what they read. If little or no meaning comes from reading, students lose motivation to read. Furthermore, meaning is essential for long-term retention of what they have read. Strategies designed to improve reading comprehension have been shown to improve students' interest in reading and their success.

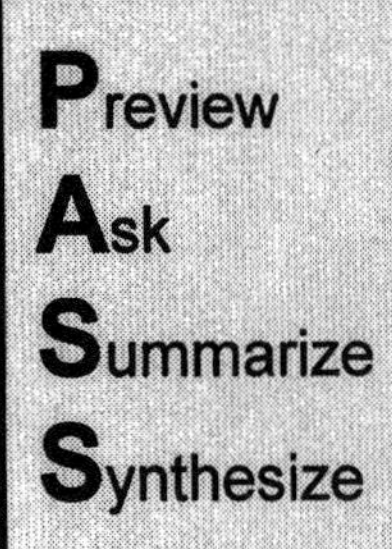

The PASS Process. One such successful strategy, suggested by Deshler, Ellis, and Lenz (1996), is a four-step process called by the acronym PASS (Preview, Ask, Summarize, and Synthesize). The teacher guides the students through the four steps, ensuring that they respond orally or in writing to the activities associated with each step. Grouping formats, such as cooperative learning, can be used to encourage active student participation and reduce anxiety over the correctness of each student's response.

1. **P**review, Review, and Predict:
   - Preview by reading the heading and one or two sentences.
   - Review what you already know about this topic.
   - Predict what you think the text or story will be about.
2. **A**sk and Answer Questions:
   - Content-focused questions:
   - Who? What? Why? Where?
   - How does this relate to what I already know?
   - Monitoring questions:
     Does this make sense?
     Is my prediction correct?
     How is this different from what I thought it was going to be about?
   - Problem-solving questions:
     Is it important that it make sense?
     Do I need to reread part of it?
     Can I visualize the information?
     Does it have too many unknown words?
     Should I get help?
3. **S**ummarize:
   - Explain what the short passage you read was all about.
4. **S**ynthesize:
   - Explain how the short passage fits in with the whole passage.
   - Explain how what you learned fits in with what you knew.

If students have difficulty with any particular step, they can go back to the previous step to determine what information they need in order to proceed.

Collaborative Strategic Reading

Another excellent technique for helping students comprehend what they read and build vocabulary is called Collaborative Strategic Reading (CSR). It is particularly effective in classrooms where students have many different reading abilities and learning capabilities. The strategy is compatible with all types of reading programs.

Collaborative Strategic Reading is particularly effective in classrooms where students have many different reading abilities and learning capabilities.

CSR uses direct teaching and the collaborative power of cooperative learning groups to accomplish two phases designed to improve reading comprehension (Klingner, Vaughn, and Schumm, 1998). The first phase is a teacher-led component that takes students through four parts of a reading plan: Preview, Click and Clunk, Get the Gist, and Wrap-Up. The second phase involves using cooperative learning groups to provide an interactive environment where students can practice and perfect their reading comprehension skills.

PHASE ONE
Teacher-Led Activities

✓ *Preview the reading.* Students know that previews in movies give some information about coming events. Use this as a hook to the new reading. The learners preview the entire reading passage in order to get as much as they can about the passage in just a few minutes time. The purpose here is to activate their prior knowledge about the topic and to give them an opportunity to predict what they will learn.

Refer to student experiences about a movie, television program, or prior book that might contain information relevant to the new reading. Also, give clues to look for when previewing. For example, pictures, graphs, tables, or call-out quotes provide information to help predict what students already know about the topic and what they will learn.

✓ *Click and clunk.* Students with reading problems often fail to monitor their understanding while they read. Clicks and clunks are devices to help students with this monitoring. Clicks are parts of the reading that make sense; clunks are parts or words that don't.

Ask students to identify clunks as they go along. Then the class works with the teacher to develop strategies to clarify the clunks, such as

- Rereading the sentences while looking for key words that can help extract meaning from the context
- Rereading previous and following sentences to get additional context clues
- Looking for a prefix or suffix in the word that could help with meaning
- Breaking the word apart to see if smaller words are present that provide meaning

✓ *Get the gist.* The goal of this phase is twofold. First, ask the readers to state in their own words the most important person, place, or thing in the passage. Second, get them to tell in as few words as possible (i.e., leaving out the details) the most important idea about that person, place, or thing. Because writing often improves memory, occasionally ask the students to write down their gists. Students can then read their gists aloud and invite comments from the group about ways to improve the gist. This process can be done so that all students benefit by enhancing their skills.

✓ *Wrap-up.* Wrap-up is a closure activity that allows students to review in their mind what has been learned to ensure that it makes sense and has meaning. Focus students on the new learning by asking them to generate questions whose answers would show what they learned from the passage. They should also review key ideas.

Start with questions that focus on the explicit material in the passage, such as who, what, where, and when. Afterward, move to questions that stimulate higher-order thinking, such as, "What might have happened if . . .?" and "What could be another way to solve this problem?" Writing down the response will help students sort out and remember the important ideas.

PHASE TWO
Cooperative Learning Groups

This phase puts the students into cooperative learning groups to practice CSR in an interactive environment. True cooperative learning groups are usually made up of about five students of mixed ability levels who learn and perform certain roles in the group to ensure completion of the learning task (Johnson and Johnson, 1989). The roles rotate among the group members so that every student gets the opportunity to be the leader and use the various skills needed to perform each task. Although there are many roles that students can perform, here are the most common (assuming five members per group):

- **Leader.** Leads the group through CSR by saying what to read next and what strategy to use.
- **Clunk expert.** Reminds the group what strategies to use when encountering a difficult word or phrase.
- **Announcer.** Calls on different group members to make certain that everyone participates and that only one person talks at a time.
- **Encourager.** Gives the group feedback on behaviors that are to be praised and those that need improvement.

- **Reporter.** Takes notes and reports to the whole class the main idea that the group has learned and shares a question that the group generated during its wrap-up.

Here are suggestions for using the cooperative learning groups with this strategy:

✓ *Cue sheets.* Giving all group members a cue sheet to guide them through the CSR provides a structure and focus for the group. The cue sheet should be specific for each role. For example, the leader's sheet contains statements that steer the group through each step of CSR (e.g., "Today's topic is . . ." "Let's predict what we might learn from this." "Let's think of some questions to see if we really understand what we learned.") and also direct other group members to carry out their role (e.g., "Announcer, please call on others to share their ideas." "Encourager, tell us what we did well and what we need to do better next time.").

✓ *CSR learning logs.* Recording in logs helps students to keep track of what was learned. Students can keep separate logs for each subject. The log serves as a reminder for follow-up activities and can be used to document a student's progress as required by the individualized education plan.

✓ *Reading materials.* CSR was originally designed for expository text, but has also been used successfully with narrative text. For the strategy to be successful, select reading passages that are rich in clues, that have just one main idea per paragraph, and that provide a context to help students connect and associate details into larger ideas.

Additional Strategies

Some of the models for teaching reading discussed in Chapter 3 that involve repeated oral reading are appropriate to use with older struggling readers. Paired (or partner) reading and readers' theatre are particularly effective classroom strategies. Reading aloud helps students of all ages gain confidence in their developing reading skills. This is especially important around the fourth grade where there is a large increase in vocabulary words with irregular pronunciations. Struggling readers need considerable practice with these words to develop fluency and avoid the well-known drop in reading performance that occurs in fourth grade. Two of the main sources of irregular pronunciation problems are:

1. Words that contain the same root but are pronounced differently. Examples are *bough, cough, dough* and *rough; have* and *gave;* or *bead* and *dead.*

2. Words where the same letters get different pronunciations, as in the following pairs: *electric–electricity, grade–gradual, nation–national, muscle–muscular,* and *sign–signature.*

These words must be learned and overlearned by repeated practice as part of the fluency exercises given in class.

Attention Therapy to Improve Comprehension

Successful reading requires sustained attention to the printed text. Researchers now recognize that attention is a complex process that requires the brain to focus, shift, sustain, and encode relevant stimuli while simultaneously impeding the processing of irrelevant stimuli (Mirsky, 1996). In reading, visual attention (the eyes scanning the page) must be sustained long enough for the visual processing system (in the rear of the brain) to perceive the text so that the cognitive processing system (frontal lobe) can comprehend the text. Visual attention, therefore, is the catalyst that links perception to comprehension.

Students with attention deficits often have reading difficulties as well. Because visual attention is a learned skill, the research question here is: Can giving students with reading difficulties attention therapy that improves visual attention lead to better reading comprehension? In a recent study (Solan, Shelley-Tremblay, Ficarra, Silverman, and Larson, 2003), 30 grade 6 students with reading problems were split into two groups. One group received 12 one-hour sessions of individually monitored, computer-based attention therapy programs. The second group served as the control and was given no therapy during the 12-week period. The therapy program consisted of computer-based activities designed to improve perceptual accuracy, visual efficiency, visual search, visual scan, and visual span. Each session was followed with paper-and-pencil exercises for additional practice. The program also emphasized improving visual memory.

After completing the program, the mean reading comprehension scores improved significantly, from the 23rd to the 35th percentile, and a grade equivalent increase from 4.1 to 5.2. Because this improvement is well over one standard deviation, it is unlikely that the results can be attributed to the practice that occurred as part of the program. This study is significant because it showed that (1) attention skills are malleable and measurable, (2) attention therapy improves attention duration, and (3) students who receive attention therapy score better in tests of reading comprehension than controls.

Although the sample in this study was small, the results were intriguing. If further studies support these findings, then computer-based attention therapy programs may someday become another tool that teachers of remedial reading may consider in their efforts to improve their students' reading comprehension.

Answer to Test Question # 8

Question: Many poor readers have attention problems that schools are not equipped to handle.

Answer: *False.* Many poor readers expend a great deal of effort at first trying to decode text, but their struggle leads to frustration and eventually to inattentiveness.

Tutoring in Reading for Fluency

Tutoring can be a significant enhancement to fluency in reading (Snow et al., 1998). Tutors can be volunteers, older students, or parents. Essentially, tutors provide individual guided practice and corrective feedback to a student while the student reads aloud from meaningful text at a suitable level of difficulty. To be effective, it is important that the tutors have a specific approach to the tutoring session. All tutors should be provided training in basic tutoring techniques and in the selection of appropriate materials. These materials should be closely related to the reading materials that the students are using in their classes.

Parker, Hasbrouck, and Denton (2002a) suggest three types of tutoring interventions: (1) repeated reading with a model, (2) oral reading with monitoring and feedback, and (3) error monitoring and reading practice.

Repeated Reading With a Model

Simultaneous, repeated reading with a tutor is an effective method for improving the fluency of reluctant readers. By carefully adjusting the timing and control of the repeated readings, the tutor helps the student foster independent reading skills. Here are the three steps to this approach.

✓ *Step One: Introduction*

- Start with a passage that will take 3 to 5 minutes for the student to read aloud.
- Read the title.
- Give a general description of the topic.
- Ask if the student knows anything about the topic.
- Give a reason or purpose for reading the topic.
- Explain that the passage may be difficult so you will read it together.

✓ *Step Two: Simultaneous reading*

- Read the passage with the student, sitting slightly behind so as not to be a visual distraction.
- Read slowly in a clear, soft voice as the student reads aloud at the same time.
- Regulate your speed of reading to allow the student to keep up.
- The student and you should move your fingers under the printed text as you read.
- Listen carefully as to whether the student is following, with, or leading your reading of difficult words. Most students will initially follow the tutor. But with greater confidence, they will read more nearly with the tutor, and eventually will lead.
- As the student comes closer to your reading speed, soften your voice. As the student leads more, soften your voice further and slow your pace slightly to allow the student to lead even more.

✓ *Step Three: Simultaneous repeated readings*

- After a short break, begin rereading. From two to five readings will be beneficial, depending on the student's motivation and age.
- With each rereading, maintain a smooth pace and encourage the student to read with you and to lead by softening your voice and slowing your pace slightly.

Oral Reading With Monitoring and Feedback

This process uses a text that the student can read with 90 to 95 percent oral reading accuracy, and at a moderate level of difficulty. The tutor provides direct feedback on difficult words encountered in the text. The aim here is for the student to avoid long pauses while attempting to decode unfamiliar words and to build fluency and confidence in reading. Here are the two steps in this process.

✓ *Introduction*

- Ask the student to read the passage aloud as smoothly, quickly, and accurately as possible.
- Reassure the student that, although you do not want to interrupt the reading, you will help with words that are unfamiliar or misread.
- Show the student how to use a finger or marker to pace the reading and to keep on track.

✓ *Providing feedback*

- Sit slightly behind the student so as not be a visual distraction.

- Immediately pronounce correctly any mispronounced word, and have the student quickly repeat it without breaking stride in reading.
- Strive for minimal interruption, but immediately correct each error. If the student is making more than one error every 10 words or so, then the passage is too difficult.
- Have the student use a finger or marker to pace the reading.
- Take note of any pattern in the student's errors, such as any specific words that are missed with high frequency, missing specific letter or sound patterns, and violations of phonics rules. This is an advanced tutoring skill and should only be done by tutors who have a good knowledge of phonics and word structure.

Error Monitoring and Reading Practice

This approach gives students the opportunity to practice difficult words not connected to text. Students practice reading word patterns, words, and sentences from flashcards. The flashcard practice proceeds rapidly, without interruption, for 15 to 25 cards, or 3 to 5 minutes, depending on the student's age. If the student gets stuck on a word, wait only 1 to 3 seconds before saying it. Stick the more difficult words back in the deck toward the front so the student has more practice with them. Here are three different variations of this reading practice.

✓ *Word patterns*

- Write the words to be practiced on index cards. The student can help make the cards, if appropriate.
- Consider writing the word on both sides of the card to make it easier for you to see it.
- Group flashcards with similar error patterns for later, focused practice.

✓ *Word practice*

- As the student is reading a passage aloud, mark any word reading errors with a pencil check or underline them on a separate copy.
- Allow the reading to continue until the student has made 5 to 15 errors. Stop the reading at the end of a sentence or paragraph.
- Prepare flashcards with selected missed words on them. Avoid the names of characters, places, or vocabulary specific to the story as well as unusual or rarely used words. Select words that are commonly used by the student and that reflect useful phonemic and structural patterns.

✓ *Sentence practice (in context)*

- As the student is reading a passage aloud, mark on a separate copy any word reading errors with a pencil check or underline.

- Allow the reading to continue until the student has made 5 to 15 errors. Stop the reading at the end of a sentence or paragraph.
- Point out the student's first error and ask, "What is this word?" If the student cannot read it, identify the word.
- Have the student read the entire sentence again until it can be done without hesitation or error. Continue this process with all the original errors.
- When completed, have the student continue reading the passage until another 5 to 15 errors are made. Repeat the above steps.

Evaluating the Effectiveness of Tutoring

Effective tutoring should enable the student to read meaningful, connected text at that student's instructional reading level. Reading performance can be evaluated by three indexes: oral reading accuracy (ORA), oral reading fluency (ORF), and through questions on comprehension presented after the student has read a passage. These evaluations should be carried out periodically to provide feedback to the tutor.

Oral Reading Accuracy (ORA). This is calculated by a simple formula in which the number of word errors (not counting repetitions or self-corrected errors) is subtracted from the total number of words read, and then dividing that result by the total number of words. The resulting decimal is multiplied by 100 to yield a percentage.

Have the student read a previously practiced passage without the tutor and calculate the student's ORA. For example, if the student reads a passage of 150 words and makes 15 errors while reading all the words, the calculation would be 150 minus 15, which is 135, divided by 150. The result is 0.9, which is then multiplied by 100 to yield 90 percent. The goal is for a 95 percent ORA. If the goal is not met, the student continues to practice on that passage with the tutor, attempting to reach the goal.

$$\frac{\text{(Total Number of Words Read)} - \text{(Number of Word Errors)}}{\text{(Total Number of Words)}} \text{ X } 100 = \text{ \% Oral Reading Accuracy}$$

Oral Reading Fluency (ORF). Because time is involved, this is also known as the student's *reading rate,* and is the same as the calculation of words correct per minute (WCPM) discussed in Chapter 3 (see Table 3.1).

For example, a third-grade student reads a passage of 150 words with 17 errors in one-and-a-half minutes. Subtracting the 17 errors from the 150 words yields a total of 133 words that were correctly read in 1.5 minutes. Dividing the 1.5 minutes into 133 words yields a

WCPM of 89. Comparing the 89 to the average reading rates listed in Table 3.2 shows that this student is reading at the lower end of the range for third grade.

First calculate the ORF for an unpracticed reading and compare that to the ORF after the student has practiced with the passage. The change in ORF values will be a measure of the student's progress toward fluency. It is also helpful to compare the student's ORF with a chart of average reading rates for students in grades 2 through 12 (see Table 3.2).

Both the ORA and the ORF can be charted on a bar or line graph to provide additional motivation for the student (see Figure 3.7). Having the students participate in creating the chart will also increase their sense of accomplishment.

Tutoring in Reading for Comprehension

Poor readers often fail to comprehend what they have read. This may occur because they failed to comprehend key words or sentences, or how the sentences related to each other, or simply because they did not maintain concentration or interest. It is also possible that the readers lack the background knowledge necessary to comprehend the text. Tutoring in reading comprehension starts with carefully selecting reading materials and with improving understanding and motivation. Here are some suggestions for how to accomplish this (Parker, Hasbrouck, Denton, 2002b).

✓ *Selecting reading passages or books*

- To select readable text, ask the student to read a 100-word segment of the selected text and calculate the student's oral reading accuracy (ORA), as explained earlier. An ORA score of 80 or less means that the text is too frustrating for the reader. Scores of 85 to 90 percent are acceptable when the tutoring involves close monitoring and feedback from the tutor and multiple practices with the same text. An ORA score of 90 to 95 percent is considered best for closely monitored tutoring. A text with ORA scores of 95 percent and higher can be used with little tutor guidance and should be considered for independent reading practice by the student.
- To select comprehensible text, ask the student to read a passage. Then ask three or four brief open-ended questions that cannot be answered by common knowledge alone. The questions should cover most of the content of the passage and should not rely on trivial details. For example, "Why did that happen?" "What did he mean when...?" "What do you think will happen if...?" If the student can answer two or three questions correctly, the text can be used in tutoring. On the other hand, if the student can answer none or just one question, the text is not appropriate for tutoring.

✓ *Improving understanding*

- What did it say? Recognize that comprehension problems are often caused by problems with fluency. In their attempt to read smoothly and accurately, students lose the meaning at the sentence level and beyond. Sit beside the student with a 4" x 6" card. After the student reads one or two sentences, cover them and ask, "What did that say?" The student should paraphrase the meaning of what was just read. Praise the student's response and either elaborate on the response or offer a model summary, such as "I would add..." or "I would say..." Ensure the student that many different responses are acceptable.

  Move on to the next few sentences and repeat the process. As the student develops summarizing skills, ask the student to summarize longer selections of three or four sentences or a full paragraph. With this approach, the student's comprehension progresses from single sentence, to multisentence, to paragraph, and on to several paragraphs. As the text selection gets longer, remind the student to keep the oral summary to just one or two sentences.
- Read to find out. This approach for improving understanding requires you to read the text and prepare ahead of time. Ask the student to read a certain amount of text (depending on the reader's skill level) and to find out a certain amount of information. The answer should not be found through common knowledge alone and should not rely on trivial details. The student can refer back to the text to substantiate the answer. Listen to the student's response, provide supportive feedback, and augment the student's response or offer a model one of your own, if necessary.

✓ *Improving motivation*

- Students become motivated when they see achievement and greater understanding as a result of their efforts. By teaching students how to learn, rather than just specific skills, you help them apply a set of skills to solve tasks more effectively and efficiently in school as well as in nonacademic settings.
- Students are also motivated when you give them a reason to read. Most students really want to succeed in school. Knowing how to read fluently and with understanding can be a powerful motivator for reading more and for pleasure.

The READ 180 Program

Among the commercial programs available to help older struggling readers, the READ 180 program, now published by Scholastic, Inc., has yielded some impressive results. The research behind this program began in 1985 at Vanderbilt University where computer software was developed that used student performance data to adjust and differentiate the path of reading instruction. The software program continued to be revised and was eventually field-tested with more than 10,000 students in the Orange County, Florida schools from 1994 through 1997. Designed for low-achieving readers in grades 4 and above, the software program emphasizes direct, explicit, and systematic instruction in word analysis, phonics, spelling, reading comprehension, and writing.

Because of its success in raising the reading scores of older struggling readers in Orange County, the Council of Great City Schools piloted the program during 1998-1999 in the Department of Defense schools and in some of its largest urban schools, including Boston, Columbus, Dallas, Houston, and Los Angeles. Most students in the pilot schools who participated in the program showed significant improvements in reading and overall school performance as well as the development of more positive attitudes and behaviors. See the **Resources** section for more information on READ 180.

REWIRING THE BRAINS OF STRUGGLING READERS

Can the human brain be rewired for certain tasks? If so, is it possible to reroute the auxiliary circuits used by struggling readers to utilize the left posterior regions that are predisposed to rapid and automatic reading? Perhaps the most exciting news from neuroscience about reading has been the studies to determine whether such rewiring can occur as a result of using reading interventions. These imaging studies looked at children with difficult reading problems before and after they were subjected to an extensive phonologically-based reading program.

In Chapter 4, Figure 4.7 shows the fMRI images before the interventions. Note the activation in the frontal areas of the brain typical of dyslexic readers. In a study sponsored by Syracuse University, specially-trained teachers provided second-grade and third-grade struggling readers with 50 minutes of individualized tutoring daily in activities related to the alphabetic principle. The tutoring, which lasted eight months (105 hours) was in addition to the students' regular reading instruction. At the end of the year-long intervention, all of the children improved their reading in varying degrees. The fMRI images taken immediately after the program showed the emergence of primary processing systems on the left side of the brain (like those used by good readers) in addition to the auxiliary pathways on the right side common to dyslexic and struggling readers. Furthermore, one year after the program intervention, fMRIs indicated there was additional development of the primary neural systems on the left rear side of the brain while the right front areas were less prominent (Figure 5.3). In other words, the program intervention appeared to have rewired the brains of struggling readers to more closely approximate the reading circuitry in the brains of typical readers, resulting in accurate and *fluent* readers (Shaywitz, 2003; Shaywitz et al., 2003).

Changes in Brains of Struggling Readers

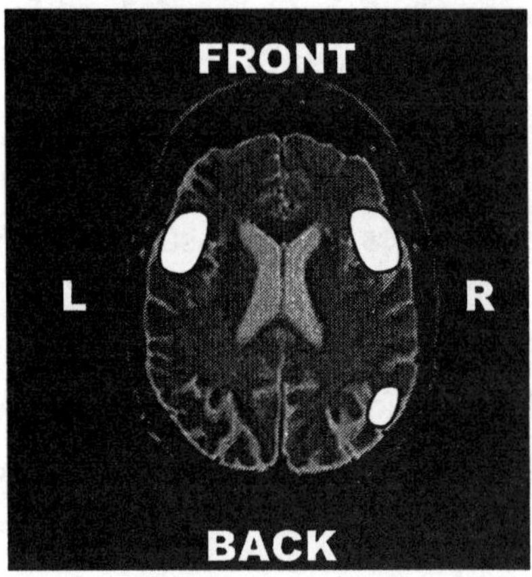

Before Reading Interventions

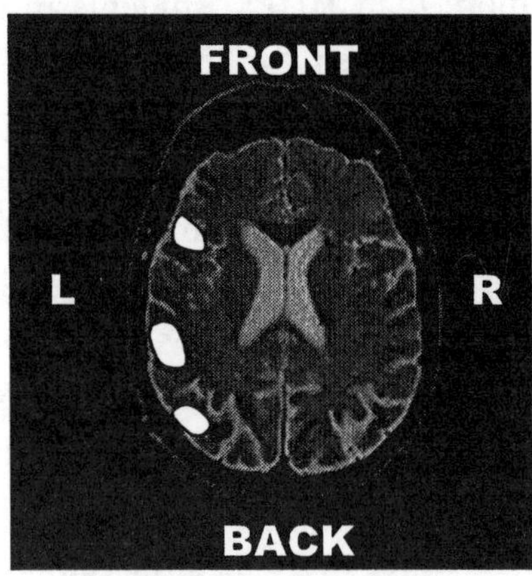

After Reading Interventions

Figure 5.3 These representative scans show the changes evident in the brains of struggling readers about one year after their involvement with effective reading interventions. Note that the interventions have helped the children develop reading areas (shown in white) that more closely resemble the areas used by typical readers, as shown in Figure 4.3 (Shaywitz et al., 2003).

A University of Washington fMRI study of shorter duration used a program based on phoneme and morpheme mapping with 10 dyslexic children and 11 normal readers. After 28 hours of instruction, the fMRI scans showed changes in the brain functions of the dyslexic children that closely resembled the neural processing characteristics of typical readers (Aylward et al., 2003).

Another study addressed the question of how much time the auditory system needs to correctly process the onset (or beginning) phoneme in a word. The only way to hear the difference between the words *bear* and *pear* is in the first 40 milliseconds of the onset of those sounds. You will recall from Chapter 4 that if the visual and auditory processing systems are not synchronized during reading, a child will have difficulty correctly matching phonemes to the letters that represent them. As a result, other brain regions are called into play in an effort to decode the words. Dyslexic students are thus required to use a more labor-intensive set of neural pathways to recognize, decode, and comprehend the words they are reading.

The study involved 20 dyslexic children aged 8 to 12 years (Temple et al., 2003). Their brains were scanned with functional MRIs before and after participating in a eight-week training program that focused on developing the alphabetic principle and phonemic practice. A control group of 12 students with normal reading abilities also had their brain scanned but did not participate in the training.

The pretraining scans were taken while the children were asked to identify letters that rhymed. During this exercise, children with typical reading abilities showed activity in the left temporal area (Broca's area) as well as in the occipito-temporal region typical of skilled readers. Dyslexics, however, struggled with the task and showed activation mainly in the left and right frontal areas, similar to those shown for the dyslexic reader in Figure 4.7.

The dyslexic students then used a computer program called *Fast ForWord* for 100 minutes a day, five days a week. The program was designed to help students recognize the differences between onset sounds, especially those in words that rhyme. For example, the computer would show a picture of a boy and a toy. The computer voice would ask the student to point to the boy. At first, the computer voice asked the questions in a slow, exaggerated manner to help the student hear the differences in the */b/* and */t/* onset sounds. As the student progressed, the speed of the computer voice slowly increased.

After eight weeks of training, the dyslexic children were again given fMRIs while performing the rhyming activities. Their brain scans showed increased activity after remediation in the same areas that were activated in the typical reading children performing this task. As in other similar studies, the intense training in phonological awareness stimulated areas in the dyslexic brain that were not activated while reading prior to the training. There was also increased activity in right frontal brain regions not used by typical reading children. Apparently, the recovery of a more typical pathway also reactivated frontal areas that are used in dyslexic children to compensate for their decoding difficulties. The researchers speculate that this activation pattern in the right frontal area might continue to change over time and come closer to that of typical readers (Habib, 2003).

The dyslexic children were retested after the training in several reading and language skills. In Figure 5.4, it is evident that the posttraining scores of the dyslexic children went up in the three reading areas tested by the Woodcock-Johnson Reading Mastery Test, namely, word identification, word attack, and passage comprehension.

Studies using fMRI indicate that intensive research-based interventions can change the brain functions of struggling readers to more closely match that of typical readers.

These and subsequent studies seem to indicate that research-based reading programs that use computers to help students build phonemic awareness can substantially—and perhaps permanently—benefit struggling readers. The changes due to remediation brought the brain function of dyslexic children closer to that seen in children without reading problems. Apparently, the commonly observed dysfunction in the brains of dyslexic children can be at least partially improved through programs that focus on auditory processing and oral language training, resulting in improved language and reading ability. Three effective computer programs are *Earobics* by Cognitive Concepts, Inc., *Fast ForWord* by the Scientific Learning Corporation, and the *Lindamood Phoneme Sequencing Program (LiPS)* by the Lindamood-Bell Learning Processes Company. See the **Resources** section for more information.

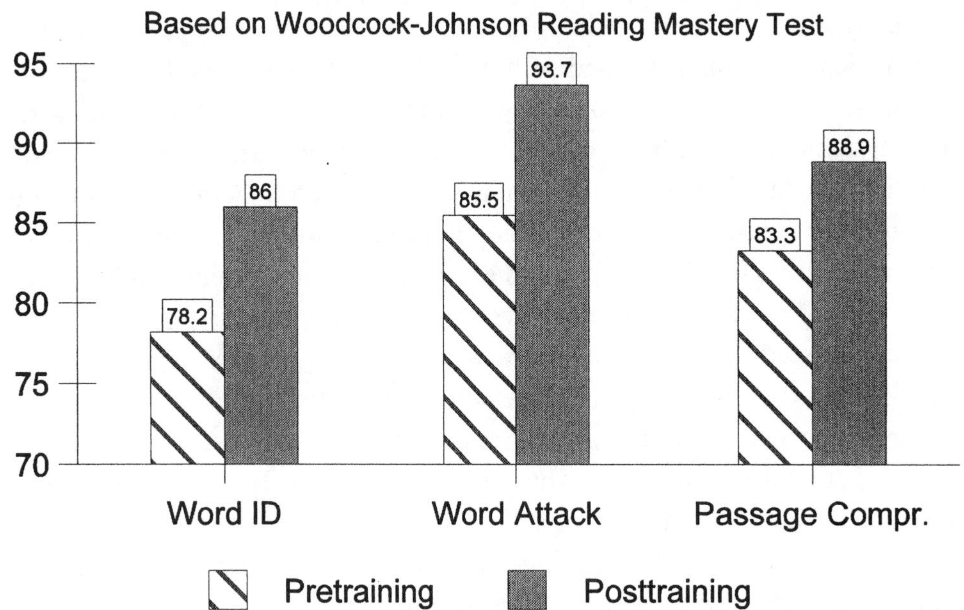

Figure 5.4 The graph shows the pretraining and posttraining average scores of the dyslexic students on the word identification, word attack, and reading comprehension sections of the Woodcock-Johnson Mastery Test (Temple et al., 2003).

READING PROBLEMS AND TAKING TESTS

Tests are a difficult undertaking for students with reading problems, regardless of age. Teachers and schools, however, can make appropriate allowances and modifications that allow these students to show what they really know. Here are some accommodations to consider. Tailor the accommodations to meet the specific needs and age level of each student (Sams, 2003).

✓ When designing a test for these students, stick to a large simple type font (e.g., Arial), put key words in boldface, and provide plenty of space for answers.

✓ Make the purpose of the test clear to the student. If appropriate, also note that spelling, grammatical errors, and handwriting will not affect the test grade.

✓ Make sure you give clear and concise instructions.

✓ Allow additional time so that the test is a measure of what they know, not of the speed of their reading or writing.

- ✓ For essay exams, provide a model answer that shows the layout, paraphrasing, and conclusions expected in the answer. This helps students understand what is expected of them.
- ✓ Read out the questions, if needed, in areas such as mathematics and science since those are the areas being tested, not reading.
- ✓ For some children, have an adult record the child's answers thereby allowing the child to focus on responses rather than on writing.
- ✓ Consider allowing the student to use a word processor to record answers.
- ✓ Use visual aids where appropriate since many struggling readers and dyslexic students often have strong visual-spatial skills.
- ✓ Test in a location where students can work without being self-conscious about their work pace, rest breaks, or additional time.
- ✓ Consider alternative testing formats, such as an oral examination, PowerPoint presentations, or allowing the student to submit an audiotape with responses.

ADVICE TO STUDENTS WITH READING PROBLEMS

Here are some suggestions that parents and teachers can give to students with reading problems that can help them overcome many of the difficulties associated with this condition. Note that some of the advice is more appropriate for older children in that it relates to at-home situations where poor readers and dyslexic students need practice in organizing and managing their affairs (DITT, 2001; Shaywitz, 2003).

At home

- Pack your school bag before you go to bed, assuring a calm start to the next day.
- Put copies of your school schedule around the house, especially in the area where you do your homework. Make extra copies in case you lose them.
- Write down important information, such as class assignments, due dates for class work, tests, extra-curricular activities, and other appointments.
- Know your body's rhythm. Avoid doing homework when you are hungry, tired, or feeling low.

- Keep the telephone numbers of at least two classmates who can tell you the homework assignment if you failed to record it accurately.
- When doing long assignments, break them down into smaller chunks and take frequent breaks to maintain your interest. Recognize that it will take you longer to read a passage than other students because your brain uses a pathway that is slower. But take the time you need and use your intellect and reasoning to understand the material fully and accurately.
- Do your homework in an area that is quiet and free from distractions.

In school

- Avoid taking too many courses that include a large amount of reading.
- Sit in the front of the class and away from windows to avoid being distracted.
- Develop your own shorthand so you can take notes during class to help you remember important information.
- If possible, tape-record your classes and listen to the recording when you are more relaxed and can absorb more.
- Many textbooks are now available on audiotape from Recording for the Blind and Dyslexic. Check out their book list at www.rfbd.org.
- Get extra help from your teacher to develop your study skills, especially before tests.
- Ask your teacher if you can take a short essay test in place of a multiple-choice test. Multiple-choice tests do not give you enough context to decode unfamiliar words. Also, short essay responses give you a better opportunity to show what you have learned.
- Visualizing images probably comes easily to you. Whenever possible, design concept maps and use other types of graphic organizers to help you organize your work.
- Do not be afraid to tell your teacher that you do not understand something. Other students are likely to be in the same situation.
- Giving oral responses in the class may be difficult for you. Share this with your teachers to determine if there are other ways you can demonstrate your knowledge.
- Work on your computer skills because typing is a lot easier than writing. Be sure to proof-read and spell-check your work.
- Being dyslexic may make your school work seem hard, but it is no excuse for not putting forth the effort. Many dyslexics are successful.
- Use the Internet to find out more about dyslexia and to get ideas on how to develop your study skills.

ADVICE FOR PARENTS OF CHILDREN WITH READING PROBLEMS

Parents who learn that their child has reading problems, such as dyslexia, often experience blame, denial, guilt, fear, isolation, and anger. But by accepting that their child has a specific learning difficulty, they will be able to work on those strategies needed to allow their child to reach full potential. Here are some thoughts for parents of a child with reading problems to consider (DITT, 2001; Shaywitz, 2003):

- You know your child better than anyone else. If you suspect a reading problem, there probably is.
- Get professional help as soon as possible. Knowing exactly what is wrong will help you decide the best course of action for your child. Remember that not all struggling readers have dyslexia.
- Make your home an encouraging and safe place. To a child with reading problems, school can be a disheartening experience.
- Do not discuss your children's learning problems in front of them without including them in the discussion.
- Even if diagnosed with dyslexia, remember that your child is more normal than different. Explain to the child that dyslexia means having a hard time learning to read. Emphasize that this has nothing to do with intelligence. Many people with this condition have learned to read and have become successful students and adults. With effort and practice, the child will learn to read.
- Tell the child that struggling readers and people with dyslexia often have trouble hearing all the sounds in a word. They may only hear two sounds in a three syllable word. Reassure the child that other children have this problem and that it can be overcome with proper instruction.
- You might even explain about the different pathways that normal and dyslexic brains take when learning to read (see Chapter 4). Dyslexic children will learn to read, but it will take longer.
- Encourage the child to pursue areas of strength, such as music or sports, to experience the feelings of success in other areas of life.
- Teach your child how to pack the school bag for each day.
- Give your child the opportunity to tell you in a calm environment what happened in school and during the day. Sharing problems and concerns with a sympathetic listener can make them much less burdensome.
- Keep a record of how long it takes your child to do homework. Share this information with teachers who may be unaware of how much time your child needs to complete these tasks.

- Get in touch with the school periodically to discuss what strategies are being used to help your child. Use similar strategies at home when reading with your child.
- Read assigned books and other materials to or with your child, explaining the meaning of new words and checking if your child understands what has been read.
- If the child asks questions about grammar or spelling when writing, give the answer so the child can move on. Dyslexic children often have problems with short-term memory, so supply the answer if they know the process.
- Seek out support groups for families with dyslexic children. They often can provide a lot of useful information about how to deal with learning difficulties.

What's Coming?

The strategies and considerations presented in this chapter are designed to teach poor readers how to overcome their difficulties and become better readers. Such progress is particularly important as students in elementary school move up to middle and high school where reading of the course content becomes a vital part of successful learning. The strategies and techniques that teachers can use to help all students cope with the vast amount of reading required in secondary school content areas are the focus of the next chapter.

CHAPTER 6
Reading in the Content Areas

This chapter addresses several basic questions about improving reading in the content areas. They include:

- *What are some successful strategies for helping students comprehend content material?*
- *In what sequence should these strategies be used?*
- *What are some patterns that exist in the organization of content in different subject areas?*

Students entering the intermediate grades, middle school, and high school are faced with an increased amount of reading and the expectation that they are able to comprehend the content in their texts. Yet, little effort is made to determine either the reading ability of the students entering the class or the difficulty of the reading materials. Consequently, some students are doomed to failure from the start because they cannot read the course material, and they end up frustrated at both the teacher and the subject.

Many secondary teachers express concern about the reading and reading-related problems of their struggling students. Yet, except in English and Language Arts, most content area teachers do not view themselves as reading teachers, and they often express doubts about their ability to provide effective instruction in reading strategies. Studies show, however, that when content area teachers take the time to teach and use reading strategies regularly, student achievement in the content area rises, especially in middle schools (Bryant, Linan-Thompson, Ugel, Hamff, and Hougen, 2001).

In their earlier years, students were taught developmental reading through the use of multilevel texts. However, content teachers usually teach from a single text written at a certain reading level. Furthermore, developmental reading emphasizes the process (learning to read) while content area reading emphasizes application (reading to learn). In any particular class, the range of reading achievement among students often spans several grade levels. The challenge for the teacher, then, is to determine what strategies will help students acquire the content knowledge while trying to manage the wide range of differences in reading achievement.

> The challenge for the content area teacher is to determine what strategies will help students acquire the content knowledge while managing the wide range of differences in reading achievement.

For some students, the text itself is intimidating. High school science and history texts can easily run over 1,000 pages. Content teachers often assume that students come to their classes with the reading skills necessary to use the required text successfully. Moreover, these teachers may not recognize three major differences between the developmental reading that students had in earlier grades with the expository reading required for their course. The first difference is in learning new vocabulary. In developmental reading, vocabulary is taught in context, meaning is clarified, and words are rehearsed and practiced at a pace that most children can accomplish. In content courses, the vocabulary used in basic texts is highly specialized and technical, and often presented so quickly that students have little time to fully comprehend its meaning.

The second difference lies in the way concepts are introduced and explored. In developmental reading, teachers present concepts that are familiar, and they cover them at a pace that is appropriate for most children. In content courses, teachers present concepts that are unfamiliar and complex, usually at a rapid pace because there is so much to cover. The third difference is in the specialized type of reading that is needed for some courses, such as the ability to read charts, tables, graphs, maps, globes, and technical instruments (Baer and Nourie, 1993). Table 6.1 summarizes the main differences between developmental reading and reading in content areas.

It is important for content area teachers to determine the level of reading difficulty in their course materials and the ability of their students to read them. By making some accommodations in materials and selecting appropriate strategies, all teachers can help more students succeed in learning the course content.

STRATEGIES FOR HELPING STUDENTS READ CONTENT MATERIAL

The strategies described here are compiled from a variety of sources (Baer and Nourie, 1993; NIFL, 2001; OPS, 2003; Slavin, 1995) and are intended to help students acquire course content successfully through reading and other methods. They are not intended to imply that

Table 6.1 Differences Between Developmental and Content Area Reading

	Developmental	Content Area
Texts	Several multilevel texts	Usually a single text at a fixed reading level
Teaching Approach	Learning the process of reading (learning to read)	Learning to apply what has been read (reading to learn)
Range of Reading Abilities	Usually limited to a span of one or two grade levels	Can span five or more grade levels
Vocabulary Acquisition	Mostly general in nature. Presented at modest pace so students have time to practice words, clarify meanings, and reinforce comprehension.	Highly specific and technical. Presented quickly, so students have little time to practice words and develop meaning.
Presentation of Concepts	Concepts are usually familiar and presented at a modest pace.	Concepts are unfamiliar and complex, and presented at rapid pace with little time for thorough processing.
Specialized Reading	Limited mostly to printed text.	Can include reading charts, tables, graphs, maps, globes, and technical instruments.

Source: Baer and Nourie, 1993

the school can abdicate its ongoing responsibility to help students improve their reading skills at all grade levels. To some extent, every content teacher is also a teacher of reading, not of developmental reading, but by virtue of using a variety of techniques that allow students with reading problems to learn content. The strategies are:

- Using direct instruction
- Conquering vocabulary
- Helping with comprehension
- Rewriting content material
- Incorporating supplemental textbooks
- Establishing in-class vertical files
- Using audiovisual aids
- Promoting cooperative learning groups

Using Direct Instruction

Students who have reading problems usually rely heavily on teacher explanations to grasp concepts and to identify what is essential to learn. Therefore, direct instruction can be a critical factor in their achievement. During direct instruction

✓ Clearly identify important concepts

✓ Explain why we are learning them

✓ Present the concepts in an organized manner

✓ Define and use unusual vocabulary words in context

✓ Recommend a limited and specific reading textbook assignment that covers your presentation

✓ Ask students to summarize orally the main points you presented in the direct instruction segment

✓ Consider asking the students to write out the summary as well

✓ Suggest other print sources (of a lower reading level) that also explain the content

Conquering Vocabulary

Technical, unfamiliar, and unusual words are often stumbling blocks for students when reading course content. Familiar words used in a specialized context can also cause problems. Students encountering such words can learn them in any of four different ways (NIFL, 2001)..

✓ *Learning a new meaning for a known word.* The student recognizes the word but is learning a new meaning for it. For example, the student knows what a tree *branch* is, but is learning that the word can also describe a *branch* of government or *branch* of a river.

✓ *Learning the meaning of a new word to describe a known concept.* The student knows the concept but not this particular word to describe it. For example, the student has had experience with globes and baseballs but does not know they are examples of *spheres.*

✓ *Learning the meaning of a new word for an unknown concept.* The student is not familiar with the concept or the word that describes it, and must learn both. For example, the student is not be familiar with the process or the word *osmosis.*

✓ *Clarifying and enriching the meaning of a known word.* The student is learning finer distinctions or connotations in the usage of what may seem like similar words. For example, understanding the distinctions among *dashing, jogging, running, sprinting,* and *trotting.*

All these types of learning vary in difficulty. The third type, learning the meaning of a new word for an unknown concept, is one of the most common, yet challenging. Much learning in the content areas involves this type of word learning. As students learn about *photosynthesis, secants,* and *oligarchies,* they may be learning new concepts as well as new words. Learning concepts and words in mathematics, social studies, and science may be even more difficult because each major concept is often linked to other new concepts. For example, the concept *oligarchy* can be associated with other unfamiliar concepts, such as *monarchy, plutocracy,* and *dictatorship. Photosynthesis* can be associated with *phototropism* and *osmosis.*

Identify these types of words in advance of assigning the reading. Work to develop students' word consciousness by calling their attention to the way writers choose words to convey meaning. Help them research a word's origin or history and to see if they can find examples of that word's usage in their everyday lives.

Decoding New Words

Older students acquire more than half of the approximately 3,000 new words they learn each year through reading (Stahl, 2000). For English language learners, vocabulary knowledge is one of the most critical factors affecting their achievement in the content areas. Teachers cannot assume that English language learners possess the vocabulary needed to decode and comprehend the numerous word meanings they encounter in the course materials. Even though these students may possess proficient listening and speaking skills in English, it takes time and rereading to understand the formal aspects of English as used in secondary level texts. Because knowledge of vocabulary is so closely linked to reading comprehension, students need to learn strategies for decoding new words that they encounter in the content texts. These strategies include decoding multisyllabic words and getting the meaning of unfamiliar words from context (OPS, 2003).

Decoding Multisyllabic Words. One strategy for decoding multisyllabic words takes just six steps. The teacher guides the student through the steps. Using a worksheet to analyze the word facilitates the process. Figure 6.1 illustrates one possible worksheet format with an example.

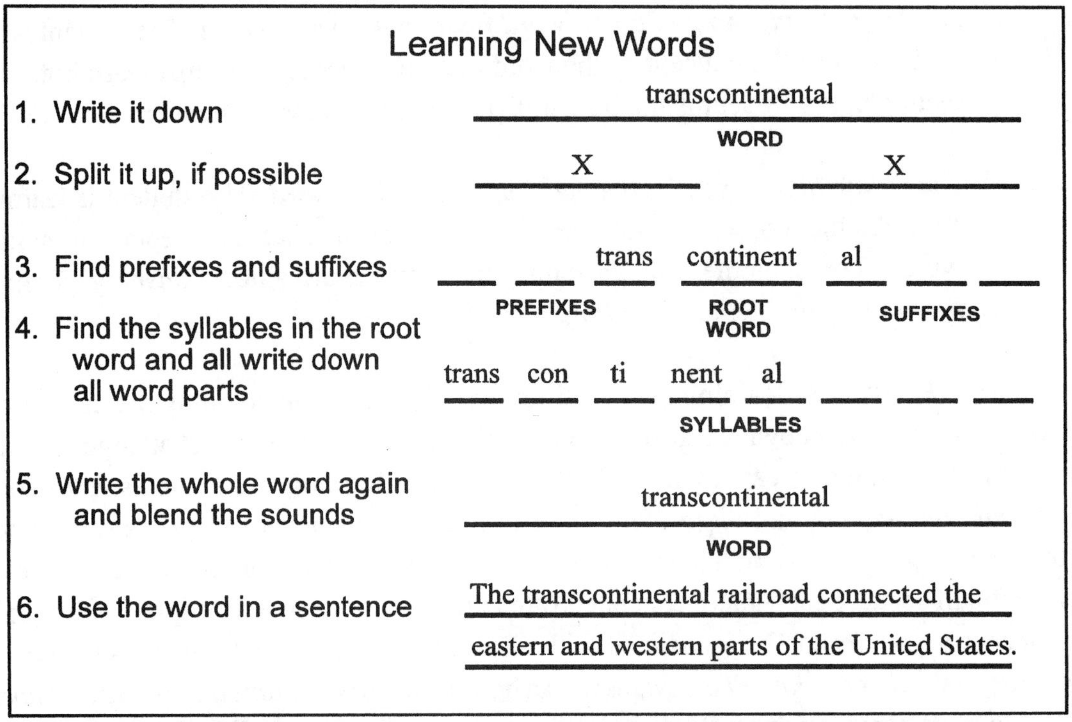

Learning New Words

1. Write it down	transcontinental (WORD)
2. Split it up, if possible	X / X
3. Find prefixes and suffixes	trans (PREFIXES) / continent (ROOT WORD) / al (SUFFIXES)
4. Find the syllables in the root word and all write down all word parts	trans con ti nent al (SYLLABLES)
5. Write the whole word again and blend the sounds	transcontinental (WORD)
6. Use the word in a sentence	The transcontinental railroad connected the eastern and western parts of the United States.

Figure 6.1 This chart helps students to decode new words through a six-step process. The word "transcontinental" is used here as an example (Adapted from OPS, 2003).

1. The student first writes the whole word down, *transcontinental.*
2. If it is a compound word, such as *butterfingers,* the student writes down each word part, *butter* and *fingers.*
3. If it is not a compound word, the student puts an "x" on these lines and moves to the nest step which is to write down the root word and any prefixes and suffixes so that *transcontinental* becomes *trans, continent, al.*
4. Next, the student breaks down the root word into its syllables (*continent = con, ti, nent*) and writes down all the word parts, *trans, con, ti, nent, al.*
5. Now the student writes the whole word again while saying it aloud and blending the syllable sounds, *transcontinental.*
6. Finally, the student uses the new word in a sentence, *The transcontinental railroad connected the eastern and western parts of the United States.*

Using Context Clues. The context in which an unfamiliar word is used can often give hints as to its meaning. Help students use context clues by doing the following:

✓ Select an authentic text passage containing the unfamiliar words that can be defined through context. Ensure that the students have enough prior knowledge that they can reasonably determine the words' meanings.

- ✓ Model the process of using context clues to determine meaning by going through the steps of the Context Clues Strategy (See box).
- ✓ Think aloud as you use the strategy so that students can follow your reasoning.
- ✓ Explain how you used the clues to arrive at the meaning of the word.
- ✓ Identify the key words surrounding the target word that helped you decide on its meaning.
- ✓ Verify the word's meaning in the dictionary.
- ✓ Have students practice the model by giving them a page of text with three unknown words highlighted.

Context Clues Strategy

1. When you come to a word you don't know, continue reading to a good stopping place.
2. Use the context to figure out the meaning of the new word.
3. Guess what the meaning might be.
4. Test your guess by asking if the meaning:
   Looks right
   Sounds right
   Makes sense
5. Check your guess in the dictionary.

Helping With Comprehension

Students who are struggling readers often have difficulty comprehending what they are reading. Strategies that help students to relate the content to their prior knowledge, to practice mental imagery, and to locate the main idea can be very effective aids to comprehension. Here is some general advice you can give students to help them with comprehension.

- ✓ Look over what you will be reading, noting words and phrases that are in bold face or italics. Look also for any charts, graphs, and pictures. Review any chapter summaries and related questions that are useful to guide your reading. Not everything in the text is equally important, so read to capture the main ideas.

- ✓ Take notes or draw diagrams while reading to help you remember main phrases and ideas. Use graphic organizers and mind maps, too.
- ✓ Read the text more than once.
- ✓ When you encounter an unknown word, try to guess its meaning by looking at the context. The sentences immediately before and after can give you good clues to determine meaning.
- ✓ Try to make connections between main ideas and their supporting details.
- ✓ Each time you finish a paragraph, stop and try to summarize it in your own words.
- ✓ Discuss what you have read with others who have read the same text.

Narrative and Expository Text. Some strategies need to be modified depending on the nature of the text. Narrative text is commonly associated with literature instruction and focuses on settings, characters, plots, conflicts, conflict resolution, and themes. Expository text is more commonly found in science and social studies texts and focuses on acquiring and processing information related to comparisons, cause and effect, and sequencing. In mathematics, expository text relates to the semantic and linguistics structures necessary to translate word problems into mathematical expressions.

Using Prior Knowledge

Students bring with them a wide range of knowledge and experiences about many topics. Prior knowledge significantly influences a reader's comprehension of new topics, concepts, and vocabulary found in content area texts. Comprehension of those texts relies heavily on the students' prior knowledge and their ability to apply it to the topics being covered in the content area. Reading difficult content text can be made easier if students can relate the reading to what they already know. Before assigning a difficult text selection,

- ✓ Preview the text with them
- ✓ Ask them what they already know about the content of the selection (a concept, time period, or topic)

✓ Discuss and explain any unusual or technical words

✓ Use visual aids whenever possible

Using Mental Imagery

Readers often form mental images or pictures while reading. These visualizations help them remember and understand what they have read. Encourage students to form visual images of what they are reading by urging them to picture a character, setting, a model in motion, or an event described in the text.

Imagery runs the gamut from simple concrete pictures to complex motor learning and multistep procedures. Because imagery is still not a common instructional strategy, it should be implemented early and gradually. These guidelines are adapted from Parrott (1986) and West, Farmer, and Wolff (1991) for using imagery as a powerful aid to understanding text and retention.

✓ *Prompting.* Use prompts for telling students to form mental images of the content being learned. They can be as simple as "form a picture in your mind of..." to more complex directions. Prompts should be specific to the content or task and should be accompanied by relevant photographs, charts, or arrays, especially for younger children.

✓ *Modeling.* Model imagery by describing your own image to the class and explaining how that image helps your recall and use of the current learning. Also, model a procedure and have the students mentally practice the steps.

✓ *Interaction.* Strive for rich, vivid images where items interact. The richer the image, the more information it can include. If there are two or more items in the images, they should be visualized as acting on each other. If the recall is a ball and a bat, for example, imagine the bat hitting the ball.

✓ *Reinforcement.* Have students talk about the images they formed and get feedback from others on the accuracy, vividness, and interaction of the images. Talk provides mental rehearsal and helps students to remember the image for an extended period of time.

✓ *Add context.* Whenever possible, add context to the interaction to increase retention and recall. For example, if the task is to recall prefixes and suffixes, the context could be a parade with the prefixes in front urging the suffixes in the rear to catch up.

- ✓ *Avoid overloading the image.* Although good images are complete representations of what is to be remembered, they should not overload the working memory's capacity in older students of about seven items.

Locating the Main Idea

Help students develop a strategy for locating the main idea in fiction and nonfiction passages (OPS, 2003).

- ✓ Model the procedure used in the Strategy for Locating the Main Idea (see box on the next page).
- ✓ After modeling, lead the students through guided, then independent practice.
- ✓ Use graphic organizers that are appropriate for the passage.
- ✓ The paragraph summaries can take several forms, depending on whether you are using narrative or expository text. Have students identify which type of text they are reading, since they are different in form and intent.
- ✓ Narrative text:

  Start by giving them some sentence fragments, such as
  "This story takes place ________________________________."
  "________________ is a character who ________________________."
  "A problem occurs when ________________________________."
  "The problem is finally solved when ________________________."
  "At the end of the story ________________________________."

- ✓ Expository text:

  Main idea/Topic: ________________________________.
  Subtopic: ____________________________.
  Detail 1 ________________________.
  Detail 2 ________________________.
  Subtopic: ____________________________.
  Detail 1 ________________________.
  Detail 2 ________________________.

- ✓ Consider using cooperative learning for this activity, because it gives students opportunities to share and critique their summaries. This oral rehearsal aids in retention of important ideas, concepts, and details.

✓ If students have difficulty, provide summaries that are partially filled in and let the students furnish the missing details.

Strategy for Locating the Main Idea

1. Look at the title, headings, and picture. What do you already know about this topic?
2. Predict what the author might say about this topic.
3. Read the passage to find out the significant details or facts. Reread the passage to clarify any questions.
4. Modify your thoughts about the main idea as you review each detail.
5. Think about what the details or facts have in common.
6. Decide on the main idea.
7. Write a summary paragraph that includes the author's essential points and supporting details.

(Adapted from OPS, 2003)

Paraphrasing for Comprehension

Paraphrasing is commonly thought of as copying information from a text source and changing a few words. That process rarely results in retention of learning because the copying act can be done almost automatically and without much conscious thought. If the purpose of paraphrasing is to give students opportunities to get a deeper understanding of the text, to make connections to what they already know, and to enhance remembering, then a much more systematic process must be followed.

Effective paraphrasing incorporates reading, writing, listening, and speaking, thereby activating the brain's frontal lobe and leading to a fuller comprehension of the course material. It can be used in all content areas and with students in the upper elementary grades and beyond, and it can help students learn from many different types of texts, including fiction and nonfiction.

The process encourages active student participation, provides for mental, oral, and written rehearsal of newly-learned material, and enhances comprehension and retention. At the same time, it develops reading, communication, and creative skills (Fisk and Hurst, 2003). See the box on the next page for the guidelines and steps for using paraphrasing successfully in the classroom.

Paraphrasing for Comprehension

Guidelines:

This strategy is appropriate for upper elementary grades and beyond. It can be used in all content areas and with all types of texts, including fiction and nonfiction. It is effective because it uses all modes of communication: reading, writing, listening, and speaking. The process encourages active student participation, provides for mental, oral, and written rehearsal of newly-learned material, and enhances comprehension and retention. At the same time, it develops reading, communication, and creative skills.

A good paraphrase must convey the original meaning of the author but in the student's own words and phrasing. The voice of the author also should be maintained. If the original work is humorous, satirical, sarcastic, or melancholy, the paraphrase should be also. Students should therefore identify the author's meaning and voice before they start writing.

The teacher should explain the purpose and benefits of paraphrasing. Students already do some paraphrasing when they take notes in class, write a book report, or give a speech. Outside examples can include telling someone about a trip taken, or a news reporter summarizing an interview.

Steps:

This general scheme has four steps. Modify the steps as appropriate for the age level of the students and the nature of the material being read.

1. *First reading and discussion.* Read aloud the text to be paraphrased while students follow along in their own texts. Have the students suggest possible definiitions for any unfamiliar words. After clarifying the vocabulary, ask the students to identify the main idea and the author's tone.
2. *Second reading and note-taking.* Students read the text on their own and take detailed notes when they finish a paragraph. The notes should capture the main idea and supporting details, but should be in the student's own words. Students may want to use a thesaurus to help them with difficult or technical words.
3. *Written paraphrase.* When finished with the note-taking, the students put the original text away so it will not to influence the next step. Using only their notes, the students write their paraphrased version that communicates the main ideas with the same voice of the original text.
4. *Sharing paraphrases.* When the paraphrases are completed, the students form pairs and compare the similarities and differences between their respective paraphrases. They are also asked to decide how the author's voice is communicated in their versions.

(Adapted from Fisk and Hurst, 2003)

Reading Aloud to the Class

Consider reading certain parts of the text to the class, especially those parts that use difficult or highly technical words or describe complex situations. Remember that many students can understand something when they hear it even though they may not be able to read about it themselves. Reading aloud can also be used to make connections between texts, to develop background information, or for enjoyment. Where appropriate, the oral reading can be done by other students, school volunteers, or parents. Another option is for you or a student to record certain text sections on audiotapes and have them available for student use in the school's media center.

Rewriting Content Material

Consider the possibility of rewriting some of the course materials that may have a particularly high level of reading difficulty. Rewriting the material at a reading level closer to that of the students who are having problems, allows those students to gain confidence in their ability to understand the content despite their reading difficulties. Another possibility is to have students who do understand the course material rewrite it for their classmates. This approach reinforces both reading and writing skills.

Incorporating Supplemental Textbooks

Identify textbooks that cover the same material as the course text but are written at a lower reading level. This may require using several books because it is unlikely that one book will cover all the course content. Trade books are another possibility. They also present concepts covered in the primary textbook but are generally at a lower reading level. Furthermore, trade books help students recognize that the study of content subjects is not limited to school textbooks. By presenting concepts in many different ways, supplemental texts enhance student learning.

Establishing In-Class Vertical Files

Students will often read a magazine or newspaper article about a subject more readily than a textbook. Establish and maintain a file of such articles that relate to the course content. Update the file periodically and encourage students to contribute to the file when they come across an appropriate article.

Using Audiovisual Aids

Audiovisual aids are a great help to students with reading problems. Many students today have grown up in and become acclimated to a multimedia environment. Whenever possible, use videotapes, audiotapes, television, computer programs, overhead transparencies, and other technology to supplement and accompany direct instruction. All students benefit from the use of these materials.

Promoting Cooperative Learning Groups

Cooperative learning (Johnson and Johnson, 1989) is a particularly effective strategy in classes that have a wide range of student abilities, including reading. This approach allows students to work in teams and to be assigned tasks that match their ability and that contribute to the whole group effort. As the team members interact, students have opportunities to share and learn the concepts being studied.

SEQUENCING THE READING STRATEGIES

Now that we have discussed some of the strategies content area teachers can use to help their students comprehend course materials, the next step is to look at the sequence in which the strategies should be presented for maximum effect on student comprehension. The sequence can be divided into three phases: activities before, during, and after reading the content text (Cibrowski,1993; Paterno, 2001).

Phase 1: Before Reading

The purpose of these activities is to activate prior knowledge and to stimulate the brain's memory recall and imagery systems to spark curiosity, to motivate, and to facilitate retention of learning. Deciding which strategies to use depends on the material to be read and the background knowledge of the students.

✓ *Questions to ask.* Using questions to engage students in a dialogue about something they are about to read can clarify their thinking and help them determine what to expect from reading the material.

- Make connections between the learner's background knowledge and the reading. "This passage is about______. What do you already know about this?"

State a purpose for reading the passage. "This section is about_____. What are some things we could learn about this?"

- Make predictions. "This passage is about_____. What do you think this could be about? What might happen to you if you________?"

✓ *Select core vocabulary.* Choose the words that are likely to be unfamiliar and difficult and present them on the board or on paper. Ask students to write a definition, even if it is only a guess. Collect and return the papers at the end of Phase 3 to complete by filling in the correct definitions.

✓ *Write out the predictions.* Have students write out what they think the passage will be about and what they might learn from it.

✓ *Analogies and visual images.* Relate the material in the new reading to knowledge the students already possess. Ask them to think about what they know that is similar to what they think will be in the passage.

✓ *Concept maps.* Concept maps used before reading help students identify important concepts and ideas and how they are related to each other. By understanding these relationships in advance, students are more likely to comprehend their text readings.

Phase 2: During Reading

These strategies are designed to address two difficulties that poor readers have with content area texts: (1) The students spend far more time struggling with individual words than in constructing meaning from text. (2) The texts often have main ideas deeply embedded in text and too many concepts are superficially presented at once.

✓ *Questions to ask.* These questions help students review what they are learning while reading, confirm or change their predictions, and make connections to prior readings.

- Clarify and review what has happened so far. "What are some things you have already learned about________?"
- Confirm or create new predictions. "Now that you have learned_________, will you keep or change your predictions?"
- Make connections to other readings.

✓ *Reciprocal teaching techniques.* As explained earlier, this is a powerful technique because students assume a dominant role in their own learning. It includes the four strategies of questioning, clarifying, summarizing, and predicting. Teachers and students become partners in improving the students' understanding of the content material and their ability to monitor their own comprehension. Although the technique was developed more than 20 years ago, it is not part of the common practice of secondary content area teachers. When it is used, however, research studies have demonstrated that students who worked with reciprocal teaching increased their group participation and use of the strategies taught, learned from the passages studied, and increased their learning when reading independently. Furthermore, the studies showed that the technique could be used in various settings and that the students maintained the reading gains they achieved (Slater and Horstman, 2002).

The technique takes about 10 days to teach, during which time the teacher is doing a lot of modeling. Eventually, the teacher increasingly hands over responsibility to the students who take assume the roles of teacher/leader and lead the discussions with the other students. The teacher monitors the group and intervenes to keep the students on task and to facilitate the discussion. See the box on the next page for an explanation of the steps and procedures involved in reciprocal teaching.

✓ *Summary notes.* Students write down a summary of each section of the passage as soon as they finish it. The summary should include the main idea and supporting details. Concept maps can help.

Phase 3: After Reading

The strategies here are to help students rehearse, analyze, and extend their reading to increase the chances they will remember what they have read. Questioning and vocabulary prediction are important parts of this process.

✓ *Questions to ask.* These questions foster retention of learning by reinforcing the concepts in the reading and encouraging critical thinking and personal response.

- Reinforce the concept. "Have you had any of the experiences mentioned in the passage? If so, how did you feel about them?"
- Model ways of thinking through the information they have read. "What events are described in this passage? What caused them? How do you know that?"
- Encourage critical thinking and personal response. "What do you think might have happened if ___? Why did the author ___?"

Reciprocal Teaching

Guidelines:

The teacher explains the four supporting strategies used in this technique: *Questioning* focuses the students' attention on main ideas and provides a means for checking their understanding of what they are reading. *Clarifying* requires students to work on understanding confusing and ambiguous sections of text. *Summarizing* requires students to determine what is important in the text and what is not. *Predicting* requires students to rehearse what they have learned and to begin the next section of text with some expectation of what is to come.

The teacher models the sequence of strategies. Eventually, the teacher increasingly hands over responsibility to the students who now assume leadership roles in the discussion. The teacher monitors the group to keep students on task and to facilitate the discussion.

Specific Steps:

1. The leader reads aloud a short segment of text.
2. Questioning: The leader or other group members generate several questions related to the passage just read, and group members answer the questions. Ex: What was the problem here? What was the cause? What was the solution? What was the chain of events?
3. Clarifying: The leader and group members clarify any problems or misunderstandings. Ex: What does the word____mean? What did the author mean when he said______?
4. Summarizing: After all problems have been clarified, the leader and group members summarize the text segment.
5. Predicting: Based on the discussion and the reading thus far, the leader and group members make predictions about the contents of the upcoming text.
6. This sequence is repeated with subsequent sections of the text. With daily practice, struggling readers will master the four supporting strategies and will use them for all their independent reading in other content area courses.
7. Some cautions:

   Start with simple questions at the beginning. But as students gain more practice, model open ended questions that are thought-provoking:

   Explain why ___.
   Explain how ___.
   What is a new example of ___?
   What conclusions can you draw from ___?
   What do you think causes ___? Why?
   What evidence do you have to support your answer?
   What are the strengths and weaknesses of ___?
   Compare ___ and ___ with regard to ___.

   Do not hesitate to provide more modeling and direct explanation, when needed, throughout the reciprocal teaching process.

(Adapted from Cibrowski, 1993; Slater and Horstman, 2002)

- Build awareness of common themes. "What else have we read that is similar to this? What parts are the same and what parts are different?"

✓ *Vocabulary prediction.* Redistribute the vocabulary prediction forms from Phase 1 and have the students write in the definitions based on their reading. Ask them to discuss what they learned about the meaning and use of the vocabulary words.

✓ *Analyze good and bad examples of writing.* Have the students view, analyze, and discuss good and bad examples of chapter summaries. Ask them to explain the characteristics of good and bad summaries and to write their own, using the criteria for the good summaries.

✓ *Other readings related to the course text.* Suggest other resources for the students to read that relate to the text. Trade books or magazines at the appropriate reading level should be available in class or at the school's library media center.

GRAPHIC ORGANIZERS AND COMPREHENSION OF CONTENT AREA READING

Graphic organizers have been mentioned in previous chapters as valuable tools for organizing and representing knowledge and for illustrating relationships between concepts. Even though graphic organizers have been mentioned in pedagogical literature for over 30 years, content area teachers have been slow to incorporate them as a routine instructional tool. Yet, research studies have shown them to be particularly effective in helping students with reading problems and other learning disabilities to learn content area material. The studies also have found that reading assignments that require students to complete graphic organizers in lieu of answering traditional study guide questions can significantly increase reading comprehension as well (Chmielewski and Dansereau, 1998; Katayama and Robinson, 2000). With this evidence in mind, let's spend some time discussing the reasons why graphic organizers can be effective and present some different types of organizers for consideration.

Graphic organizers are effective because they (Ellis, 1998)

- Show the organization or structure of concepts as well as relationships between concepts
- Make it more clear to students what they are expected to do and allow students to focus on what is important
- Provide a mental framework for helping students to organize knowledge and build the framework piece by piece, linking it to other learned frameworks

- Show how each item on the graphic can serve as a link to remembering related information discussed in class
- Reduce the cognitive demands on the learner by showing (as opposed to just telling) students how the information is structured, allowing the teacher to present information at more sophisticated and complex levels
- Develop literacy and thinking skills because the quality of the students' writing improves not only in the organization of ideas, but also in fluency and in other areas such as writing mechanics (punctuation, spelling, capitalization, etc.)
- Encourage students to use information processing and higher-order thinking skills, such as using cues to recognize important information, making decisions about what is important or essential, consolidating information, identifying main ideas and supporting details, and making decisions about the best way to structure the information
- Stimulate students who have constructed different organizers to discuss their diagrams and debate the importance of various points, draw conclusions, make connections to other ideas, and form inferences, predictions, or forecasts
- Result in an almost immediate improvement in performance on classroom tests for many students, whereas increased scores on standardized achievement tests occur more gradually as students gain skills using graphic organizers strategically

Some teachers resist using graphic organizers because they believe it takes too much class time to draw them. But now there are inexpensive computer programs (e.g., Inspiration Software) that help students construct and print different types of organizers in just minutes.

Types of Organizers

Graphic organizers come in several different forms, depending on the nature of the associated material to be learned. Among the most common types of graphic organizers are the following:

- Concept mapping
- Flowchart
- Matrix
- Webbing

Concept Mapping

One of the first types of graphic organizers to be developed, concept maps were originally used in the late 1970s to help students learn complex concepts in science. As research studies revealed how much more science children learned through using concept maps, they spread slowly to other subject areas (Novak and Musonda, 1991). More recent studies show that concept mapping also improves content area text comprehension and summarization for intermediate, middle, and high school students (Chang, Sung, and Chen, 2002; Chmielewski and Dansereau, 1998). Concept maps are now becoming more popular. There are multiple Internet sites that offer numerous examples of concept maps in all subject areas.

Concept maps are used to

- Develop an understanding of a body of knowledge
- Explore new information and relationships
- Access prior knowledge.
- Gather new knowledge and information.
- Share knowledge and information generated.

Share the guidelines included in the box on tips for making concept maps. Computer programs that build graphic organizers would be more efficient than paper-and-pencil versions, but both are equally effective at improving learning. Cooperative learning teams find Post-its

Tips for Making a Concept Map

Before students get started with their concept map, they should answer the following questions:

- What is the central word, concept, research question, or problem around which to build the map?
- What are the concepts, items, descriptive words, or important questions that one can associate with the concept, topic, research question, or problem?

Here are some suggestions that will help them construct the map:

✓ Consider using a computer program, such as *Inspiration,* to construct the map. If that is not available, Post-its are handy and allow you to move the concepts around a board easily.

✓ Use either a top-down approach, working from general to specific, or use a free association approach by brainstorming items and then develop the links and explain the relationships.

✓ If possible, use different colors and shapes for items and links to identify different types of information.

✓ Use different colored items to identify prior and new information.

✓ Experiment with a variety of different layouts until you find one that is compelling, understandable, and attractive .

✓ Be prepared to revise the map several times. This is another reason why computer software is helpful.

are very useful because they allow items to be moved around on a board or chart until the team is satisfied that they have the best arrangement. The Post-its also make revisions easy.

Before getting started on their concept maps, the students should get their research materials, class notes, and related articles together to use as their database for constructing the map. They should also ask themselves questions about the learning, such as:

- What is the central word, concept, research question, or problem around which to build the map?
- What are the concepts, items, descriptive words, or important questions that I can associate with the concept, topic, research question, or problem?

Procedure. Classroom instruction about the major topic usually takes place first. Armed with their new knowledge, the students gather their resources. Working independently, in teams, or as a whole class, the students start selecting the items, identifying the relationships, and choosing the descriptive words that will describe the relationships. After making the first chart, they review it to determine if the relationships are correctly labeled, and whether some other arrangement would make the map clearer or more attractive. Remember, there is rarely only one way to do a concept map. Later, students with different maps can discuss their variations and debate their differences. Figure 6.2 shows a concept map built around the process of photosynthesis. All the basic steps are included. The map can be made more attractive with pictures of plants, a sun, or a glass of water placed near the appropriate item.

Flowchart

A flowchart is used typically to depict a sequence of events, stages, phases, actions and outcomes. This version is good to use with young children and as a first step in developing linear relationships. The questions to ask before completing the chart are:

- What is the name of the event, procedure, or person that will be described?
- What are the specific stages, steps, phases, or events?
- Are the events in the correct sequence?
- How do the stages, steps, phases, or events relate to one another?
- What is the final outcome?

After the important steps have been identified, the students fill in the flowchart in the proper sequence. In some situations the flowchart can represent a part of a cycle, as in the case of the example on the left side of Figure 6.3. The flowchart shows the five steps in reciprocal teaching for a passage of text read aloud. After completing the steps in the first passage, the process is repeated for the second passage, and so on.

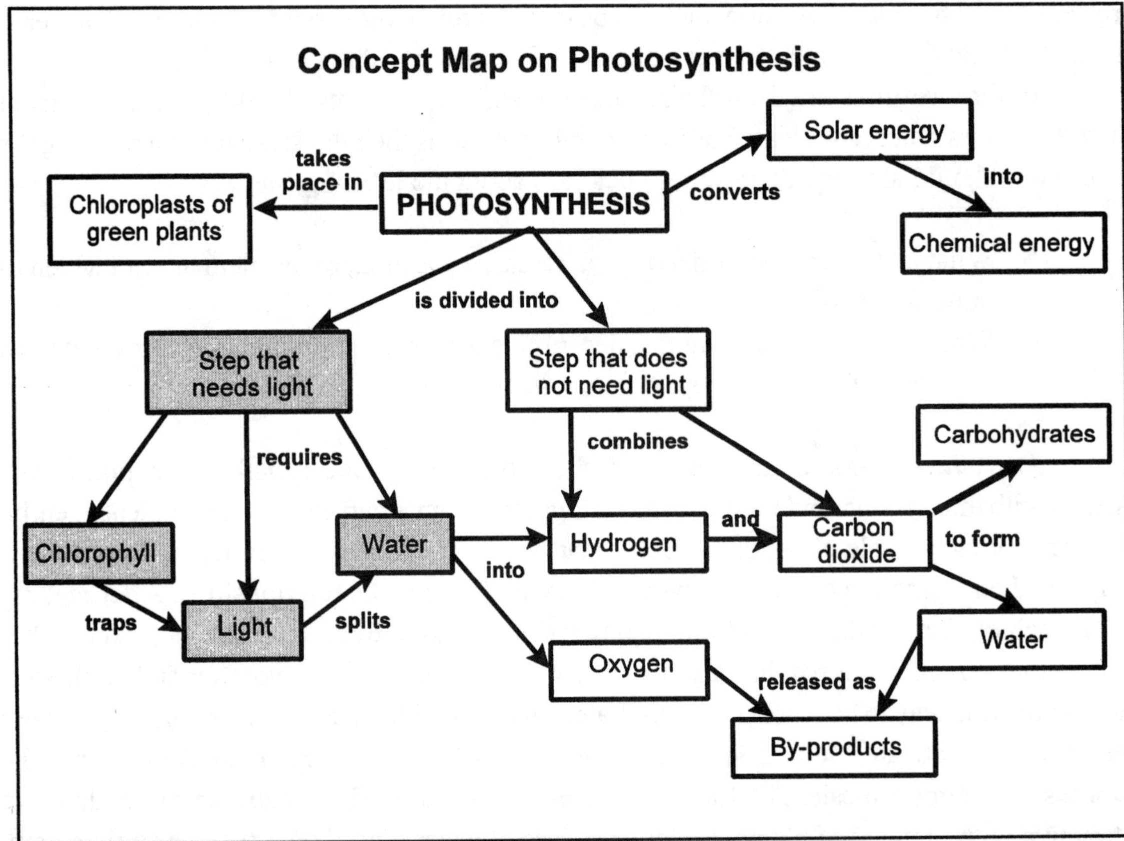

Figure 6.2 This is an example of a concept map built around the process of photosynthesis. As long as the basic steps are included, there are many different configurations that this map could take. It is important that the student write the relationship between any two items near the arrow that links them.

Venn Diagrams

John Venn first used these diagrams in the late 1800s to show relationships in mathematics. They are now used across many content areas to compare and contrast the qualities of two or three items, such as people, places, events, stories, ideas, situations, and things. Use a double Venn diagram to work with two items and a triple Venn diagram for three items. The questions to ask when preparing to use a Venn diagram are:

- What items do you want to compare?
- What characteristics do the items have in common (intersecting portions)?
- What characteristics do the items not have in common (nonintersecting portions)?

The Venn diagram on the right in Figure 6.3 compares some of the similarities and differences between fish and whales. Characteristics that are common to both fish and whales are shown in the area where the two circles overlap.

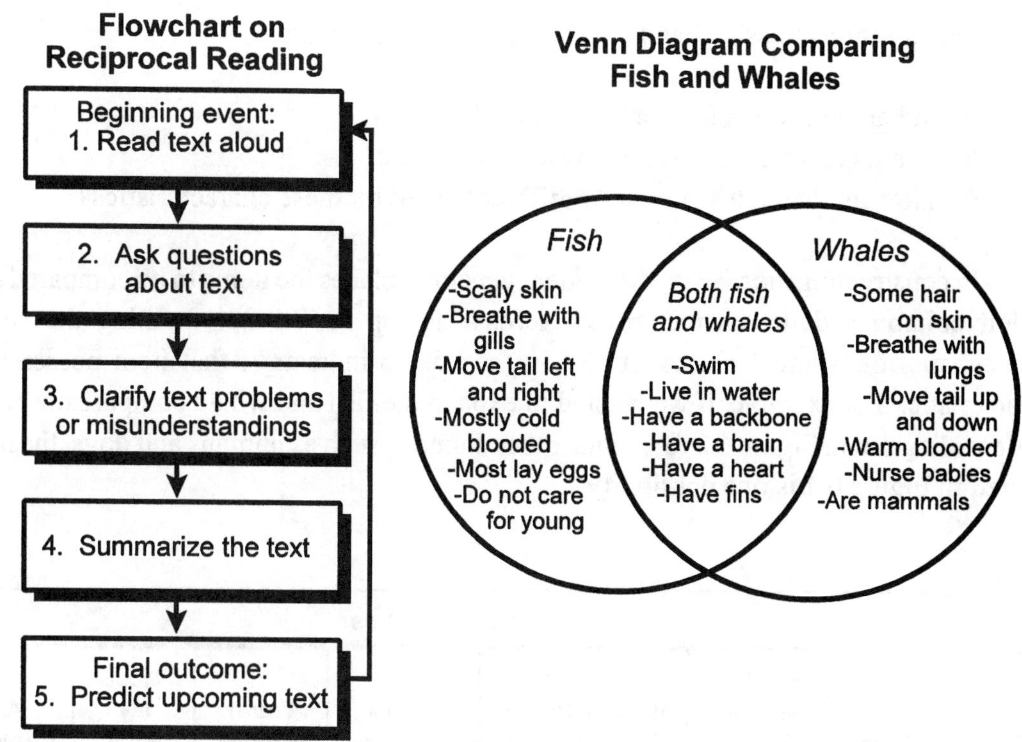

Figure 6.3 On the left is a flowchart organizer depicting the steps in the reciprocal reading process. The arrow from Step 5 to Step 1 shows the process is repeated for each passage of text. On the right is a Venn diagram comparing characteristics of fish and whales. Common characteristics are in the area where the circles overlap.

Matrixes

When comparing the characteristics of more than three items, Venn diagrams become too difficult to construct. In this instance, the matrix is a much easier organizer to use and it can be adapted to a variety of learning activities. Among the most common types are the following three:

- Comparison matrix
- K-W-H-L hart
- Content grids

Comparison Matrix. This matrix is used to describe and compare attributes and characteristics of two or more items, such as people, places, events, stories, ideas, situations, and things. One distinct advantage of this matrix is that there is no limit to the number of items or characteristics that can be included.

The questions to ask when preparing the matrix chart are:

- What items do you want to compare?
- What characteristics do you want to compare?
- How are the items similar or different based on these characteristics?

In constructing the matrix, the student generally places the items to be compared down the left column and the characteristics across the top row. After defining the specific characteristic, the student places an "X" in the box to indicate if that item possesses the characteristic. For example, if we wanted to expand the fish and whale comparisons used in the Venn diagram in Figure 6.3 to include other animals, such as humans and dogs, the matrix pictured in Figure 6.4 is one possibility.

	Characteristics							
Animal	**Swim**	**Breathe air with lungs**	**Have fins**	**Have a brain**	**Have a backbone**	**Warm blooded**	**Most lay eggs**	**Are mammals**
Fish	X		X	X	X		X	
Whales	X	X	X	X	X	X		X
Humans	X	X		X	X	X		X
Dogs	X	X		X	X	X		X

Figure 6.4 A comparison matrix of different characteristics belonging to several types of animals.

K-W-H-L Chart. This is an expansion of the more familiar K-W-L matrix in that it includes a step whereby the students identify how they plan to find out the needed information. The K-W-H-L chart's familiarity does not detract from its usefulness. Although it is more commonly used in elementary schools, it is an effective memory device at all grade levels (Figure 6.5). With this matrix, students plan and gather initial information on a topic or theme, identify primary and secondary resources they need to access, develop a plan for accessing resources, and identify the attributes and characteristics they will need to research.

The questions to ask when preparing to use a K-W-H-L chart are:

- What do we already know?
- What do we want to find out?
- How are we going to find out? What primary and secondary resources can we access?

- What attributes or characteristic should we focus on?
- What have we learned?

After reading the text and learning the material, the students go back to the "K" column to determine if any of their prior knowledge was inaccurate. They should note any of the statements that are inaccurate, according to the text, and rewrite them so that they are correct. Then they go to the "W" column and check any of their questions that the text did not answer. Students should be prepared to bring these unanswered questions up in class, or tell how they will find answers to them and where they will look to get the answers.

K	W	H	L
What do we **K**now?	What do we **W**ant to find out?	**H**ow can we find out what we need to learn?	What did we **L**earn?
Plants are living things.	What do plants need to live?	Biology books	Plants need sunlight, water, and nutrients to survive.
Many plants are green.	Why are plants green?	Biology books Internet search	Plants are green because they contain chlorophyll.
Some plants grow tall.	What are some plants that grow tall?	Internet search Field trips	Sunflowers and corn are plants that grow tall.
Some animals eat plants.	What do we call animals that eat just plants?	Biology books Encyclopedia	Animals that eat only plants are called herbivores.
Attributes we need to use: plant size, color, location			

Figure 6.5 This type of matrix takes advantage of the students' prior knowledge and encourages them to monitor their own learning. This example is a lesson on the characteristics of plants. (Adapted from Bender and Larkin, 2003)

Content Grids. This type of matrix helps students to think about and evaluate certain characteristics of people, places, events, and things. It may include making a decision about who was the bravest person in recent history, the best type of computer to buy, or the greatest environmental threat of the 21st century. Before beginning, the class should decide on the items to be included as well as the set of criteria that will be used to determine their decisions. Then they write in each block their judgment and rationale about how well or how poorly each item (person, place, thing, etc.) meets each criterion. Students can complete this matrix alone first and discuss their decisions later in groups, or they can complete the matrix together as part of a cooperative learning activity. Either way, the process leads students to higher-order thinking in that they must analyze and judge competing items against the same set of criteria. Figure 6.6 shows examples of different types of course content matrices.

Who Was the Bravest Leader in Recent History?				
	Fought against evil	Improved people's lives	Persistent	Trustworthy
Mahatma Ghandi				
Winston Churchill				
Franklin Roosevelt				

What Is the Greatest Environmental Threat of the 21st Century?				
	Economic impact	Number of people affected	Degree of danger	Length of danger
Ozone layer depletion				
Dumping toxic chemicals in the ground				
Global warming				
Acid rain				

Figure 6.6 These are two examples of content grids. The class must first decide on the items and criteria before filling in the matrix with their judgments and rationale.

Webs

Webs come in many varieties but they are generally used for brainstorming ideas about something that has been read and for solving problems in content areas. They are effective memory devices because they translate printed words into vivid visual images of relationships between items that the slower reader may not detect in the text. Brainstorming webs integrate the language components of the brain's left hemisphere with the visual and spatial talents of the right hemisphere—a "whole brain" approach that is important in learning and remembering. Creativity is also an essential component here because the brain's frontal lobe makes free associations and begins to build a holistic picture from seemingly isolated items. As the process continues, the brain reorganizes concepts into images that can be communicated to others. Thus, brainstorming webs are excellent discussion tools that stimulate higher-order thinking and processing.

Although brainstorming webs involve free associations, they are not unguided activities that just consume time, as some teachers think. Rather, the brainstorming process is always guided by specific questions, such as

- What is the topic to be brainstormed?
- Is the process of brainstorming clear?
- What should be the final product?

Brainstorming webs are usually made individually when a student is mapping out relationships that appear in the content reading. When working individually, students produce a wider range of ideas and patterns than when working in the group. They do not have to worry about other people's opinions and can therefore be more creative.

For problem solving, brainstorming in cooperative learning groups is very effective because it uses the brain power and experiences of everyone in the group. When individual members reach their limit on an idea, another member's background knowledge or experience may take the idea to another stage. In this manner, group brainstorming tends to produce web diagrams that include more subtle and deeper relationships. Figure 6.7 is an example of a web developed by a cooperative learning group based on some of the characteristics of vertebrates.

READING PATTERNS IN CONTENT AREAS

Recall from earlier chapters that the human brain seeks patterns in order to interpret its environment. This same pattern-seeking trait applies to reading content area material. As the brain reads content area text, such as science or social studies, it looks for patterns of thought that can be connected with past experience and comprehended. Each content areas is comprised of unique patterns of organized knowledge that the reader must identify in order to successfully understand that particular subject. When content area teachers clearly identify the types of patterns that students should be looking for when they read the subject text, they help their students establish the mind-set their brains need to make sense of the printed text. Here

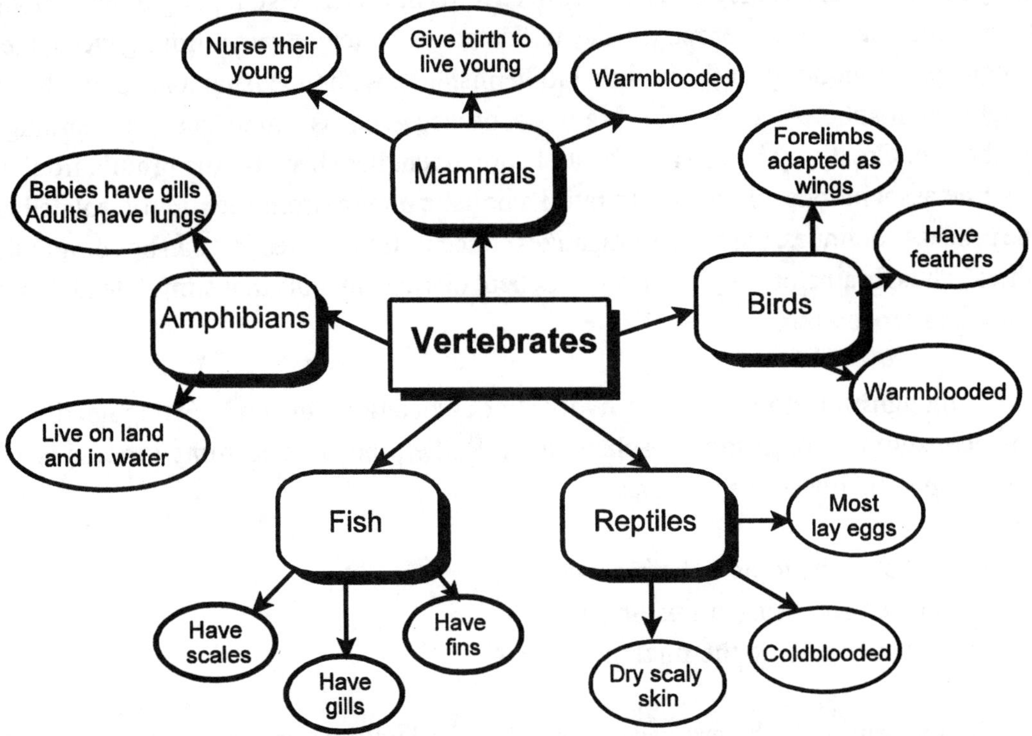

Figure 6.7 This web diagram depicts some of the characteristics of vertebrates. The web could be expanded by adding more characteristics and giving specific examples of each type.

are some of the patterns of organized knowledge that comprise some of the school's curriculum areas.

Art/Music/Drama

- Dialogue that describes, visualizes, and portrays actions
- Interpreting language through movement
- Readers' theatre to link oral and written language
- Role-playing to practice and interpret dialogue
- Understanding the perspective of the artist , composer, or writer

Literature

- Describing and visualizing the setting
- Character development of main and supporting characters, their authenticity and their relationships
- Distinguishing plot and episodes
- Understanding the literary piece's genre
- Discovering the moral, theme, or message

Mathematics

- Patterns and key words for solving word problems
- Symbolic relationships and operators
- Searching for evidence and reasoning
- Understanding graphic relationships

Science

- Types of classification
- Experimental procedures
- Cause and effect
- Steps in problem solving
- Definitions and explanations, with or without diagrams

Social Studies

- Definitions and explanations
- Cause and effect
- Chronological or sequential events
- Comparing and contrasting
- Distinguishing fact and opinion

Studies indicate that a large number of students of all ethnic backgrounds are functioning below grade level in their reading. This is a particularly difficult problem for students reading in the content areas where they are reading to acquire knowledge and skills in subjects such as mathematics, health, science, and social studies. In these subjects, the vocabulary used in the texts is often technical and written at a more difficult readability level. In this chapter, I have offered numerous tested strategies that could be used to aid these students in acquiring and understanding vocabulary, and in gaining a more accurate and deeper comprehension of the content they read. My hope is that teachers willing and determined to make "reading to learn" a successful experience for their students will consider adding these strategies to their repertoire.

Answer to Test Question # 9

Question: There is little that secondary school content area teachers can do to improve the comprehension skills of their students who are poor readers.

Answer: *False*. Content area teachers can use numerous tested strategies that aid poor readers in understanding vocabulary and in gaining a more accurate and deeper comprehension of the content they read.

What's Coming?

The next and last chapter looks at the basic components of a successful reading program. It summarizes what students need to know as they learn to read and what teachers need to do to make that process more successful for all students. The chapter also suggests professional development activities for teachers and school principals, presents some ways of closing the reading achievement gap, and discusses the importance of implementing action research in schools and classrooms.

CHAPTER 7
Putting It All Together

This chapter addresses several basic questions about what parents and educators can do to help more children learn to read successfully. They include:

- *What are the basics of a successful reading program?*
- *What do beginning readers need to learn?*
- *What do teachers need to know about teaching reading?*

THE BASICS OF A SUCCESSFUL READING PROGRAM

Surely by now it is clear that learning to read is no easy task. Unlike spoken language, there are no areas of the brain prewired for reading. Thus, there is no reason to consider reading to be a natural ability like speaking. Human beings have been talking for thousands of years, while reading is a relatively recent and quite artificial accomplishment. Toddlers seem to be preprogrammed to talk, and they usually learn to do so without formal instruction. On the other hand, the fact that large numbers of adults never do learn to read suggests that this ability is not in the same category.

Of course, some children learn to read with minimal instruction. These children, however, do not as a result read stories in a qualitatively different way from children taught via systematic phonics. The only difference seems to be that they have managed to crack the phonetic code on their own, without much teaching. How they learned the letter-sound correspondences seems to make no difference to the end result. Children who have become good readers though the whole-language approach have no advantage over children who have become good readers through systematic phonics. There is no harm in some children learning to read on their own. The problem is that the vast majority do not. Consequently, one of the major long-term goals of schools is to graduate students who are lifelong and highly competent readers.

Successfully achieving that long-term goal is not easy, because some barriers need to be overcome. These include teachers uninformed about the new understandings of how the brain learns to read, outdated materials for teaching reading, outdated methods for teaching reading, and the overemphasis on test scores. Moreover, to accomplish a long-term goal, short-term goals must first be achieved. I offer here some suggested short-term goals that I hope educators will consider. They are based on the current state of research on how we learn to read and on studies of effective instruction in reading.

Expose Teachers to Current Scientific Knowledge About How the Brain Learns to Read

During the past 10 years, research developments in neuroscience and cognitive psychology have added greatly to our understanding of how the brain learns to read and the nature of the problems that can arise during that process. We now know enough from this research to put many myths about reading to rest. We have a better idea which instructional strategies will increase the likelihood that more children can learn to read successfully. The research supports the continued use of some strategies while doubting the effectiveness of others. Armed with this knowledge, teachers can make better choices in reading programs and in their own instructional methods. That is the good news. The bad news is that the implications of this research for our practice are not getting to many classroom teachers fast enough. Nevertheless, teachers of early reading are aware that there is a growing body of newer research on reading, so word is slowly getting out.

One recent survey of nearly 550 kindergarten and first-grade teachers (Bursuck, Munk, Nelson, and Curran, 2002) was designed to examine their attitudes toward, and knowledge of, beginning reading practices that are research supported. Most teachers believed that many reading problems could be prevented with early intervention. On the other hand, teachers rated themselves low on their knowledge of effective literacy practices and on their ability to identify at-risk readers. Teachers are listening to the research but apparently need to be more involved in those teacher-training efforts that translate the research into effective classroom practices.

Teachers of reading must have access to the summaries of findings from a broad base of research on reading-related topics. They also need to recognize different types of studies. For example:

- *Experimental studies* provide generalizations that offer sound advice based on trends.
- *Correlational studies* usually provide reasoned hypotheses about how two variables can affect each other.
- *Case studies* help teachers consider new methods for instruction and assessment.

The responsibility of the school district is to engage teachers in ongoing study of the changing knowledge base produced by discoveries in scientific research on the reading process. Teachers need to be a vital part of the decision-making process in schools because it is through their work that children learn to read. With this approach, teachers recognize that teaching is not just an art form anymore; it is now a *science* and an art form. By staying abreast of scientific developments, they can make informed decisions and contribute to locally developed, scientifically-based programs of instruction and assessment in reading.

Teaching is not just an art form anymore; it is now a science and an art form.

Develop a Scientifically-Based Reading Program and Stick With It

The scientific evidence is clear: Learning to read successfully requires the ability to manipulate sounds into words, to break down words into their component sounds, and to match sounds with the letters that represent them. A scientifically-based reading program, therefore, will focus on developing phonological awareness, and then on to the more sophisticated phonemic awareness. Children need to know and recognize the alphabet in print and be able to match those letters with the sounds they represent. Mastering the alphabetic principle is essential to becoming a proficient reader, and instructional methods that explicitly teach this principle are more effective than those that do not. Learning phonics is especially important for children who are at risk for not learning to read. In addition to phonics instruction, using whole-language activities as a *supplement* helps to make reading enjoyable and meaningful. The reading program should emphasize vocabulary building, and the rules of grammar and syntax, and include activities that lead to reading fluency and comprehension.

Reading programs that overemphasize extensive and repetitive drills in phonics will bore students, and programs that overemphasize guessing how words sound and what they mean will be a source of frustration for students, especially those at risk of not learning to read. Phonological awareness, phonemic awareness, and the alphabetical principle should be taught in interesting and innovative ways, using a variety of materials. Usually, the program begins with coded texts to reinforce letter-sound correspondences. But teachers should select other high-interest sources of reading that maintain student attention and demonstrate that learning to read can be enjoyable.

Concerns about whether the technologically-centered toys that children play with today, including computers, will lessen their motivation to read are unfounded.

Concerns abound about whether the technologically-centered toys that children play with today, including computers, will lessen their motivation to read. The concerns are unfounded, because a major portion of computer interactions still involves reading and writing, and that will continue to be the case for the near future. Parents and teachers need to find ways of using the attraction of the technology to lure children into working with programs that will help them learn to read.

Once a program with these components has been developed or selected, stick with it. Too much energy, teacher good will, and resources are wasted when districts leap from one reading program to another, based on the latest political favorite or on which publisher has made the greatest offer. Consistency is essential if we expect the program to have a lasting impact on developing the reading skills of students in the early grades.

What Skills Should Be in Place by Grade 3?

Most researchers agree that reading skills have to be in place by the end of third grade if the student is to cope successfully with the increasing reading requirements of the ensuing grades. What reading skills should our students have acquired at that time to demonstrate that they can continue to progress as successful readers? Calfee and Norman (1998) suggest that by the end of third grade, students should acquire critical literacy, which includes the skill and will to use language in all its forms as well as to solve problems and communicate effectively. To do so, children need to

- Master the alphabetic principle
- Read fluently
- Understand what they are reading
- Have strategies to sound out unfamiliar words
- Be confident in spelling
- Read almost any book in the elementary school library
- Write almost anything that falls within the child's knowledge and experience
- Have an appetite for reading and writing

Offer Ongoing Professional Development That Includes Teaching Strategies Based on the New Research

Because all reading programs are not the same, teachers must be educated in how to evaluate the different programs to determine which ones are based on strong evidence. Preservice and inservice programs need to provide teachers with the training necessary to select, develop, and implement the most appropriate reading program. Systematic phonics instruction is a necessary and vital component of learning to read, but it is not the only component. A total reading program should include instruction in phonemic awareness, vocabulary development, fluency, and comprehension (NRP, 2000).

Beginning teachers are in extra need of inservice support. Too often their preservice courses did not provide them with sufficient knowledge and skills to help all children become successful readers. Studies of teacher preparation programs show that too little time is allocated to the teaching of reading and that there is wide variance in the content of these programs (NRP, 2000; Snow et al., 1998).

Every day teachers try to help students learn to read. For some children, learning to read comes quickly, usually because of exposure to frequent language experiences during the preschool years. But for other children, learning to read is a struggle, and this is when teachers really *do* make a difference. Recent studies bear this out. Torgesen and his colleagues (2001) conducted two separate studies of children with reading disabilities using the same instructional methods. However, the researchers found that the outcomes were different. The students in the study that used highly skilled and knowledgeable teachers with considerable experience in teaching showed the greater improvement in reading achievement compared to the other study that had largely inexperienced teachers with little understanding of scientifically-based methods.

> Teachers make a difference. Students of experienced teachers with knowledge of scientifically-based methods had higher reading achievement scores that students of inexperienced teachers.

When early literacy teachers do participate in training to learn about research-based practices, the results can be impressive. For example, Abbott and her colleagues implemented a three-year project designed to train kindergarten and first-grade teachers in phonemic

What Beginning Readers Need to Learn

- *Phonological awareness:* Rhyming, alliteration, deleting, and substituting sounds, sound patterns
- *Phonemic awareness:* Segmenting words into individual sounds, manipulating phonemes
- *Visual perception of letters:* Understanding the names of the letters of the alphabet and recognizing them in print
- *Alphabetic principle*: Correlating letter-sound patterns with specific text
- *Word recognition:* Learning words that occur most often in language and that are needed in writing
- *Orthographic awareness*: Understanding spelling rules and writing conventions
- *Syntax:* Understanding rules affecting the word order in phrases and sentences
- *Fluency in oral reading:* Rereading texts to develop fluency

awareness concepts (Abbott, Walton, and Greenwood, 2002). The training for kindergarten teachers included onset fluency, rapid letter naming, and phonemic segmentation fluency. For first-grade teachers, the training expanded on phonemic segmentation. Research procedures were translated into step-by-step classroom procedures with teacher input. Students of the kindergarten teachers trained in the research-into-practice program scored remarkably well on all three areas tested. These same students also made impressive gains in phoneme segmentation the following year in first grade.

Children who come to school with phonics skills already developed and who can apply them correctly do not need the same intensity and level of phonics instruction as children who are just beginning to learn to read. Professional development should help teachers assess the needs of individual children and tailor instruction to meet these needs.

Remember the Content Area Teachers

To some degree, all teachers are teachers of reading. Yet, we often overlook content area teachers when designing professional development programs to enhance reading instruction. Districts should provide meaningful training to content area teachers that includes simple yet effective strategies they can use to help their students better comprehend their content material (see Chapter 6 for suggested strategies).

Even modest training times can be effective. Ten middle school content area teachers participated in a four-month professional development program to enhance the reading outcomes of the struggling readers in their classrooms (Bryant et al., 2001). The professional development program examined the teachers' knowledge of reading instruction and reading difficulties, and the training helped the teachers integrate three reading strategies (word identification, fluency, and comprehension) into their content area instruction. At the conclusion of the study, three findings emerged:

1. Content area teachers were not cognizant of the reading difficulties their students had and were overwhelmed by these challenges.
2. The content area teachers welcomed the inservice training on the comprehension strategies, insisted on substantial modeling, engaged in biweekly support meetings, and took time in class to implement the strategies.
3. Teachers saw positive effects from the strategies through improvements in vocabulary decoding and use, reading comprehension, and graph interpretations.

Middle school is the last chance for struggling readers to get the support they need in reading to learn. Content area teachers at this level who are knowledgeable in how to use research-based interventions can have a major impact on the reading success of their students.

Teach Reading Through the Students' Strengths

Difficulties with reading frequently mask a student's strengths in other cognitive areas. Because struggling readers have problems with their phonologic module's ability to interpret the meaning of individual words, they will miss details in the text. Furthermore, they have difficulty remembering extended lists of unfamiliar words long enough to comprehend complex sentences. You will recall from Chapter 3 that dyslexics deal with this situation by calling upon their brain's right frontal lobe during reading to interpret the overall meaning of a passage. Consequently, the dyslexic students' reliance on the right frontal lobe develops other cognitive strengths, such as creativity, problem solving, critical thinking, concept formation, and reasoning (Shaywitz, 2003).

Difficulties with reading frequently mask a student's strengths in other cognitive areas.

Although overall cognitive ability may not influence the acquisition of phonemic awareness or of understanding phonics, reasoning and verbal skills can help dyslexic children and other struggling readers comprehend what they are reading. By using their bank of vocabulary words, personal experiences, and other knowledge, these students can use their cognitive skills to identify unfamiliar words in text. Teachers can work with these students to

What Teachers Need to Know About Teaching Reading

- How the brain learns to read
- The relationship between spoken language and reading
- How to provide direct instruction in phonics
- How to provide direct instruction in the alphabetic principle
- The relationship between phonology and morphology in relation to spelling
- How to diagnose spelling and reading skills
- How to use strategies that help students gain fluency
- How to help students understand the rules of syntax
- The dependence of reading comprehension on other aspects of reading and on language skills
- Procedures for ongoing in-class assessment of children's reading abilities
- How to modify instructional strategies based on in-class assessments
- Understanding the needs of students with disabilities and those with limited English proficiency
- How to use a variety of reading intervention strategies to address different learning styles and cultures
- How to apply research judiciously to their practice and how to update their knowledge base

expose them to opportunities that bolster their strengths through enhancing their vocabularies, expanding their storehouse of knowledge, and enriching their worldly experiences. This approach allows students with reading difficulties to use their other strengths to overcome their phonological weakness.

Offer Professional Development in Reading to Building Principals

Principals are the instructional leaders of their school. They need to become familiar with the latest scientific research on reading. Learning to read is far too important a goal to be left to discretionary programs and individual teacher decisions about what approach to take. The challenge for the principal is to maintain consistency of instruction while still encouraging the unique contributions of teachers. In the end, however, principals must insist that the district select a scientifically-based reading program, ensure that all teachers of beginning reading follow it, and stress the development of phonological awareness.

Effective reading instruction in kindergarten and the primary grades should be one of the principal's top priorities. Below is a brief survey that may help principals and teachers determine the extent to which the school's reading program is meeting the needs of all children. (For a much more comprehensive program evaluation survey, see Simmons and Kame'enui, 2003.)

Components of Our Reading Program

Directions: Circle the number that most closely describes the extent to which a component is present in your school's reading program. When finished, connect the circles with straight lines to get a profile of your reading program. Add up the values of the circled numbers (highest score is 63). Discuss the importance of any individual component that receives a score of 1.

Component	Little or None 1	Some 2	Significant 3
Program is research based	1	2	3
Teachers have been trained in research-based strategies related to the program	1	2	3
Emphasis on phonemic awareness	1	2	3
Systematic instruction and practice in phonics	1	2	3
Systematic instruction in the alphabetic principle	1	2	3
Activities and practice to enhance word decoding	1	2	3

Component	Little or None 1	Some 2	Significant 3
Activities and practice on word recognition	1	2	3
Activities and practice on semantics	1	2	3
Activities and practice on syntax	1	2	3
Writing activities are coordinated with reading instruction	1	2	3
Activities for building vocabulary growth	1	2	3
Strategies that use morphology to build spelling skills and enhance vocabulary growth	1	2	3
Instructional practices develop the children's ability to monitor their reading comprehension	1	2	3
Activities for improving reading fluency	1	2	3
Activities for improving reading comprehension	1	2	3
Strategies for improving content area reading	1	2	3
Inservice opportunities connected to the program	1	2	3
Other literature sources are integrated into the program	1	2	3
Instructional practices in middle grades build on reading and literacy growth in the primary grades	1	2	3
Interventions for helping teachers diagnose and address reading difficulties	1	2	3
Constructive communication about the program is maintained with parents	1	2	3

When you have completed the chart, add up the values of the circled numbers to get a total score. The highest possible score is 63. Take a close look at any component with a score of 1. Why is that the case? What can you do about it?

Working With Parents and Students

Principals provide a great community service when they talk to parents of newborns and alert them to the importance of the early preschool years in developing a child's literacy. Given the evidence that the brain's ability to acquire spoken language is at its peak in the early years, parents should create a rich environment that includes lots of communication activities, such as talking, singing, and reading aloud. In schools, this means addressing any language-learning problems quickly to take advantage of the brain's ability to rewire improper connections during this important period of growth. It also means that parents and teachers should not assume that children with language-learning problems are going to be limited in cognitive thought processes as well.

Principals can also ensure that the school's reading program will help students associate reading with pleasure. For readers having difficulties, principals can develop a library of specially recorded books that have a slow pace, clear phrasing, and small amounts of material per tape side. Struggling readers need to listen to the audiotape and to follow along.

Close the Achievement Gap in Reading

We hear a lot these days about closing the achievement gap between low-income and minority children, and other students. Despite the continuing concern, money, and effort, the gap in reading scores refuses to narrow. What causes this unfortunate situation depends on who you ask. Adults often say these students achieve poorly because they don't eat breakfast, they are too poor, their parents don't care, and they don't have any books at home. This focuses blame on the children and their families. But talking with students often produces different reasons. They talk about teachers who are not qualified in what they are teaching, about counselors who underestimate their potential, about principals who dismiss their concerns, and of a curriculum that is boring and irrelevant to their needs.

No one argues that issues like poverty, family stability, and home environment do not matter, because clearly they do. But if educators assume that unfortunate social and economic conditions will affect how *much* a child learns, then we end up not challenging the child. As a result, these students become the object of a self-fulfilling prophesy: We expect less of them, so we give them less, and they produce less in return.

Educators are not usually able to change what happens to children outside of school, but they can ensure that what happens *in school* really matters. Closing the achievement gap, in my opinion, requires concerted effort in four areas.

- *Establish and maintain high standards, and expect all students to meet them.* People rise and fall to the level of expectations we set for them. Too often in high-poverty schools there is little expectation that students can meet the reading standards. We misinterpret their lack of literacy as an inability to acquire literacy. Schools must be clearly committed to the notion that standards are for everyone and that everyone *can* reach them with appropriate instruction and, if needed, systematic interventions.

- *Design a challenging reading curriculum that is aligned with the standards.* Assume that all students can learn phonemic awareness and the alphabetic principle, although some students may take longer. Keep the practice consistent and challenging and introduce interesting literature as appropriate to enhance comprehension.

- *Provide systematic research-based additional help for struggling readers.* Many schools have programs, such as Title 1, designed to offer additional help in reading and mathematics. But these sessions can subject the students to more of the same outdated strategies that did not work in their regular classrooms. For some children, the school day just does not provide enough time to include the activities they need to catch up. More effort should be made to provide help through an extended school day, on weekends, before school, during vacation periods, and in the summer. Districts that have implemented these extended instructional times for struggling readers are reporting significant improvements in reading achievement.

- *Ensure that teachers thoroughly know the subjects they are teaching.* In many states, more than 20 percent of middle school and high school teachers are teaching outside their areas of college study (NCES, 2002). That number increases dramatically in high-poverty schools because fully-qualified teachers often find those positions less desirable and succeed in avoiding them. Numerous research studies over decades have shown that the classroom teacher remains the single greatest factor that determines most students' success in learning. As I have stated in my earlier books, the quality of learning rarely exceeds the quality of teaching. When we have fully-qualified teachers with high expectations and an updated knowledge base of how to teach reading, we can make great headway in closing the reading achievement gap.

The quality of learning rarely exceeds the quality of teaching.

Encourage Teachers to Be Researchers

Teachers cannot be mere consumers of the knowledge emerging from scientific research. They must position themselves as active participants in the research community. One way to do this is through action research. Action research gives the practitioner a chance to be a researcher and to investigate specific problems that affect teaching and learning. Unlike traditional education research, where teachers are studied by outsiders, action research is conducted by teachers themselves to study their own classroom practices. It is a systematic investigation into some aspect of the school pursued by educators out of a desire to improve what they do. Action research expands the role of a teacher as an inquirer into teaching and learning through systematic classroom research.

> Action research expands the role of the teacher as an inquirer into teaching and learning through systematic research.

Teachers of reading can test whether a particular strategy they want to use is effective by trying it with some students and not with others. By setting up a small research project in the classroom, teachers can determine how well the students using the strategy (test group) learned compared with those that did not use the strategy (control group).

Action research is well suited to schools because of its democratic methodology, inclusiveness, flexibility of approach, and potential for changing practice. Action research uses a solution-oriented approach that is characterized by cycles (Figure 7.1) of

- Identifying the problem ("Will this strategy be more effective than other ones I have used?")
- Systematically collecting data ("How will I know if it worked?")
- Analyzing the data ("Did it improve their learning? How?")
- Taking action on the data ("What changes should I make?")
- Redefining the problem, if necessary ("Is there something else I should try?")
- Sharing the results with colleagues

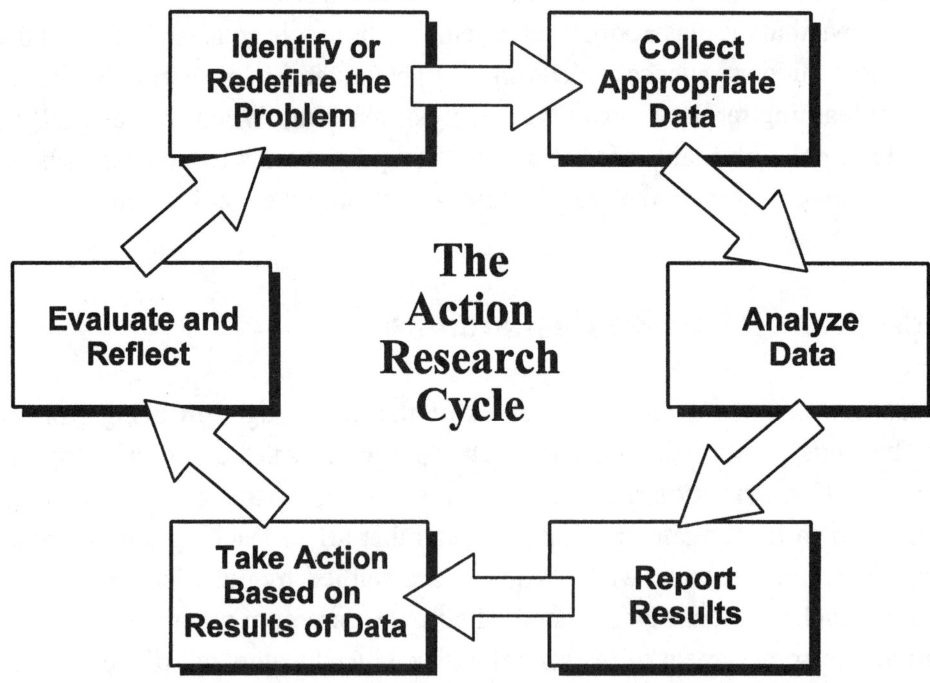

Figure 7.1 The diagram illustrates the six steps in the action research cycle, starting with identifying or redefining the problem.

Because the teacher who is responsible for implementing changes also does the research, a real fit is created between the needs of a specific learner and the action taken. Teachers of reading should understand that their own honing of proven instructional strategies through reflection and systematic monitoring of their students' progress is a critical component of a scientifically-based reading program. Action research provides a means to that end.

Action research also provides teachers with opportunities to gain knowledge and skills in research methods and applications and to become more aware of the possibilities and options for change. Teachers using action research are likely to be receptive and supportive of systemic changes that school leaders may be seeking. We teach our students that inquiry is a tool of scientists. By engaging in action research, teachers extend their knowledge of reading instruction through inquiry. They carefully observe, generate and test hypotheses, collect data, and draw conclusions based on evidence that are shared with other reading teachers and researchers.

CONCLUSION

One point I have made in this book is that teaching children to read is not an easy task. This is especially true in the typical primary classroom where teachers welcome children from an ever-increasing variety of home situations, cultures, and native languages. Given these variables, successful teachers of reading are flexible rather than rigid in their approach, and they know through experience what they need to do to make learning to read exciting and meaningful. They also acknowledge that the findings of scientific studies are clear: explicit instruction in phonemic awareness is essential because it helps the beginning reader understand the alphabetic principle and apply it to reading and writing. Enriched text complements this process to provide relevant and enjoyable reading experiences.

This balanced approach avoids the seemingly endless reading wars and recognizes that learning to read and write are complex activities requiring at least seven levels of brain processing that must eventually be integrated:

- Phonological - knowing the sound system of language, phonemic awareness, and sound-letter correspondences
- Graphic - visually perceiving letters and symbols
- Lexical - recognizing words and their component parts, such as prefixes and suffixes
- Syntactic - understanding rules of grammar and discourse
- Semantic - comprehending meaning and detecting thematic structures
- Communicative - expressing purposes and intentions
- Cultural - communicating shared beliefs and knowledge

Effective reading programs and reading teachers should address all these levels of processing because each level supports the others. At the same time, children must be encouraged to use all the resources available to them in their efforts to decode, comprehend, and compose text. During this process, teachers need to have the skills to quickly recognize reading problems that arise and be able to select tested strategies to help students overcome those problems. Studies show that effective classroom instruction alone can reduce reading failure to about 6 percent (Foorman et al., 1998).

Researchers recently reported that effective classroom instruction coupled with targeted small-group instruction reduced the proportion of students with IQs of 77 to122 who were performing below the 30th percentile in early reading skills to less than 2 percent (Denton and Mathes, 2003; Torgesen, 2002, 2004). The importance of quality professional development became clear when studies of nearly 4,900 children in high-poverty schools found reading improvement to be significantly related to professional development within a coaching and mentoring model in the classroom, irrespective of the reading method used (Foorman and Moats, 2004; Moats and Foorman, 2003). There is little doubt that the knowledge, strength, and sophistication of the teacher is what really matters in helping children learn to read successfully. It is to that end that this book was written, and it is my hope that teachers and parents who read it will feel more empowered to help their children gain the literacy skills they need to be productive citizens of the world.

There is little doubt that the knowledge, strength, and sophistication of the teacher is what really matters in helping children learn to read successfully.

Glossary

Acoustic analysis. The process that separates relevant word sounds from background noise, decodes the phonemes of the word, and translates them into a phonological code that can be recognized by the mental lexicon.

Affix. Letters attached to the beginning (prefix) or end (suffix) of a word.

Alphabetic principle. The understanding that spoken words can be broken down into phonemes, and that written letters represent the phonemes of spoken language.

Aphasia. The impairment or loss of language abilities following damage to the brain.

Automaticity. The instant decoding of letters (and other stimuli), such that the brain processing involved in the decoding process is automatic.

Balanced approach. An approach that advocates the incorporation of both phonics instruction and enriched text to teach beginning readers.

Blending. Combining the phonemes of a spoken word into a whole word, as in blending */d/ /o/ /g/* into *dog.*

Blocking. A linguistic principle that prevents a rule from applying to a word that already has an irregular form, such as the existence of *stood* blocks a rule from adding *-ed* to *stand,* thus preempting *standed.*

Broca's area. A region of the brain located behind the left temple that is associated with speech production, including vocabulary, syntax, and grammar.

Chunking. The ability of the brain to perceive a coherent group of items as a single item or chunk.

Collaborative strategic reading (CSR). A technique to improve reading comprehension by using heterogeneous groups in multilevel classes.

Comprehension. The ability to understand and attribute meaning to what is heard or read.

Content area reading. Reading in curriculum areas where students learn course content, such as facts and concepts, rather than learning skills.

Corpus callosum. The bridge of nerve fibers that connects the left and right cerebral hemispheres and allows communication between them.

Decoding. The ability to use the alphabetic principle to sound out a word by recognizing which phonemes are represented by the letters, and then blending those phonemes into a legitimate word.

Deep orthography. A language writing system, such as English, which does not have a one-to-one correspondence between the spoken phonemes and the letters that represent them. The same phoneme can be represented by different letters in words.

Digraph. A phoneme consisting of two successive letters that is pronounced as a single sound, as the *-ea* in *clean,* the *ch-* in *child,* or the *-ng* in *song.*

Dyslexia. A persistent developmental problem in learning to read. In 2002, the International Dyslexia Association adopted the following definition: "Dyslexia is a specific learning disability that is neurobiological in origin. It is characterized by difficulties with accurate and/or fluent word recognition and by poor spelling and decoding abilities. These difficulties typically result from a deficit in the phonological component of language that is often unexpected in relation to other cognitive abilities and the provision of effective classroom instruction. Secondary consequences may include problems in reading comprehension and reduced reading experience that can impede growth of vocabulary and background knowledge."

Event-related potential (ERP). An electrical signal emitted by the brain in response to a stimulus such as a picture or a word. The signals are detected by electrodes pasted to the scalp.

Fixation. The period of time when our eyes stop after making rapid movements across the page during reading. It is during these fixations of about 200 to 250 milliseconds that the eyes actually acquire information from the text.

Frontal lobe. The front part of the brain that monitors higher-order thinking, directs problem solving, and regulates the excesses of the emotional system.

Functional magnetic resonance imaging (fMRI). A process that measures blood flow to the brain to record areas of high and low neural activity.

Gist. An interpretation and mental representation of the meaning of a phrase, sentence, paragraph, passage, and so on.

Grapheme. The smallest part of written language that represents a single phoneme in the spelling of a word. A grapheme may be just one letter, such as *b, d, g,* and *s,* or several letters, as in *ck, sh, igh,* and *th.*

Immediate memory. A temporary memory where information is processed briefly (in seconds) and subconsciously, then either blocked or passed on to working memory.

Invented spelling. The creation of plausible spellings of real words using one's knowledge of letter names and sounds.

Lexicon. A person's mental dictionary consisting of words and their meanings.

Long-term storage. The areas of the brain where memories are stored permanently.

Millisecond (ms). A unit of time that represents one one-thousandth of a second.

Morpheme. The smallest units into which words can be cut that have meaning, as in *un-in-habit-able* (four morphemes).

Morphology. The component of grammar that studies how words are built from pieces called morphemes, and that affixes change the meaning of words in predictable ways.

Magnetic resonance imaging(MRI). A process that uses radio waves to disturb the alignment of the body's atoms in a magnetic field to produce computer-processed, high-contrast images of internal structures.

Nonword. A string of letters that cannot be pronounced and that have no meaning, such as *ndwsb* or *tgzaq*.

Occipito-temporal area. The area of the brain that overlaps portions of the occipital and temporal lobes where all the important information about a word is stored, including its spelling, pronunciation, and meaning.

Onset. The initial consonant sound of a syllable, such as the *t-* sound in *tag,* or the *sw-* sound in *swim.*

Oral reading accuracy. This is calculated by subtracting the number of word errors during reading (not counting repetitions or self-corrected errors) from the total number of words read, and dividing that result by the total number of words. The resulting decimal is multiplied by 100 to yield a percentage.

Oral reading fluency. Also known as **words correct per minute,** this measure is calculated by subtracting the number of word errors during one minute of reading (not counting repetitions or self-corrected errors) from the total number of words read.

Orthography. The written system that describes a spoken language. Spelling and punctuation represent the orthographic features of written English.

Overlearning. The ability to perform a task with little attention or conscious thought.

Parieto-temporal area. The area of the brain that overlaps portions of the parietal and temporal lobes where word analysis is thought to occur during reading.

Positron emission tomography (PET). A process that traces the metabolism of radioactively-tagged sugar in brain tissue, producing a color image of cell activity.

Phoneme. The smallest units of sound that make up a spoken language. For example, the word *go* has two phonemes, *guh* and *oh.* The English language has about 44 phonemes. Some phonemes are represented by more than one letter.

Phonemic awareness. The ability to hear, identify, and manipulate phonemes in spoken syllables and words.

Phonics. The understanding that there is a predictable relationship between the sounds of *spoken* language (phonemes) and the letters that represent those sound in *written* language (graphemes).

Phonologic memory. The ability to retain verbal bits of information (phonemes) in working memory.

Phonological awareness. In addition to phonemic awareness, it includes the ability to recognize that sentences are comprised of words, words are comprised of syllables, and syllables are comprised of onsets and rimes that can be broken down into phonemes.

Phonology. The component of grammar that studies the sound patterns of a language, including how phonemes are combined to form words, as well as patterns of timing, stress, and intonation.

Prosody. The rhythm, cadence, accent patterns, and pitch of a language.

Pseudoword. A string of letters that can be pronounced but has no meaning (also called nonsense or invented words), such as *gebin* or *splor.*

Regression. The movement of the eyes backwards over a written line to re-read text.

Rehearsal. The reprocessing of information in working memory.

Rime. A part of a syllable that contains the vowel and all that follows it, as the *-ag* sound in *tag* or the *-im* sound in *swim.*

Schema theory. This theory suggests that mental structures resulting from our experiences help us interpret and predict new situations.

Semantics. The study of how meaning is derived from words and other text forms.

Shallow orthography. A language writing system, such as Spanish or Finnish, that has a consistent correspondence between the spoken phonemes and the letters that represent those phonemes in writing.

Silent sustained reading (SSR). A strategy in which students are assigned to do silent reading for a specified number of minutes each day. Its effectiveness has not been proved.

Syllable. A word part that contains a vowel or vowel sound pronounced as a unit: *speak-er, a-lone.*

Syntax. The rules and conventions that govern the order of words in phrases, clauses, and sentences.

Wernicke's area. The region of the brain, usually located in the left hemisphere, thought to be responsible for sense and meaning in one's native language.

Whole-language. An approach to reading instruction that emphasizes the recognition of words as wholes and de-emphasizes letter-sound relationships.

Word-blindness. The inability to read words even when a person's eyes are optically normal.

Word form. The neural model that encompasses the spelling, pronunciation, and meaning of a word.

Working memory. The temporary memory of limited capacity where information is processed consciously.

References

Abbott, M., Walton, C., and Greenwood, C. R. (2002). Phonemic awareness in kindergarten and first grade. *Teaching Exceptional Children, 34,* 20-26.

Ahmed, S. T., and Lombardino, L. J. (2000). Invented spelling: An assessment and intervention protocol for kindergarten children. *Communication Disorders Quarterly, 22,* 19-28.

Allington, R. L., and Woodside-Jiron, H. (1998). Decodable text in beginning reading: Are mandates and policy based on research? *ERS Spectrum, 16,* 3-11.

Amitay, S., Ben-Yehudah, G., Banai, K., and Ahissar, M. (2002). Disabled readers suffer from visual and auditory impairments but not from a specific magnocellular deficit. *Brain, 125,* 2272-2285.

Anglin, J. M. (1993). Vocabulary development: A morphological analysis. *Monographs of the Society for Research in Child Development, 58,* 10.

Armbruster, B. (1996). Schema theory and the design of content-area textbooks. *Educational Psychologist, 21,* 253-276.

Aylward, E., Richards, T., Berninger, V., Nagy, W., Field, K., Grimme, A., Richards, A., Thomson, J., and Cramer, S. C. (2003). *Instructional treatment associated with changes in brain activation in children with dyslexia.* Paper presented at the conference of the Organization for Human Brain Mapping, June, 2003, New York, NY.

Baer, G. T., and Nourie, B. L. (1993). Strategies for teaching reading in the content areas. *The Clearing House, 67,* 121-122.

Bailey, G. (1993). A perspective on African-American English. In D. Preston (Ed.), *American dialect research* (pp. 287-318). Philadelphia: Benjamins.

Beaton, A. (1997). The relation of planum temporale asymmetry and morphology of the corpus callosum to handedness, gender, and dyslexia: A review of the evidence. *Brain and Language, 60,* 255-322.

Beatty, J. (2001). *The human brain: Essentials of behavioral neuroscience.* Thousand Oaks, CA: Sage Publications.

Bender, W. N., and Larkin, M. J. (2003). *Reading strategies for elementary students with learning difficulties.* Thousand Oaks, CA: Corwin Press.

Berninger, V. W., Vaughan, K., Abbott, R., Abbott, S., Rogan, L., Brooks, A., et al. (1997). Treatment of handwriting problems in beginning writers: Transfer from handwriting to composition. *Journal of Educational Psychology, 89,* 652-666.

Bischoff-Grethe, A., Proper, S. M., Mao, H., Daniels, K. A., and Berns, G. S. (2000). Conscious and unconscious processing of nonverbal predictability in Wernicke's area. *Journal of Neuroscience, 20,* 1975-81.

Bolton, F., and Snowball, D. (1993). *Ideas for spelling.* Portsmouth, NH: Heinemann.

Brady, S., and Moats, L. (1997). *Informed instruction for reading success: Foundations for teacher preparation.* Baltimore, MD: International Dyslexia Association.

Brady, S. and Moats, L. (1998). Buy books, teach reading. *The California Reader, 31,* 6-10.

Brown, R., Pressley, M., Van Meter, P., and Schuder, T. (1996). A quasi-experimental validation of transactional strategies instruction with low-achieving second grade readers. *Journal of Educational Psychology, 88,* 18-37.

Brown, W. E., Eliez, S., Menon, V., Rumsey, J. M., White, C. D., and Reiss, A. L. (2001). Preliminary evidence of widespread morphological variations of the brain in dyslexia. *Neurology, 27,* 781-783.

Brun, M., Bouvard, M., Chateil, J., Bénichou, G., Bordessoules, M., and Allard, M. (2003). *Phonological treatment in dyslexic children: Neural network in fMRI.* Paper presented at the conference of the Organization for Human Brain Mapping, June, 2003, New York, NY.

Bryant, D. P., Linan-Thompson, S., Ugel, N., Hamff, A., and Hougen, M. (2001). The effects of professional development for middle school general and special education teachers on implementation of reading strategies in inclusive content area classes. *Learning Disabilities Quarterly, 24,* 251-264.

Burdette, J. H., Hairston, W. D., Flowers, D. L., and Wallace, M. T. (2003). *Cross-modal temporal integration in developmental dyslexia.* Paper presented at the Annual Conference of the Society for Neuroscience, November 8, 2003, New Orleans, LA.

Burnham, D., Kitamura, C., and Vollmer-Conna, U. (2002). What's new pussycat? On talking to babies and animals. *Science, 296,* 1435.

Bursuck, W. D., Munk, D. D., Nelson, C., and Curran, M. (2002, Fall). Research on the prevention of reading problems: Are kindergarten and first grade teachers listening? *Preventing School Failure,47,* 4-9.

Byrne, B. (1991). Experimental analysis of the child's discovery of the alphabetic principle. In L. Riehen and C. Perfetti (Eds.), *Learning to read: Basic research and its implications* (pp. 75-84). Hillsdale, NJ: Erlbaum.

Calderón, M., Hertz-Lazarowitz, R., and Slavin, R. (1998). Effects of Bilingual Cooperative Integrated Reading and Composition on students making the transition from Spanish to English reading. *The Elementary School Journal, 99,* 153-166.

Calderón, M., and Minaya-Rowe, L. (2003). *Designing and implementing two-way bilingual programs.* Thousand Oaks, CA: Corwin Press.

Calfee, R. C., and Norman, K. A. (1998). Psychological perspectives on the early reading wars: The case of phonological awareness. *Teachers College Record, 100,* 242-274.

Camilli, G., and Wolfe, P. (2004, March). Research on reading: A cautionary tale. *Educational Leadership, 61,* 26-29.

Carbo, M. (2003, September). How principals can do it all in reading — Part III. *TEPSA Instructional Leader, 16,* 1-3.

Carnine, D. W., Silbert, J., and Kame'enui, E. J. (1997). *Direct instruction reading.* Upper Saddle River, NJ: Prentice Hall.

Chang, K., Sung, Y., and Chen, I. (2002). The effect of concept mapping to enhance text comprehension and summarization. *Journal of Experimental Education, 71,* 5-23.

Chard, D. J., and Dickson, S.V. (1999, May). Phonological awareness: Instructional and assessment guidelines. *Intervention in School and Clinic, 34,* 261-270.

Chard, D. J., and Osborn, J. (1998). *Suggestions for examining phonics and decoding instruction in supplementary reading programs.* Austin, TX: Texas Education Agency.

Cheour, M., Ceponiene, R., Lehtokoski, A., Luuk, A., Allik, J., Alho, K., & Näätänen, R. (1998, September). Development of language-specific phoneme representations in the infant brain. *Nature Neuroscience, 1,* 351–353.

Chmielewski, T., and Dansereau, D. F. (1998). Enhancing the recall of text: Knowledge mapping training promotes implicit transfer. *Journal of Educational Psychology, 90,* 407-413.

Chomsky, C. (1979). Approaching reading through invented spelling. In L. Resnick and P. Weaver (Eds.), *Theory and practice of early reading* (Vol. 2, pp. 43-65). Hillsdale, NJ: Erlbaum.

Cibrowski, J. (1993). *Textbooks and students who can't read them.* Cambridge, MA: Brookline Books.

Cole, P. G., and Mengler, E. D. (1994). Phonemic processing of children with language deficits: Which tasks best discriminate children with learning disabilities from average readers? *Reading Psychology, 15,* 223-243.

Coles, G. (2004). Danger in the classroom: "Brain glitch" research and learning to read. *Phi Delta Kappan, 85,* 344-351.

Collins, A. M. and Loftus, E. F. (1975). A spreading-activation theory of semantic processing. *Psychological Review, 82,* 407-428.

Cooper, G. (Ed.) (1987). *Red tape holds up bridge, and more flubs from the nation's press.* New York: Perigee Books.

Coyne, M. D., Kame'enui, E. J., and Simmons, D. C. (2001). Prevention and intervention in beginning reading: Two complex systems. *Learning Disabilities Research and Practice, 16,* 62-73.

Cunningham, A. E., and Stanovich, K. E. (1997). Early reading acquisition and its relation to reading experience and ability. *Developmental Psychology, 33,* 934-945.

Cunningham, A. E., and Stanovich, K. E. (1998, Spring/Summer). What reading does for the mind. *American Educator,* pp. 8-17.

Damasio, H., Grabowski, T. J., Tranel, D., Hichwa, R. D., and Damasio, A. (1996). A neural basis for lexical retrieval. *Nature, 380,* 499-505.

Dapretto, M., and Bookheimer, S. Y. (1999). Form and content: Dissociating syntax and semantics in sentence comprehension. *Neuron, 2,* 427.

Dehaene-Lambertz, G. (2000). Cerebral specialization for speech and non-speech stimuli in infants. *Journal of Cognitive Neuroscience, 12,* 449-460.

Demb, J. B., Boynton, G. M., and Heeger, D. J. (1998). Functional magnetic resonance imaging of early visual pathways in dyslexia. *Journal of Neuroscience, 18,* 6939-6951.

Denton, C. A., and Mathes, P. G. (2003). Intervention for struggling readers: Possibilities and challenges. In B. Foorman (Ed.), *Preventing and remediating reading difficulties.* Baltimore, MD: York Press.

Deshler, D.D., Ellis, E.S., and Lenz, B.K. (1996). *Teaching adolescents with learning disabilities: Strategies and methods.* Denver, CO: Love Publishing.

Driscoll, M. (1994). *Psychology of learning for instruction.* Boston: Allyn and Bacon.

Dyslexia International – Tools and Technology (DITT). (2001). *Language shock – Dyslexia across cultures.* Brussels: Author.

Eckert, M. M., Leonard, C. M., Richards, T. L., Aylward, E. H., Thomson, J., and Berninger, V. W. (2003). Anatomical correlates of dyslexia: Frontal and cerebellar findings. *Brain, 126,* 482-494.

Edelen-Smith, P.J. (1998). How now brown cow: Phoneme awareness activities for collaborative classrooms. *Intervention in School and Clinic, 33,* 103-111.

Ehri, L. (1998). Grapheme-phoneme knowledge is essential for learning to read words in English. In J. Metsala and L. Ehri (Eds.), *Word recognition in beginning literacy* (pp.3-40). Mahwah, NJ: Erlbaum.

Ehri, L., Shanahan, T., and Nunes, S. (2002). Response to Krashen. *Reading Research Quarterly, 37,* 128-129.

Ellis, E. S. (1998). *The framing routine.* Tuscaloosa, AL: Masterminds.

Escamilla, K. (1994). Descubriendo la Lectura: An early intervention literacy program in Spanish. *Literacy, Teaching, and Learning, 1,* 57-70.

Fisher, S. E., and DeFries, J. C. (2002). Developmental dyslexia: Genetic dissection of a complex cognitive trait. *Nature Reviews Neuroscience, 30,* 767-780.

Fisk, C., and Hurst, B. (2003). Paraphrasing for comprehension. *The Reading Teacher, 57,* 182-185.

Fitzgerald, J., and Noblit, G. (2000). Balance in the making: Learning to read in an ethically diverse first-grade classroom. *Journal of Educational Psychology, 92,* 3-22.

Foorman, B. R., Francis, D. J., Fletcher, J. M., Schatschneider, C., and Mehta, P. (1998). The role of instruction in learning to read: Preventing reading failure in at-risk children. *Journal of Educational Psychology, 90,* 37-55.

Foorman, B. R., and Moats, L. C. (2004). Conditions for sustaining research-based practices in early reading instruction. *Remedial and Special Education, 25,* 51-60.

Francis, N., and Kucera, H. (1982). *Frequency analysis of English usage: Lexicon and grammar.* Boston: Houghton Mifflin.

Galuske, R. A. W., Schlote, W., Bratzke, H., and Singer, W. (2000). Interhemispheric asymmetries of the modular structure in human temporal cortex. *Science, 289,* 1946-1949.

Gazzaniga, M. S. (1998). *The mind's past.* Berkeley, CA: University of California Press.

Gazzaniga, M. S., Ivry, R. B., and Mangun, G. R. (2002). *Cognitive neuroscience: The biology of the mind* (2nd ed.). New York: Norton.

Gernsbacher, M. A. (1990). *Language comprehension as structure building.* Hillsdale, NJ: Erlbaum.

Goldberg, E. (2001). *The executive brain: Frontal lobes and the civilized mind.* New York: Oxford University Press.

Gough, P. B., and Juel, C. (1991). The first stages of word recognition. In L. Rieben and C. A. Perfetti (Eds.), *Learning to read: Basic research and its implications* (pp. 47-56). Hillsdale, NJ: Erlbaum.

Graham, S., Harris, K. R., and Fink, B. (2000). Is handwriting causally related to learning to write? Treatment of handwriting problems in beginning writers. *Journal of Educational Psychology, 92,* 620-633.

Gunn, B., Biglan, A., Smolkowski, K., and Ary, D. (2000). The efficacy of supplemental instruction in decoding skills for Hispanic and non-Hispanic students in early elementary school. *The Journal of Special Education, 34,* 90-103.

Habib, M. (2003). Rewiring the dyslexic brain. *Trends in Cognitive Science, 7,* 330-333.

Hanushuk, E. A., Kain, J. F., and Rivkin, S. G. (1998). Does special education raise academic achievement for students with disabilities? *National Bureau of Economic Research,* Working Paper No. 6690, Cambridge, MA.

Harm, M. W., and Seidenberg, M. S. (1999). Phonology, reading acquisition, and dyslexia: Insights from connectionist models. *Psychological Review, 106,* 491-528.

Hart, B, and Risley, T. R. (2003). The early catastrophe: The 30 million word gap by age 3. *American Educator, 27,* 4-9.

Hart, E. R. and Speece, D. L. (1998). Reciprocal teaching goes to college: Effects of postsecondary students at risk for academic failure. *Journal of Educational Psychology, 90,* 670.

Hasbrouck, J. E., and Tindal, G. (1992). Curriculum-based oral reading frequency norms for students in grades 2 through 5. *Teaching Exceptional Children, 24,* 41-44.

Helenius, P., Salmelin, R., Richardson, U., Leinonen, S., and Lyytinen, H. (2002). Abnormal auditory cortical activation in dyslexia 100 msec after speech onset. *Journal of Cognitive Neuroscience, 14,* 603-617.

Howes, N., Bigler, E. D., Burlingame, G. M., and Lawson, J. S. (2003). Memory performance of children with dyslexia: A comparative analysis of theoretical perspectives. *Journal of Learning Disabilities, 36,* 230-246.

Idol, L. (1987). Group story mapping.: A comprehensive strategy for both skilled and unskilled readers. *Journal of Learning Disabilities, 20,* 196-205.

Indefrey, P., Kleinschmidt, A., Merboldt, K. D., Kruger, G., Brown, C., Hagoot, P., and Frahm, J. (1997). Equivalent responses to lexical and nonlexical visual stimuli in occipital cortex: A functional magnetic resonance imaging study. *NeuroImage, 5,* 78-81.

International Dyslexia Association (IDA). (2003). *Common signs of dyslexia.* Baltimore, MD: Author.

Johnson, D.W., and Johnson, R.T. (1989). Cooperative learning: What special educators need to know. *The Pointer, 33,* 5-10.

Joseph, J., Noble, K., and Eden, G. (2001). The neurobiological basis of reading. *Journal of Learning Disabilities, 34,* 566-579.

Kaminen, N., Hannula-Jouppi, K., Kestila, M., Lahermo, P., Muller, K., Kaaranen, M., Myllylouma, B., Voutilainen, A., Lyytinen, H., Nopola-Hemmi, J., and Kere, J. (2003, May). A genome scan for developmental dyslexia confirms linkage to chromosome 2pl1 and suggests a new locus on 7q32. *Journal of Medical Genetics, 40,* 340-345.

Katayama, A. D., and Robinson, D. H. (2000). Getting students partially involved in note-taking using graphic organizers. *Journal of Experimental Education, 68,* 119-133.

Kim, K. H. S., Relkin, N. R., Lee, K. M., and Hirsch, J. (1997). Distinct cortical areas associated with native and second languages. *Nature, 388,* 171-174.

Klingner, J. K., Vaughn, S., and Schumm, J. S. (1998). Collaborative strategic reading during social studies in heterogeneous fourth grade classrooms. *Elementary School Journal, 99,* 3-22.

Krashen, S. (2001). More smoke and mirrors: A critique of the National Reading Panel report on fluency. *Phi Delta Kappan, 83,* 119-123.

Krashen, S. (2002). Phonemic awareness training necessary? *Reading Research Quarterly, 37,* 128.

Labov, W. (2003). When ordinary children fail to read. *Reading Research Quarterly, 38,* 128-131.

Lai, C. S., Fisher, S. E., Hurst, J. A., Vargha-Khadem, F., and Monaco, A. P. (2001). A forkhead-domain gene is mutated in a severe speech and language disorder. *Nature, 413,* 519-523.

Leonard, C. M. (2001). Imaging brain structure in children: Differentiating language disability and reading disability. *Learning Disability Quarterly, 24,* 158-176.

Londin, E. R., Meng, H., and Gruen, J. R. (2003). A transcription map of the 6p22.3 reading disability locus identifying candidate genes. *BMC Genomics, 4.* Available online at http://www.biomedcentral.com/1471-2164/4/25.

Lyon, G. R. (2002). Reading development, reading difficulties, and reading instruction: Educational and public health issues. *Journal of School Psychology, 40,* 3-6.

Mahony, D., Singson, M., and Mann, V. A. (2000). Reading ability and sensitivity to morphophonological situations. *Reading and Writing: An Interdisciplinary Journal, 12:3/4,* 191-218.

Mann, V. A. (2000). Introduction to special issue on morphology and the acquisition of alphabetic writing systems. *Reading and Writing: An Interdisciplinary Journal, 12:3/4,* 143-147.

Martinez, M., Roser, N., and Strecker, S. (1999). "I never thought I could be a star": A readers' theatre ticket to fluency. *The Reading Teacher, 52,* 326-334.

Mather, N. and Goldstein, S. (2001). *Learning disabilities and challenging behaviors: A guide to intervention and classroom management.* Baltimore, MD: Brookes.

McCandliss, B. D., Cohen, L., and Dehaene, S. (2003, July). The visual word form area: Expertise for reading in the fusiform gyrus. *Trends in Cognitive Sciences, 7,* 293-299.

Michigan Department of Elementary and Secondary Education (MDESE). (2003). *Missouri parents as teachers graphs.* Available online at http://dese.mo.gov/divimprove/fedprog/earlychild/ECDA/PAT%20FACT%20Sheet.pdf.

Mirsky, A. F. (1996). Disorders of attention: A neuropsychological perspective. In G. R. Lyon and N. A. Krasnegor (Eds.), *Attention, memory, and executive function* (pp. 71-95. Baltimore, MD: Brookes.

Moats, L. C., and Foorman, B. R. (2003). Measuring teachers' content knowledge of language and reading. *Annals of Dyslexia, 53,* 23-45.

Moats, L. C., Furry, A. R., and Brownell, N. (1998). *Learning to read: Components of beginning reading instruction.* Sacramento, CA: Comprehensive Reading Leadership Center.

Morris, D., Bloodgood, J. W., Lomax, R. G., and Perney, J. (2003). Developmental steps in learning to read: A longitudinal study in kindergarten and first grade. *Reading Research Quarterly, 38,* 302-328.

Munakata, Y., McClelland, J. L., Johnson, M. H., and Siegler, R. S. (1997). Rethinking infant knowledge: Toward and adaptive process account of success and failures in object permanence tasks. *Psychological Review, 104,* 686-713.

Nandy, R., Cordes, D., Berninger, V., Richards, T., Aylward, E., Stanberry, L., Richards, A., and Maravilla, K. (2003). *An fMRI approach to the diagnosis of dyslexia using CCA and a phoneme matching task.* Paper presented at the conference of the Organization for Human Brain Mapping, June, 2003, New York.

National Assessment of Educational Progress (NAEP). (2003). *The nation's report card: Reading 2003.* Washington, DC: Author.

National Association for the Education of Young Children (NAEYC). (1998). *Learning to read and write: Developmentally appropriate practices for young children.* Available online at http://www.naeyc.org/resources/position_statements/psread4.htm.

National Center for Educational Statistics (NCES). (2002). *Qualifications of the public school teacher workforce: Prevalence of out-of-field teaching 1987-88 to 1999-2000.* Available online at http://nces.ed.gov/programs/coe/2003/section4/indicator28.asp.

National Institute for Literacy (NIFL). (2001). *Put reading first: The research building block for teaching children to read.* Jessup, MD: Author.

National Reading Panel (NRP). (2000). *Teaching children to read: An evidence-based assessment of the scientific research literature and its implications for reading instruction.* Washington, DC: National Institute of Child Health and Human Development.

Nicolson, R. I., Fawcett, A. J., and Dean, P. (2001, September). Developmental dyslexia: The cerebellar deficit hypothesis. *Trends in Neuroscience, 24,* 508-511.

Novak, J. D., and Musonda, D. (1991). A twelve-year longitudinal study of science concept learning. *American Educational Research Journal, 28,* 117-153.

O'Connor, R. E., and Jenkins, J. R. (1995). Improving the generalization of sound/symbol knowledge: Teaching spelling to kindergarten children with disabilities. *The Journal of Special Education, 29,* 255-275.

Omaha Public Schools (OPS). (2003). *Reading tips: Secondary content teachers.* Available online at www.ops.org/reading.

Palincsar, A. S., and Brown, A. L. (1984). The reciprocal teaching of comprehension-fostering and comprehension-monitoring activities. *Cognition and Instruction, 1,* 117-175.

Parker, R., Hasbrouck, J. E., and Denton, C. (2002a). How to tutor students with reading problems. *Preventing School Failure, 47,* 42-44.

Parker, R., Hasbrouck, J. E., and Denton, C. (2002b). How to tutor students with comprehension problems. *Preventing School Failure, 47,* 45-47.

Parrott, C. A. (1986). Visual imagery training: Stimulating utilization of imaginal processes. *Journal of Mental Imagery, 10,* 47-64.

Paterno, J. (2001). *Secondary reading strategies.* Available online at www.angelfire.com/wa2/buildingcathedrals/SecondaryReadingStrategies.

Pearson, P. D., and Duke, N. K. (2002). Comprehension instruction in the primary grades. In C. C. Block and M. Pressley (Eds.), *Comprehension instruction: Research-based best practices.* New York: Guilford.

Peereman, R., Content, A., and Bonin, P. (1998). Is perception a two-way street: The case of feedback consistency in visual word recognition. *Journal of Memory and Language, 39,* 151-174.

Pennington, B. F. (1990). The genetics of dyslexia. *Journal of Child Psychology and Psychiatry, 31,* 193-201.

Pinker, S. (1994). *The language instinct: How the mind creates language.* New York: William Morrow.

Pinker, S. (1999). *Words and rules: The ingredients of language.* New York: Basic Books.

Pressley, M. (1998). *Reading instruction that works: The case for balanced teaching.* New York: Guilford.

Pressley, M., and Afflerbach, P. (1995). *Verbal protocols of reading: The nature of constructively responsive reading.* Hillsdale, NJ: Erlbaum.

Price, C., Moore, C., and Frackowiak, R. S. J. (1996). The effect of varying stimulus rates and duration of brain activity during reading. *Neuroimage, 3,* 40-52.

Rawson, M. B. (1995). *Dyslexia over the life span: A 55 year longitudinal study.* Cambridge, MA: Educator's Publishing Service.

Rayner, K., Foorman, B. R., Perfetti, C. A., Pesetsky, D., and Seidenberg, M. S. (2001, November). How psychological science informs the teaching of reading. *Psychological Science in the Public Interest, 2* , 31-74.

Reading Recovery Council (2002). *What evidence says about Reading Recovery.* Columbus, OH: Author.

Renvall, H., and Hari, R. (2002). Auditory cortical responses to speech-like stimuli in dyslexic adults. *Journal of Cognitive Neuroscience, 14,* 757-768.

Richards, T. (2001, Summer). Functional magnetic resonance imaging and spectroscopic imaging of the brain: Application of fMRI and fMRS to reading disabilities and education. *Learning Disability Quarterly, 24,* 189-204.

Rumsey, J., Horwitz, B., Donohue, B. C., Nace, K. L., Maisog, J. M., and Andreason, P. (1999). A functional lesion in developmental dyslexia: Left angular gyral flow predicts severity. *Brain and Language, 70,* 187-204.

Sams, G. (2003). *Dyslexia and exams.* Available online at http://www.dyslexia-parent.com.

Scientific Learning Corporation (SLC). (2000). *Fast ForWord reading: Why it works.* Oakland, CA: Author.

Share, D. L., and Stanovich, K. E. (1995). Cognitive processes in early reading development: Accommodating individual differences into a model of acquisition. *Issues in Education, 1,* 1-57.

Shaywitz, S. E. (2003). *Overcoming dyslexia: A new and complete science-based program for reading problems at any level.* New York: Knopf.

Shaywitz, S. E. (1996, November). Dyslexia. *Scientific American,275,* 98-104.

Shaywitz, B., Shaywitz, S., Blachman, B., Pugh, K. R., Fulbright, R., Skudlarski, P., Mencl, E., Constable, T., Holahan, J., Marchione, K., Fletcher, J., Lyon, R., and Gore, J. (2003). *Development of left occipito-temporal systems for skilled reading following a phonologically-based intervention in children.* Paper presented at the conference of the Organization for Human Brain Mapping, June, 2003, New York.

Shaywitz, B. A., Shaywitz, S. E., and Gore, J. (1995). Sex differences in the functional organization of the brain for languages. *Nature, 373,* 607-609.

Simmons, D. C., and Kame'enui, E. J. (2003). *A consumer's guide to evaluating a core reading program grades K-3: A critical elements analysis.* Institute for the Development of Educational Achievement, University of Oregon. Available online at http://reading.uoregon.edu/appendices/con_guide_3.1.03.pdf.

Simos, P. G., Breier, J. I., Fletcher, J. M., Bergman, E., and Papanicolaou, A. C. (2000). Cerebral mechanisms involved in word reading in dyslexic children: A magnetic source imaging approach. *Cerebral Cortex, 10,* 809-816.

Singson, M., Mahony, D., and Mann, V. A. (2000). The relation between reading ability and morphological skills: Evidence from derivational suffixes. *Reading and Writing: An Interdisciplinary Journal, 12:3/4,* 219-252.

Sipe, L. R. (2001). Invention, convention, and intervention: Invented spelling and the teacher's role. *The Reading Teacher, 55,* 264-273.

Slater, W. H., and Horstman, F. R. (2002). Teaching reading and writing to struggling middle school and high school students: The case for reciprocal teaching. *Preventing School Failure, 46,* 163-166.

Slavin, R. E. (1995). *Cooperative learning: Theory, research and practice* (2nd ed.). Boston: Allyn & Bacon.

Slavin, R. E., and Cheung, A. (2003). *Effective programs for English language learners: A best-evidence synthesis.* Baltimore, MD: Johns Hopkins University, CRESPAR.

Smith, F., and Goodman, K. S. (1971). On the psycholinguistic method of teaching reading. *Elementary School Journal, 71,* 177-181.

Snow, C. E., Burns, M. S., and Griffin, P. (Eds.). (1998). *Preventing reading difficulties in young children.* Washington, DC: National Academy Press.

Solan, H. A., Shelley-Tremblay, J., Ficarra, A., Silverman, M., and Larson, S. (2003). Effect of attention therapy on reading comprehension. *Journal of Learning Disabilities, 36,* 556-563.

Sousa, D. A. (2001a). *How the brain learns.* Thousand Oaks, CA: Corwin Press.

Sousa, D. A. (2001b). *How the special needs brain learns.* Thousand Oaks, CA: Corwin Press.

Southwest Educational Development Laboratory (SEDL). (2001). *The cognitive foundations of learning to read.* Austin, TX: Author.

Speece, D. L., and Mills, C. (2003). Initial evidence that letter fluency tasks are valid indicators of early reading skill. *Journal of Special Education, 36,* 223-233.

Squire, L. R., & Kandel, E. R. (1999). *Memory: From mind to molecules.* New York: W. H. Freeman.

Stahl, S. A. (2000). *Promoting vocabulary development.* Austin, TX: Texas Education Agency.

Stinson, E. (2003). *Best practices in reading instruction.* Nashville, TN: NPT Educational Services.

Stone, G. O., Vanhoy, M., and Van Orden, G. C. (1997). Perception is a two-way street: Feedforward and feedback phonology in visual word recognition. *Journal of Memory and Language, 36,* 337-359.

Swaab, T. Y., Baynes, K., and Knight, R. T. (2002, September). Separable effects of priming and imageability on word processing: An ERP study. *Cognitive Brain Research, 15,* 99-103.

Swanborn, M. S. L., and de Glopper, K. (1999). Incidental word learning while reading: A meta-analysis. *Review of Educational Research, 69,* 261-285.

Tallal, P., Miller, S. L., Bedi, G., Byma, G., Wang, X., Nagarajan, S., Schreiner, C., Jenkins, W. M., and Merzenich, M. M. (1996, January). Fast-element enhanced speech improves language comprehension in language-learning impaired children. *Science, 271,* 81–84.

Tan, A., and Nicholson, T. (1997). Flashcards revisited: Training poor readers to read words faster improves their comprehension of text. *Journal of Educational Psychology, 89,* 276-288.

Taylor, B. M., Pearson, P. D., Clark, K. F., and Walpole, S. (2000). Effective schools and accomplished teachers: Lessons about primary reading instruction in low-income schools. *Elementary School Journal, 101,* 121-166.

Temple, E., Deutsch, G. K., Poldrack, R. A., Miller, S. L., Tallal, P., Merzenich, M. M., and Gabrieli, J. D. E. (2003, March). Neural deficits in children with dyslexia ameliorated by behavioral remediation: Evidence from functional MRI. *Proceedings of the National Academy of Sciences, 100,* 2860-2865.

Tiu, R. D., Jr., Thompson, L. A., and Lewis, B. A. (2003). The role of IQ in a component model of reading. *Journal of Learning Disabilities, 36,* 424-436.

Torgesen, J. K. (1999). Phonologically-based reading disabilities: Toward a coherent theory of one kind of learning disability. In R. Sternberg and L. Spear-Swerling (Eds.), *Perspectives on learning disabilities* (pp. 106-135). Boulder, CO: Westview Press.

Torgesen, J. K. (2001). Individual differences in response to early intervention in reading: The lingering problem of treatment resisters. *Learning Disabilities Research and Practice, 15,* 55-64.

Torgesen, J. K. (2002). The prevention of reading difficulties. *Journal of School Psychology, 40,* 7-26.

Torgesen, J. K. (2004). Lessons learned from research on interventions for students who have difficulty learning to read. In P. McCardle and V. Chhabra (Eds.), *The voice of evidence in reading research.* Baltimore, MD: Brookes.

Torgesen, J. K., Alexander, A. W., Wagner, R. K., Rashotte, C. A., Voller, K. K. S., and Conway, T. (2001). Intensive remedial instruction for children with severe reading disabilities. *Journal of Learning Disabilities, 34,* 33-58.

Treiman, R. A., and Cassar, M. (1997). Spelling acquisition in English. In C. A. Perfetti, L. Rieben, and M. Fayol (Eds.), *Learning to spell: Research, theory, and practice across languages* (pp. 61-80). Mahwah, NJ: Erlbaum.

Uhry, J. (1999). Invented spelling in kindergarten: The relationship with finger-point reading. *Reading and Writing, 11,* 441-464.

Vandervelden, M. C., and Siegel, L. S. (1997). Teaching phonological processing skills in early literacy: A developmental approach. *Learning Disability Quarterly, 20,* 63-81.

Van Petten, C., & Bloom, P. (1999, February). Speech boundaries, syntax, and the brain. *Nature Neuroscience, 2,* 103–104.

Vaughn, S., Linan-Thompson, S., and Hickman, P. (2003). Response to instruction as a means for identifying students with reading/learning disabilities. *Exceptional Children, 69,* 391-409.

Vaughn, S., Moody, S. W., and Schumm, J. S. (1998). Broken promises: Reading instruction in the resource room. *Exceptional Children, 64,* 211-225.

Vellutino, F., Scanlon, D., Sipay, E. R., Small, S. G., Pratt, A., Chen, R., and Denckla, M. B. (1996). Cognitive profiles of difficult-to-remediate and readily remediated poor readers: Early intervention as a vehicle for distinguishing between cognitive and experiential deficits as basic causes of specific reading disability. *Journal of Educational Psychology, 88,* 601-638.

Weiler, J. (1998). *Success for All: A summary of evaluations.* (ERIC/CUE Digest Number 139). New York: ERIC Clearinghouse on Urban Education.

West, C. K., Farmer, J. A., and Wolff, P. M. (1991). *Instructional design: Implications from cognitive science.* Englewood Cliffs, NJ: Prentice Hall.

Wilson, A. M., and Lesaux, N. K. (2001). Persistence of phonological processing deficits in college students with dyslexia who have age-appropriate reading skills. *Journal of Learning Disabilities, 34,* 394-400.

Wise, B. W., Ring, J., and Olson, R. K. (1999). Training phonological awareness with and without attention to articulation. *Journal of Experimental Child Psychology, 72,* 271-304.

Wright, B. A., Bowen, R. W., and Zecker, S. G. (2000). Nonlinguistic perceptual deficits associated with reading and language disorders. *Current Opinion in Neurobiology, 10,* 482-486.

Yatvin, J. (2003, April 30). I told you so! The misinterpretation of the National Reading Panel Report. *Education Week, 22,* 56, 44, 45.

Yopp, H. K., and Yopp, R. H. (2000). Supporting phonemic awareness development in the classroom. *The Reading Teacher, 54,* 130-143.

Zigmond, N., and Jenkins, J. (1995). Special education in restructured schools. *Phi Delta Kappan, 76,* 531-535.

Resources

Note: All internet sites were active at time of publication.

Content Area Reading Online

Web site: www.content-reading.org

A subgroup of the International Reading Association, this site was formed to provide information on research and successful practices related to content area reading. The site offers valuable suggestions in several different subject areas.

The Council for Exceptional Children

1110 North Glebe Road
Suite 300
Arlington, VA 22201-5704
Tel.: 1-888-CEC-SPED
Web site: www.cec.sped.org

The Council's site has many suggestions for teachers and parents of children with learning disabilities as well as those who are gifted.

The Dyslexia Parents Resource

Web site: www.dyslexia-parent.com

Lots of hints and tips on how to deal with children who have been diagnosed with dyslexia.

The Dyslexia Teacher Online

Web site: www.dyslexia-teacher.com

This site offers plenty of information for teachers on research and practices related to working with dyslexic students.

Earobics Literacy Launch

Cognitive Concepts, Inc.

Web site: www.earobic.com

A research-based supplemental reading program for students in pre-kindergarten through grade 3. A combination of computer technology, multimedia tools, and print materials support components in phonological awareness, vocabulary, fluency, phonics, and reading comprehension.

Fast ForWord Reading Language Program

Scientific Learning Corporation

Web site: www.scientificlearning.com

A scientifically-based computer program that is designed for helping beginning readers develop phonemic awareness, letter-sound correspondences, fluent word recognition, vocabulary, and an appreciation of literature. Programs for older struggling readers are also available.

Florida Center for Reading Research

Web site: www.fcrr.org

This center was established by the state of Florida to analyze reading curricula and materials. The site offers assessment reports on various reading programs.

Graphic Organizers

Web site: www.graphic.org

This site has examples of different types of graphic organizers and suggestions on how to use them in lessons at all grade levels.

Inspiration Software, Inc.

Web site: http://inspiration.com

This company produces software that helps students construct all types of visual organizers for improving comprehension and building thinking skills. *Kidspiration* is designed for grades K through 5, and *Inspiration* is for grade 6 and higher. Demonstration versions can be downloaded from the site.

International Dyslexia Association

Chester Building, Suite 382

8600 LaSalle Road

Baltimore, MD 21286-2044

Tel.: 1-800-223-3123

Web site: www.interdys.org

International Reading Association
800 Barkdale Road
P.O. Box 8139
Newark, DE 19714-8139
Tel.: 1-800-336-READ
Web site: www.reading.org
The world's largest association devoted to reading maintains a rich source of information, including useful advice to parents and teachers who are helping children learn to read. This site also offers access to research articles and studies related to reading.

Kid's Health Web Site - Dyslexia:
Web site: www.kidshealth.org/parent/medical/learning/dyslexia.html
Information on the nature and treatment of dyslexia, written mainly for parents.

Lindamood Phonemic Sequencing Program (LiPS)
Lindamood Bell Learning Processes
Web site: www.lindamoodbell.com
The LiPS program is based on the interventions that researchers used to help struggling readers develop phonemic awareness and improve their reading achievement.

Literacy Connections
Web site: http://literacyvolunteer.homestead.com/index.html
The Literacy Connections Web site provides information on reading aloud, tutoring techniques, ESL literacy, and adult literacy. This site is a good resource for all reading teachers, literacy volunteers, and program directors.

Literacy and Technology
Web site: www.oswego.org/staff/cchamber/literacy/index.cfm
Developed by the Oswego City School District in New York, USA, this Web site includes links to resources that support the new literacies of the Internet as well as more traditional literacies.

Literature Circles Resource Center
Web site: http://fac-staff.seattleu.edu/kschlnoe/LitCircles/Overview/overview.html
Maintained by Seattle University's School of Education, this site offers educators many resources, suggestions, and sample lessons for using literature circles as part of a balanced literacy program.

National Association for the Education of Young Children

1509 16th Street NW
Washington, DC 20036
Tel.: 1-800-4242460
Web site: www.naeyc.org
This long-standing organization supports efforts to improve professional practice and opportunities in the education of children from birth through third grade.

National Clearinghouse for English Language Acquisition and Language Instruction Educational Programs.

Web site: www.ncela.gwu.edu/library/curriculum/index.htm#READING
This site has information, articles, and Web resources for reading instruction and other important topics in the education of English language learners.

National Institute for Literacy

1775 I Street, NW
Suite 730
Washington, DC 20006-2401
Tel.: 202-233-2025
Web site: www.nifl.gov
An agency supported by the U.S. government that promotes activities to strengthen literacy for people of all ages. It has several reports available online that review scientific research studies in reading.

National Reading Panel (NRP).

Web site: www.nationalreadingpanel.org
Its report is available in its entirety or as an abbreviated 33-page summary from the panel's Web site.

National Reading Styles Institute

P.O. Box 737
Syosset, NY 11791
Tel.:1-800-331-3117
Web site: www.nrsi.com/nrsi.htm
This site has information about reading styles and the research-based reading program developed by Marie Carbo.

Organization for Human Brain Mapping

Web site: www.humanbrainmapping.org

An organization of scientists and clinicians involved in using brain imaging to understand more about the structures and functions of the brain. The site provides information about the organization as well as research abstracts from some of their seminars.

The Partnership for Reading

Web site: www.nifl.gov/partnershipforreading

This site has a database of the abstracts of over 450 research studies related to the teaching of reading in grades K to 3. The studies have met a high standard of research and are categorized by phonemic awareness, phonics, fluency, vocabulary, text comprehension, computer instruction, and teacher education.

READ 180

Scholastic, Inc.

Web site: http://teacher.scholastic.com/read180

This scientifically-researched computer program, designed for struggling readers in grades 4 and above, has shown considerable success in raising reading and overall achievement in urban school districts.

Reading Recovery Council of North America

1926 Kenny Road, Suite 100

Columbus, OH 43210-1069

Tel.: 614-292-7111

Web site: www.readingrecovery.org

This is the official site of the Reading Recovery program which has been used in numerous school districts for over a decade to help beginning struggling readers.

Road to Reading

Web site: http://208.183.128.8/read

The Road to Reading Web site offers elementary teachers information on valuable classroom strategies for reading and writing with students.

Students Achieving Independent Learning (SAIL)

Web site: www.sail2comprehension.com

SAIL is a text comprehension strategies instruction program that was originally designed to help low-achieving students in reading but has been found to be effective in enhacing reading comprehension in students at all ability levels.

Success for All Foundation

200 West Towsontown Boulevard

Baltimore, MD 21204-5200

Tel.: 1-800-584-4998

Web site: www.successforall.net

Here is all the information one needs to understand the history, components, implementation, and effectiveness of the Success for All program.

U.S. Department of Education

600 Maryland Avenue SW

Washington, DC 20202

Tel.: 1-800-USA-LEARN (872-5327)

Web site: www.ed.gov

This site includes access to the ERIC databases, explanations of the requirements of the No Child Left Behind legislation, and descriptions of all the other activities that are the responsibility of the Department of Education.

Index

HOW THE Special Needs Brain Learns

Treat people as if they were
what they ought to be and
you help them to become
what they are capable of being.

— Johann von Goethe

David A. Sousa

HOW THE Special Needs Brain Learns

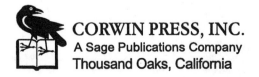
CORWIN PRESS, INC.
A Sage Publications Company
Thousand Oaks, California

For information:

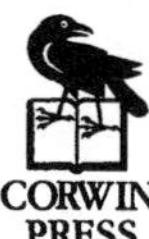
CORWIN PRESS

Corwin Press, Inc.
A Sage Publications Company
2455 Teller Road
Thousand Oaks, California 91320
E-mail: order@corwinpress.com

Sage Publications Ltd.
6 Bonhill Street
London EC2A 4PU
United Kingdom

Sage Publications India Pvt. Ltd.
M-32 Market
Greater Kailash I
New Delhi 110 048 India

Printed in the United States of America

Library of Congress Cataloging-in-Publication Data

Sousa, David A.
How the special needs brain learns / David A. Sousa.
p. cm.
Includes bibliographical references and index.
ISBN 0-7619-7850-X (cloth) — ISBN 0-7619-7851-8 (pbk.)
1. Learning disabled children—Education. 2. Learning.
3. Cognition in children. I. Title.
LC4704.5.S68 2001
370.15′23—dc21 2001001280

This book is printed on acid-free paper.

05 06 07 7 6

Acquiring Editor: Robb Clouse
Editorial Assistant: Kylee Liegl
Cover Designer: Tracy E. Miller

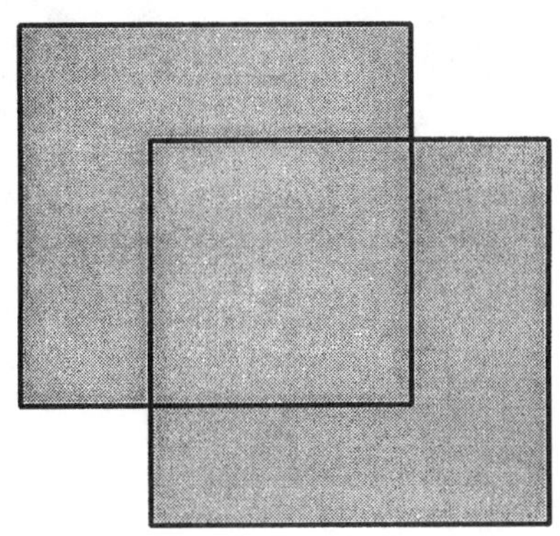

CONTENTS

LIST OF STRATEGIES TO CONSIDER

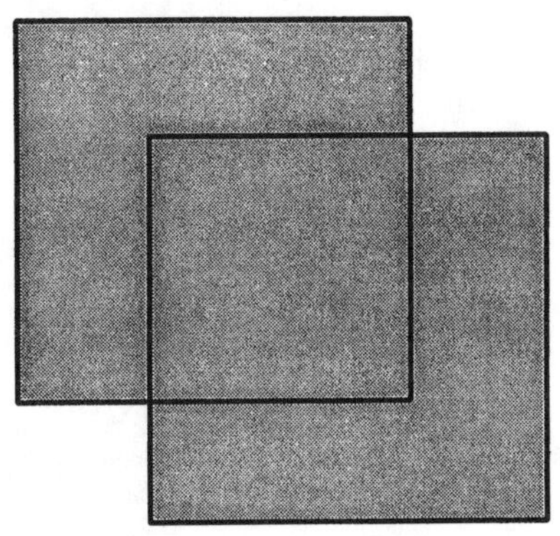

About the Author

David A. Sousa, Ed.D., is an international educational consultant. He has made presentations at national conventions of educational organizations and has conducted workshops on brain research and science education in hundreds of school districts and at several colleges and universities across the United States, Canada, and Europe.

Dr. Sousa has a bachelor's degree in chemistry from Massachusetts State College at Bridgewater, a master of arts in teaching degree in science from Harvard University, and a doctorate from Rutgers University. His teaching experience covers all levels. He has taught junior and senior high school science, served as a K–12 director of science, and was Supervisor of Instruction for the West Orange, New Jersey, schools. He then became superintendent of the New Providence, New Jersey, public schools. He has been an adjunct professor of education at Seton Hall University, and a visiting lecturer at Rutgers University. He was president of the National Staff Development Council in 1992.

Dr. Sousa has edited science books and published numerous articles in leading educational journals on staff development, science education, and brain research. He is listed in *Who's Who in the East* and *Who's Who in American Education* and has received awards from professional associations and school districts for his commitment to research, staff development, and science education.

He has been interviewed on the NBC *Today* show and on National Public Radio about his work with schools using brain research. He makes his home in Florida.

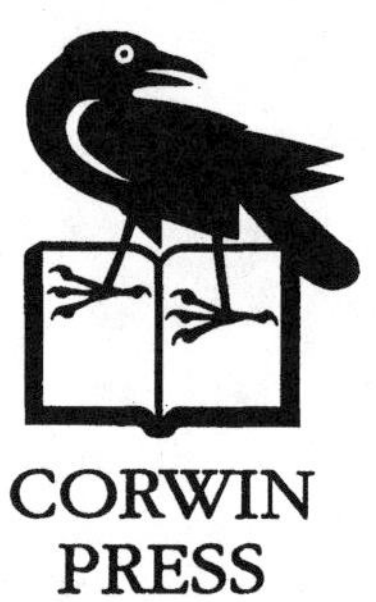
CORWIN
PRESS

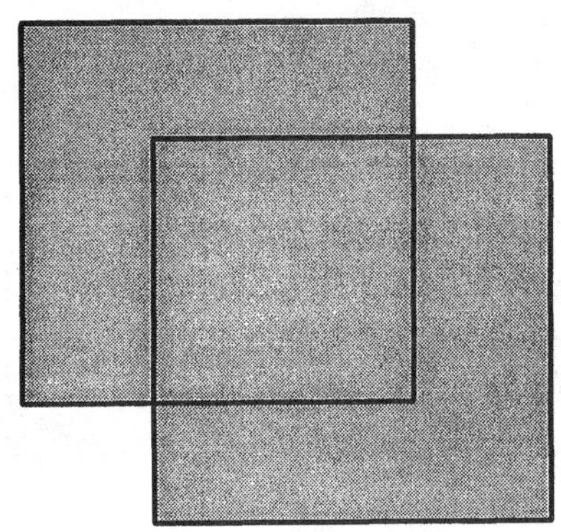

INTRODUCTION

Teachers and students get up every school-day morning hoping to succeed. That hope is not always realized because many factors exist that affect the degree of success or failure in a teaching and learning situation. Some of these factors are well beyond the control of the teacher and the school staff. What teachers *do* control, of course, are the decisions they make about what to teach and about how to present the lesson so that student learning is most likely to occur. In making these decisions, teachers draw on their knowledge base and experience to design activities, ask questions, and respond to the efforts of their students.

Educators are finding themselves searching for new strategies and techniques to meet the needs of an ethnically, culturally, and socially diverse student population. Some tried-and-true strategies do not seem to be as successful as they were in the past, and more students seem to be having difficulty acquiring just the basic skills of reading, writing, and computation. The number of public school students being diagnosed with specific learning disabilities is growing. The total public school population classified as having specific learning disabilities between the 1988-89 and 1997-98 school years rose from 4.90 to 5.91 percent, a 20.6 percent increase (USDE, 1999).

This situation is generating frustration in different parts of the educational community. As a result, educators are searching for new approaches, parents are seeking alternative schooling formats (charter schools and vouchers), and legislators are demanding more standards and testing. It remains to be seen whether any of these efforts will result in more effective services to students with special needs.

Meanwhile, more students diagnosed with learning disabilities are being mainstreamed into regular classrooms and teachers continue to search for new ways to help these struggling students achieve. The percentage of students classified with specific learning disabilities who receive instruction in regular classrooms between the 1988-89 and 1995-96 school years rose from 17.6 percent to 42.4 percent, a dramatic 141 percent increase. As more students with learning difficulties are mainstreamed into regular classes, general education teachers are finding that they need help adjusting to the added responsibility of meeting the varied needs of these students. Consequently, special education teachers will need to collaborate more than ever with their general education colleagues on ways to differentiate instruction in the mainstreamed classroom.

General and special education teachers will need to collaborate more than ever on ways to differentiate instruction.

Who Are Special Needs Students?

For the purposes of this book, the term "special needs" refers to students

- diagnosed and classified as having specific learning problems, including speech, reading, writing, and mathematics disorders
- enrolled in Title I programs
- not classified for special education nor assigned to Title I, but still struggling with problems affecting their learning, such as those with sleep deprivation

The term does not refer to students with learning problems resulting primarily from hearing, visual, or physical handicaps, or from economic or environmental disadvantage.

Can Brain Research Help?

Teachers may face significant challenges when meeting the needs of children who have learning problems. Trying to figure out what is happening in the brains of these children can be frustrating and exhausting. Until recently, science could tell us little about the causes of learning disorders and even less about ways to address them successfully.

The nature of the difficulties facing students with learning problems vary from maintaining focus, acquiring language, learning to read and write, solving mathematical problems, and remembering important information, to just plain staying awake. Thanks to the development of imaging and other technologies, neuroscientists can now look inside the live brain and, as a result, are gaining new knowledge about its structure and functions. Some of this research may reveal enough clues to help guide the decisions and practices of educators working with students who have special needs.

Because of the efforts of scientists over the years to cure brain disorders, we know more about troubled brains than we do about healthy ones. Early ventures into the brain involved extensive risks which were justified by the potential for curing or improving the patient's condition. But now, essentially risk-free imaging technologies (such as functional magnetic resonance imaging) are giving us greater knowledge about how the normal brain works. For instance, a program created in 1999, called the Interagency Education Research Initiative (IERI), has been established to fund scientific research to study the brain activity of children with and without learning disabilities. IERI is a joint project of the National Science Foundation, the U.S. Department of Education, and the National Institute of Child Health and Human Development. The initiative supports a variety of programs. One study, based at the University of Texas at Houston, uses brain imaging technology to detect the activity patterns in the brains of kindergartners as they learn to read. Researchers meet periodically to discuss their progress and results. IERI's goal is to establish a new research community that uses the results of hard science to influence educational decisions and practice (Viadero, 2001).

Another promising approach to working with diverse learners is being directed by the National Center for Accessing the Curriculum (NCAC). Funded by the Office of Special Education and Programs in the U.S. Department of Education, the NCAC focuses on Universal Design for Learning (UDL), an evolving approach that combines brain research and a digitized curriculum to provide individualized and differentiated instruction in the classroom. Teachers can use the technology to ease the burden of selecting multiple UDL teaching strategies that address different learning styles, abilities, and disabilities in a variety of learning contexts. Although no universally designed curriculum is currently available, NCAC is encouraging publishers to develop digital companions for all printed curriculum materials that they publish.

Because all students with learning problems comprise such a heterogeneous group, no one strategy, technique, or intervention can address all their needs. Today, more than ever, neuroscientists, psychologists, computer experts, and educators are working together in a common crusade to improve our understanding of the learning process. Comparing the functions of brains without deficits to the functions of brains with deficits is revealing some remarkable new insights about learning and behavioral disorders. Some of the findings are challenging long-held beliefs about the cause, progress, and treatment of specific learning disorders. Educators in both general and special education should be aware of this research so that they can decide what implications the findings have for their practice.

Comparing the functions of brains without deficits to the functions of brains with deficits is revealing some remarkable new insights about learning and behavioral disorders.

What Is in This Book?

This book provides research information about common learning disabilities to prospective and current teachers and administrators so that they may consider alternative instructional approaches. Basic brain structures and their functions, as well as a brief description of learning and retention are the subjects of the first chapter. The second chapter provides an overview of factors that can affect brain development and a general discussion of learning disabilities. Subsequent chapters focus on specific learning difficulties, ranging from attention disorders to autism. Putting it all together is the purpose of the final chapter, which summarizes the types of interventions that can address the learning difficulties found in today's classrooms.

Practical applications of the research can be found in the chapter sections called *Strategies to Consider*, which suggest how educators might translate the research into school and classroom practice so that students with learning difficulties can be more successful. Obviously, some of the strategies would be appropriate for all learners. However, the suggestions have been written specifically to address the special needs of students with learning difficulties.

The book will help answer such questions as:

- How different are the brains of today's students?
- What kinds of strategies are particularly effective for students with learning disabilities?
- What progress is brain research making in discovering the causes of different learning disorders?
- Will brain research help us make more accurate diagnoses of learning problems?
- Can schools inadvertently exacerbate ADHD-like behavior in students?
- Can students with native language problems learn a second language?
- How does the brain learn to read?
- How much does lack of sleep affect student performance in schools?
- How can we address the emotional needs of students in the classroom?
- What more do we know about autism?

Some of the information and suggestions found here came from advocacy organizations, including the National Institute of Mental Health, the National Information Center for Children and Youth With Disabilities, and the Learning Disability Association of America (see the resources section). Where possible, I have sought out original medical research reports, and these are included in the references section of the book. A few of the strategies are derived or adapted from the second edition of my previous book, *How the Brain Learns*, also published by Corwin Press.

This book is not intended to be a comprehensive text describing all the types of barriers that can affect learning. Rather, it focuses on the common difficulties and disorders that any teacher is likely to encounter in the general or special education classroom. On a broader scale, the updates on research and some of the suggested strategies may benefit all who work to educate children.

As we gain a greater understanding of the human brain, we may discover that some students designated as "learning disabled" may be merely "schooling disabled."

As we gain a greater understanding of the human brain, we may discover that some students designated as "learning disabled" may be merely "schooling disabled." Sometimes, these students are struggling to learn in an environment that is designed inadvertently to frustrate their efforts. Just changing our instructional approach may be enough to move these students to the ranks of successful learners. My hope is that this book will encourage all school professionals to learn more about how the brain learns so that they can work together for the benefit of all students.

A Word of Caution

Several chapters contain lists of symptoms that are used to help identify specific disorders. The symptoms are included only for informational purposes and they should not be used as a basis for diagnosis. Any individual who exhibits persistent learning problems should be referred to qualified clinical personnel for assessment.

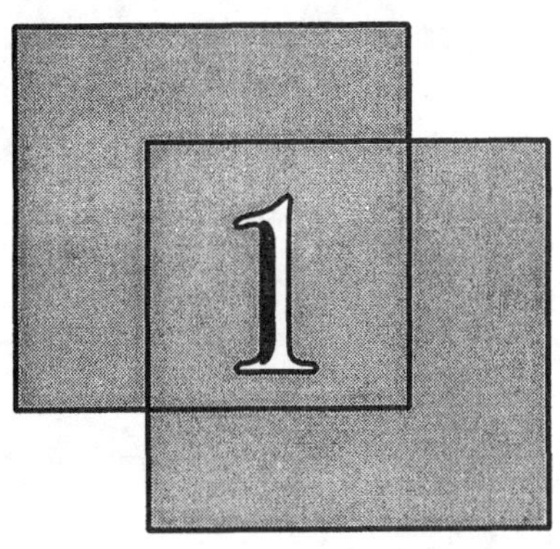

How the Brain Learns

The human brain is an amazing structure. At birth, it is equipped with over 100 billion nerve cells designed to collect information and learn the skills necessary to keep its owner alive. Although comparatively slow in its growth and development compared to the brains of other mammals, it can learn complex skills, master any of over 6,000 languages, store memories for a lifetime, and marvel at the glory of a radiant sunset. Early in life, the brain's cells grow and connect with each other—at the rate of thousands per second—to store information and skills. Most of the connections result in the development of neural networks that will help the individual successfully face life's challenges. But sometimes, certain connections go awry, setting the stage instead for problems.

To understand the complexity of human brain growth and development, let's review some basic information about its structure. For our purposes, we will first look at major parts of the outside of the brain (Figure 1.1): the frontal, temporal, occipital, and parietal lobes; the motor cortex; and the cerebellum. Although the minor wrinkles are unique in each brain, several major wrinkles and folds are common to all brains. These folds form a set of four lobes in the largest part of the brain, called the *cerebrum* (Latin for brain). Each lobe specializes in performing certain functions.

The frontal lobe contains almost 50 percent of the volume of each cerebral hemisphere and is often referred to as the executive control center. The temporal lobe is the speech center. Visual processing is the main function of the occipital lobe, while the parietal lobe is responsible for sensory integration and orientation. Table 1.1 lists the functions of the four lobes as well as of the motor cortex.

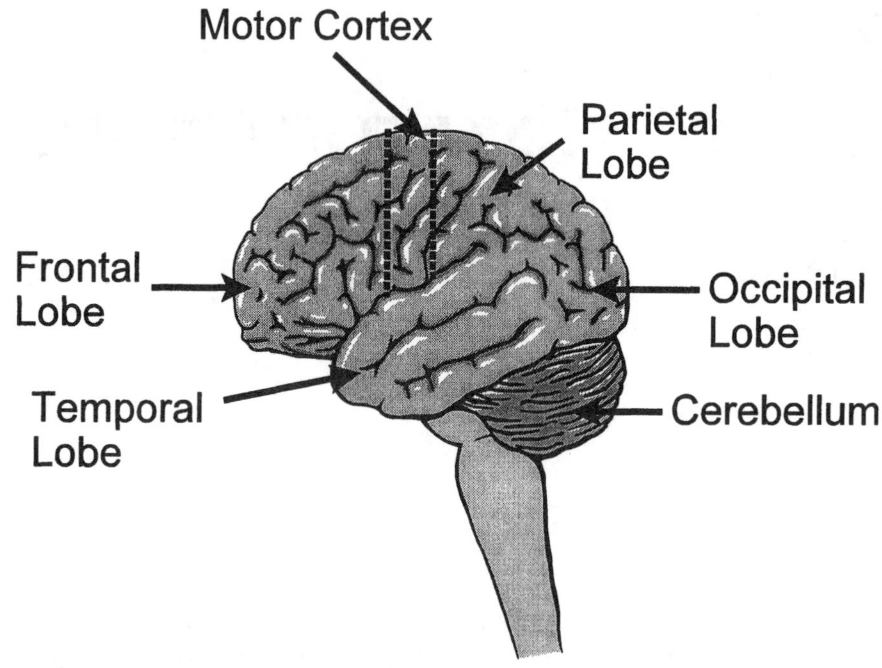

Figure 1.1 *This diagram shows the four major lobes of the brain (cerebrum) as well as the motor cortex and the cerebellum.*

Table 1.1 Some Exterior Parts of the Brain		
Structure		Function
Cerebrum	Frontal Lobe (often referred to as the *executive control center*)	Personality, curiosity, planning, problem solving, higher-order thinking, and emotional restraint
	Temporal Lobe	Interpretation of sound, speech (usually on the left side only), and some aspects of long-term memory
	Occipital Lobe	Visual processing
	Parietal Lobe	Orientation, calculation, and certain types of recognition
	Motor Cortex	Control of body movements

Next, we will look at the inside of the brain and at some of its major structures (see Figure 1.2). Table 1.2 lists the functions of some of the interior parts of the brain: the brain stem, limbic area, cerebrum, and cerebellum.

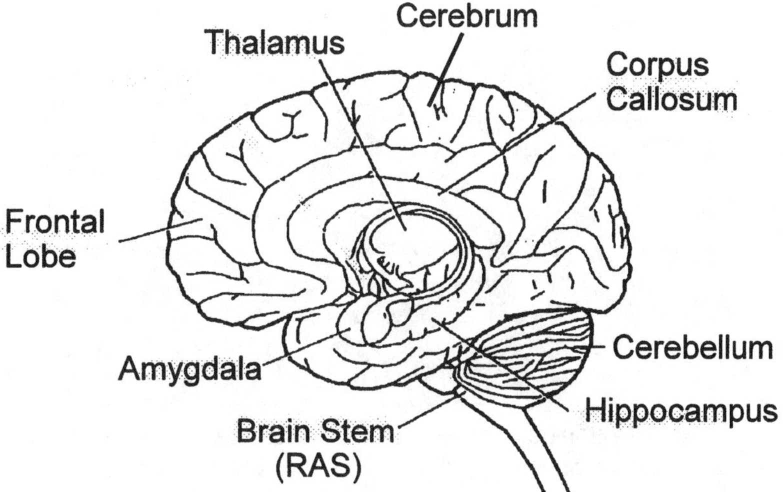

Figure 1.2 *A cross section of the human brain.*

Table 1.2 Some Interior Parts of the Brain	
Structure	**Function**
Brain Stem	The oldest and deepest area of the brain, this is often referred to as the reptilian brain because it resembles the entire brain of a reptile. Here is where vital body functions (such as respiration, body temperature, blood pressure, and digestion) are monitored and controlled. The brain stem also houses the reticular activating system (RAS), responsible for the brain's alertness.
Limbic Area	Above the brain stem lies the limbic area, whose structures are duplicated in each hemisphere of the brain. Three parts of the limbic area are important to learning and memory: *Thalamus.* All incoming sensory information (except smell) goes first to the thalamus. From here it is directed to other parts of the brain for additional processing. *Hippocampus.* Named for the Greek word for a sea monster resembling a seahorse, because of its shape, it plays a major role in consolidating learning and in converting information from working memory via electronic signals to the long-term storage regions, a process that may take from days to months. This brain area constantly checks information relayed to working memory and compares it to stored experiences. This process is essential for the creation of meaning. *Amygdala.* Attached to the end of the hippocampus, the amygdala (Greek for almond) plays an important role in emotions, especially fear. Because of its proximity to the hippocampus and its activity on PET scans, researchers believe that the amygdala encodes an emotional message, if one is present, whenever a memory is tagged for long-term storage.

Table 1.2 Some Interior Parts of the Brain — Continued	
Cerebrum	The cerebrum represents over 80 percent of the brain by weight. For some still unexplained reason, the nerves from the left side of the body cross over to the right hemisphere, and those from the right side of the body cross over to the left hemisphere. The two hemispheres are connected by a thick cable, called the *corpus callosum*, composed of over 250 million nerve fibers. The hemispheres use this bridge to communicate with each other and to coordinate activities. The hemispheres are covered by a thin but tough laminated *cortex* (Latin for tree bark). The cortex is composed of six layers of cells meshed in approximately 10,000 miles of connecting fibers per cubic inch! Here is where thinking, memory, speech, and muscular movement are controlled.
Cerebellum	The cerebellum (Latin for little brain) coordinates every movement. Because the cerebellum monitors impulses from nerve endings in the muscles, it is important in the learning, performance, and timing of complex motor tasks, including speaking. The cerebellum may also store the memory of rote movements, such as touch-typing and tying a shoelace. A person whose cerebellum is damaged cannot coordinate movement, has difficulty with speech, and may display the symptoms of autism.

The Control Functions of the Brain

The Frontal Lobe

The frontal lobe is the executive control center of the brain, monitoring higher-order thinking, directing problem solving, and regulating the excesses of the emotional system. Because emotions drive attention, the efficiency of this area is linked to the limbic centers. The frontal lobe also contains our self-will area—what some might call our personality. Trauma to the frontal lobe can cause dramatic—and sometimes permanent—behavior and personality changes. (One wonders why we allow 10-year-olds to play football and soccer where the risk of trauma to the frontal lobe is so high.)

The brain's executive system matures slower than the emotional system, so adolescents may resort to high-risk behavior.

Because most of the working memory is located in the frontal lobe, it is the area where focus occurs. The frontal lobe, however, matures slowly. MRI studies of postadolescents reveal that the frontal lobe continues to mature into early adulthood. Thus, the emotional regulation capability of the frontal lobe is not fully operational during adolescence (Sowell, Thompson, Holmes, Jernigan, and

Toga, 1999). This is one reason why adolescents are more likely than adults to submit to their emotions and may resort to high-risk behavior.

Brain Cells

The control functions and other activities of the brain are carried out by signals traveling along brain cells. The brain is composed of a trillion cells of at least two known types: nerve cells and their support cells. Nerve cells are called *neurons* and represent about one-tenth of the total number of cells—roughly 100 billion. Most of the cells are support cells, called *glial* (Greek for glue) cells, that hold the neurons together and act as filters to keep harmful substances out of the neurons.

Neurons are the functioning core for the brain and the entire nervous system. They come in different sizes, but it takes about 30,000 brain neurons to fit on the head of a pin. Unlike other cells, the neuron (Figure 1.3) has tens of thousands of branches or *dendrites* (from the Greek word for tree) emerging from its center. The dendrites receive electrical impulses from other neurons and transmit them along a long fiber, called the *axon* (Greek for axis). Each neuron has only one axon. A layer called the *myelin* (related to the Greek word for marrow) *sheath* surrounds each axon. The sheath insulates the axon from the other cells and increases the speed of impulse transmission. The impulse travels along the neurons through an electrochemical process and can move the entire length of a 6-foot adult in 2/10ths of a second. A neuron can transmit between 250 and 2,500 impulses per second.

Neurons have no direct contact with each other. Between each dendrite and axon is a small gap of about a millionth of an inch called a *synapse* (from the Greek meaning to join together). A typical neuron collects signals from others through the dendrites. The neuron sends out spikes of electrical activity (impulses) through the axon to the synapse where the activity releases chemicals stored in sacs (called *synaptic vesicles*) at the end of the axon.

The chemicals, called *neurotransmitters*, either excite or inhibit the neighboring neuron. Nearly 100 different neurotransmitters have been discovered so far. Some of the common neurotransmitters are acetylcholine, epinephrine, serotonin, and dopamine.

Learning and Retention

Learning occurs when the synapses make physical and chemical changes so that the influence of one neuron on another also changes. For instance, a set of neurons "learns" to fire together. Repeated firings make successive firings easier and, eventually, automatic under certain conditions. Thus, a memory is formed.

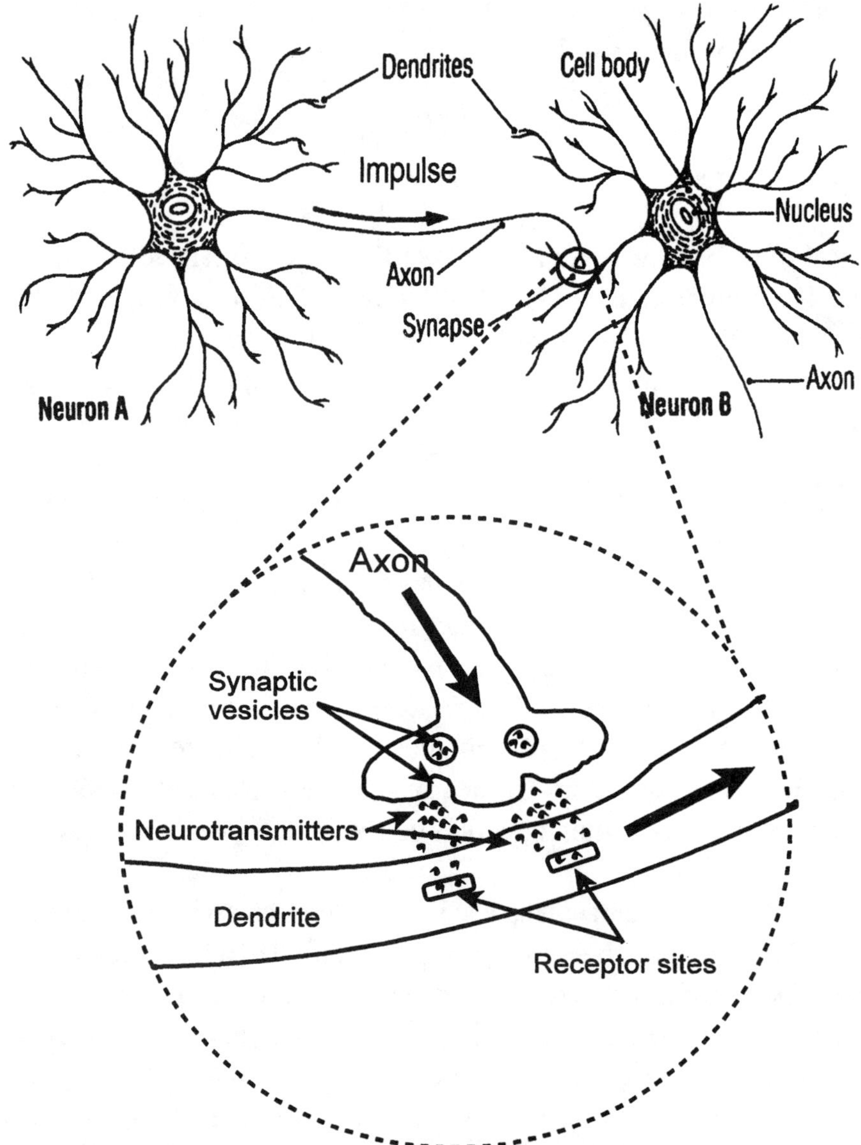

Figure 1.3 *Neurons, or nerve cells, transmit impulses along an axon and across the synapse to the dendrites of the neighboring cell. The impulse is carried across the synapse to receptor sites by chemicals called neurotransmitters that lie within synaptic vesicles (Sousa, 2001, p. 21).*

For all practical purposes, the capacity of the brain to store information is unlimited. That is, with about 100 billion neurons, each with thousands of dendrites, the number of potential neural pathways is incomprehensible. The brain will hardly run out of space to store all that an individual learns in a lifetime. Learning is the process by which we *acquire* new knowledge and skills; memory is the process by which we *retain* knowledge and skills for the future.

Investigations into the neural mechanisms required for different types of learning are revealing more about the interactions between learning new information, memory, and changes in brain structure. Just as muscles improve with exercise, the brain seems to improve with use. Although learning does not increase the number of brain cells, it does increase their size, their branches, and their ability to form more complex networks.

> *Learning is the process by which we acquire knowledge; memory is the process by which we retain it.*

The brain goes through physical and chemical changes when it stores new information as the result of learning. Storing gives rise to new neural pathways and strengthens existing pathways. Hence, every time we learn something, our long-term storage areas undergo anatomical changes that, together with our unique genetic makeup, constitute the expression of our individuality (Beatty, 2001).

Learning and retention also occur in different ways. Learning involves the brain, the nervous system, and the environment, and the process by which their interplay acquires information and skills. Sometimes, we need information for just a short period of time, like the telephone number for a pizza delivery, and then the information decays after just a few seconds. Thus, learning does not always involve long-term retention.

A good portion of the teaching done in schools centers on delivering facts and information to build concepts that explain a body of knowledge. We teach numbers, arithmetic operations, ratios, and theorems to explain mathematics. We teach about atoms, momentum, gravity, and cells to explain science. We talk about countries and famous leaders and discuss their trials and battles to explain history, and so on. Students may hold on to this information in working memory just long enough to take a test, after which the knowledge readily decays and is lost. Retention, however, requires that the learner not only give conscious attention but also build conceptual frameworks that have sense and meaning for eventual consolidation into long-term storage networks.

Implications for Students With Learning Disabilities. Because students with learning disabilities can have difficulty focusing for very long, they are even more likely to perceive learning facts as a temporary effort just to please the teacher or to pass a test. It becomes increasingly important, then, for teachers of these students to emphasize *why* they need to learn certain material. Meaning (or relevancy) becomes the key to focus, learning, and retention.

Retention is the process whereby long-term memory preserves a learning in such a way that the memory can be located, identified, and retrieved accurately in the future. This is an inexact process influenced by many factors including the degree of student focus, the length and type of rehearsal that occurred, the critical attributes that may have been identified, the student's learning style, any learning disabilities, and, of course, the inescapable influence of prior learning.

Rehearsal

The brain's decision to retain a learning seems to be based primarily on two criteria: *sense* and *meaning*. Sense refers to whether the student understands the learning, "Does this fit my perception of how the world works?" Meaning, on the other hand, refers to relevancy. Although the student may understand the learning, the more important question may be, "So what? What's this got to do with me?" Attaching sense and meaning to new learning can occur only if the learner has adequate time to process and reprocess it. This continuing reprocessing is called *rehearsal* and is a critical component in the transference of information from working memory to long-term storage.

Learning is likely to be remembered if it makes sense and has meaning to the learner.

Two major factors should be considered in evaluating rehearsal: the amount of time devoted to it, which determines whether there is both initial and secondary rehearsal, and the type of rehearsal carried out, which can be rote or elaborative.

Time for Initial and Secondary Rehearsal

Time is a critical component of rehearsal. Initial rehearsal occurs when the information first enters working memory. If the learner cannot attach sense or meaning, and if there is no time for further processing, the new information is likely to be lost. Providing sufficient time to go beyond initial processing to secondary rehearsal allows the learner to review the information, to make sense of it, to elaborate on the details, and to assign value and relevance, thus increasing significantly the chance of long-term storage.

Scanning studies of the brain indicate that the frontal lobe is very much involved during the rehearsal process and, ultimately, in long-term memory formation. This makes sense because working memory is also located in the frontal lobe. Several studies using fMRI scans of humans showed that, during longer rehearsals, the amount of activity in the frontal lobe determined whether items were stored or forgotten (Buckner, Kelley, and Petersen, 1999; Wagner, Schacter, Rotte, Koutstaal, Maril, Dale, Rosen, and Buckner, 1998).

Students carry out initial and secondary rehearsal at different rates of speed and in different ways, depending on the type of information in the new learning and on their learning styles, including any learning disabilities. As the learning task changes, learners automatically shift to different patterns of rehearsal.

Rote and Elaborative Rehearsal

Rote Rehearsal. This type of rehearsal is used when learners need to remember and store information exactly as it is entered into working memory. This involves a simple strategy necessary to learn information or a skill in a specific form or sequence. We employ rote rehearsal to remember a poem, the lyrics and melody of a song, multiplication tables, telephone numbers, and steps in a procedure. This rehearsal usually involves direct instruction. However, students with learning disabilities often perceive rote rehearsal as intensely boring, forcing the teacher to find creative and interesting ways to accomplish the rehearsal while keeping students on task.

Elaborative Rehearsal. This type of rehearsal is used when it is unnecessary to store information exactly as learned, and when it is important to associate new learnings with prior learnings to detect relationships. This is a complex thinking process, in which the learners reprocess the information several times to make connections to previous learnings and assign meaning. Students use rote rehearsal to memorize a poem, but elaborative rehearsal to interpret its message, for example. When students get very little time for, or training in, elaborative rehearsal, they resort more frequently to rote rehearsal. Consequently, they fail to make the associations or discover the relationships that only elaborative rehearsal can provide. Also, they continue to believe that the value of learning is merely the recalling of information as learned rather than the generating of new ideas, concepts, and solutions.

Students with learning disabilities need more time and guidance than others to rehearse the new learning in order to determine sense and recognize meaning.

Students with learning disabilities need more time and guidance than others to rehearse the new learning in order to determine sense and recognize meaning. They need help with both types of rehearsal, including a rationale for each. When deciding how to use rehearsal in a lesson, teachers need to consider the time available as well as the type of rehearsal appropriate for the specific learning objective. Keep in mind that rehearsal only contributes to, but does not guarantee, information transfer into long-term storage. However, there is almost no long-term retention *without* rehearsal.

How Different Are the Brains of Today's Students?

We often hear teachers remark that students of today are more different in the way they learn. They seem to have shorter attention spans and become bored more easily than ever before. Why is that? Is something happening in the environment of learners that alters the way they approach the learning process? Does this mean that more students will have learning problems?

Students *are* different today and so are their brains. They have grown up in an environment different from their parents'. Beginning at birth (some say earlier), the brain is collecting information and learning from its environment. The home environment of a child several decades ago was usually quiet—some might say boring compared to today. Parents and children did a lot of talking and reading, often together. The occasional radio program was an exciting event. For these children, school was an interesting place because it had television, films, field trips, and guest speakers—experiences not usually found at home. With few cultural distractions, school was an important influence in a child's life and the primary source of new information.

> *The brains of today's students are attracted more than ever to the unique and different—what is called novelty.*

Today, children have become accustomed to rapid sensory and emotional changes in their environment and respond by engaging in all types of activities of short duration at home and in the malls. By acclimating itself to these changes, the brain is attracted more than ever to the unique and different—what is called *novelty*. This attraction to novelty is not the result of any changes in the physical structures of the brain, but the result of neural associations and networks responding to the multiplicity of today's input.

Adult skeptics need but watch MTV for just a few minutes to discover that the images change every few seconds and play heavily on emotions. Better yet, compare the toys of the millennium with the toys of the 1950s and 1960s. The major difference is advancing technology. School children can now play an inexpensive yet mentally challenging electronic game while riding on the school bus only to be met with a paper-and-pencil, fill-in-the-blank worksheet in the classroom.

Furthermore, school is but one of *many* factors influencing our children. Even the younger students are wrestling with the need to be unique while under pressure to conform. As preteens enter puberty, they have to develop and deal with relationships, identify peer groups, and respond to religious influences without adequate maturity. Add to this mix the changes in family patterns and lifestyles, as well as the sometimes drastic effects of modern diets, drugs, and sleep deprivation (see Chapter 8), and we can realize how very different the environment of today's child is from that of just a few years ago.

Changing Sensory Preferences of Students

Our five senses collect enormous amounts of information from the environment. This information is filtered by the brain so that important data (e.g., your favorite television show) is processed while unimportant stimuli (e.g., background noise) is ignored. For most of us, the five primary senses do not all contribute equally to our learning. We have preferences. Just as most of us are either left-handed or right-handed, most of us also have sensory preferences, that is, we tend to favor one or two senses over the others when gathering information to deal with a complex learning situation. The preferences tend to be among the senses of sight, hearing, and kinesthetic-tactile (the expanded concept of touch).

Although no one knows for sure *exactly* what causes sensory preferences, the current explanation is that it is a mix of both mild genetic and strong environmental influences, especially in an individual's early years. Preferences, of course, are just that: *preferences*. They do not mean that the individual is not able to process with other senses. Just as a right-handed person can certainly use the left hand with competence, a visually preferred person is able to use all the other senses when needed. But when faced with a complex task, most of us will rely more on our preferences to accomplish that task.

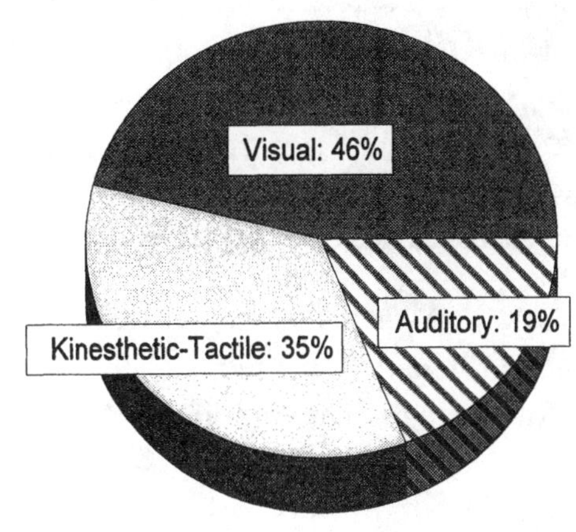

Figure 1.4 *The sensory preferences of the U.S. student population in grades 3-12 for the mid- 1990s. (Swanson, 1995; Sousa, 1997)*

Studies of sensory preferences in school children over the past 40 years have shown shifts among the percentage of students with particular preferences. Figure 1.4 shows the best estimates for the sensory preferences of the student population in grades 3 to 12 in the mid-1990s (Sousa, 1997). Other studies have found similar results (Swanson, 1995). Note that nearly one-half of this population has a visual preference and just under one-fifth has an auditory preference. Yet, in too many secondary school classrooms, talk is the main mode of instruction, often accompanied by minimal overheads or charts. Over one-third of students have a kinesthetic-tactile preference, indicating that movement helps their learning. But think of how much kids in secondary schools just sit at their desks, moving only to change classrooms.

Have Schools Changed to Deal With This Different Brain?

Schools and teaching really haven't changed that much. The computers used in many schools provide few of the options that students get with their more powerful computers at home. In high schools, lecturing continues to be the main method of instruction, and the overhead projector is often the most advanced technology used. Many students remark that school is a dull, nonengaging environment that is much less interesting than what is available outside of school.

They have a difficult time focusing for extended periods and are easily distracted. Because they see little novelty and relevancy in what they are learning, they keep asking the eternal question, "Why do we need to know this?" Some teachers interpret this attitude as alienation from school while other teachers see it as a sign of a learning disability. In both instances, they are likely to refer the student for counseling and diagnosis. Consequently, it is possible that more children are being referred for special education evaluation not because they have true learning difficulties but because an inflexible (though well-meaning) school environment has not adapted to their changing brains.

By rethinking what we do in schools and classrooms, perhaps more children will get the education they need and deserve.

Rather than disparaging the changing brain and culture, perhaps we should recognize that we must adjust schools to accommodate these changes. As we gain a more scientifically based understanding about today's novel brain and how it learns, we must rethink what we do in classrooms and schools. Maybe then more children will stay in the educational mainstream rather than be sidelined for labeling.

Some students, of course, do develop learning disabilities that need to be accurately diagnosed and addressed. The following chapters will discuss several types of learning disabilities, review recent research about them, and suggest ways of helping students who demonstrate them.

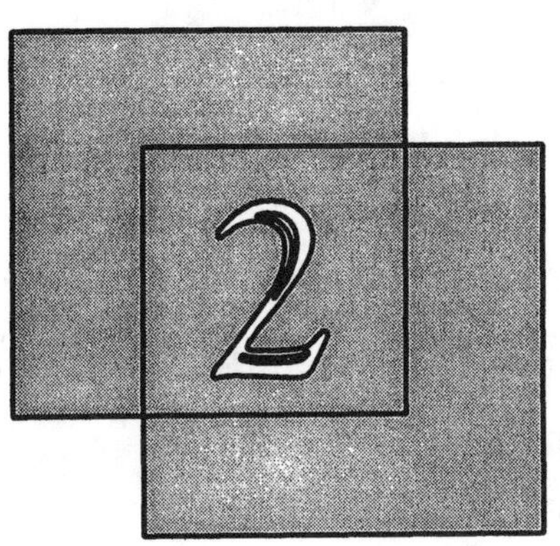

When Brains Differ

Neuron development starts in the embryo shortly after conception and proceeds at an astonishing rate. Between 50,000 and 100,000 new brain cells are generated *each second* from the fifth to the twentieth week of life. Genetic instructions govern the rate of growth and direct the migration of neurons to different levels, forming the six layers of the fetus's cerebral cortex. In the first four months of gestation, about 200 billion neurons are formed, but about half will die off during the fifth month because they fail to connect with any areas of the growing embryo. This purposeful destruction of neurons (called *apoptosis*) is genetically programmed to ensure that only those neurons that have made connections are preserved, and to prevent the brain from being overcrowded with unconnected cells. Sometimes apoptosis gets out of control and connections that might otherwise have imparted certain intuitive skills—such as photographic memory—may be pruned as well. Defective apoptosis may also explain both the amazing abilities and deficits of autistic savants, and the impaired intelligence associated with Down syndrome. Any drugs or alcohol that the mother takes during this time can interfere with the growing brain cells, increasing the risk of fetal addiction and mental defects. Neuron growth in the fetus can also be damaged if the mother is under continual stress.

The neurons in a child's brain make many more connections than do those in an adult's brain. A newborn's brain makes connections at an incredible pace as the child absorbs its environment. The richer the environment, the greater the number of interconnections that are made; consequently, learning can take place faster and with greater meaning.

As the child approaches puberty, the pace slackens and two other processes begin: Connections the brain finds useful become permanent; those not useful are eliminated (apoptosis) as the brain selectively strengthens and prunes connections based on experience. This process continues throughout our lives, but it appears to be most intense between the ages of 3 and 12.

Thus at an early age experiences are already shaping the brain and designing the unique neural architecture that will influence how it handles future experiences in school, work, and other places.

Research Examines Learning Disabilities

Possible Causes of Learning Disabilities

Neuroscientists once believed that all learning disabilities were caused by a single neurological problem. By contrast, recent research has shown that learning disabilities do not stem from a single cause but from difficulties in bringing together information from different regions of the brain. These difficulties can arise during the fetal development of the child.

During pregnancy, the development of the brain is vulnerable to all kinds of disruptions. If the disruption occurs later in the pregnancy, errors may occur in the makeup of brain cells, their location, or the connections they make with neighboring cells. Some researchers believe that these errors may show up later as learning disorders.

> *Some children may exhibit behavior that looks like a learning disability but may simply be a delay in maturation.*

Experiments with animals have shown that other factors can disrupt brain development as well. Table 2.1 shows some of the factors currently under investigation and their potential impact on the development of the young brain. Problems in brain development that occur before, during, or after the birth of a child may eventually lead to learning difficulties. But not all learning difficulties are technically disabilities. For example, many children are just slower in developing certain skills. Therefore, some children may exhibit behavior that *looks like* a learning disability but may simply be a delay in maturation.

Learning disabilities are characterized by a significant difference between a child's achievement and that individual's overall intelligence. Students with learning disabilities often exhibit a wide variety of traits including problems with spoken and written language, reading, arithmetic, reasoning ability, and organization skills. These may be accompanied by inattention, hyperactivity, impulsivity, motor disorders, perceptual impairment, and a low tolerance for frustration. Because each of these traits can run the gamut from mild to severe, it is necessary to assess each student's disabilities carefully to determine the best approach for effective teaching.

Table 2.1 Some Factors That Affect Brain Development
(Adapted from NIMH, 1995)

Genetic Links	Because learning disabilities tend to run in families, there may be a genetic link. However, the parent's learning disability often takes a slightly different form in the child. This may indicate that directly inheriting a specific learning disability is unlikely. It is possible that the child inherits a subtle brain dysfunction that can lead to a learning disability. It is also possible that some learning difficulties may stem from the family environment. Parents with an expressive language disorder, for example, may talk less to their children, or their language may be atypical. Hence, the child lacks a good model for acquiring language and, consequently, may seem learning disabled.
Tobacco, Alcohol, and Other Drug Use	The mother's use of cigarettes, alcohol, or other drugs may damage the unborn child. Mothers who smoke during pregnancy often bear smaller babies who tend to be at risk for problems including learning disorders. Alcohol can distort neural growth and result in fetal alcohol syndrome, which often leads to hyperactivity and intellectual impairment. Even small amounts of alcohol during pregnancy can affect the frontal lobe and lead later to problems with attention, learning, and memory. Drugs like cocaine (especially crack) seem to affect the development of the receptor cells that transmit incoming information from our senses. This receptor damage may cause children to have difficulty understanding speech sounds or letters, a common problem found in the offspring of crack-addicted mothers.
Problems During Pregnancy or Delivery	Sometimes the mother's immune system attacks the fetus causing newly formed brain cells to settle in the wrong part of the brain. This migration may disturb the formation of neural networks needed for language and cognitive thought. During delivery, the umbilical cord may become twisted and temporarily cut off oxygen to the brain, which can damage or kill neurons and lead to learning disorders.
Toxins in the Child's Environment	Environmental toxins may disrupt brain cell growth and development in the early years. Lead and cadmium are getting particular research attention. Lead was once common in gasoline and paint and is still found in some homes and water pipes. Exposure to lead can cause learning difficulties. Cadmium is used for making some steel products and can get into the soil. Moreover, evidence exists showing that children with cancer can develop learning difficulties if treated with radiation or chemotherapy at an early age.
Stress in the Child's Environment	Prolonged and inappropriate stress in the environment can harm the brain at any age. Corticosteroids released into the bloodstream during stress can damage the hippocampus and thus interfere with the coding of new information into memory. These chemicals also damage neurons in other brain areas, thereby increasing the risk of stroke, seizure, and infections (Restak, 2000).

Gender Differences

Of increasing concern is the observation that more than twice as many boys as girls are diagnosed with learning difficulties; over four times as many boys are diagnosed with dyslexia and autism. What accounts for these gender differences? No one knows for sure. Some neuroscientists believe that male fetuses are more likely than female fetuses to invoke a foreign-body response by the mother's immune system. The response may induce a hostile environment that leads to fetal brain damage and eventual brain disorders.

Other researchers contend that an unknown factor present during the last trimester of pregnancy slows the formation of the brain's cortex, especially in the left hemisphere. Because girls are not influenced by this mysterious factor, their brains mature normally and are therefore better able to handle the stresses of pregnancy and birth. This may explain why females recover better than males from fetal brain damage (Restak, 2000). The research continues.

A third possibility is that certain brain deficits affecting learning result from genetic mutations on the X chromosome. Females have two X chromosomes, so they are protected if the healthy chromosome can prevent the effects of the mutated one. Males, on the other hand, possess only one X chromosome, so they suffer the full consequences of any mutations on that chromosome.

What Forms of Instruction Are Most Effective?

An analysis of almost 30 years of research indicates that the following interventions are most effective with learning disabled students:

- The most effective form of teaching was one that combined direct instruction (e.g., teacher-directed lecture, discussion, and learning from textbooks) with teaching students the strategies of learning (e.g., memorization techniques, study skills).

- The component that had the greatest effect on student achievement was *control of task difficulty*, in which, for example, the teacher provided the necessary assistance or sequenced tasks from easy to difficult. Working in small groups (five or less) and using structured questioning were also highly effective.

- When groups of students with learning disabilities were exposed to strategy instruction (i.e., how to learn), their achievement was greater than that of groups exposed solely to direct instruction.

Misconceptions About Learning Disabilities

Table 2.2 deals with some common misconceptions about the causes and implications of learning disabilities.

Table 2.2 Misconceptions About Learning Disabilities

MISCONCEPTION	EXPLANATION
Learning disabilities are common and therefore easy to diagnose.	Although common, learning disabilities are often hidden and thus difficult to diagnose. Brain imaging shows promise in the diagnosis of some learning disabilities, but no X-ray-type imaging at this time can definitively reveal a brain defect that causes a specific learning problem. Thus, diagnosis needs to result from extensive observation and testing by a clinical team.
Children outgrow their learning disabilities.	Most learning disabilities last throughout life. However, many adults have devised strategies to cope successfully with their disabilities and lead productive lives.
Learning disabilities are caused by poor parenting.	No definitive association exists between the child rearing skills of parents and the presence or absence of permanent learning disabilities in their children. However, home discipline, the degree of parental interaction, and other factors may affect a child's self-image and enthusiasm for success in school. Physical abuse *can* cause permanent changes in the brain.
All students with learning disabilities will attend special education classes.	Many students with learning disabilities can have their problems addressed in the regular classroom. However, students who are classified typically have an individualized education plan that specifies how certain interventions will be implemented.
Medication, diet, or other treatments can cure learning disabilities.	No quick fix exists to cure learning disabilities. Even medication given to ADHD children acts by mediating the symptoms and does not cure the disorder. Because most learning disabilities are considered lifelong, the support and understanding of, and attention to the child's needs are basic to long-term treatment.
Students with learning disabilities don't try hard enough in school.	Ironically, brain scans show that many students with learning disabilities are working harder at certain tasks than other students, but the result is less successful. Students with learning disabilities often give up trying at school because of their fear of failure.
Learning disabilities affect everything the child does at school.	Some learning disabilities are very specific. Thus, a student's weakness may affect performance in one classroom setting but not in another, or only at a particular grade level.
Children with learning disabilities are just "slow."	Most learning disabilities are independent of cognitive ability. Children at all intellectual levels—including the gifted—can have learning problems.

Helping Students Become Strategic Learners

What actually makes learning difficult for students with learning disabilities has been the subject of research for many years. Examining the challenges of these students yields clues about the way they interact with their environment and possible interventions that may help them be more successful. Neil Sturomski has proposed that learners will benefit from strategies to help them learn. This section presents some of the findings and suggestions he included in an article for the National Information Center for Children and Youth with Disabilities (Sturomski, 1997).

What Is Learning?

Learning is an active process of acquiring and retaining knowledge so it can be applied in future situations. The ability to recall and apply new learning involves a complex interaction between the learner and the material being learned. Learning is likely to occur when a student has opportunities to practice the new information, receive feedback from the teacher, and apply the knowledge or skill in familiar and unfamiliar situations with less and less assistance from others.

Students bring to each new learning task a varied background of their own ideas, beliefs, opinions, attitudes, motivation, skills, and prior knowledge. They also bring the strategies and techniques they have learned in order to make learning more efficient. All these aspects contribute directly to students' ability to learn, and to remember and use what has been learned.

Teachers can facilitate a lifetime of successful learning by equipping students with a repertoire of strategies and tools for learning. These might include ways to organize oneself and new material; techniques to use while reading, writing, and studying mathematics or other subjects; and systematic steps to follow when working through a learning task or reflecting upon one's own learning.

Learning Difficulties of Students With Learning Disabilities

Sturomski (1997) stresses that students who have learning disabilities may have problems because they

- Are often overwhelmed, disorganized, and frustrated in new learning situations.
- Have difficulty following directions.
- Have trouble with the visual or auditory perception of information.
- Have problems performing school tasks, such as writing compositions, taking notes, doing written homework, or taking paper-and-pencil tests.
- Have a history of academic problems. Such students may believe that they

cannot learn, that school tasks are just too difficult and not worth the effort, or that, if they do succeed at a task, it must have been due to luck.

- Do not readily believe that there is a connection between what they do, the effort they make, and the likelihood of academic success. These negative beliefs about their ability to learn, and the nature of learning itself, can lower self-esteem and have far-reaching academic consequences.

Coping With the Difficulties

> *Students with learning disabilities need to know what strategies are useful in a learning situation and be able to use them effectively.*

Acquiring the necessary knowledge, skills, and strategies for functioning independently in our society is as important to students with learning disabilities as it is to their peers without disabilities. Perhaps one of the most fundamental skills for everyone to learn is *how to learn*. Students can become effective, lifelong learners when they master certain techniques and strategies to assist learning and know which techniques are useful in different kinds of learning situations.

We all use various methods and strategies to help us remember new information or skills. Yet, some of us are more conscious of our own learning processes than others. For instance, many students know little about the learning process, their own strengths and weaknesses in a learning situation, and what strategies and techniques they naturally tend to use when learning something new.

Hence, students with learning disabilities need to become strategic learners, and not haphazardly use whatever strategies or techniques they have developed on their own. To be able to decide which strategies to use, for example, students need to observe how others think or act when using various strategies. Learning skills develop when students receive opportunities to discuss, reflect upon, and practice personal strategies with classroom materials and appropriate skills. Through feedback, teachers help students refine new strategies and monitor their choices. Over time, teachers can diminish active guidance as students assume more responsibility for their own strategic learning.

What Are Learning Strategies?

Learning strategies are efficient, effective, and organized steps or procedures used when learning, remembering, or performing. These tools and techniques help us to understand and to retain new material or skills, to integrate this new information with what we already know in a way that makes sense, and to recall the information or skill later. When we are trying to learn new information or perform a task, our strategies include both cognitive and behavioral aspects.

Strategies can be simple or complex. Simple learning strategies are cognitive activities usually associated with less challenging learning tasks. Some examples of simple strategies are the following:

- Taking notes
- Making a chart or outline
- Asking the teacher questions
- Asking ourselves questions
- Using resource books or the Internet
- Re-reading what we don't understand
- Asking someone to check our work
- Developing a mnemonic device

Complex strategies help us accomplish more complex tasks involving multiple steps or higher-order thinking, such as analysis or answering "What if...?" questions. The following are examples of complex strategies:

- Planning, writing, and revising an essay
- Identifying sources of information
- Stating main ideas and supporting our position
- Distinguishing fact from opinion
- Searching for and correcting errors in our work
- Keeping track of our progress
- Being aware of our thought processes
- Evaluating the validity of sources

The research literature is full of suggestions for strategy interventions designed to make learners more aware of what they are doing. Some of these suggestions are found at the end of this chapter.

Types of Learning Strategies

Sturomski (1997) also notes the different ways learning strategies can be categorized. One way, for example, is to classify strategies as either cognitive or metacognitive.

Cognitive Strategies. These help a person process and manipulate information to perform tasks such as taking notes, asking questions, or filling out a chart. They tend to be task specific, that is, certain cognitive strategies are useful when learning or performing certain tasks.

Metacognitive Strategies. These are more executive in nature and are used when planning, monitoring, and evaluating learning or strategy performance. They are often referred to as self-regulatory strategies, helping students become aware of learning as a process and of what actions will facilitate that process. For example, taking the time to plan before writing assists students in writing a good composition. The ability to evaluate one's work, the effectiveness of learning, or even the use of a strategy is also metacognitive, demonstrating that a learner is aware of and thinking about how learning occurs.

Students who use metacognitive strategies frequently tend to become self-regulated learners. They set goals for learning, coach themselves in positive ways, and use self-instruction to guide themselves through learning problems. Further, they monitor their comprehension or progress and reward themselves for success. Just as students can be taught cognitive, task-specific strategies, so can they be taught self-regulatory, metacognitive ones. In fact, the most effective interventions combine the use of cognitive and metacognitive strategies.

Strategies have also been categorized by their purpose or function for the learner. Lenz, Ellis, and Scanlon (1996) suggest three types of functional strategies:

1. Acquisition strategy: Used initially to learn new information or skills
2. Storage strategy: Used to manipulate or transform information so that it can effectively be placed in memory
3. Knowledge strategy: Used to recall or to show what has been learned

Research About the Effectiveness of Learning Strategies

> *Learning and retention are more likely to occur when students can observe, engage in, discuss, reflect upon, and practice the new learning.*

Research into strategies of learning has been going on for over 30 years, long before the availability of brain scanning technologies. Since the 1970s, researchers at the University of Kansas have investigated the benefits of strategy instruction, especially for individuals with learning disabilities. Their work produced one of the most well researched and well articulated models for teaching students to use learning strategies. Known as the Strategies Integration Model, or SIM, this method outlines a series of steps so that educators can effectively teach any number of strategies or strategic approaches. See the model at the end of this chapter in Strategies to Consider.

Recent cognitive research supports the notion that learning and retention are more likely to occur when students can observe, engage in, discuss, reflect upon, and practice the new learning. When teachers help students to use learning strategies and to generalize their strategic knowledge to other academic and nonacademic situations, they are promoting student independence in the process of learning.

For students who have learning disabilities, learning strategy instruction holds great educational promise for the following reasons:

- Instruction helps students learn how to learn and become more effective in the successful performance of academic, social, or job-related tasks. Students can better deal with immediate academic demands as well as cope with similar tasks in different settings under different conditions throughout life. The strategies are particularly powerful in the face of new learning situations.

- Instruction makes students aware of how strategies work, why they work, when they work, and where they can be used. To assist students, teachers will need to
    - talk about strategies explicitly,
    - name and describe each strategy,
    - model how each strategy is used by thinking aloud while performing tasks relevant to students,
    - provide students with multiple opportunities to use the strategies with a variety of materials, and
    - provide feedback and guidance while students refine and internalize the use of each strategy.

Ultimately, responsibility for strategy use needs to shift from teachers to students. This promotes independent learners with the cognitive flexibility necessary to address the many learning challenges they will encounter in their lives.

> *Learning strategies help students become better equipped to face current and future learning tasks.*

Although no single technique or intervention can address all the varied needs of students with learning disabilities, teaching the strategies of learning will help these students become better equipped to face current and future learning tasks. By learning how to learn, they can become independent, lifelong learners—one of the primary goals of education.

The Importance of Positive Self-Statements

Students with learning disabilities often have negative feelings about learning and about themselves. Because of past experiences, these students believe they cannot learn or that the work is simply too difficult. As a result, they may believe they cannot achieve success in learning through their own efforts. Teachers need to address this issue when presenting information on the strategies of learning. By modeling positive self-statements, teachers can convince students to attribute success in learning to their own efforts and to the use of appropriate learning strategies. For learning strategies to be successful, students need to have a positive self-image and recognize the connection between effort and success. See the Strategies to Consider for suggestions on how to build student self-esteem.

Gifted Children With Learning Disabilities

Albert Einstein is considered one of the greatest scientists of the twentieth century. His great mind was able to discuss the quantum nature of light, provide a description of molecular motion, and introduce the special theory of relativity. Einstein was famous for continually reexamining traditional scientific assumptions and coming to straightforward, elegant conclusions no one else had reached. Yet for all his brilliance, he was considered a slow student in school because he could not sit still, would go off on abstract tangents during discussion, and rarely obeyed the rules. Given all the accounts of his early school behavior, in modern times we would most likely have diagnosed him as having attention-deficit hyperactivity disorder.

It is only in recent years that educators have accepted that high ability and learning problems can exist in the same person.

The notion that a gifted child can have learning disabilities strikes some people as bizarre, something like an oxymoron. Consequently, many children who are gifted in some ways and deficient in others go undetected and unserved by their schools. They tend to fall through the cracks because the system is not designed to deal with such widely different conditions occurring in the same student. In fact, it is only in recent years that educators have even begun to accept that high abilities and learning problems can exist together in the same person.

Variations Within These Students

Researchers in this area have identified three subgroups of children with this dual exceptionality (Baum, 1994):

1. The first group includes students identified as gifted but who exhibit learning difficulties in school. Through poor motivation, laziness, or low self-esteem, they perform poorly and are often labeled as underachievers. As a result, their learning disabilities remain unrecognized until they fall far behind their peers.

2. The second group includes students who have already been diagnosed with learning disabilities but whose high abilities have never been recognized. This may be a larger group than one might believe at first. If their high ability remains unrecognized, then it never becomes part of their educational program and these children never benefit from services to gifted children.

3. The third—and perhaps largest—group represents those children whose abilities and disabilities mask each other. They often function at grade level, are considered average students, and do not seem to have problems or any special needs. Although they may be seem to be performing well, they are in fact functioning well below their potential. In later high school years, as course work becomes more difficult, learning difficulties may become apparent, but their true potential will not be realized.

Children in all three groups are at risk for social and emotional problems when either their potential or learning disabilities go unrecognized. The problem is further compounded by the identification process because the activities used to select students for either learning disability or gifted services tend to be mutually exclusive. Consequently, these students fail to meet the criteria for either type of services.

The Difficulties of Identification

Researchers have not been successful to date in finding measurement activities that will accurately identify children with both talents and learning disabilities. Further, the number of possible combinations of intellectual giftedness and learning disabilities is so great that any attempt to devise a single set of reliable measures is probably futile. Nonetheless, researchers agree that a battery of measurements should be developed to assess these students. The battery should include an achievement battery, an intelligence test, indicators of cognitive processing, and behavioral observations (Brody and Mills, 1997). The goal is early identification and intervention for gifted students with learning disabilities so that their needs and talents are recognized and appropriately addressed by the school staff.

Strategies to Consider

Guidelines for Working With Special Needs Students

Teachers should consider these guidelines to help students with special needs succeed. The following general strategies are appropriate for all grade levels and subject areas (NICHCY, 1997).

- **Capitalize on the student's strengths.** This is more likely to give the student a feeling of success and lessen any feelings of inadequacy that flow from the disability.

- **Provide high structure and clear expectations.** These students do better in an organized environment and need to know what is expected of them. Take nothing for granted and make sure the student is aware of acceptable and unacceptable types of behavior.

- **Use short sentences and simple vocabulary.** These students often have difficulty processing complex sentence structures and usually have a limited vocabulary. Behavior problems can arise when the student is unclear about what the teacher said.

- **Provide opportunities for success in a supportive atmosphere to help build self-esteem.** Students with learning problems often have low self-esteem. Any opportunity the teacher provides to improve self-esteem may convince the student to pay more attention to learning and to be more persistent.

- **Allow flexibility in classroom procedures.** For example, permit students with written language difficulties to use tape recorders for note taking and test taking.

Guidelines for Working With Special Needs Students—Continued

- **Make use of self-correcting materials that provide immediate feedback without embarrassment.** Because many of these students have a short attention span, activities that give immediate feedback are desirable. Students can assess their own progress quickly and without knowing each other's results.

- **Use computers for drill and practice and for teaching word processing.** Computers are patient devices for drill and practice. Many programs provide varied opportunities to practice and usually give a running score of the student's progress. Word processing programs can often convince students to try creative writing despite any problems with written language.

- **Provide positive reinforcement of appropriate social skills.** Appropriate social behavior at school is likely to be repeated if it is positively reinforced. Look for opportunities to "catch the student being good."

- **Recognize that students with learning disabilities can greatly benefit from the gift of time to grow and mature.** These students often progress slowly, but many progress nonetheless. Patience with them can be rewarding for both teachers and students.

Strategies to Consider

Strategies for Involvement and Retention

Students with attention difficulties need help to maximize their engagement and to improve their retention of learning. The following strategies are appropriate for all students, and especially those who have learning problems (Fulk, 2000).

- **Get Their Attention.** Use humor, unexpected introductions, and various other "attention grabbers" to stimulate student interest in the lesson.

- **Make It Relevant.** Relevancy (or meaning) is one of the major factors affecting retention. Students are not likely to retain what they perceive as irrelevant. Keep in mind that it is *their* perception of relevancy that matters, not *yours*.

- **Model, Model, Model.** Show students how to do it. Use models, simulations, and examples for simple as well as complex concepts. Ask them to develop original models.

- **Use Teams.** The research indicates that these students are particularly successful when working in teams. The opportunity to discuss what they are learning keeps them actively engaged and helps them to practice interpersonal skills.

- **Set Goals.** Success is a key factor in maintaining involvement. Set realistic goals with the students (e.g., "Let's try to solve three problems this time.").

- **Find Out What They Already Know.** Take the time to assess what students already know about the topic being taught. Building on this prior knowledge is an effective way of helping students establish relevancy.

Strategies for Involvement and Retention—Continued

- **Use Visuals.** We live in a visually oriented culture and students are acclimated to visual stimuli. Graphs, pictures, diagrams, and visual organizers are very effective learning and retention devices.

- **Go for the Big Picture.** The brain is a pattern seeker. Use graphics to put together the big picture, showing how concepts are connected. Discuss the patterns that emerge and link them to what students have already learned.

- **Think and Talk Aloud.** When teachers think aloud, they model the steps in cognitive processing and reveal what information or skills can be used to approach and solve a problem. Talking aloud is an excellent memory enhancer, especially when students discuss open-ended questions, such as "What might have happened if...?" or "What would you have done instead?"

- **Suggest Mnemonic Devices.** All memory tricks are valuable. Teach mnemonic devices, such as acronyms (ROY G BIV for colors of the spectrum, HOMES for the Great Lakes), keywords, and imaging to help students remember factual information or steps in a procedure.

- **Use a Variety of Practice Formats.** Practice is the key to retention but can be perceived as boring when the teacher uses only one practice format. Try small dry-erase boards, computer programs, or simulations to keep practice interesting and varied. And, if students can correctly solve five problems, do we need to give them 20?

- **Explain the Value of Note-Taking.** Writing is not only a good memory tool, but it also helps students organize their thoughts and focus on what is important. Gradually decrease the amount of information you give in an outline so that students need to provide more input.

- **Use Closure Strategies Regularly.** Closure strategies, such as journal writing and group processing ("Tell your partner two things you learned today."), enhance retention of learning.

Strategies to Consider

Teaching Students to Use Learning Strategies

Much has been learned through research regarding effective learning-strategy instruction. As mentioned earlier, a well-articulated instructional approach known as the Strategies Integration Model (SIM) has emerged from research conducted at the University of Kansas (Ellis, Deshler, Lenz, Schumaker, and Clark, 1991). Based on cognitive behavior modification, the SIM is one of the field's most comprehensive tools for providing strategy instruction. It can be used to teach virtually any strategic intervention (Sturomski, 1997).

Strategies Integration Model (SIM)

Select the Strategy, then

1. Determine prior knowledge and generate interest in learning the strategy
2. Describe the strategy
3. Model the strategy
4. Practice the strategy
5. Provide feedback
6. Promote application to other tasks

Selecting the Strategy. First, the teacher selects a strategy that is clearly linked to the tasks students need to perform at the place they need to perform them. When the strategy is matched to student needs, they perceive relevancy and tend to be motivated to learn and use the strategy. After selecting the strategy or approach to teach, the six steps of the SIM guide the actual instruction.

Step 1. Determine Prior Knowledge and Generate Interest in Learning the Strategy. It is important to use a type of pretest to determine how much students already know about using the strategy. This information provides a starting point for instruction. Younger students, for example, may have no understanding of how they learn; older students may have already encountered their learning weaknesses. Motivate students by letting them know that gains in learning can occur when the strategy is used effectively. Studies have shown that it is important to tell students directly that learning this strategy using effort and persistence will help them achieve whatever skill is being addressed.

Teaching Students to Use Learning Strategies—Continued

Use a pretest that centers on the materials and tasks that students actually encounter in class. Following the pretest, the class should discuss the results by asking questions such as:

- How did we do?
- Were we able to perform the task successfully?
- What types of errors did we make? Why?
- What did we do, or think about, to help ourselves while taking the pretest?
- What difficulties did we have? How did we address those difficulties?

If students did not perform particularly well, then discuss a strategy or technique that will help them perform that task more successfully in the future.

According to the SIM model, it is important to obtain a commitment from students to learn the strategy. To accomplish this, teachers can discuss the value of the strategy and the fact that they are committed to helping the students. Teachers should point out the likelihood that success may not be immediate, but that success will come if the student perseveres and practices the strategy.

Student-teacher collaboration in use of the strategy is especially important with elementary school students. Teachers need to discuss and practice strategies with these young students frequently. The commitments can be verbal or in writing, but the idea here is to get the students involved and to make them aware that their participation in learning and in using the strategy is vital to their eventual success.

Step 2. Describe the Strategy. In this step, teachers clearly define the strategy, give examples, discuss the benefits of learning the strategy, and ask students to determine various ways the strategy can be used. The teacher should also identify real-life assignments in specific classes in which students can apply the strategy and ask students if they can think of other work for which the strategy might be useful. Students should also be told the various stages involved in learning the strategy, so they know what to expect.

After this overview, the students are ready to delve more deeply into hearing about and using the strategy. Instruction becomes more specific so that

– Continued –

Teaching Students to Use Learning Strategies—Continued

each step of the strategy is described in detail and presented in such a way that students can easily remember it. Acronyms can help students remember the various steps involved. An example is the COPS strategy, which helps students detect common writing errors (Shannon & Polloway, 1993).

Displaying a poster or chart about the strategy and its steps will also help memory and retention. During this phase, the class also discusses how this new approach to a specific task differs from what students are currently using. For closure, conclude with a review of what has been learned.

Acronyms Help Students Remember the Steps in Using a Strategy

COPS is the acronym for a strategic approach that helps students detect and correct common writing errors. Each letter stands for an aspect of writing that students need to check for accuracy.

C	Capitalization of appropriate letters
O	Overall appearance of paper
P	Punctuation used correctly
S	Spelling accuracy

Step 3. Model the Strategy. Modeling the strategy is an essential component of strategy instruction. In this step, teachers overtly use the strategy to help students perform a relevant classroom or authentic task, talking aloud as they work so that students can observe how a person thinks and what a person does while using the strategy. For example, you could model

- deciding which strategy to use to perform the task at hand;
- working through the task using that strategy;
- monitoring performance (i.e., is the strategy being applied correctly, and is it helping the learner effectively complete the work?);
- revising one's strategic approach; and,
- making positive self-statements.

The self-talk that the teacher provides as a model can become a powerful guide for students as responsibility for using the strategy transfers to them.

Step 4. Practice the Strategy. Practice leads to retention. The more students and teachers collaborate to use the strategy, the more likely the strategy will become part of the students' strategic repertoire. Initial guided practice is designed to check for understanding and first applications.

Teaching Students to Use Learning Strategies—Continued

Students should be encouraged to think aloud as they work through their practice tasks, explaining the problems they are having, the decisions they are making, or the physical actions they are taking. These student "think alouds" should increasingly reveal the specific strategy being used to help them complete the task successfully. Initially, the "think alouds" should be part of teacher-directed instruction. Later, the students benefit greatly from practicing in small groups, where they listen and help each other understand the task, why the strategy might be useful in completing the task, and how to apply the strategy to the task. Eventually, the practice sessions become self-mediated as students work independently to complete tasks while using the strategy.

As practice continues, the level of difficulty of the materials being used should gradually increase. In the beginning, students practice using the strategy with materials that are at or slightly below their comfort level, so they do not become frustrated by overly difficult content. The materials must be well matched to the strategy so that students can readily understand the strategy's value. As students become more proficient in using the strategy, introduce materials that are more difficult.

Step 5. Provide Feedback. The feedback that teachers give students on their use of the strategy is a critical component of the SIM model. It helps students learn how to use a strategy effectively and how to change what they are doing when a particular approach is unsuccessful. It is also important for students to reflect upon their approach to and completion of the task and to self-correct when necessary. What aspects of the task did they complete well? What aspects were hard? Did any problems arise, and what did they do to solve the problems? What might they do differently the next time they have to complete a similar task?

Step 6. Promote Application to Other Tasks (Generalization). The value of using learning strategies increases greatly when students are able to apply the strategy in new situations. It may not become obvious to many students that the strategy they have been learning and practicing may be ideal for helping them to complete a learning task in a different classroom or learning situation; this is particularly true of students with learning disabilities (Borkowski, Estrada, Milstead, and Hale, 1989). Thus, merely exposing the students to strategy training

– Continued –

Teaching Students to Use Learning Strategies—Continued

is not sufficient for both strategy learning and strategy utilization to occur (Wood, Rosenburg, and Carran, 1993). Guided and consistent practice in generalizing how the strategies can transfer to various settings and tasks is vital for students with learning disabilities (Pressley, Symons, Snyder, and Cariglia-Bull, 1989), as are repeated reminders that strategies of learning can be used in new situations (Borkowski et al., 1989).

Therefore, teachers need to discuss with students what transfer is all about (Sousa, 2001, pp. 136-165) and how and when students might use the strategy in other settings. An important part of this discussion will be getting students to review the actual work that they have in other classes and discussing with students how the strategy might be useful in completing that work. Actually going through the steps of the strategy with specific work assignments can be very effective.

Students can generate their own examples of contexts in which to apply the strategy. For example, they could use the COPS strategy discussed in Step 2 for homework assignments, job applications, friendly letters, English papers, written problems in mathematics, and spelling practice. Additionally, teachers within a school may wish to coordinate among themselves to promote student use of strategies across settings, so that the strategies being taught in one classroom are mentioned and supported by other teachers as well. All of these approaches will promote student generalization of the strategy.

Strategies to Consider

Building Self-Esteem

The following strategies can be used to help students build their self-esteem:

- Use students' names when addressing them.
- Have conversations with *every* student.
- Have student work occasionally assessed by other audiences (students, other teachers, parents).
- Avoid making assumptions about student behavior, and separate the behavior from the person.
- Point out positive aspects of your students' work.
- Shake hands with students, especially when you greet them.
- Allow students to explore different learning options (Internet, resource works, interviews, etc.).
- Display student work (with the student's permission).
- Give each student a responsibility in the classroom.
- Avoid criticizing a student's question.
- Provide multiple opportunities for students to be successful in your classroom (especially when giving tests).

– Continued –

Building Self-Esteem—Continued

- ☻ Help students turn failure into a positive learning experience.
- ☻ Celebrate your students' achievements, no matter how small.
- ☻ Allow students to make decisions about some aspects of class work (what kind of report to do, what color something can be, etc.).
- ☻ Try to get to know about the student's life outside of school (without prying).
- ☻ Provide opportunities for students to work in productive groups.
- ☻ Spend extra time with struggling students.
- ☻ Ask students about their other activities (sports, music and drama groups, etc.).
- ☻ Encourage students to take *appropriate* risks.
- ☻ Allow students to suffer the consequences of their behavior and avoid being overprotective.

Strategies to Consider

Working With Special Needs Students in Groups

Chapter 1 discusses the value of rehearsal. Group activities are effective means for students to rehearse by talking to each other about their learning. However, teachers are often concerned that special needs students may remain passive, drift off-task, or disrupt the group process.

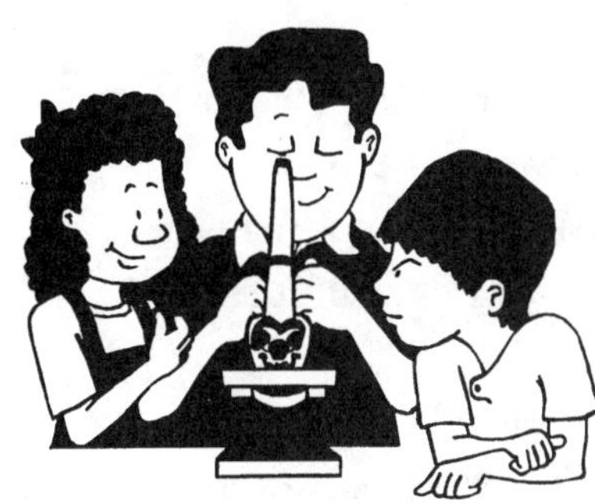

Wood and Jones (1998) report that group activities, especially if they include cooperative learning strategies, are particularly effective in getting struggling students to participate in the regular classroom setting. Group work is often a more effective alternative to the more traditional assignment of having a student read the text and answer questions at the end of the chapter—a practice that special needs students find frustrating. For example, speaking in front of a small group is less intimidating than speaking in front of the entire class. These students also find that their own experiences can be triggered when others in the group remember an event.

The following suggest some of the many ways to implement this strategy. Remember to make appropriate adjustments for the age of the students.

- **Assign Students to Heterogeneous Groups**
  - Divide the class into three sections—high, middle, and low—based on their mastery of the subject matter. Assign one student from each section to a group.
  - If necessary, switch students so that each group is made up of students who can benefit from each other, but not so different that they are intimidated by other members of the group.
  - Give the group assignment and stress the importance of working together. Students can read to each other, answer questions, discuss what they already know, or show a partner how to do something. The object is for all members of the group to accomplish the learning objective successfully.

– Continued –

Working With Special Needs Students in Groups—Continued

- **Use the Retelling Strategy in Each Group**
  - Ask the students to read a portion of their text, either silently or whispering to their partners. When finished, allow some think time and ask them to tell their partners what they learned and what they remembered about the text.
  - If necessary, model this retelling strategy by telling aloud something you have read. Include analogies, personal anecdotes, and other imagery to embellish your retelling. Demonstrate how imaging and metaphors help in memory. This establishes a clear model for students to follow.
  - Keep moving among the groups while they are retelling, asking questions to assess their progress and to assist where needed.
  - After the students complete their retelling sessions, call on them to relate what they have read and learned. Look for opportunities to ask "What if...?" questions.
  - Write the student responses on the board or overhead transparency so that all can see. Point out any differences in the responses and ask students to discuss them.

- **Some Options to Consider**
  - Encourage students to gather information from other sources in addition to the text, such as the Internet, pictures, and charts.
  - Within groups, give struggling students material to use that is written at an easier level.
  - Follow-up activities can include going on a field trip, watching a video, observing an experiment, or listening to a guest speaker.

Using strategies in addition to reading is especially helpful to struggling learners whose difficulties with reading may become overly frustrating and turn them away from the learning experience.

Strategies to Consider

Assisting Gifted Students With Learning Disabilities

Educators who study the effectiveness of strategies on the education of gifted students with learning disabilities offer the following suggestions (Brody and Mills, 1997).

❑ **Use technology.** Technology helps talented students overcome their disabilities. For example:

- Students who are capable of high-level mathematics but have difficulty with computation can use calculators to move ahead in their area of strength
- A microcomputer with a word processing program and a spell checker can be very helpful to a student who has difficulties with writing or spelling
- Students with reading problems but having high auditory processing abilities can use tape recorders and other sources of information, such as films, that are not dependent on reading

❑ **Taking responsibility for their own learning.** This is a powerful strategy because it forces these students to use their gifts to recognize and shore up their weaknesses. It can include:

- Teaching them self-assessment techniques
- Exposing them to new and interesting methods of inquiry
- Assisting them in locating information
- Exposing them to a broad range of topics to stimulate new interests
- Providing experiential learning

❑ **Other considerations.**

- Gear curriculum to their strengths rather than their weaknesses
- Divide big tasks into small tasks and make them meaningful
- Give genuine praise where appropriate
- Use peer tutoring to compensate for areas of weakness
- Provide cooperative learning activities regularly

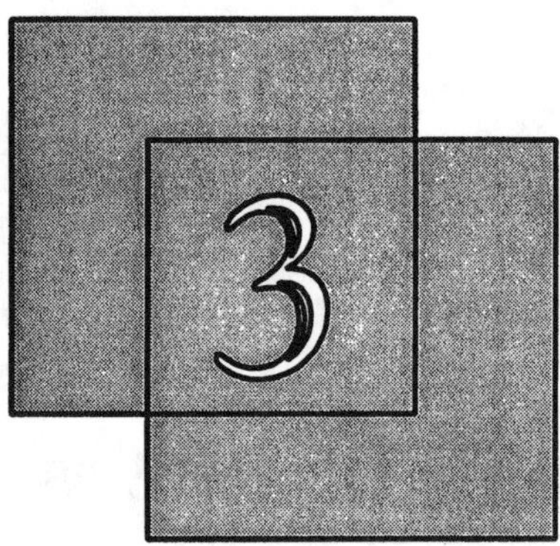

ATTENTION DISORDERS

As brain research slowly reveals more of how the brain learns, educators gain renewed hope in understanding problems that can arise during this complex process. Most learning requires the brain's attention (also called *focus*). Because emotions often drive attention, this activity occurs first in the brain's limbic area (Chapter 1) and requires the coordinated effort of three neural networks: *alerting*, *orienting*, and *executive control* (Posner and Raichle, 1994). Alerting helps the brain to suppress background stimuli and inhibit ongoing activity. Orienting

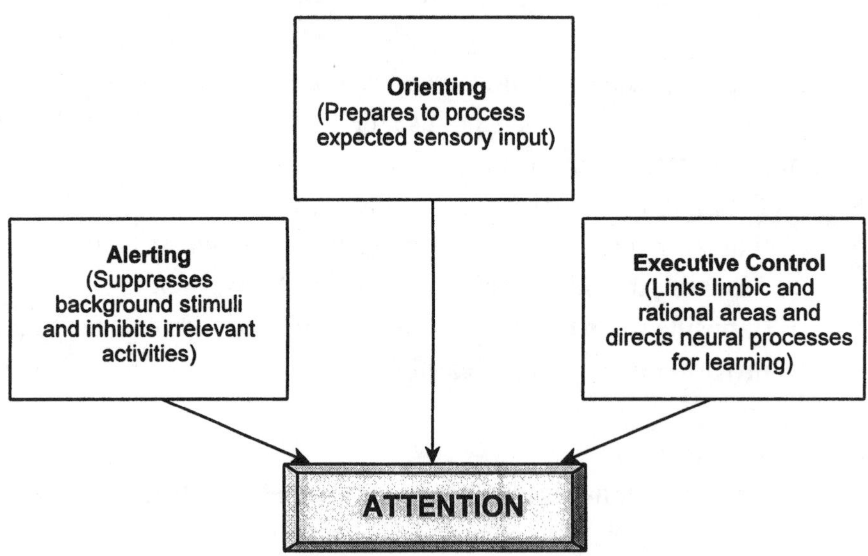

Figure 3.1 *Attention for learning requires the coordinated efforts of three neural networks: alerting, orienting, and executive control.*

mobilizes neural resources to process the expected input and inhibit all other input. Executive control links the limbic centers with the rational areas of the cerebrum, directing the various neural processes needed to respond to a specific learning objective. Problems can arise anywhere within the brain, and the resulting loss of attention may be accompanied by hyperactivity and impulsivity (see Figure 3.1).

Research Findings

What Is Attention-Deficit Hyperactivity Disorder (ADHD)?

Attention-deficit hyperactivity disorder (ADHD) is a syndrome that interferes with an individual's ability to focus (inattention), regulate activity level (hyperactivity), and inhibit behavior (impulsivity). It is one of the most common learning disorders in children and adolescents. It affects an estimated 4.1 percent of youths ages 9 to 17 for a period of at least six months. About 2 to 3 times more boys than girls are affected. ADHD usually becomes evident in preschool or early elementary years, frequently persisting into adolescence and occasionally into adulthood.

> **Some Indicators of ADHD**
>
> (Not all indicators may be present in the same individual. Indicators should appear before the age of 7 and persist for at least six months in at least two of the child's environments.)
>
> *Inattention:* Fails to attend to details; difficulty sustaining attention; does not seem to listen; fails to finish; has difficulty organizing tasks; avoids sustained effort; loses things; is distracted by extraneous stimuli; is forgetful.
>
> *Hyperactivity:* Talks incessantly; leaves seat in classroom; may dash around or climb; difficulty playing quietly; fidgets with hands or feet; motor excess.
>
> *Impulsivity:* Blurts out answers; difficulty waiting for turn; interrupts or intrudes.

Although most children have some symptoms of hyperactivity, impulsivity, and inattention, there are those in whom these behaviors persist and become the rule rather than the exception. These individuals need to be assessed by health care professionals with input from parents and teachers. No specific test exists for ADHD. The diagnosis results from a thorough review of a physical examination, a variety of psychological tests, and the observable behaviors in the child's everyday settings. These behaviors are compared to a list of symptoms contained in the fourth edition of the *Diagnostic and Statistical Manual of Mental Disorders* (DSM-IV). A diagnosis of ADHD requires that 6 or more of the symptoms for inattention or for hyperactivity-impulsivity be present for at least six months, appear before the age of 7, and be evident across at least two of the child's environments (e.g., at home, in school, on the playground, etc.). Recently, ADHD has been classified into three subtypes: Predominantly inattentive, predominantly hyperactive-impulsive, and the combined type.

Differences Between ADHD and ADD. Some children have no trouble sitting still or inhibiting their behavior, but they are inattentive and have great difficulty focusing. They tend to be withdrawn, polite, and shy. Because they lack the hyperactivity symptom, these children are often referred to as having Attention Deficit Disorder (ADD) without hyperactivity. The two conditions are categorized as different disorders because there are some symptomatic differences.

Table 3.1 shows some of the behavioral differences observed in students diagnosed with ADHD compared with those diagnosed with ADD. The descriptions may seem simplistic, but they do help to discriminate between two conditions that are very closely related. Although ADHD and ADD are separate disorders, many of the strategies suggested in this chapter can apply to both groups of students.

Table 3.1 Some Behavioral Differences Between ADHD and ADD

	ADHD	ADD
Decision Making	Impulsive	Sluggish
Attention Seeking	Show off Egotistical Relishes in being the worst	Modest Shy Often socially withdrawn
Assertiveness	Bossy Often irritating	Underassertive Overly polite and docile
Recognizing Boundaries	Intrusive Occasionally rebellious	Honors boundaries Usually polite and obedient
Popularity	Attracts new friends but has difficulty bonding	Bonds but does not easily attract friends
Associated Diagnoses	Oppositional Defiance Conduct Disorder	Depression

What Causes ADHD?

The exact causes of ADHD are unknown. Scientific evidence indicates that this is a neurologically based medical problem for which there may be several causes. Some research studies suggest that the disorder results from an imbalance in certain neurotransmitters (most likely dopamine and serotonin) that help the brain regulate focus and behavior. One thing seems certain:

Parents and teachers do not *cause* ADHD. However, how they react to a child with ADHD symptoms may lessen or worsen the effects of the disorder.

ADHD has been associated with symptoms in children after difficult pregnancies and problem deliveries. Maternal smoking as well as exposure to environmental toxins, such as dioxins, during pregnancy also increase the risk of an ADHD child. Other studies indicate that the ADHD brain consumes less glucose—its main fuel source—than the non-ADHD brain, especially in the frontal lobe regions (Zametkin, Mordahl, Gross, King, Semple, Rumsey, Hamburger, and Cohen, 1990). Brain imaging studies have revealed structural differences in adults with ADHD, suggesting that the disorder may have a genetic component.

Is ADHD Inherited?

Probably. Genetic predispositions for ADHD are likely because the disorder tends to run in families. Children with ADHD usually have at least one close relative who also has ADHD, and at least one-third of all fathers who had ADHD as a youth have children with ADHD. Stronger evidence of a genetic connection comes from studies showing that if one identical twin has the disorder, the other is likely to have it also. One suspect cause is the gene responsible for coding the neuron receptors for the key neurotransmitter dopamine. A significant function of dopamine is to help the brain focus with intent to learn.

> *ADHD has probably been in the gene pool for thousands of years.*

The genetic marker for ADHD behavior probably has been present in the gene pool for thousands of years, indicating that ADHD individuals had important roles to play in the survival of early societies. In prehistoric times, for example, individuals with ADHD behavior could have been valuable as scouts to protect a hunting party from sneak attack by predators. Success in this role required people who could rapidly scan a wide area looking for danger. Impulsiveness and quick-thinking were decided advantages in a hunting society. A scout who was too deeply focused on just one interesting tree or fixated on an attractive vista would likely miss the approaching predator and get eaten. ADHD traits became a mixed blessing, however, when societies became agrarian.

Although there may be a genetic predisposition for ADHD, this does not imply that parenting and schooling don't matter. On the contrary, these are likely to be susceptibility—rather than dominant—genes, so the child's environment plays a major role in determining whether the genetic traits appear. How the parents and school cope with a "problem" child will shape that child's development and interaction with the world (DeGrandpre and Hinshaw, 2000).

Can Brain Scans Reveal ADHD?

Maybe. Several neuroimaging studies have shown that the brains of those diagnosed with ADHD differ consistently from non-ADHD individuals. For example, two structures in the limbic area (the cordate nucleus and the globus pallidus) and one in the cerebellum (the vermis) are smaller in adults diagnosed with ADHD than in adults without the disorder (see Figure 3.2). Further, it seems that these structural differences are strongly associated with a genetic defect. The two limbic structures appear to be involved in the dopamine network. Dopamine is a neurotransmitter that, among other things, helps to control attention. In the ADHD individual, the smaller size of the globus pallidus and the cordate nucleus may decrease the effectiveness of dopamine, resulting in difficulty sustaining attention (Barkley, 1998). Another recent study reported that adults diagnosed with ADHD had abnormally low levels of an enzyme (DOPA decarboxylase) that produces dopamine (Swanson, Castellanos, Murias, LaHoste, and Kennedy, 1998).

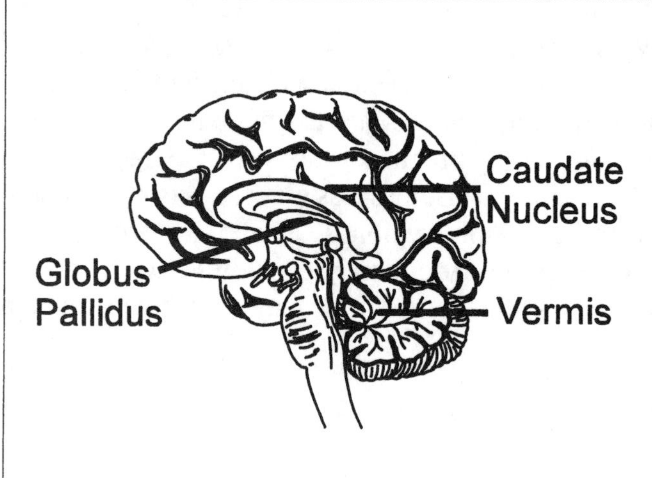

Figure 3.2 *Brain scans have shown the globus pallidus, caudate nucleus, and vermis to be smaller in many ADHD adults. (Barkley, 1998)*

Scans also show that the overall brain size of children with ADHD is about 5 percent smaller than normal. However, this size difference, while consistent, is too small to make a diagnosis of ADHD in a particular individual (Swanson et al., 1998). Besides, brain imaging techniques are expensive and thus will not likely be used as a standard diagnostic tool for ADHD in the foreseeable future.

Is ADHD on the Increase?

No one knows for sure. Although the number of children identified with the disorder has risen, no clear indication exists that the rise is due to greater prevalence of the disorder, to better diagnosis and identification, or both. Certainly, heightened media interest has led to increased awareness of the disorder and the availability of effective treatments. Some scientists suggest that the changing family patterns and child-rearing problems of today may have more to do with the rise in children labeled ADHD than any biological factors. As more children are raised by total strangers, video games, and television, ADHD-like behavior may become the norm rather than the exception.

As more children are raised by total strangers, video games, and television, ADHD-like behavior may become the norm rather than the exception.

Is It Possible to Have ADHD-Like Behavior and Not ADHD?

Yes. Some children diagnosed with ADHD early in life simply have the symptoms which mimic disorder but do not have the disorder. There are other factors that produce ADHD-like symptoms: Some children have not learned the acceptable and unacceptable rules of behavior in certain environments, such as school. Their behavior, therefore, looks like ADHD, but these children may benefit more from being taught the appropriate behavior than from medication. Other children sometimes develop allergic reactions to certain foods that result in, among other things, hyperactive behavior. Again, these children will benefit more from diet modification than medication to control behavior. Additional factors could be stress reactions, other medical conditions, or intolerant schools.

Can Schools Inadvertently Enhance ADHD-Like Behavior?

As discussed in Chapter 1, most children are growing up in an environment that is very different from just a few years ago. But many schools haven't changed their instructional approaches to accommodate the resulting new brain. The possibility exists, therefore, that school and classroom operations can inadvertently create or enhance ADHD-like behavior in students when

- teachers under pressure to *cover* curriculum move too fast (even with the realization that some students need more time)
- the main mode of instruction is teacher talk (when we know that more students have visual and kinesthetic learning preferences)
- room arrangements allow students to hide from the teacher and create mischief (the classic row-by-row formation is more conducive to isolation than collaboration)
- discipline is arbitrary and perceived as unfair (students in secondary schools encounter 6 to 8 teachers daily, each with a different set of rules and expectations)
- there are few or no opportunities to get up and move around (too much stuff to cover, so students just sit and listen)
- the classroom is too hot or too dark (studies show students achieve more in rooms that are well-lit with plenty of natural light)
- there are few opportunities for students to interact with each other (interactive learning reduces boredom and increases retention)
- the classroom emotional climate is neutral or tense (positive emotional climate enhances learning).

Modifying the preceding situations can often change ADHD-like behavior into more positive student participation and academic success.

What Is the Future of ADHD Research?

Promising. Additional studies will need to be conducted to differentiate true ADHD individuals from those whose symptoms mimic the disorder. Brain scans may eventually be an important part of this diagnosis. Brain imaging studies before and after the use of different medications may also help identify the behavioral and cognitive networks that cause the disorder, thereby leading to more effective treatment. Recently, a committee of the National Institutes of Health recommended a study to determine the long-term benefits and risks of stimulant medications, such as methylphenidate (known as Ritalin®), currently used to treat ADHD. Studies looking at the influence of certain risk factors as well as possible genetic links to the disorder are also underway.

What Do Educators Need to Consider?

Teachers need to pinpoint areas in which each student's difficulties occur. Otherwise, valuable intervention resources may be spent where they are not effective. For example, one ADHD student may have difficulty starting a task because the directions are not clear, while another may understand the directions but may have difficulty getting organized to begin a task. These two students need different types of interventions. Also, the sooner educational interventions begin, the better. They should be started when educational performance is affected and problems persist.

Teachers of these students need to be positive, upbeat, and highly organized problem solvers. Unpredictability is a classroom constant, but teachers who use praise liberally and who are willing to put in extra effort will often experience success with ADHD students. After all, most of these students want to succeed.

Impact on Learning

ADHD can affect a student in one or more of the following performance tasks:

- Starting tasks
- Staying on task
- Completing tasks
- Making transitions
- Interacting with others
- Following directions
- Producing work at consistently normal levels
- Organizing multistep tasks

Strategies to Consider

Avoiding School-Created ADHD-Like Behavior

Directions: Complete the profile below to determine whether some of your classroom or school structures can inadvertently create ADHD-like behavior in students. On a scale of 1 (lowest) to 5 (highest), circle the number that indicates the degree to which your teaching/school does the following. Connect the circles to see a profile.

1.	I/We move quickly during instruction because I/we have a lot of curriculum to cover.	1----2----3----4----5
2.	I/We use lecture as the main method of instruction.	1----2----3----4----5
3.	I/We have classrooms arranged so it is possible for some students to be hidden from the teacher.	1----2----3----4----5
4.	Each teacher determines the rules of behavior for the classroom.	1----2----3----4----5
5.	I/We tend to keep students in their seats during lessons to avoid opportunities for behavior problems.	1----2----3----4----5
6.	I/We usually turn down the lights when using the overhead projector or other visual aid.	1----2----3----4----5
7.	I/We generally use the textbook as the main focus of instruction and classroom activity.	1----2----3----4----5
8.	Copying information from the board is one of the main methods I/we use to give students information.	1----2----3----4----5
9.	I/We tend to give more time to presenting information than to concern over students' emotional needs.	1----2----3----4----5

– Continued –

Avoiding School-Created ADHD-Like Behavior—Continued

Scoring. If most of the circles are in the 3 to 5 range, there is a reasonable probability that some students who do not have true ADHD could be displaying ADHD-like behaviors. Here's why:

Response 1: Moving too quickly can lose some students who are deep processors. They want to spend more time playing with a concept before going on to the next. If the teacher doesn't allow time for processing, these students may nonetheless stay with the first idea and would thus be off task or become defiant about moving on. Slowing down and allowing processing time is more likely to lead to retention of learning.

Response 2: Fewer of today's students learn best by listening. They have been raised in a culture that emphasizes rapidly changing visual impact. Too much teacher talk will drive some students to create visual representations of their own (doodling) and thus they will appear off task. Using a multisensory approach is more likely to keep more students focused.

Response 3: When some students are hidden from the teacher's sight, they can resort to off-task behavior or get into mischief, especially if there are no chances for student participation in the lesson. Classroom seating arrangements should ensure that every student can be seen by the teacher.

Response 4: When each teacher determines the rules of behavior in each classroom, chances are high for rules to change from one teacher to the next (elementary) or from classroom to classroom (secondary). Students may then perceive the application and enforcement of discipline as arbitrary, which can result in defiance. Schools with low disciplinary problems are generally those with a few rules that all teachers enforce.

Response 5: Brain research is showing the importance of movement in opening neural pathways. More students today need movement to focus. Keeping them in their seats for long periods of time may encourage some students to fidget, squirm, or get up on their own, typical signs of ADHD-like behavior.

Response 6: Many secondary students come to school with less sleep than they need. Low lights will cause them to get drowsy and thus appear inattentive. How many sleep-deprived teachers might nod off under the same circumstances? Would that mean that the teachers have ADHD? Keep the lights on!

Avoid School-Created ADHD-Like Behavior—Continued

Response 7: Textbooks are helpful instructional tools, but they are rarely novel. When they are the main focus of instruction, students can drift and resort to other off-task behaviors. Using a variety of information sources, including the textbook, is far more interesting.

Response 8: Many of today's students see the copying of information from a board as boring busywork. Discussing the information in groups with "What if...?" scenarios is far more intriguing and will less likely lead to off-task behavior.

Response 9: More students are coming to school hoping to get their emotional needs met, mainly because this is not happening at home. Educators must recognize the importance of maintaining a purposeful, positive emotional climate in schools and classrooms. Brain research is showing us that survival ("Am I *safe* here?") and emotional needs ("Am I *wanted* here?") must be met before we can expect students to focus on the curriculum.

Changes in school operations and teacher behavior that adjust those responses in the 3 to 5 range toward the 1 to 2 range may decrease the incidence of ADHD-like behavior in students.

Strategies to Consider

General Guidelines for Working with ADHD/ADD Students

✓ **Provide the student with a structured, predictable, and welcoming environment.** As part of this environment,

- Display rules and make sure students understand them
- Post daily schedules and assignments in a clear manner
- Call attention to any schedule changes
- Set specific times for specific tasks
- Design a quiet workspace that students can use on request
- Seat problem students near positive peer models
- Plan academic subjects for the morning hours
- Provide regularly scheduled and frequent breaks during which students can stretch
- Use attention-getting devices, such as secret signals, color codes, etc.
- Do a countdown for the last several minutes of an activity
- If a student starts getting disruptive, ask the student to read or answer a question
- Sincerely praise students for constructive things they have done during the day
- Shift the focus away from competition to contribution, enjoyment, and satisfaction
- Contact parents to report good news and build a supportive relationship

✓ **Modify the Curriculum.** ADHD/ADD students (as all students) can often benefit from the notion that less is more. If a student can demonstrate proficiency after 10 problems, then don't assign 20. Curriculum modification can also include the following:

- Mixing activities of high and low interest
- Avoiding more than 20 minutes of seatwork or inactivity
- Providing computerized learning materials
- Simplifying and increasing visual presentations
- Teaching organization and study skills
- Using memory strategies, such as mnemonic devices
- Using visual references for auditory instruction
- Giving students simple decisions to make during the day to build this skill
- Explaining your decision to students and having them explain theirs to you
- Writing tests with easier questions dispersed throughout to keep motivation high

Strategies to Consider

Getting, Focusing, and Maintaining Attention

The greatest challenges for the teacher of ADHD/ADD students are to get their attention, focus it towards a learning objective, and maintain that attention during the learning episode. The following are some suggested activities for each of these steps (Rief, 1998).

Getting Student Attention

✓ Use auditory signals, such a ringing a bell, using a beeper or timer, or playing a bar of music on the piano.

✓ Use visual signals, such as raising your hand or flashing the lights, to indicate the time for silence; or say "Everybody...ready."

✓ Use color. Use colored markers on white board or on overhead transparencies. Colored paper can be used to highlight key words, steps, or patterns.

✓ Use eye contact. Students should face you when you are speaking to them, especially when you give instructions.

✓ Use story-telling and humor. Add a bit of mystery to your story and ask students to guess the ending (orally or in writing). Use props to pique interest.

✓ Start a lesson with an interesting question or problem, and model enthusiasm and excitement about the upcoming lesson.

✓ If using an overhead, place an object on it to get attention. Frame important points with your hands or a colored box.

– Continued –

Getting, Focusing, and Maintaining Attention—Continued

Focusing Student Attention

- Use the overhead projector frequently when giving direct instruction. It helps focus attention and you can write on it without turning your back to the students. You can write in color, place objects on it for interest, frame important points, and cover up irrelevant information. Be sure to remove any distracting material from the screen to avoid confusion. Use a stick or laser pointer to draw attention to the material on which you want students to focus.
- Use multisensory strategies during your presentation. Maintain your visibility and make sure you can be heard by all students.
- Be aware of competing sounds in your environment, such as noisy ventilators or outside traffic, and try to limit their distraction.
- Use illustrations and encourage students to draw as much as possible. The drawings do not have to be accurate or sophisticated, just clear enough to understand a concept. Have fun with this. Even silly illustrations can help students remember a series of events, key points, steps in problem solving, or abstract information.
- Use graphic organizers that are partially filled in. Have students enter information as you proceed through the lesson. Carefully choose the organizer that appropriately shows relationships between and among ideas contained in the lesson.
- Incorporate demonstrations and hands-on activities whenever possible.
- Position all students so they can easily see the board or screen. Encourage them to readjust their seating whenever their view is blocked.

Getting, Focusing, and Maintaining Attention—Continued

Maintaining Student Attention

- Present with a lively, brisk pace and keep moving to maintain your visibility. Avoid lag time in instruction.
- Talk less. Talk is a powerful memory device so give students opportunities to converse with each other about what they are learning. Maintain accountability by asking them to share with you what they learned from their partner.
- Use pictures, diagrams, manipulatives, gestures, and high-interest materials.
- Ask higher-order thinking questions that are open-ended, require reasoning, and stimulate critical thinking and discussion.
- Vary the way you call on students so they cannot predict who is next. Encourage them to share answers orally with a partner or a group, or write them down in a journal.
- Use the proper structure of cooperative learning groups. ADHD students do not usually function well without the clearly defined structures and expectations that cooperative learning techniques provide.
- Allow students to use individual chalk or dry-erase boards, which are motivating and effective in checking for understanding and in determining who needs extra help and practice.
- Use motivating computer programs that provide frequent feedback and self-correction for skill-building and practice.

Strategies to Consider

Strategies for Specific ADHD/ADD Behaviors

<table>
<tr><th>For Excessive Activity</th><th>For Inability to Wait</th><th>For Failure to Sustain Attention to Routine Tasks and Activities</th></tr>
<tr><td>Channel activity into acceptable avenues. For example, rather than attempting to reduce a student's activity, encourage directed movement in classrooms when this is not disruptive. Allow standing during seatwork, especially at the end of a task.</td><td>Give the student substitute verbal or motor responses to make while waiting. This might include teaching the student how to continue on easier parts of the task (or a substitute task) while waiting for the teacher's help.</td><td>Decrease the length of the task. There are many ways to do this, including breaking one task into smaller parts to be completed at different times, or just assigning fewer tasks or problems.</td></tr>
<tr><td>Use activity as a reward. For example, to reward appropriate behavior, allow the student to run an errand, clean the board, or organize the teacher's desk.</td><td>When possible, permit daydreaming or planning while the student waits. For example, the student might be allowed to doodle or play with some objects while waiting. Another option is to show the student how to underline or record relevant information.</td><td rowspan="2">Make tasks interesting. For example, allow students to work with partners or in small groups; use an overhead projector or other device; or alternate high and low interest activities.
Novelty can often sustain interest. Make a game out of checking students' work, and use games to help in learning rote material.</td></tr>
<tr><td>Use active responses in instruction. Teaching activities that encourage active responses (e.g., moving, talking, organizing, writing in a diary, painting, or working at the board) are helpful to ADHD students.</td><td>When inability to wait becomes impatience, encourage leadership. Do not assume that impulsive statements or behavior are aggressive in intent. Cue the student when an upcoming task will be difficult and extra control will be needed.</td></tr>
</table>

Strategies for Specific ADHD/ADD Behaviors—Continued

For Noncompliance and Failure to Complete Tasks	For Difficulty at the Beginning of Tasks	For Completing Assignments on Time
Make sure the tasks fit within the student's learning abilities and preferred response style. Students are more likely to complete tasks when they are allowed to respond in various ways, such as with a computer, on an overhead, on tape. Make sure that disorganization is not the reason the student is failing to complete tasks.	Increase the structure of the tasks and highlight the important parts. This includes encouraging more note-taking, giving directions orally as well as in writing, clearly stating the standards for acceptable work, and pointing out how tasks are structured (e.g., topic sentences, headers, table of contents, index).	Increase the student's use of lists and assignment organizers (notebook, folders). Write assignments on the board and make sure that the student has copied them.
Find ways to increase the choice and specific interest of tasks for the student. Consider allowing the student with ADHD a selection of specific tasks, topics, and activities. Determine which activities the student prefers and use these as incentives.	Ask the student to write down the steps needed to get the task started and have the student review the steps orally.	Establish routines to place and retrieve commonly used objects, such as books, assignments, and clothes. Pocket folders are helpful because new work can be placed on one side and completed work on the other. Parents can be encouraged to establish places for certain things (e.g., books, homework) at home. Students can be encouraged to organize their desk or locker with labels and places for certain items.
		Teach students that, upon leaving one place for another, they will ask themselves, "Do I have everything I need?"

(Adapted from Fowler, 1994)

Strategies to Consider

Using Mnemonics to Help Retention

Mnemonics (from the Greek *to remember*) are very useful devices for remembering unrelated information, patterns, or rules. They were developed by the ancient Greeks to recall dialogue in plays and for passing information to others when writing was impractical. There are many types of mnemonic schemes that will assist memory challenged ADHD/ADD students. Here are two examples that can be easily used in the classroom. Work with students to develop schemes appropriate for the content.

✓ **Rhyming Mnemonics.** Rhymes are simple yet effective ways to remember rules and patterns. They work because if you forget part of the rhyme or get part of it wrong, the words lose their rhyme or rhythm and signal the error. To retrieve the missing or incorrect part, you start the rhyme over again, which helps you relearn it because each line serves as the auditory cue for the next line.

Common examples of rhymes we have learned are "*I* before *e*, except after *c* ...," "Thirty days hath September ...," and "Columbus sailed the ocean blue ...." Here are some rhymes that can help students learn information in other areas:

The Spanish Armada met its fate
In fifteen hundred and eighty-eight.

Divorced, beheaded, died;
Divorced, beheaded, survived.
(the fate of Henry VIII's six wives, in chronological order)

The number you are dividing by,
Turn upside down and multiply.
(rule for dividing by fractions)

Using Mnemonics to Help Retention—Continued

This may seem like a clumsy system, but it works. Make up your own rhyme, alone or with the class, to help you and your students remember more information faster.

✓ **Reduction Mnemonics:** In this scheme, you reduce a large body of information to a shorter form and use a letter to represent each shortened piece. The letters are either combined to form a real or artificial word or are used to construct a simple sentence. For example, the real word **HOMES** can help us remember the names of the great lakes (Huron, Ontario, Michigan, Erie, and Superior). The name **ROY G BIV** aids in remembering the seven colors of the spectrum (red, orange, yellow, green, blue, indigo, and violet). The artificial word **NATO** recalls North Atlantic Treaty Organization. The sentence **My Very Earnest Mother Just Served Us Nine Pizzas** can help us remember the nine planets of the solar system in order from the sun (Mercury, Venus, Earth, Mars, Jupiter, Saturn, Uranus, Neptune, and Pluto). Here are other examples:

Please Excuse My Dear Aunt Sally.
(the order for solving algebraic equations: Parenthesis, Exponents, Multiplication, Division, Addition, Subtraction)

Frederick Charles Goes Down And Ends Battle.
(F, C, G, D, A, E, B: the order that sharps are entered in key signatures; reverse the order for flats)

In Poland, Men Are Tall.
(the stages of cell division in mitosis: Interphase, Prophase, Metaphase, Anaphase, and Telophase)

Krakatoa Positively Casts Off Fumes, Generally Sulfurous Vapors.
(the descending order of zoological classifications: Kingdom, Phylum, Class, Order, Family, Genus, Species, Variety)

King Henry Doesn't Mind Drinking Cold Milk.
(the descending order of metric prefixes: Kilo-, Hecto-, Deca-, (measure), Deci-, Centi-, and Milli-)

Note: This strategy is adapted from Sousa, D.A. (2001). *How the Brain Learns* (2nd ed.). Thousand Oaks, CA: Corwin Press, pp. 131-132.

Strategies to Consider

Tips for Parents of ADHD/ADD Children

Parents of children with ADHD/ADD sometimes feel overwhelmed by the challenges associated with these disorders. However, the following tips, suggested by the National Information Center for Children and Youth with Disabilities (Fowler, 1994), may give parents some help in dealing with their children. Teachers and parents should work together to develop a consistent plan for responding to the child's needs.

- ❑ Learn about ADHD/ADD. The more you know, the more you can help yourself and your child.

- ❑ Praise your child when he or she does well. Talk about your child's strengths and talents.

- ❑ Be clear, consistent, and positive. Set clear rules that tell your child what *to do*, not just what *not* to do. Be clear about what will happen if the rules are not followed. Praise good behavior and reward it.

- ❑ Learn about strategies for managing your child's behavior. These include the techniques of charting, having a reward program, ignoring behaviors, natural consequences, logical consequences, and time-out. Using these strategies will lead to more positive behaviors and cut down on problem behaviors.

- ❑ Talk with your doctor about whether medication will help your child, getting second opinions if your questions go unanswered. **Caution:** Some people claim that ADHD/ADD can be treated primarily with megavitamins, chiropractic scalp massage, allergy treatments, and unusual diets. Be aware that these treatments have not yet stood up to scientific scrutiny. However, as new evidence emerges, an integrated approach of various treatments might be considered.

- ❑ Pay attention to your child's mental health—and your own! Be open to counseling. It can help you deal with the challenges of raising a child with

Tips for Parents of ADHD/ADD Children—Continued

ADHD/ADD. It can also help your child deal with frustration, have greater self-esteem, and learn more about social skills.

- ❑ Talk to other parents whose children have ADHD/ADD and share practical advice and emotional support. Look at the resources and organizations at the end of this book for more help.

- ❑ Meet with school officials to develop an educational plan to address your child's needs. Both you and your child's teacher should get a written copy of this plan.

- ❑ Keep in touch with your child's teacher to find out how your child is doing in school. Offer support. Tell the teacher how your child is doing at home.

- ❑ Remember that as researchers continue their investigations, we may gain new knowledge that could change some of our current understandings and beliefs about the nature of ADHD and ADD, resulting in the development of alternative treatments. Keep abreast of what is happening in this field through some of the organizations listed in the resources section of this book.

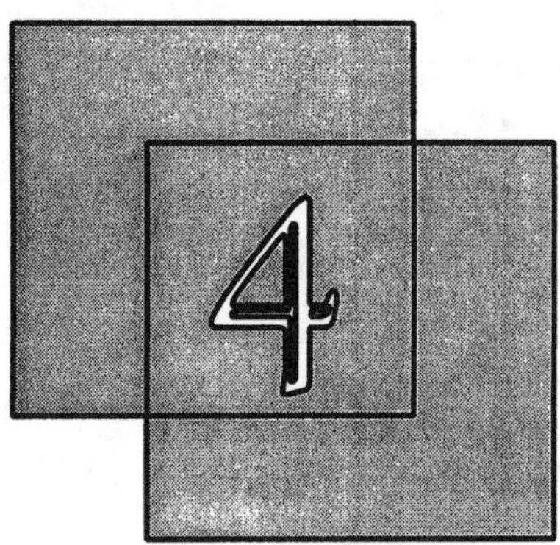

4 Speech Disabilities

Human beings have developed an elaborate and complex means of spoken communication that many say is largely responsible for our place as the dominant species on this planet. Spoken language is truly a marvelous accomplishment for many reasons. At the very least, it gives form to our memories and words to express our thoughts. The human voice can pronounce about 200 vowel and 600 consonant sounds that allow it to speak any of the estimated 6,500

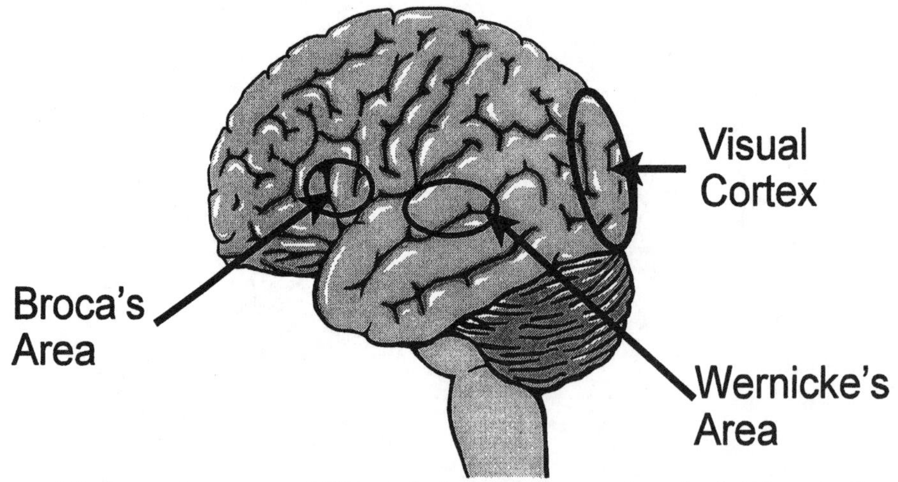

Figure 4.1 *Broca's area and Wernicke's area, located in the left hemisphere, are the two major language processing centers of the brain. The visual cortex, across the back of both hemispheres, processes visual stimuli.*

languages (not counting dialects) that exist today. With practice, the voice becomes so fine-tuned that it makes only about one sound error per million sounds and one word error per million words.

Before the advent of scanning technologies, we explained how the brain produced spoken language on the basis of evidence from injured brains. In 1861, French surgeon Paul Broca noted that damage to the left frontal lobe induced language difficulties generally known as *aphasia*, wherein patients muttered sounds or lost speech completely. Broca's area (just behind the left temple) is about the size of a quarter (Figure 4.1). A person with damage to Broca's area, for example, could understand language but could not speak fluently. In 1871, German neurologist Carl Wernicke described a different type of aphasia—one in which patients could not make sense of words they spoke or heard. These patients had damage in the left temporal lobe. Wernicke's area (above the left ear) is about the size of a silver dollar. Those with damage to Wernicke's area could speak fluently, but what they said was quite meaningless. The inferences, then, were that Broca's area stored vocabulary, grammar, and probably syntax of one's native language, while Wernicke's area was the site of native language sense and meaning.

But more recent research, using scanners, indicates that spoken language production is a far more complex process than previously thought. When preparing to produce a spoken sentence, the brain uses not only Broca's and Wernicke's areas, but also calls on several other neural networks scattered throughout the left hemisphere. Nouns are processed through one set of patterns; verbs are processed by separate neural networks. The more complex the sentence structure, the more areas that are activated, including the right hemisphere.

Learning Spoken Language

Is Language Prewired in the Brain?

In the 1950s, MIT linguist Noam Chomsky theorized that young children could not possibly learn the rules of language grammar and syntax merely by imitating adults. He proposed that nature endowed humans with the ability to acquire their native language by attaching what they hear to a language template that is prewired in the brain by birth—just as baby tigers are prewired to learn how to hunt. Other linguists now suggest that language acquisition may be the result of some genetic predisposition coupled with the baby brain's incredible ability to sort through the enormous amount of information it takes in—including language—and to identify regular patterns. Although the debate over how much language is prewired is far from over, researchers are gaining remarkable insights into how and when the young brain masters

> *The human brain is prewired at birth to learn all the languages on this planet.*

language. Figure 4.2 shows some of the major milestones of spoken language development during the first 36 months.

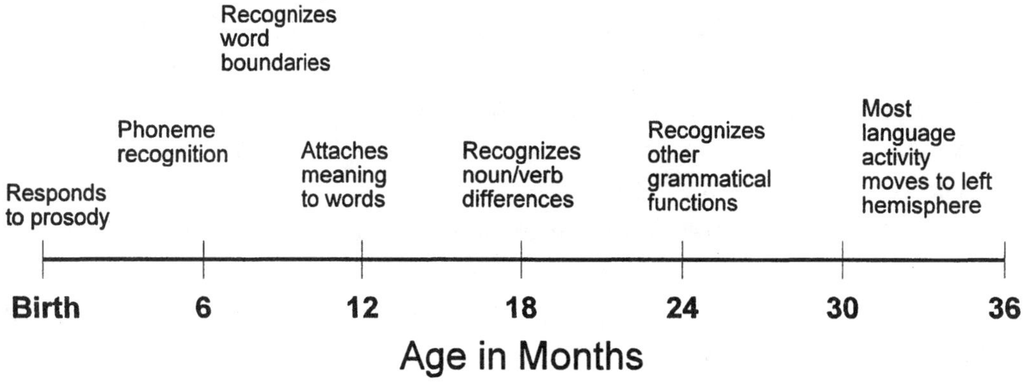

Figure 4.2 *An average timeline of spoken language development during the child's first 3 years. Considerable variation exists among individual children. (Sousa, 2001, p. 179)*

Learning Sounds Called Phonemes. The neurons in a baby's brain are capable of responding to the sounds of all the languages on this planet. At birth (some say even before) babies respond first to the *prosody*—the rhythm, cadence, and pitch—of their mother's voice, not the words. Spoken language consists of minimal units of sound, called *phonemes*, which combine to form syllables. For example, in English, the consonant sound "p" and the vowel sound "o" are both phonemes that combine to form the syllable *po-* as in *potato*.

Each language has its own set of phonemes. Surprisingly, however, the total number of phonemes used by all the world's languages is only about 90. This number represents the maximum number of sounds that the human vocal apparatus can produce. Although the infant's brain can perceive this entire range of phonemes, only those that are repeated get attention, and the neurons reacting to the unique sound patterns get continually stimulated and reinforced.

By the age of 10 to 12 months, the toddler's brain has begun to distinguish and remember phonemes of the native language and to ignore foreign sounds. For example, one study (Cheour, Ceponiene, Lehtokoski, Luuk, Allik, Alho, and Näätänen, 1998) showed that at the age of 6 months, American and Japanese babies are equally good at discriminating between the "l" and "r" sounds, even though Japanese has no "l" sound. However, by age 10 months, Japanese babies have a tougher time making the distinction, while American babies have become much better at it. During this and subsequent periods of growth, the ability to distinguish native sounds improves, while one's ability to distinguish nonnative speech sounds diminishes.

From Phonemes to Words. The next step for the brain is to detect words from the stream of sounds it is processing. This is not an easy task because people don't pause between words when speaking. Yet the brain has to recognize differences between, say, *green house* and *greenhouse*. Remarkably, babies begin to distinguish word boundaries by the age of 8 months even though they don't know what the words mean (Van Petten and Bloom, 1999). They begin to acquire new vocabulary words at the rate of about 10 a day. At the same time, memory and Wernicke's areas are becoming fully functional so the child can now attach meaning to words. Of course, learning words is one skill; putting them together to make sense is another, more complex skill.

Learning Grammar. Chomsky believed that all languages contain some common rules that dictate how sentences are constructed, and that the brain has preprogrammed circuits that respond to these rules. Modern linguists think that the brain may not be responding so much to basic language rules as to statistical regularities heard in the flow of the native tongue. They soon discern that some words describe objects while others describe actions. Toddlers detect patterns of word order—person, action, object—so they can soon say, "I want cookie." Other grammar features emerge, such as tense, and by the age of 3, over 90 percent of sentences uttered are grammatically correct. Errors are seldom random, but usually result from following perceived rules of grammar. If "I batted the ball" makes sense, why shouldn't "I holded the bat?" Regrettably, the toddler has yet to learn that nearly 200 of the most commonly used verbs in English are irregularly conjugated.

> *The more that children are exposed to spoken language in the early years, the more quickly they can discriminate between phonemes and recognize word boundaries.*

During the following years, practice in speaking and adult correction help the child decode some of the mysteries of grammar's irregularities and a sophisticated language system emerges from what once was babble. No one knows how much grammar a child learns just by listening, or how much is prewired. What is certain is that the more children are exposed to spoken language in the early years, the more quickly they can discriminate between phonemes and recognize word boundaries.

Effects of Television. Just letting the toddler sit in front of a television does not seem to accomplish this goal, probably because the child's brain needs live human interaction to attach meaning to the words. Moreover, television talk is not the slow, expressive speech that parents use with their infants, which infants like and want to hear. Although toddlers may be attracted to the rapidly changing sounds and images on a television, little or no language development is in progress. Further evidence indicates that prolonged television watching can impair the growth of young brains. Susan Johnson, a pediatrician at the University of California, San Francisco, cites several studies that raise concerns over the effects of television viewing on young minds (Johnson, 1999). These studies point out that the visual system is not stimulated properly by television viewing in that there is no pupil dilation and the eyes stare at the screen and do not move from one point to the next—a skill critical for reading. The images change every 5 to 6 seconds (even faster during commercials) robbing the higher-thought areas of the brain (in the frontal lobe) of time to process the images. The wavelengths of light produced by the television tube's phosphors are very limited compared to the full spectrum of light we receive when viewing objects outdoors. Furthermore, television reduces the opportunities for the child's brain to create internal images.

Putting It All Together. The successful use of oral language requires the brain to produce sounds that follow a certain set of patterns and rules for

- phonology—phonemes (the smallest sounds of language)
- morphology—word formation
- syntax—sentence formation
- semantics—word and sentence meaning, especially idioms
- prosody—intonation and rhythm of speech
- pragmatics—effective use of language for different purposes, following rules of conversation, and staying on topic

Amazingly, most brains get it right. But problems can occur anywhere along the way. Some problems may just be a matter of time, i.e., the brain needs more time to discern the patterns and figure out the rules. More persistent problems may be due to physiological difficulties (e.g., hearing loss), childhood trauma (physical or psychological), genetic influences, or other factors not yet understood.

Problems in Learning Spoken Language

Language Problems With Children and Pre-Adolescents

Language Delay. Most toddlers begin to speak words around the age of 10 to 12 months. However, in delayed speech, children may not speak coherent words and phrases until nearly 2 years of age. The evidence

Language Delay

Symptoms Around Age 1 ½ to 2:

- Uses only a few words during speech
- Uses only a few phrases during speech
- Speech is not coherent

suggests that a language delay to 2 years is inherited, thus representing a distinct disorder not easily remedied by environmental interventions (Dale, Simonoff, Bishop, Eley, Oliver, Price, Purcell, Stevenson, and Plomin, 1998). This revelation diminishes the claim some people make that environmental influences cause most language delay. However, certain environmental factors, such as stress, *can* cause language delay in some children.

Specific Language Impairment. A broad range of problems in learning language are grouped in the category often referred to as specific language impairment (SLI). It describes a general condition in which a child's spoken language does not develop at the expected and acceptable rate, even though the person's sensory and cognitive systems appear normal and there is no apparent environmental problem. Parents may first become aware of SLI when their children fail to demonstrate the normal bursts of language development that occur around the age of two years. Many of these children will eventually achieve normal levels of language development during the subsequent two years. However, some will continue to display language difficulties at school age, having difficulty building vocabulary as well as difficulty acquiring written language.

Specific Language Impairment

Symptoms:

- Complexity of speech not developing with age
- Little or no growth in vocabulary
- Consistently poor grammar with little or no improvement
- Difficulty remembering recently used words

Although most of the cognitive functions of children with SLI are normal, verbal memory deficits often occur. Montgomery (2000) tested the verbal memory of a group of SLI and non-SLI children on word recall and sentence comprehension. He found that children with SLI had less functional verbal working memory capacity and greater difficulty managing their working memory abilities than their non-SLI peers. A study by Weismer, Evans, and Hesketh (1999) also found similar verbal working memory deficits in word recall. However, the students with SLI showed no performance difference on language processing tasks involving true/false test items.

The question is whether SLI has a biological or an environmental basis, or some combination of both. Studies with a large group of SLI children tend to support the notion of a biological basis through genetic influences and seem to point to deficits in the brain systems responsible for grammar and vocabulary processing (Leonard, 1998; Tomblin and Buckwalter, 1998). Therefore, care must be taken in ascribing environmental factors or identifying a single intervention as a cure for SLI. Because many

Expressive Language Disorder

Symptoms:

- Below average vocabulary skills
- Difficulty producing complex sentences
- Improper use of correct tenses
- Problems in recalling words

of the children with SLI have little or no cognitive deficit, it would seem that interventions should focus on cognitive strategies that help explain and practice the rules of grammar as well as acquire vocabulary in context.

Some children with SLI also display the symptoms of attention-deficit hyperactivity disorder (ADHD). Recent studies (Williams, Stott, Goodyer, and Sahakian, 2000), however, suggest that these two disorders are not directly connected and originate from deficits in different cerebral systems.

Expressive Language Disorder. Children with this disorder have trouble expressing themselves in speech. They often have a weak vocabulary and difficulty recalling words and constructing complex sentences. Although the cause is unknown, cerebral damage, head trauma, and malnutrition have been associated with the disorder. Treatment usually involves language therapy that focuses on increasing the number of phrases a child can use. The phrases are presented as blocks and the child practices building complex sentences from these blocks. Language therapy and similar treatments show an encouraging recovery rate, especially if interventions are started soon after diagnosis.

Receptive Language Disorder. Those with receptive language disorder have trouble understanding certain aspects of speech. They may not respond to their names, have difficulty following directions, or point to a bell when you say ball. Their hearing is fine, but they can't make sense out of certain sounds, words, or sentences they hear. Sometimes, they may appear inattentive.

Because receiving and using speech are closely related, many people with receptive language disorder also have symptoms of expressive language disorder. The combined symptoms are referred to as Receptive-Expressive Language Disorder.

Receptive-Expressive Language Disorder

Symptoms:

- Impairment in language comprehension
- Impairment in language expression
- Speech contains many articulation errors
- Difficulty recalling early visual or auditory memories

Language Problems With Adolescents

Problems with language can be particularly troublesome for adolescents because language plays such a major role in all secondary school subjects. The elementary years emphasize language development. The middle school grades begin to focus on specific subjects where mastery of language is assumed. But in high school, teachers expect students to have an increased vocabulary, more advanced sentence structure, and the ability to use different kinds of language for different situations.

Much effort goes into identifying and remediating language problems in young children. Yet less effort seems to be directed toward identifying adolescents with language problems. Such problems can lead to feelings of failure, low self-esteem, poor academic and social success, and a high drop-out rate. Adolescents with language disorders can be those

- who received no interventions;
- who initially received treatment through early intervention programs, but who still have some language difficulties;
- who had normal language development, but experienced a disruption because of some mental, physical, emotional, or traumatic event; and,
- who have some other learning disability.

Adolescent Language Disorder

Symptoms:

- Failure to understand or follow rules of conversation, such as taking turns and staying on topic
- Difficulty using different language for different needs of the learner or situation
- Difficulty requesting further information to aid understanding
- Incorrect use of grammar
- Poor or limited vocabulary
- Difficulty with instructions, especially those that are long or grammatically complex
- Extreme forgetfulness
- Difficulty understanding puns, idioms, jokes, riddles

Working with adolescents with language difficulties requires more direct instruction aimed at treating the identified language weakness. Consistent practice is important, but the practice should not be so repetitive as to be perceived as boring. Practice using computer programs creates interest, and success in mastering these programs can enhance self-esteem.

Language and Cognitive Thought. Several studies are providing strong evidence that language and cognitive thought are separated in the brain. One study involved patients with Williams syndrome, a rare genetic disorder first described in 1961. Children with this disorder have difficulty with simple spatial tasks, and many have IQ scores in the 40 to 50 range and cannot read or write above the first-grade level.

Because evidence exists that language and cognitive thought are separated in the brain, we should not assume that students with language problems are not intelligent.

Despite these inadequacies, they develop extraordinary spoken language skills. They amass large vocabularies, can speak in complex, grammatically correct sentences, and often have the gift of gab, and engaging personalities. Coincidently, many children with Williams syndrome exhibit extraordinary musical talent (Lenhoff, Wang, Greenberg, and Bellugi, 1997).

Implications at Home. Given the evidence that the brain's ability to acquire spoken language is at its peak in the early years, parents should create a rich environment that includes lots of communication activities, such as talking, singing, and reading. However, the acquisition of speech and language can be affected by a number of factors, including muscular disorders, hearing problems, or developmental delays. These factors should be investigated if a child demonstrates significant delay or difficulty in speech.

Can Students With Language Deficits Learn a Second Language?

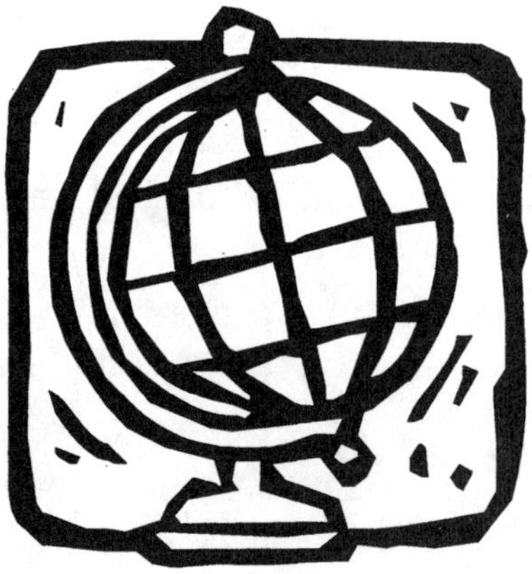

As foreign language study becomes more common in our schools, the question arises: Should students with language difficulties be expected to learn a second language? For students without language difficulties, learning another language can be a rewarding experience that can enrich their lives forever. But for students with language problems, it can be a stressful, if not painful, experience.

Continued research on how the brain learns is revealing some insights into the neural systems responsible for language acquisition. During the 1960s, Kenneth Dinklage (1971) at Harvard University was investigating why some of the brightest students at Harvard could not pass their foreign language classes. The students were highly motivated and devoted enormous amounts of time and effort to studying their languages, but many were still failing. Furthermore, their anxiety over the situation only made the situation worse. After interviews and testing, Dinklage found that some of these students had been diagnosed with language disabilities which they had overcome with considerable effort and tutoring; others had undiagnosed language problems. Taking the university's language classes revealed these problems.

In an unorthodox experiment, Dinklage convinced native language speakers with learning disabilities to teach the troubled students. Most of the students taught in this experiment were able to pass their foreign language classes. Dinklage's work highlighted the basic problem facing language disabled students in foreign language classrooms: The problem is related to being learning disabled, not to any lack of motivation or effort or even to the anxiety produced by the situation. Anxiety was not the cause of failure but the result. Students not previously diagnosed as having language difficulties showed up as such in the foreign language classroom. However, once the instructional methods addressed the language difficulties issues, the students could learn.

In the 1980s, Leonore Ganschow (1995) and Richard Sparks (1993) studied Dinklage's work as well as related research that described language as having three component parts or linguistic codes: phonological, semantic, and syntactic. From this, they developed their own theory, called the Linguistic Coding Deficit Hypothesis. It states that difficulties with the acquisition of foreign language originate from problems in one or more of these linguistic codes in the student's native language system. These problems can result in mild to extreme deficiencies with specific oral and written aspects of language. Not surprisingly, Ganschow and Sparks assert that most learners who experience difficulty with foreign language learning have problems with phonological awareness—the ability to recognize and manipulate the basic sounds of language, called phonemes. Consequently, students who have difficulty recognizing phonemes will also have problems with the interpretation and production of language that is needed for basic understanding, speaking, and spelling.

Language deficits that arise when learning a first language are very likely to arise when learning a second language.

Ganschow and Sparks maintain that individuals who are very strong in all three linguistic codes will be excellent language learners. Conversely, those who are weak in all three codes will be very poor language learners. In between these extremes lies a spectrum of students who may be very good at spoken language but poor at written language, and other students with the opposite characteristics, and still others with combinations of all the possible linguistic variations.

Because of these great variations in the capabilities of students with language deficits, the following question arises: What do we mean when we say they have *learned* the second language? Some students may become excellent readers of the language but not be able to carry on a simple conversation. Others may have difficulty reading the language but be very fluent in conversation and have a near-native accent. Still others may be able to speak correctly but with an accent that is not even close to that of native speakers.

The important point, nonetheless, is that the difficulties these students have in acquiring a foreign language stem from deficits in their first language. With this knowledge in hand, Ganschow and Sparks developed two approaches to foreign language instruction that have been effective (see **Strategies to Consider** at the end of this chapter).

What Is the Future of Language Disorders Research?

Brain imaging technology is revealing much more about the relationship between exposure to speech and language, brain development, and communication skills. Genetic studies are investigating whether at least some language problems may be inherited. The effect of frequent ear infections on the development of speech and language is also under investigation.

Scientists are trying to distinguish those language problems that may be overcome by maturation alone from those that may require some type of intervention or therapy. Some research is focusing on characterizing dialects that belong to certain ethnic and regional groups. This knowledge will help professionals distinguish a language dialect from a language disorder. The success of these efforts would spare children who are merely slower in developing or speaking a dialect the embarrassment of unnecessary labeling, while concentrating treatment on those who really need it. Another area of study is the effect of language development on later school performance.

Finally, some studies are exploring how the brain acquires a second language either during or after learning one's native language. Understanding which neural systems are involved in learning native and second languages can guide the development of instructional practices that will make it easier for all students to learn more than one language.

What Do Educators Need to Consider?

Educators need to do all of the following:

- Address any language-learning problems quickly to take advantage of the brain's ability to rewire improper connections during this important period of growth.
- Give more attention to the language problems of adolescents and train secondary school teachers in identifying and addressing language weaknesses.
- Accept the notion that students with language difficulties may still be able to learn a second language when taught with the appropriate instructional approaches.
- Not assume that children with language-learning problems are going to be limited in cognitive thought processes as well.

The acquisition of oral language is a natural ability that comes more easily to some children than to others. Functional imaging technologies, such as PET and fMRI scans, are allowing a more detailed study of the parts of the brain that are activated during the processing of spoken language. As research reveals more about the amazing process by which we learn to speak languages, parents, educators, and other professionals will be better able to give help to those with language-learning problems.

Impact on Learning

Language disorders can affect learning in the following ways:

- Some language delays are simply the result of delayed maturation and do not represent a permanent disorder.
- Language deficits affecting the acquisition of a native language will likely affect the acquisition of a second language.
- Language deficits will not usually affect a student's cognitive thought processes.

Strategies to Consider

Speech and Language Patterns by Age

The human brain is programmed to learn spoken language during the child's earliest years. As language learning progresses, certain behavior patterns emerge over time forming the building blocks to continued language growth and development. Early language development occurs in context with other skills, such as cognition (thinking, understanding, and problem solving), gross and fine motor coordination (stacking, throwing, catching, and jumping), social interaction (peer contact and group play), and taking care of one's self (washing, eating, and dressing).

The National Institute on Deafness and Other Communication Disorders (NIDCD, 2000) and the Learning Disabilities Association of America (LDA, 2000) have compiled from the research a list of speech and language behaviors that emerge for most children from birth through the age of six years. Each child is different, but the list is a good indicator of speech and language progress for most children.

Birth to 5 Months

- ☻ Reacts to loud sounds
- ☻ Turns head towards a sound source
- ☻ Watches your face when you speak
- ☻ Vocalizes pleasure and displeasure sounds (laughs, giggles, or cries)
- ☻ Makes noise when talked to

Between 6 and 11 Months

- ☻ Recognizes name
- ☻ Says 2-3 words besides "mama" and "dada"
- ☻ Understands simple instructions
- ☻ Imitates familiar sounds
- ☻ Recognizes words as symbols for objects: cat—meows; car—points to garage

Speech and Language Patterns by Age—Continued

Between 12 and 17 Months

- Understands "no"
- Says 2-3 words to label an object (pronunciation may not be clear)
- Attends to a book or toy for about two minutes
- Follows simple directions accompanied by gestures
- Answers simple questions nonverbally
- Gives a toy when asked
- Brings an object from another room when asked
- Points to objects, pictures, and family members

Between 18 and 23 Months

- Enjoys being read to
- Uses 10-20 words, including names (pronunciation may not be clear)
- Follows simple directions without gestures
- Understands words like "eat" and "sleep"
- Imitates the sounds of familiar animals
- Correctly pronounces most vowels and *n, m, p,* and *h*, especially in the beginning of syllables and short words
- Asks for common foods by name
- Uses words like "more" to make wants known
- Begins to use pronouns such as "mine"
- Points to simple body parts such as nose

– Continued –

Speech and Language Patterns by Age—Continued

Between 2 and 3 Years

- Identifies body parts
- Converses with self and dolls
- Has a vocabulary of over 400 words. Asks questions, such as "What's that?"
- Uses two-word negative phrases such as "no want"
- Forms some plurals by adding an "s" to words
- Uses more pronouns, such as "you" and "I"
- Gives first name and holds up fingers to tell age
- Combines nouns and verbs, such as "daddy go"
- Knows simple time concepts, such as "tomorrow" and "last night"
- Refers to self as "me" rather than by name
- Tries to get adult attention with "watch me" phrases
- Likes to hear same story repeated
- Talks to other children as well as adults
- Answers "where" questions
- Matches 3-4 colors
- Understands big and little
- Names common pictures and things
- Solves problems by talking instead of hitting or crying
- Uses short sentences, such as "Me want cookie."

Between 3 and 4 Years

- Can tell a story
- Uses sentences of 4-5 words
- Has a vocabulary of about 1000 words
- Uses most speech sounds but may distort more difficult sounds such as *l, r, s, sh, ch, y, v, z,* and *th*
- Strangers begin to understand much of what is said
- Uses verbs that end in "ing," such as "walking" and "talking"
- Names at least one color
- Understands "yesterday," "tonight," "summer"
- Begins to obey requests, like "Put the toy under the chair."
- Knows last name, name of street, and several nursery rhymes

Speech and Language Patterns by Age—Continued

Between 4 and 5 Years

- Uses past tense correctly
- Uses sentences of 4-5 words
- Has a vocabulary of about 1500 words
- Defines words
- Speech is understandable but makes mistakes pronouncing long words such as "hippopotamus"
- Uses some irregular past tense verbs such as "ran"
- Names and points to colors red, blue, yellow, and green
- Identifies triangles, circles, and squares
- Understands "in the morning," "next," and "noontime"
- Can talk of imaginary conditions, such as "I hope"
- Asks many questions, including "who" and "why"

Between 5 and 6 Years

- Uses sentences of 6-8 words
- Has a vocabulary of about 2000 words
- Defines objects by their use (you eat with a fork) and can tell what objects are made of
- Understands spatial relations like "on top," "behind," "far," and "near"
- Understands time sequences (what happened first, second)
- Knows home address
- Identifies penny, nickel, and dime
- Understands common opposites like big/little and same/different
- Counts ten objects
- Asks questions for information
- Distinguishes the left and right hand
- Uses complex sentences, for example, "Let's go to the park after we eat"
- Uses imagination to create stories

As a precaution, a child who is more than a year delayed should be examined by medical professionals for possible systemic problems, such as hearing loss. Remember that many children who have early speech and language delays eventually catch up to their developmental stage by the time they enter school.

Strategies to Consider

Developing Oral Language Skills

Spoken language comes naturally to the young brain. But to master the language, the brain must first consistently *hear* it. Infants and young children hear the sounds of language and begin to make connections between words and objects or actions. At this point, speech is not necessary. The brain is acquiring vocabulary and making the associations that will give the child the words and patterns it will later need to speak the language. *Listening*, then, is the groundwork for speech and eventually for reading skills.

Recent research confirms that the young brain is fully ready to learn through tactile (touch) interaction by nine months of age. The neural networks for abstract thinking, including math and logic, are set to begin shortly thereafter. Thus, the ability to process language, sounds, music, and rhythms is functional before the age of one year. The parent is the first teacher, and what the parent does to nurture oral language skills in the early years may well set the stage for the child's future success in school. Because some language deficits are eventually overcome, the sooner the child's language skills are engaged and practiced, the greater the likelihood that the time required to correct the deficits will be reduced. Parents, teachers, and staff in early childhood centers can enhance the development of the child's oral language skills through the following activities suggested by Diamond and Hopson (1998) and the Learning Disabilities Association of America.

1. Talk to the child

- Talk to the child whenever you are together.
- Talk about the day's events, a book the child has read, a story the child has heard, or the traffic signs along the highway. Tell the child whatever you are doing.
- Ask the child to explain any activity you are doing at home, such as ironing, trimming bushes, or sorting laundry. Don't settle for single-word or short answers.
- Ask the child to point out objects in the environment and name them. Describe the characteristics of an object (long, yellow, and tasty), and ask the child to name it (banana).

Developing Oral Language Skills—Continued

2. Read to the child

- Read aloud at least 20 minutes every day while the child is sitting in your lap.
- Take turns talking about what was read.
- For a child with limited attention span, provide books with large, colorful pictures and few words.
- Ask the child to point out objects in the book as you read its name. Vary some of the phrases, like "cat in the hat" and "cat on the mat," to see if the child can hear the difference.

3. Reading books should be an interactive experience

- Discuss the book's pictures and paraphrase its story.
- Let the child make up a version of what will happen next in the story.
- If the story is familiar, allow the child to finish telling key events or to give the succeeding rhyme.
- Give the child an opportunity to correct you by purposely misreading or omitting items and events.
- Have the child point out words as you read them.
- Act out the story or create a puppet show.
- Reinforce sequential reading by starting at the beginning of the page and showing the direction of written text, from left to right and top to bottom of page.

4. Cultivate phonological awareness with auditory and visual word games

- Play rhyming games: If a child does not hear the rhyme, try a game with words that begin with the same sound.
- Play the broken record game: Say a word very slowly and break it into syllables, then have the child repeat the word at a normal speed.
- Pick a game the child enjoys, such as matching letters or copying the names of famous people.
- Have the child draw pictures and make up a story while you write it down.

– Continued –

Developing Oral Language Skills—Continued

5. Learning starts with a one-to-one match, followed by patterns and sequence	♦ Children learn to count and learn the letters of the alphabet long before they make connections to arithmetic and reading. Use activities with the child that involve counting: "Bring me one cup and two plates. Put the napkin next to one plate." Have the child repeat the instructions and match the items to the number you requested. ♦ Have the child match letters to items in the room that begin with that letter, such as *l* for lamp and *p* for pencil. Make sure the child repeats the letter and the word aloud and walks or points to the object. ♦ Move on to activities that involve patterns and sequence. Posters, checkers, dominos, and playing cards are strong symbols of patterns and sequence. The child doesn't have to learn the game to be able to identify patterns and sequences in the game pieces.
6. Provide a print-rich home and school environment	♦ Children with oral language difficulties are very likely to have problems learning to read. The sooner that they can make connections between oral language and the written word, the better. Other media, such as videotapes, audiotapes, and the computer, can help with the effort of learning to read by making it fun and worthwhile. ♦ Keep television watching to a minimum.

Strategies to Consider

Teaching Foreign Languages to Students With Language Disabilities

Research studies are identifying the problems language disabled students have with acquiring a second language. Armed with this knowledge, we can design instructional approaches that address the underlying causes and increase the chances for student success. Specifically, two approaches to foreign language instruction for language disabled students emerged from the work of Ganschow and Sparks (1995).

1. The Phonological Deficits Approach. This approach springs from the notion that most students having difficulty in acquiring a foreign language have phonological deficits in their native (first) language. Consequently, the following guidelines are suggested:

- **Teach the sound system of the foreign language explicitly.** The Orton-Gillingham method (explained in Ganschow and Sparks, 1995) is a particularly effective way to accomplish this. This method presents sounds in a highly structured fashion, accompanied by considerable visual, kinesthetic, and tactile practice and input. Studies using this method showed that students who were taught phonological skills in one language had improved their phonological awareness in English as well.
- **Teach the fundamentals of phonology in the student's native language before beginning instruction in the foreign language.** This step helps to address the students' native language deficits, which we already noted as necessary for success in acquiring the foreign language. Here students are taught to recognize phonemes, to read words efficiently, and to apply the sounds to the written language. They are learning the sounds and components of language structure and how these sounds and components are manipulated for meaning.
- **Apply the fundamentals of phonology to the foreign language.** In this step, the sounds and components of the foreign language are identified. The

– Continued –

Teaching Foreign Languages to Students With Language Disabilities —Continued

students can then transfer the knowledge they have about phonology from their first language to the second language.

2. The Course Adaptation Approach. Essentially, this approach adapts the foreign language courses to conform to those principles of instruction suitable for students with learning disabilities. It can be done in two ways:

- **Changing the Instructional Strategies.** Teachers in these courses reduce the syllabus to the essential components, slow the pace of instruction, reduce the vocabulary demand, provide constant review and practice, and incorporate as many multisensory activities as possible.
- **Designing Courses to Address Specific Deficits.** Courses can be adapted to respond to the specific requests of the foreign language students who are having difficulties in their classes. For example, one course might be designed for students who are strong in listening and speaking skills but weak in reading and writing, while another course might be more appropriate for students whose skills are in the reverse order.

For either of these approaches to work effectively, students need to undergo a realistic assessment of their language learning problems. It becomes important to ensure that the learning environment is consistent with students' needs. For example, a student who is able to do oral language well should not be placed in a situation where passing grammar and translation tests is the main requirement. Nor should a student who reads and translates proficiently be placed with a teacher who values pronunciation and conversation. Reasonable accommodations need to be made.

It is perhaps unrealistic to assume that most high schools have the capacity or will to devote foreign language classes solely to students with language disabilities. And even if the will were there, finding teachers who are trained in the methods of instruction for these students might be more of a problem. Nonetheless, the purpose of this book is to identify what current research is telling us about the learning process and to suggest ways of providing instructional settings that translate the research into educational practice.

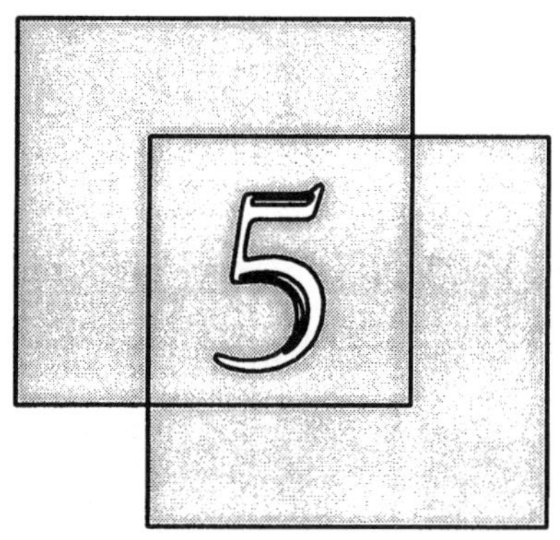

Reading Disabilities

Renewed emphasis in recent years on improving the basic skills of students has increased pressure to start reading instruction sooner than ever before. In many schools, reading instruction starts in kindergarten. Some neuropsychologists are now debating whether kindergartners are developmentally ready for this challenging task. Are we creating problems for these children by trying to get them to read before their brains are ready? Because boys' brains are physiologically one or two years less mature than girls' brains at this age, are boys at greater risk of failure? To answer these questions, let's examine what researchers have discovered about how the brain learns to read, and the problems that can develop.

Learning to Read

Is Reading a Natural Ability?

Not really. The brain's ability to acquire spoken language with amazing speed and accuracy is the result of genetic hard-wiring and specialized cerebral areas that focus on this task. But there are no areas of the brain that specialize in reading. In fact, reading is probably the most difficult task we ask the young brain to undertake. Reading is a relatively new phenomenon in the development of humans. As far as we know, the genes have not incorporated reading into their coded structure, probably because reading—unlike spoken language —has not emerged over time as a survival skill.

Many cultures (but not all) do emphasize reading as an important form of communication and insist it be taught to their children. And so the struggle begins. To get that brain to read, here's what we are saying, for example, to the English-speaking child: "That language you have been speaking quite correctly for the past few years can be represented by abstract symbols called the *alphabet*. We are going to disrupt that sophisticated spoken language protocol you have already developed and ask you to reorganize it to accommodate these symbols, which, by the way, are not very reliable. There are lots of exceptions, but you'll just have to adjust." Some children—perhaps 50 percent—make this adjustment with relative ease once exposed to formal instruction. It appears, however, that for the other 50 percent, reading is a much more formidable task, and for about 20 to 30 percent, it definitely becomes the most difficult task they will ever undertake in their lives.

> *Reading is probably the most difficult task for the young brain to do.*

How Does the Brain Read?

To read, the brain must eventually learn to connect abstract symbols to sound bits it already knows. In English, the brain must first learn the alphabet, whose letter names do not always represent their sounds in words. When are *f* or *l* ever pronounced as *ef* or *el* in English? Then the brain must connect those 26 letters to the 44 sounds of spoken English (phonemes) that the child has been using successfully for years. Thus, reading involves a recognition that speech can be broken into small sounds (phonemes) and that these segmented sounds can be represented in print (phonics). Just as the brain thinks it knows what letter represents a phoneme sound, it discovers that the same symbol can have *different* sounds, such as the *a*'s in *cat* and in *father*. Next it learns that a group of letters makes a syllable, but that the same group of letters, say *-ough*, can have multiple sounds, as in *cough*, *bough*, *dough*, and *through*. Simple, isn't it?

Unfortunately, the human brain is not born with the insight to make these sound-to-symbol connections, nor does it develop naturally without instruction. Children of literate homes may encounter this instruction before coming to school. Others, however, do not have this opportunity before coming to school. For them, classroom instruction needs to focus on making the phoneme-phonics connections before reading can be successful. If children cannot hear the "-at" sound in *bat* and *hat* and perceive that the

> *Just because some children have difficulty understanding that spoken words are composed of discrete sounds doesn't mean that they have brain damage or dysfunction.*

difference lies in the first sound, then they will have difficulty decoding and sounding out words quickly and correctly.

Researchers using brain imaging techniques are getting a clearer picture of the cerebral processes involved in reading: The word (for example, *dog*) is first recorded in the visual cortex (Figure 5.1), then decoded by a structure on the left side of the brain called the angular gyrus, which separates it into its basic sounds, or phonemes (e.g., the letters *d-o-g* are pronounced "duh, awh, guh"). This process activates Broca's area so that the word can be identified. The brain's vocabulary store and reasoning and concept formation abilities, along with activity in Wernicke's area, combine to provide meaning, producing the thought of a furry animal that barks (Shaywitz, 1996). All this occurs in a fraction of a second.

Keep in mind that although the process outlined in Figure 5.1 appears linear and singular, it is really bidirectional and parallel, with many phonemes being processed at the same time. That the brain learns to read at all attests to its remarkable ability to sift through seemingly confusing input and establish patterns and systems. For a few children, this process comes naturally; most have to be taught (Sousa, 2001).

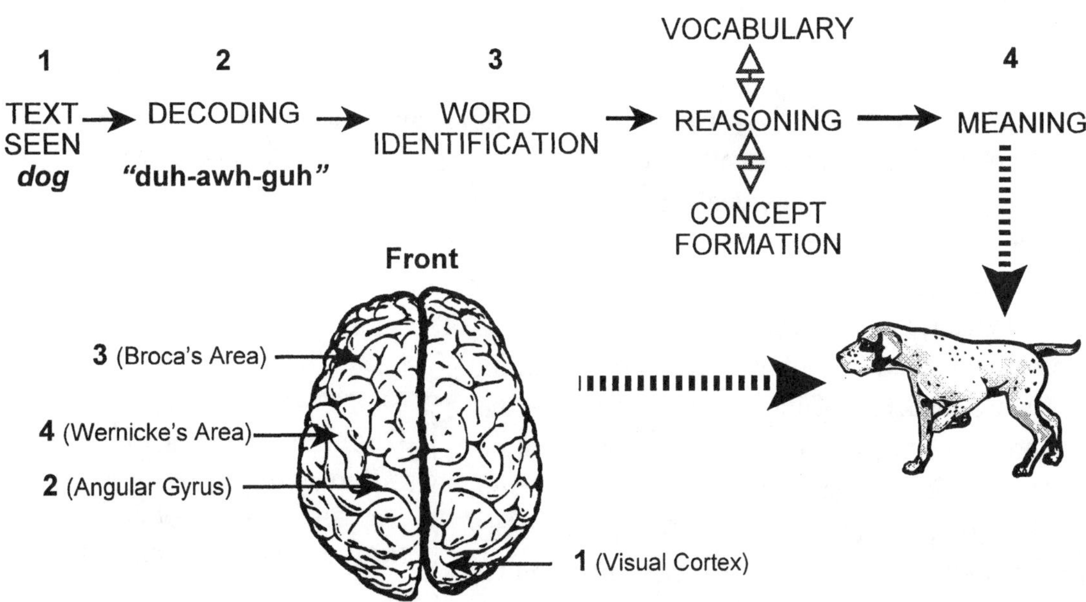

Figure 5.1 *In reading the word* dog *it is first seen (1), then decoded into its phonological elements (2), and identified (3). The higher-level functions of reasoning and concept formation provide the meaning (4) and produce the thought of a furry animal that barks. (Sousa, 2001, p. 184)*

The neural systems that perceive the phonemes in our language are more efficient in some children than in others. Just because some children have difficulty understanding that spoken words are composed of discrete sounds doesn't mean that they have brain damage or dysfunction. The individual differences that underlie the efficiency with which one learns to read can be seen in the acquisition of other skills, such as learning to play a musical instrument, playing a sport, or building a model. To some extent, neural efficiency is related to genetic composition, but these genetic factors can be modified by the environment.

Learning to read, therefore, starts with phoneme awareness, a recognition that written spellings represent sounds (called the alphabetic principle), and that this combination applies phonics to the reading and spelling of words. These skills are *necessary* but not *sufficient* to learn to read the English language with meaning. The reader must also become proficient in grasping larger units of print, such as syllable patterns, whole words, and phrases. The ultimate goal of reading is for children to become sufficiently fluent to understand what they read. This understanding includes literal comprehension as well as more sophisticated reflective understandings, such as "Why am I reading this?" and "What is the author's point?"

Phonological Awareness

What Is Phonological Awareness? Phonological awareness is the recognition that oral language can be divided into smaller components, such as sentences into words, words into syllables and, ultimately, individual phonemes. Being phonologically aware means having an understanding of all these levels. In children, phonological awareness usually starts with initial rhyming and a recognition that sentences can be segmented into words. Next comes segmenting words into syllables and blending syllables into words. The most complex level of phonological awareness is phonemic awareness—the understanding that words are made up of individual sounds and that these sounds can be manipulated to create new words.

> *Phonological awareness is different from phonics. The two are closely related, but they are not the same.*

Phonological awareness is different from phonics. Phonological awareness involves the auditory and oral manipulation of sounds. Phonics builds on the alphabetic principle and associates letters and sounds with written symbols. The two are closely related, but they are not the same. Recognition of rhyming and alliteration are usual indications that a child has phonological awareness, which develops when children are read to from books based on rhyme or alliteration. But this awareness does not easily develop into the more sophisticated phonemic awareness, which is so closely related to a child's success in learning to read (Chard and Dickson, 1999).

How Does Phonological Awareness Help in Learning to Read? New readers must recognize the alphabetic principle and that words can be separated into individual phonemes, which can be reordered and blended into words. This enables learners to associate the letters with sounds in order to read and build words. Thus, phonological awareness in kindergarten is a strong predictor of reading success that persists throughout school (Shankweiler, Crain, Katz, Fowler, Liberman, Brady, Thornton, Lunquist, Dreyer, Fletcher, Steubing, Shaywitz, and Shaywitz, 1995). Early instruction in reading, especially in letter-sound association, strengthens phonological awareness and helps in the development of the more sophisticated phonemic awareness (Snow, Burns, and Griffin, 1998).

Phonics Versus Whole-Language Approaches to Reading.

Throughout the history of teaching reading, a great debate has existed between whether it is better to start with word sounds (phonics) or to teach words as they derive their meaning from a larger context (whole language). Unfortunately, some schools that adopted the whole-language approach abandoned the teaching of phonics altogether. In fact, in any school that exclusively adopted one approach, there was always a block of students who still did not learn to read. Even those schools that purported to use a "blended" or "eclectic" approach often failed to include systematic instruction in phonological awareness, phonics, and their component skills.

Nonetheless, the research is clear: successful reading starts with phonemic awareness of sound-symbol correspondences and the blending of sound-spellings until almost any unknown word can be accurately decoded (Moats, 2000). Starting with the phonemic awareness approach is one of the few aspects of reading supported by a substantial and long-term body of research.

An exclusively whole-language approach minimizes or omits the systematic teaching of phoneme awareness, spelling patterns, and rules of grammar. Whole language appears to be primarily a system of intentions and beliefs from the late 1960s proposing that early reading instruction should focus on purpose and meaning and that word analysis skills should arise only incidently to contextual reading. However, its philosophy was derived from an analysis of how *adults* read and long before the development of brain imaging technologies. The whole language approach gained great popularity in the late 1970s, and by the early 1980s, school districts were replacing phonics-based programs with programs based on individual reading instruction with children's literature. Yet no solid body of research existed then or exists now to support the effectiveness of *exclusively* using the whole-language approach with beginning readers. Almost every basic premise that whole language advocates about how we *learn* to read is contradicted by recent scientific studies that show the following:

The research is clear: Successful reading starts with phonemic awareness.

- Learning to read is not a natural ability for the human brain.
- The alphabetic principle is not learned merely by exposure to print.
- Spoken language and written language are very different, and thus require the mastery of different skills.
- The most important skill at the beginning stages of reading is the ability to read single words accurately, completely, and fluently.
- Context is not the primary factor in beginning word recognition.

Children bring a knowledge of spoken language when they encounter the printed page. They need to learn the written symbols that represent speech, and to use them accurately and fluently. Reading instruction should begin with phonemic awareness and then move to contextual and enriched reading as the student gains competency and confidence. Thus some of the principles of whole language can be incorporated later as part of reading development (Moats, 2000).

Difficulties in Learning to Read

> *Successful reading involves the coordination of three neural networks: visual processing, sound recognition, and word interpretation.*

Reading is so complex that any small problem along the way can slow or interrupt the process. It is small wonder that children have more problems with reading than with any other skill we ask them to learn. Difficulties result essentially from either environmental or physical factors, or some combination of both. Environmental factors include limited exposure to language in the preschool years, resulting in little phoneme sensitivity, letter knowledge, print awareness, vocabulary, and reading comprehension. Physical factors include speech, hearing, and visual impairments and substandard intellectual capabilities. Any combination of environmental and physical factors makes diagnosis and treatment more difficult. Neuroimaging, however, is showing great promise as a tool for diagnosing reading and language difficulties.

As we can see from Figure 5.2, successful reading involves the coordination of three neural networks: visual processing (orthography), sound recognition (phonology), and word interpretation (semantics). In reading the word *dog*, the visual processing system puts the symbols together. The decoding process alerts the auditory processing system that recognizes the alphabetic symbols to represent the sound "dawg." Other brain regions, including the frontal lobe, search long-term memory sites for meaning. If all systems work correctly, a mental image emerges of a furry animal that barks (Patterson and Lambon Ralph, 1999). Problems can occur almost anywhere along the way. Many variations of reading disorders exist, but here are some of the more common ones that teachers encounter.

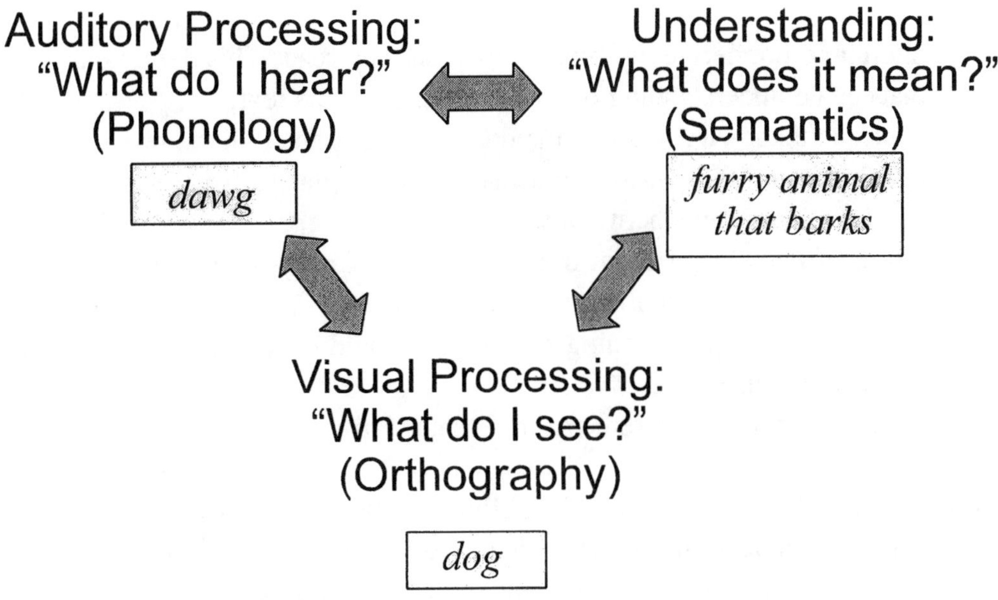

Figure 5.2 *Successful reading requires the coordination of three systems: visual processing to see the word, auditory processing to hear it, and semantic processing to understand it.*

Deficits in Phoneme Awareness and the Alphabetic Principle

> *Understanding phonemes, more than any other factor, is a critical part of successful reading.*

If the brain cannot understand that words are made up of segmented sounds that can be connected to letters (the alphabetic principle), then reading becomes extremely difficult. For children with this problem, reading is hesitant and characterized by frequent starts and stops and multiple mispronunciations. Their comprehension is low because they take too much time to read, and memory cannot retain the words long enough to understand what has been read. This condition is referred to as *phonological alexia*.

This deficit may have genetic and neurobiological origins in that the decoding process in the angular gyrus (Figure 5.1) is defective. It also may be caused by lack of exposure to spoken language patterns and usage during the preschool years. In either case, the result is the same—difficulty in linking speech sound to letters, decoding that is labored and weak, and a lack of comprehension.

Deficits in Reading Comprehension

Some children do not derive meaning from what they read. This deficit may relate to

- inadequate understanding of the words used in the text,
- inadequate knowledge about the domains represented in the text,
- a lack of familiarity with the semantic and syntactic structures that help predict relationships between words,
- a lack of knowledge about different writing conventions that are used to achieve different purposes (humor, explanation, dialogue, etc.),
- a deficit in verbal reasoning ability that would enable the reader to read between the lines, and
- a lack of the ability to remember verbal information.

This condition is referred to as *surface alexia*. Although a large number of research studies have investigated vocabulary acquisition and syntactic development, no clear answers are available at this time to explain exactly how that occurs. Thus our understanding of how to help students use reading comprehension strategies in different situations is not well developed, but new research areas seem promising.

Dysfunction in the Timing of Speech Sounds

Recent studies of young children with language-learning difficulties indicate that they may have a dysfunction in brain-timing mechanisms, which makes processing of certain speech sounds difficult. Researchers discovered that by using computer-processed language programs that pronounced words more slowly, some children (ages 5 to 10) were able to advance their reading levels by two years after just four weeks of training. This improvement was maintained for at least a year (Tallal, Miller, Bedi, Byma, Wang, Nagarajan, Schreiner, Jenkins, and Merzenich, 1996).

> *Researchers discovered that by using computer-processed language programs, some children were able to advance their reading levels by two years after just four weeks of training.*

Another revelation from brain scans is that poor readers' brains show more frontal lobe activity than do good readers' brains. This means that the poor readers are putting forth additional effort—perhaps subvocalizing—to pronounce and interpret the word correctly (Merzenich, Jenkins, Johnston, Schreiner, Miller, and Tallal, 1996; Tallal et al., 1996). So it doesn't make sense to say to a poor reader, "Try harder." The problem is not the effort, but the accuracy with which that effort is processing sounds.

Dyslexia

About 2 to 5 percent of elementary-age children have some form of developmental reading disorder known as dyslexia, which results from a defect in the ability to process graphic symbols. The disorder is not attributable to eye problems or to low intelligence.

Some Indicators of Dyslexia
(Few individuals exhibit all symptoms.)

- Difficulty recognizing written words
- Difficulty rhyming or sequencing syllables
- Difficulty determining the meaning or main idea of a simple sentence
- Difficulty encoding words--spelling
- Poor sequencing of letters or numbers
- Delayed spoken language
- Difficulty separating the sounds in spoken words
- Difficulty in expressing thoughts verbally
- Confusion about right or left handedness
- Difficulty with handwriting
- Possible family history of dyslexia

Newer research is shedding more light on dyslexia. Because dyslexics often confuse *b* and *d*, psychologists thought for many years that dyslexia was merely a vision problem. Researchers now believe that the letters can also be confused because they sound alike. This is the brain's inability to process what it *hears*, not what it *sees*. The problem seems to lie in the decoding process, which occurs in the angular gyrus (see Figure 5.1). Brain imaging studies have shown a significantly reduced blood flow to the left angular gyrus in people diagnosed with dyslexia. The studies also indicated that the amount of blood flow to this area was highly correlated with the severity of the dyslexia—the less blood flow, the worse the dyslexia (Rumsey, Horwitz, Donohue, Nace, Maisog, and Andreason, 1999).

Other imaging studies show an imperfectly functioning system for dividing words into their phonological units—a critical step for accurate reading. Letter reversals can be the result of phonological missteps in the decoding of print to sound and back to print. It is likely that the learner has problems in assigning what he says or hears in his head (the phoneme) to the letters he sees on paper (the grapheme) (Shaywitz, Shaywitz, Pugh, Fulbright, Constable, Mencl, Shankweiler, Liberman, Skudlarski, Fletcher, Katz, Marchione, Lacadie, Gatenby, and Gore, 1998). So, for many individuals, dyslexia may really be *dysphonia*—an incorrect auditory-visual association between phoneme and grapheme. If so, then remedial strategies should focus on reestablishing correct phonemic connections with intense practice.

Some people diagnosed with dyslexia probably have a form of visual impairment. One type of impairment, called *visual magnocellular-deficit* (see page 97), may cause the visual images of letters to be held longer than usual and subsequent images are superimposed onto them. Letters become blurred, causing confusion for the reader. This theory is the focus of ongoing research studies (Stein, Talcott, and Walsh, 2000).

Convincing evidence exists that dyslexia is largely inherited (Fagerheim, Raeymaekers, Tønnessen, Pedersen, Tranebjaerg, and Lubs, 1999). Thus it is a life-long chronic problem and not just a "phase." The stereotype that nearly all dyslexics are boys is not true, although it probably persists because boys are more likely to show their frustration with reading by acting out. Studies indicate that many girls are affected as well and are not getting help.

Nonlinguistic Perceptual Deficits

Recent research indicates that some people, who are otherwise unimpaired, have extreme difficulties in reading because of deficits in *nonlinguistic* auditory and visual perception. This revelation was somewhat of a surprise because conventional wisdom held that impairments in reading (and also in oral language) were restricted to problems with *linguistic* processing. Wright, Bowen, and Zecker (2000) have reviewed the research in nonlinguistic deficits. They cite six major developments that promise a better understanding of and treatment for this type of disorder.

1. **Perception of Sequential Sounds.** The inability to detect and discriminate sounds presented in rapid succession seems to be a common impairment in individuals with reading and language disorders. These individuals also have difficulty in indicating the order of two sounds presented in rapid succession. Hearing words accurately when reading or from a stream of rapid conversation (phonology, see Figure 5.2) is critical to understanding.

2. **Sound-Frequency Discrimination.** Some individuals with reading disorders are impaired in their ability to hear differences in sound frequency. This condition can affect the ability to discriminate tone and pitch in speech. At first glance, this may seem like only an oral language-related impairment. However, it also affects reading proficiency because reading involves sounding out words in the auditory processing system.

3. **Detection of Target Sounds in Noise.** The inability to detect tones within noise is another recently discovered nonlinguistic impairment. When added to the findings in 1 and 2 above, this evidence suggests that

> *Evidence is growing that auditory functions play a much greater role in reading disorders than previously thought.*

auditory functions may play a much greater role in reading disorders than previously thought.

4. **Visual Magnocellular-Deficit Hypothesis.** The interpretation of some research studies has lead to a hypothesis about the functions of the visual processing system. This proposes that certain forms of reading disorders are caused by a deficit in the visual processing system, which leads to poor detection of coherent visual motion and poor discrimination of the speed of visual motion. This part of the visual system involves large neurons and so is referred to as the magnocellular system. Impairment in this system may cause letters on a page to bundle and overlap, or appear to move—common complaints from some dyslexics.

5. **Individual Differences.** The large number of possible deficits in visual and auditory perception on various reading tasks accounts for the wide range of individual differences observed among those with reading disorders. Analyzing these differences leads to a better understanding of the multidimensional nature of reading disorders and possible treatment.

6. **Remediation.** Efforts to remediate nonlinguistic reading and language problems are showing some encouraging results. Tallal (1996) and Merzenich (1996) tested a treatment that improved the ability of children with language disorder to hear brief sounds presented in rapid succession —a skill necessary for speech perception and reading. Other studies using specially designed eyeglasses to assist eye control helped students improve their reading at twice the rate of control groups (Stein, Richardson, and Fowler, 2000).

These developments are contributing to a greater understanding of factors that contribute to nonlinguistic reading disorders and to effective remediation treatments. Research will continue to attempt to identify all nonlinguistic perceptual deficits to determine their impact on reading and language processing.

Voices of Disagreement

In fairness, it should be noted that not all researchers are in agreement that scientific evidence strongly supports a phonemic awareness approach to learning to read. Coles (2000), for example, criticizes the scientific research as subject to different interpretations and too limited in trying to explain such a complex process as reading. Although he offers no alternative, he suggests that scientific studies do not address broader questions such as, "What kind of emotions, feelings, and thinking should the teaching of reading encourage?" He also is concerned that this scientific approach will prevent the useful components of whole language from being incorporated into the teaching of reading.

What Educators Need to Consider

Because reading does not come naturally to the human brain, children learning to read have to put much effort into associating their spoken language with the alphabet and with word recognition. To do this successfully, phonemic awareness is essential. Educators should give second thought to reading programs that delay phonemic awareness or that treat it as an ancillary skill to be learned in context with general reading. All teachers are teachers of reading, and thus should have the training to strengthen the reading skills of students at every grade level.

Significant progress is being made in understanding the connection between the visual and auditory processing systems during reading. Research-based reading programs that use computers to help students coordinate these systems have substantially benefitted slower readers.

Impact on Learning

- Reading problems are the most common difficulties that children have in school and their lack of confidence in reading can affect all their school work.
- Learning to read requires a systematic process of several steps, some of which are not acquired without direct instruction.
- The visual and auditory impact of the technology (e.g., computers, toys, and games) that young children use today is subtly eroding the argument that reading is a necessary skill.

Strategies to Consider

Developing Phonological Awareness

Training in phonological awareness needs to be more intense for children with reading disabilities. Reading programs are filled with activities for separating words into phonemes, synthesizing phonemes into words, and deleting and substituting phonemes. Research suggests that the development of phonological awareness is more likely to be successful if it follows these general principles (Chard and Osborn, 1998):

- ❑ **Continuous Sounds Before Stop Sounds.** Start with continuous sounds such as *s, m,* and *f* that are easier to pronounce than the stop sounds of *b, k,* and *p.*

- ❑ **Modeling.** Be sure to model carefully and accurately each activity when it is first introduced.

- ❑ **Easy to Complex Tasks.** Move from easier tasks, such as rhyming, to more complex tasks such as blending and segmenting.

- ❑ **Larger to Smaller Units.** Move from the larger units of words and onset-rimes to the smaller units of individual phonemes.

- ❑ **Additional Strategies.** Use additional strategies to help struggling readers, such as concrete objects (e.g., bingo chips or blocks) to represent sounds.

Strategies to Consider

Phonemic Awareness and Guidelines

Research shows that early phoneme awareness is a strong indicator of later reading success. Further, the research on interventions clearly demonstrates the benefits of explicitly teaching phonemic awareness skills. No students benefit more from this instruction than those already burdened with reading problems.

The development of phonological awareness occurs over several years. It is the last step in a developmental continuum that begins with the brain's earliest awareness of rhyme. Figure 5.3 illustrates the continuum from rhyming to full phoneme manipulation (Chard and Dickson, 1999).

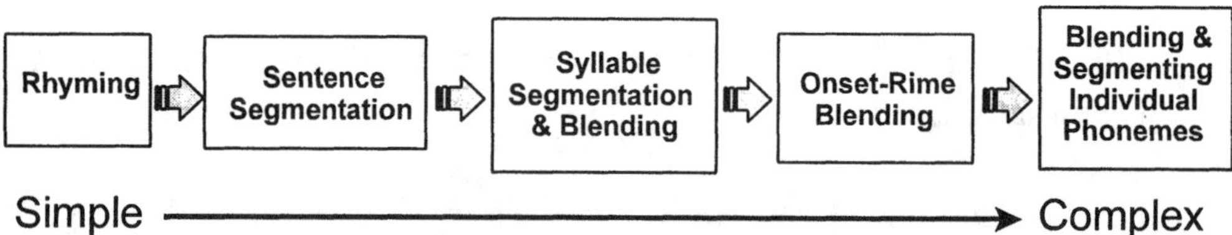

Figure 5.3 *The development of phonological awareness is a continuum that begins with simple rhyming and ends with the manipulation of individual phonemes.*

The first four steps, from rhyming to onset-rime blending, can occur during the preschool years in the appropriate environment. If the parent sings rhyming songs and reads to the child from rhyming books (e.g., Dr. Seuss' *There's a Locket in My Pocket*), the child's brain begins to recognize the sounds that comprise beginning language.

However, many children begin school with a very weak phonological base. Teachers must then assess where students lie on the phonological continuum and select appropriate strategies to move them toward phoneme awareness. Edelen-Smith (1998) offers teachers some guidelines to consider when selecting strategies to help students recognize and successfully manipulate phonemes.

Phoneme Awareness and Guidelines—Continued

General Guidelines

1. **Be Specific.** Identify the specific phonemic awareness task and select the activities that are developmentally appropriate and that keep the students engaged in the task. Select words, phrases, and sentences from curricular materials to make this meaningful. Look for ways to make activities enjoyable so students see them as fun and not as monotonous drills.

2. **Avoid Letter Names.** Use the phoneme sounds of the alphabet when doing activities and avoid letter names. Letters sounded as they are named only confuse the learner. Keep in mind that one sound may be represented by two or more letters. Target specific sounds and practice beforehand so students can hear them clearly.

3. **Treat Continuant and Stop Sounds Differently.** Continuant sounds are easier to manipulate and hear than the stop sounds. When introducing each type, treat them differently so students become aware of their differences. Exaggerate continuant sounds by holding on to them: *sssssssing* and *rrrrrrun*. Use rapid repetition with the stop consonants: */K/-/K/-/K/-/K/-/K/-/K/-athy*.

4. **Emphasize How Sounds Vary With Their Position in a Word.** Generally, the initial position in the word is the easiest sound. The final position is the next easiest and the middle position is the most difficult. Use lots of examples to make this clear, such as *mop*, *pin*, and *better*.

5. **Be Aware of the Sequence for Introducing Combined Sounds.** When introducing the combined sounds, a consonant-vowel pattern should come first, then a vowel-consonant pattern, and finally, the consonant-vowel-consonant pattern. For example: first *tie*, next *add*, and then *bed*.

– Continued –

Phoneme Awareness and Guidelines—Continued

Onset and Rime

The brain's awareness of onsets, rimes, and syllables develops before an awareness of phonemes (Goswami, 1994). Onsets are the initial consonants that change the meaning of a word; rimes are the vowel-consonant combinations that stay constant in a series. For example, in *bend*, *lend*, and *send*, the onsets are *b, l,* and *s*; the rime is *-end*. Using literature, word families, and direct instruction are strategies that focus on word play designed to enhance onset and rime recognition (Edelen-Smith, 1998).

- **Literature.** Books with rhyming patterns (like many books by Dr. Seuss) are easily recalled through repeated exposure. Almost any literary source that plays with word sounds is valuable. Books that particularly develop awareness of sound patterns associated with onset and rime are those using alliteration (the repetition of an initial consonant across several words, e.g., *Peter Piper picked a peck of peppers*) and assonance (the repetition of vowel sounds within words, e.g., *The rain in Spain stays mainly on the plain*).

- **Word Families Charts.** Using words from a story or book, construct a chart that places a different beginning letter in front of a rime. For example, start with the rime *-at* and add *f, h, b,* and *s* to form *fat, hat, bat,* and *sat*. Have the students make up a story line whenever the word changes, e.g., "The fat cat chased a hat." Encourage the students to make their own charts with different rimes and to keep them for future reference.

- **Direct Instruction.** Students who have difficulties distinguishing the sounds among rhyming words need more direct instruction. Model rhyming pairs (e.g., *sun-fun* and *hand-band*) using flash cards so students match what they see with what they hear. Be sure they repeat each rhyming pair several times to reinforce auditory input. Another activity includes three cards, only two of which have rhyming words. Ask students to pick out and say the two that rhyme, or the one that doesn't. Later, change the rhyming words to two rhyming pictures out of three (e.g., a nose, a rose, and a horse).

Strategies to Consider

Simple Phonemic Awareness

Young students are usually unaware that words are made of sounds that can be produced in isolation. This leaves it up to the teacher to find ways to emphasize the concept of speech sounds. Here are some ways to do this (Edelen-Smith, 1998):

- **Recognizing Isolated Sounds.** Associate certain speech sounds with an animal or action that is familiar to the students. For example, the buzzing sound of a bee or snoring in sleep is "zzzzzzzz–," the hissing of a snake, "ssssssss," the sound of asking for quiet, "shhhhhhhh–," or the sound of a motor scooter or motor boat, "pppppppp–."

  Alliteration, mentioned earlier, also helps with this task. Talking about Peter Piper picking a peck of peppers affords the valuable combination of sound recognition, story telling, and literary context. It also provides self-correcting cues for initial-sound isolation and for sound-to-word matching.

- **Counting Words, Syllables, and Phonemes.** It is easier for a child's brain to perceive words and syllables than individual phonemes. Thus word and syllable counting is a valuable exercise for sound recognition that can lead later to more accurate identification of phonemes. Start with a sentence from the curriculum and say it aloud. Do not write it out because the students should focus on listening. Ask the students to count the number of words they think are in the sentence. They can use markers or tokens to indicate the word number. Then show or write the sentence and have the students compare the number of words to their own count.

  Syllable counting can be done in many ways. Students can count syllables in the same way they identified the word count. Also, they can march around the room while saying the syllables, they can clap hands, tap pencils, or do any other overt activity that indicates counting.

– Continued –

Simple Phonemic Awareness—Continued

- **Synthesizing Sounds.** Sound synthesis is an essential yet easily performed skill for phonemic awareness. Start with using the initial sound and then saying the remainder of the word. For example, the teacher says, "It starts with 'b' and ends with '-and,' put it together and it says 'band'." The students take turns using the same phrasing to make up their own words. Variations include limiting the context to objects in the classroom or in the school, or to a particular story that the class has recently read.

  Guessing games can also be productive and fun activities for playing with sounds. One game involves hiding an object in a bag or some other place and then giving clues to its name sound-by-sound or syllable-by-syllable. When a student guesses the word correctly, you reveal the object. Songs can also be used. Blending the music with the sounds of words increases the chances that the phonemes will be remembered.

- **Matching Sounds to Words.** This activity asks the learner to identify the initial sound of a word, an important skill for sound segmentation. Show the student a picture of a kite and ask, "Is this a dddd-ite, or a llll-ite, or a kkkk-ite?" You could also ask, "Is there a *k* in kite?," or "Which sound does kite start with?" This allows the students to try three onsets with three rimes and to mix and match until they get it correct. Consonants make a good beginning because they are easier to emphasize and prolong during pronunciation. Have students try other words in threes. Be sure to use the phoneme sound when referring to a letter, not the letter name.

- **Identifying the Position of Sounds.** Segmenting whole words into their components is an important part of phonemic awareness. This ability is enhanced when learners recognize that sounds occur in different positions in words: initial, medial, and final. Edelen-Smith (1998) suggests explaining that words have beginning, middle, and end sounds just like a train has a beginning (engine), middle (passenger car), and end (caboose). Slowly articulate a consonant-vowel-consonant (CVC) word at this time, such a *c-a-t,* and point to the appropriate train part as you sound out each phoneme. Then have the students sound out other CVC words from a list or recent story, pointing to each train part as they say the parts of the word.

Simple Phonemic Awareness—Continued

- **Segmenting Sounds.** One of the more difficult phonemic tasks for children is to separately pronounce each sound of a spoken word in order. This process is called sound segmentation. Developing this skill should start with isolating initial phonemes. The previous activities—matching sounds to words and identifying the position of sounds—help the learner identify and recognize initial phonemes. Visual cues can also play an important part in segmenting sounds. Research on Elkonin (1973) boxes, for example, indicates that they are particularly effective in developing this important skill. Show a card with the picture of a common object, say a dog (Figure 5.4). Below the object is a series of three boxes that represent the three sounds in the word, *dog* (*duh, awh,* and *guh*). Model the process by saying the word slowly and placing a token into each box as you say the sound aloud. Then have the students practice it first with this picture and then with other pictures. Select words that are familiar to the students (or have the students select the words) so that they can use contextual clues for meaning. After sufficient practice, eliminate the cards so that students can perform the sound segmenting task without visual cues.

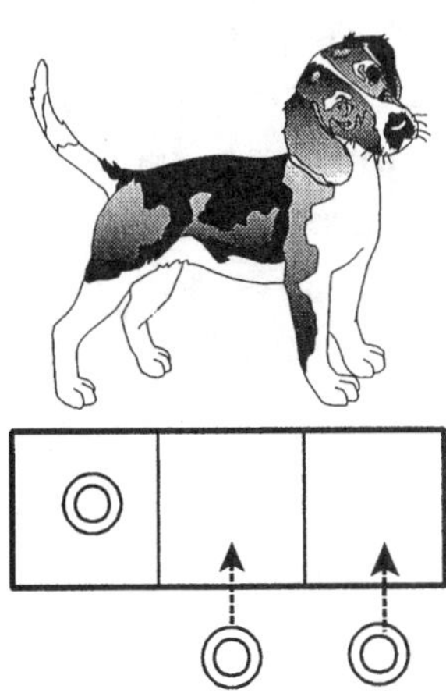

Figure 5.4 *An example of using Elkonin boxes. Students move tokens into boxes when hearing each of the phonemes. (Elkonin, 1973)*

- **Associating Sounds With Letters.** For the reading process to be successful, the brain must associate the sounds that it has heard during the prereading years of spoken language with the written letters that represent them. This is particularly difficult for students with disabilities that hamper the learning of reading. Consequently, extensive practice is essential. Nearly all of the activities mentioned above —especially those involving visual cues—can be modified to include associations between sounds and

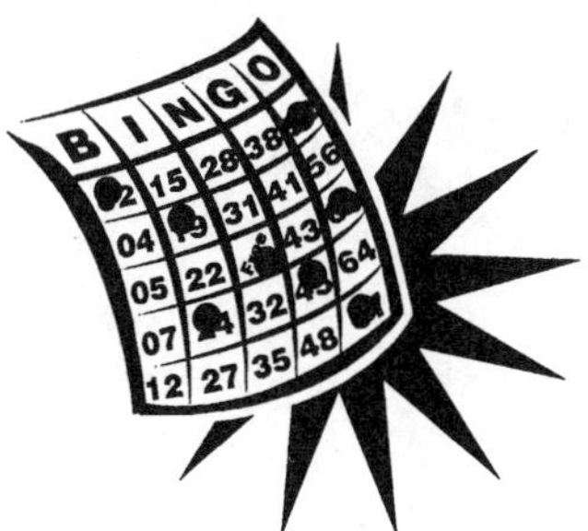

– Continued –

Simple Phonemic Awareness—Continued

letters. As the students master individual sounds, their corresponding letter names can then be introduced. A type of bingo game can also be used to practice sound-with-letter association. Each student gets a card with letters placed into a bingo grid. Draw a letter from a container and call out the phoneme. Students place tokens on the letter that corresponds to the phoneme. The student who first gets "phoneme bingo" names the letters aloud. Teachers can devise all types of variations to this bingo game to maintain the practice while keeping the task interesting and fun.

Strategies to Consider

Compound Phonemic Awareness

In compound phonemic awareness, the learner must hold one sound in memory while matching it to a second sound. For example, "Do dog and deer begin with the same sound?" The two activities that develop compound phonemic awareness involve matching one word to a second word and the deleting of sounds in a word.

❑ **Matching One Word to Another Word.** Byrne (1991) has suggested three games to develop phonemic word matching skills. The words and pictures used in each of these games should relate to themes and readings done in the classroom. One involves making a set of dominoes that have two objects pictured on each tile. The students have to join the tiles that share the same beginning or ending sounds.

A second game uses picture cards that are placed face down in a pile. Each student draws a card from the pile and places it face up. Students continue to draw cards and place them in the face-up pile. The first student to match the beginning or ending sound of a drawn card with the top card on the face-up pile says the match aloud and collects the pile.

The third game is a variation of bingo. Each bingo card contains pictures, which the students mark when their picture has the same beginning or ending sounds as the word said by the caller (student or teacher).

❑ **Deleting Sounds.** Deleting sounds from words and manipulating phonemes within words are more difficult tasks for the young brain to accomplish. Studies show that children must attain the mental age of seven years before this task can be accomplished adequately (Cole and Mengler, 1994). Furthermore, segmentation skills and letter names must be mastered before sound deletion tasks can be successfully learned.

– Continued –

Compound Phonemic Awareness—Continued

Three tasks seem to be particularly important to mastering this skill: deleting parts of a compound word, identifying a missing sound, and deleting a single sound from a word.

Deleting Parts of a Compound Word. To illustrate deleting parts of a compound word, point to a picture or an object that is a compound word and demonstrate how each word can be said with one part missing. For example, "This is a classroom. I can say *class* without the *room*. And this is a farmhouse (or greenhouse). I can say *farm* (*green*) without *house*. Now you try it. This is a playground." Use other common examples, such as *lighthouse*, *airplane, grandmother, seashore, sandbox, toothpaste,* and *nightlight.*

Identifying the Missing Sound. In this task, focus on deleting the initial and final sounds instead of the medial sounds, which is the first step to master for the young brain. Take word pairs, such as *ate-late*, and ask "What's missing in *ate* that you hear in *late*?" Other examples are *ask-mask*, *able-table*, and *right-bright*. After a few trials, have the students make up their own word pairs, preferably from lesson material.

Deleting a Single Sound From a Word. This task should begin with segmentation practice. First, separate the sound for deletion. For example, separate "g" from *glove*. "*Glove*. It starts with *g* and ends with *love*. Take the first sound away and it says *love*." Use words for which a sound deletion results in another real word. Other examples are *spot-pot*, *train-rain*, *scare-care*, and *snap-nap*. After practicing this skill, say a word aloud and ask students to say the word with the initial sound missing: "Say *mother* without the 'm'." Visual clues can help those who have difficulty saying a word with the deleted sound.

Strategies to Consider

What Teachers and Students Need to Know About Reading

Here is what the latest research is saying that teachers and students need to know for the successful teaching of reading to children with reading difficulties (Foorman et al., 1998):

What Teachers Need to Know About Teaching Reading

- How the brain learns to read
- The relationship between reading and spoken language
- Direct instruction in phonics
- Direct instruction in the alphabetic principle
- How to diagnose spelling and reading skills
- How to use a variety of reading intervention strategies

What Beginning Readers Need to Learn

- ✓ *Phonological Awareness*: Rhyming, alliteration, deleting and substituting sounds, sound patterns
- ✓ *Phonemic Awareness*: Segmenting words into individual sounds, manipulating phonemes
- ✓ *Alphabetic Principle*: Correlating letter-sound patterns with specific text
- ✓ *Orthographic Awareness*: Understanding spelling rules and writing conventions
- ✓ *Comprehension Monitoring Strategies*: Identifying the main idea, making inferences, using study skills that assist reading

Strategies to Consider

Reading Strategies for Students With Reading Difficulties

Studies have shown that both children with reading disabilities and other low achievers can master the learning strategies that improve reading comprehension skills. For students with learning problems, learning to use questioning strategies is especially important because these students do not often spontaneously self-question or monitor their own reading comprehension.

Here are three strategies that researchers and teachers have found particularly effective. Some of the strategies have been around for nearly 20 years, but their fundamental premises have been reaffirmed by recent research.

Questioning and Paraphrasing. Reciprocal Teaching is a strategic approach that fosters student interaction with the text being read. In Reciprocal Teaching, students interact deeply with the text through the strategies of questioning, summarizing, clarifying, and predicting. Organized in the form of a discussion, the approach involves one leader (students and teacher take turns being the leader) who, after a portion of the text is read, first frames a question to which the group responds. Second, participants share their own questions. Third, the leader then summarizes the gist of the text, and participants comment or elaborate upon that summary. At any point in the discussion, either the leader or participants may identify aspects of the text or discussion that need to be clarified, and the group joins together to clarify the confusion. Finally, the leader indicates that it's time to move on and solicits predictions about what might come up next in the text.

The value of paraphrasing, self-questioning, and finding the main idea are well researched strategies (Deshler, Shumaker, Alley, Clark, and Warner, 1981). Students divide reading passages into smaller parts, such as sections, subsections, or paragraphs. After reading a segment, students are cued to use a self-questioning strategy to identify main ideas and details. The strategy requires a high level of attention to reading tasks because students must alternate their use of questioning and paraphrasing after reading each section, subsection, or paragraph.

Reading Strategies for Students With Reading Difficulties—Continued

Questioning to Find the Main Idea. Wong and Jones (1982) developed a self-questioning strategy focused primarily on identifying and questioning the main idea or summary of a paragraph. Here's how it works. Students are first taught the concept of a main idea and how to do self-questioning. Students then practice, asking themselves questions aloud about each paragraph's main idea. They can use a cue card for assistance. Following the practice, the teacher provides immediate feedback. Eventually, following successful comprehension of these short paragraphs, students are presented with more lengthy passages, and the cue cards are removed. Continuing to give corrective feedback, the teacher finishes each lesson with a discussion of students' progress and of the strategy's usefulness. Wong and Jones found that students with learning disabilities who were trained in a self-questioning strategy performed significantly higher (i.e., demonstrated greater comprehension of what was read) than untrained students.

Story-Mapping. Idol (1987) studied the effectiveness of story maps. In this strategy, students read a story, generate a map of its events and ideas, and then answer questions. (Figure 5.5 is one example of a story map.) In order to fill in the map, students have to identify the setting, characters, time, and place of the story; the problem, the goal, the action that took place; and the outcome. The teacher models for students how to fill in the map, then gives many opportunities to practice the mapping technique for themselves and receive corrective feedback. The map is an effective visual tool that provides a framework for understanding, conceptualizing, and remembering important story events. Idol also found that the reading comprehension of students improved significantly when the teacher gave direct instruction on the use of the strategy, expected frequent use of the strategy, and encouraged students to use the strategy independently.

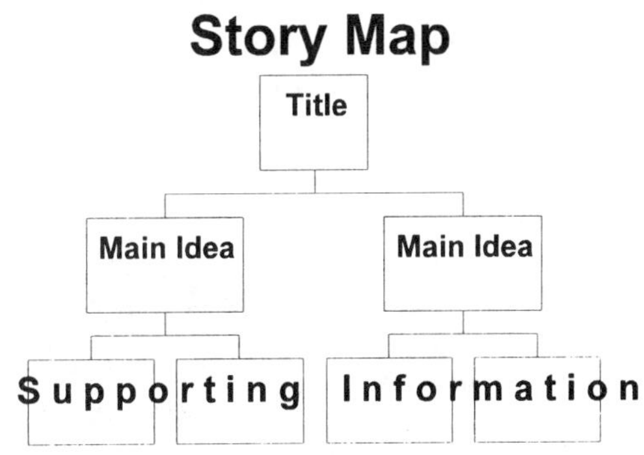

Figure 5.5 *This is just one example of a story map. (Sousa, 2001, p. 198)*

Strategies to Consider

Teaching for Reading Comprehension – Part I

Students with reading disorders often have difficulty deriving meaning from what they read. If little or no meaning comes from reading, students lose motivation to read. Furthermore, meaning is essential for long-term retention of what they have read. Strategies designed to improve reading comprehension have been shown to improve students' interest in reading and their success.

One such successful strategy, suggested by Deshler, Ellis, and Lenz (1996), is a four-step process called by the acronym **PASS** (**P**review, **A**sk, **S**ummarize, and **S**ynthesize). The teacher guides the students through the four steps, ensuring that they respond orally or in writing to the activities associated with each step. Grouping formats, such as cooperative learning, can be used to encourage active student participation and reduce anxiety over the correctness of each student's response.

1. **P***review, Review, and Predict:*
   - Preview by reading the heading and one or two sentences.
   - Review what you already know about this topic.
   - Predict what you think the text or story will be about.

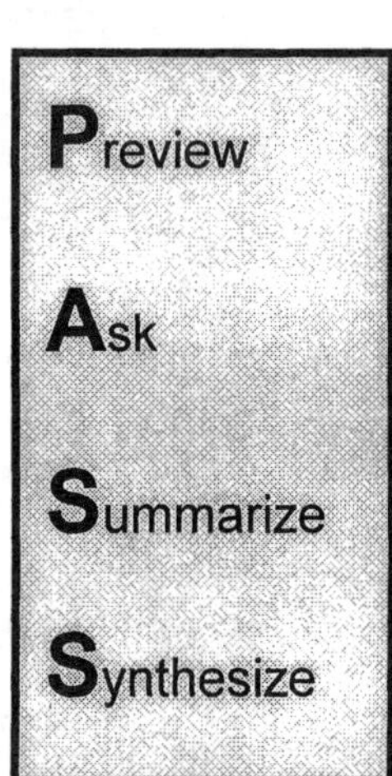

2. **A***sk and Answer Questions:*
   - Content-focused questions:
     - Who? What? Why? Where?
     - How does this relate to what I already know?
   - Monitoring questions:
     - Does this make sense?
     - Is my prediction correct?
     - How is this different from what I thought it was going to be about?

Teaching for Reading Comprehension - Part I—Continued

- Problem-solving questions:
  Is it important that it make sense?
  Do I need to reread part of it?
  Can I visualize the information?
  Does it have too many unknown words?
  Should I get help?

3. *Summarize*:

- Explain what the short passage you read was all about.

4. *Synthesize*:

- Explain how the short passage fits in with the whole passage.
- Explain how what you learned fits in with what you knew.

If students have difficulty with any particular step, they can go back to the previous step to determine what information they need in order to proceed.

Strategies to Consider

Teaching for Reading Comprehension – Part II

Another excellent technique for helping students comprehend what they read and build vocabulary is called collaborative strategic reading (CSR). It is particularly effective in classrooms where students have many different reading abilities and learning capabilities. The strategy is compatible with all types of reading programs.

CSR uses direct teaching and the collaborative power of cooperative learning groups to accomplish two phases designed to improve reading comprehension (Klingner, Vaughn, and Schumm, 1998). The first phase is a teacher-led component that takes students through four parts of a reading plan: Preview, Click and Clunk, Get the Gist, and Wrap-Up. The second phase involves using cooperative learning groups to provide an interactive environment where students can practice and perfect their reading comprehension skills.

PHASE ONE
Teacher-Led Activities

- **Preview the Reading.** Students know that previews in movies give some information about coming events. Use this as a hook to the new reading. The learners preview the entire reading passage in order to get as much as they can about the passage in a just a few minutes time. The purpose here is to activate their prior knowledge about the topic and to give them an opportunity to predict what they will learn.

  Refer to student experiences about a movie, television program, or a prior book that might contain information relevant to the new reading. Also, give clues to look for when previewing. For example, pictures, graphs, tables, or call-out quotes provide information to help predict what students already know about the topic and what they will learn.

Teaching for Reading Comprehension - Part II—Continued

- **Click and Clunk.** Students with reading problems often fail to monitor their understanding while they read. Clicks and clunks are devices to help students with this monitoring. Clicks are parts of the reading that make sense; clunks are parts or words that don't.

  Ask students to identify clunks as they go along. Then the class works with the teacher to develop strategies to clarify the clunks, such as

  - Rereading the sentences while looking for key words that can help extract meaning from the context
  - Rereading previous and following sentences to get additional context clues
  - Looking for a prefix or suffix in the word that could help with meaning
  - Breaking the word apart to see if smaller words are present that provide meaning

- **Get the Gist.** The goal of this phase is twofold. First, ask the readers to state in their own words the most important person, place, or thing in the passage. Second, get them to tell in as few words as possible (i.e., leaving out the details) the most important *idea* about that person, place, or thing. Because writing often improves memory, occasionally ask the students to write down their gists. Students can then read their gists aloud and invite comments from the group about ways to improve the gist. This process can be done so that all students benefit by enhancing their skills.

- **Wrap-Up.** Wrap-up is a closure activity that allows students to review in their mind what has been learned. Focus students on the new learning by asking them to generate questions whose answers would show what they learned from the passage. They should also review key ideas.

  Start with questions that focus on the explicit material in the passage, such as *who*, *what*, *where*, and *when*. Afterward, move to questions that stimulate higher-order thinking, such as "What might have happened if___?" and "What could be another way to solve this problem?" Writing down the response will help students sort out and remember the important ideas.

- Continued -

Teaching for Reading Comprehension - Part II—Continued

PHASE TWO
Cooperative Learning Groups

This phase puts the students into cooperative learning groups to practice CSR in an interactive environment. True cooperative learning groups are usually made up of about five students of mixed ability levels who learn and perform certain roles in the group to ensure completion of the learning task (Johnson and Johnson, 1989). The roles rotate among the group members so that every student gets the opportunity to be the leader and use the various skills needed to perform each task. Although there are many roles that students can perform, here are the most common (assuming five members per group):

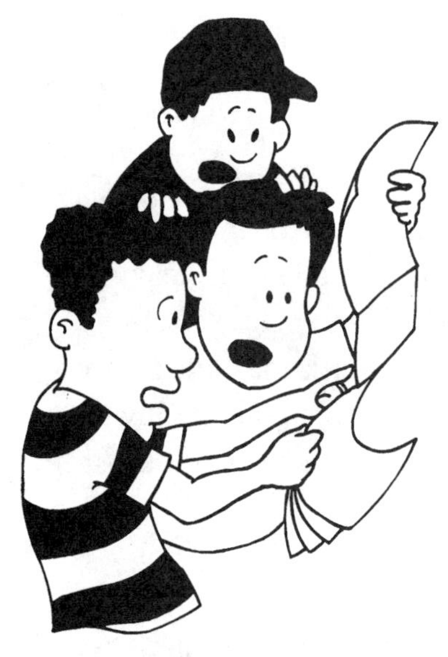

- **Leader.** Leads the group through CSR by saying what to read next and what strategy to use.
- **Clunk Expert.** Reminds the group what strategies to use when encountering a difficult word or phrase.
- **Announcer.** Calls on different group members to make certain that everyone participates and that only one person talks at a time.
- **Encourager.** Gives the group feedback on behaviors that are to be praised and those that need improvement.
- **Reporter.** Takes notes and reports to the whole class the main idea that the group has learned and shares a question that the group generated during its wrap-up.

Other suggestions for using the cooperative learning groups with this strategy are as follows:

Cue Sheets. Giving all group members a cue sheet to guide them through the CSR provides a structure and focus for the group. The cue sheet should be specific for each role. For example,

Teaching for Reading Comprehension - Part II—Continued

the leader's sheet contains statements that steer the group through each step of CSR (e.g., "Today's topic is___." "Let's predict what we might learn from this." "Let's think of some questions to see if we really understand what we learned.") and also direct other group members to carry out their role (e.g., "Announcer, please call on others to share their ideas." "Encourager, tell us what we did well and what we need to do better next time.").

CSR Learning Logs. Recording in logs helps students to keep track of what was learned. Students can keep separate logs for each subject. The log serves as a reminder for follow-up activities and can be used to document a student's progress as required by the individualized education plan.

Reading Materials. CSR was originally designed for expository text, but has also been used successfully with narrative text. For the strategy to be successful, select reading passages that are rich in clues, that have just one main idea per paragraph, and that provide a context to help students connect and associate details into larger ideas. Weekly readers are sources that often meet these needs.

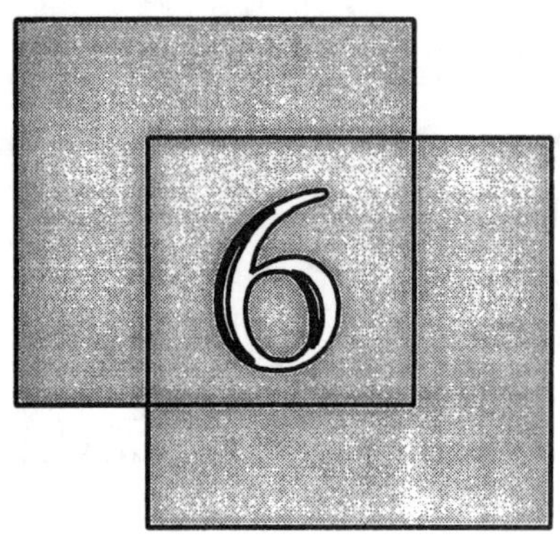

Writing Disabilities

Once the enormous challenge of learning to read is undertaken, the brain is faced with the daunting task of directing fine muscle movements to draw the abstract symbols that represent the sounds of language. For many years, researchers thought that the mental centers responsible for speech and writing were located in the same (left) side of the brain. Recent research, however, indicates that these two processes are related yet separate, sometimes residing in different cerebral hemispheres (Baynes, Eliassen, Lutsep, and Gazzaniga, 1998). This finding, which suggests that spoken and written language develop differently, is not surprising when we realize that human beings have been speaking for over 10,000 years but writing for only 3,000 years. Thus, spoken language has become innate and usually develops with ease, but writing does not develop without instruction.

Learning to Write

Writing is a highly complex operation requiring the coordination of multiple neural networks. It involves the blending of attention, fine motor coordination, memory, visual processing, language, and higher-order thinking. When an individual is writing, the visual feedback mechanisms are at work checking the output, adjusting fine motor skills, and monitoring eye-hand coordination. Meanwhile, kinesthetic monitoring systems are conscious of the position and movement of fingers in space, the grip on the pencil, and the rhythm and pace of the writing.

Cognitive systems are also busy, verifying with long-term memory that the symbols being drawn will indeed produce the sounds of the word that the writer intends. Accomplishing this task requires visual memory for symbols, whole-word memory, and spelling rules. Hence, the

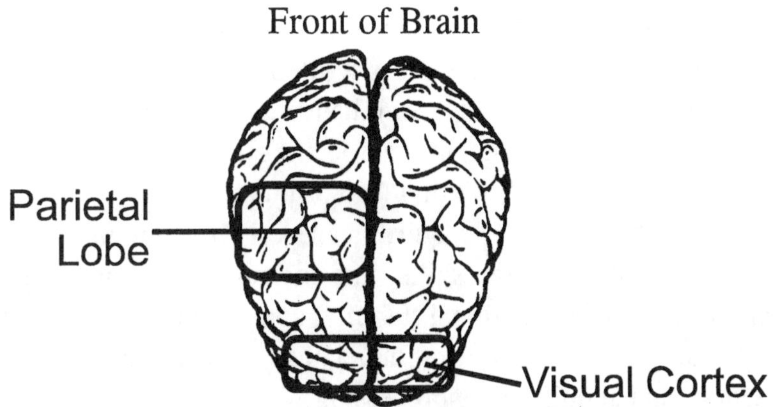

Figure 6.1 *In a right-handed individual, writing involves mainly the left parietal lobe. For a left-handed person, the right parietal lobe is the area of main activation. Regardless of which hand is used, the visual cortex involvement is the same.*

phoneme-to-grapheme match is a continuous feedback loop ensuring that the written symbols are consistent with oral language protocols the writer has previously learned.

Recent brain imaging studies have shown the labor-intensive nature of writing. The parietal lobe, which includes the motor cortex, and the occipital lobe, where visual processing occurs, were the areas of highest activity (Figure 6.1) when an individual was writing (Wing, 2000). Not surprising was the discovery that spoken language areas in the left hemisphere were also activated. Writing relies heavily on speech because most of us sound out words in our head as we write them down.

After reviewing numerous scanning studies on the writing process, Alan Wing (2000) pieced together a

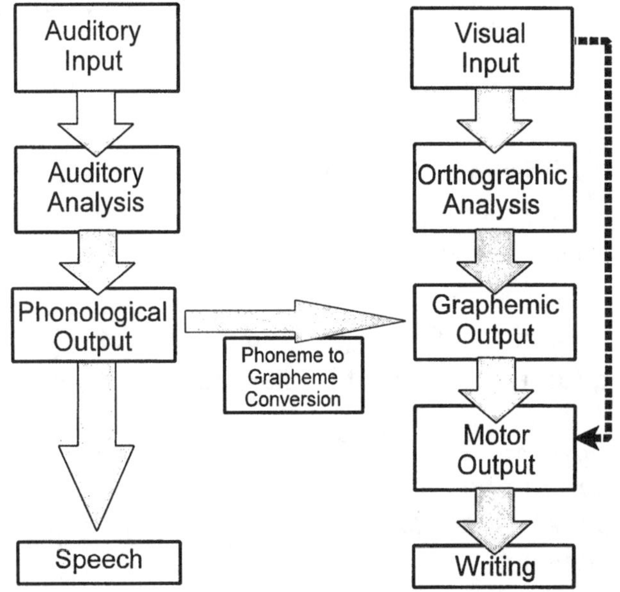

Figure 6.2 *The diagram illustrates the relationship between speech and handwriting. The writer hears the word (phonological output) and converts the sounds to the appropriate letters (graphemes). The dotted arrow shows how motor adjustments are made as the visual system judges the legibility of the writing.*

complex flow diagram illustrating the relationships between the neurological networks responsible for both speech and writing. Figure 6.2 is a simplified version of Wing's diagram. The visual systems analyze the spelling and grammar as it is written out on paper (orthography) and adjust the motor output to form the letters correctly. Simultaneously, the auditory system is sounding out the words in the brain (phonological output), associating and converting the sounds to letters (phoneme-to-grapheme conversion) for writing (motor output).

At a minimum, the ability to write requires a properly functioning central nervous system, intact receptive and expressive language skills, and the related cognitive operations. To write accurately and clearly also requires emotional stability; application of the concepts of organization and flow; an understanding of the rules of pronunciation, spelling, grammar and syntax; visual and spatial organization; and simultaneous processing.

When all these operations fall into place, writing becomes a valuable tool for learning. Writing encourages mental rehearsal, reinforces long-term memory, and helps the mind sort and prioritize information. However, for some students, the process of writing becomes an arduous task that actually interferes with learning.

Problems With Writing

Environmental Causes

Difficulties with writing can be environmental, that is, too little time was spent in the child's early years on practicing correct writing, or they can stem from deficits within one or more of the neural networks needed for legible and clear writing to occur. Let's deal first with how the school environment may contribute inadvertently to writing problems.

Teachers of writing should realize that, like reading, the brain does not perceive writing to be a survival skill. That is, the brain has no "writing centers" comparable to those for spoken language. Instead, writing requires the coordination of numerous neural networks and systems, all of which have to learn new skills. Learning to write therefore requires direct instruction—it is not innate to the brain. Hard work and lots of practice are needed just to learn the fine motor skills for reproducing the printed and cursive letters of the alphabet. In some schools, little time is given to formal instruction in writing. To conserve time, it is often taught as an ancillary activity to other learning tasks. Some of the difficulties students experience with writing may be due to an unfortunate combination of learning the difficult skills of writing with very little practice time. Further, more students are questioning the need to write well because they have access to computers at an early age and typing into a word processing program seems so much easier.

There are no areas of the brain specialized for writing.

What About Inventive Spelling and Avoiding the Teaching of Writing Mechanics? Some writing programs even advocate teaching the mechanics of writing only as student interests dictate and only in the course of writing compositions. Or, they may suggest that spelling need not be taught formally and that students will be more likely to write when they are allowed to use inventive spelling. As well-intended as that may be, long-term research findings are questioning this approach. For example,

- ❑ Descriptive research shows that the spelling and handwriting difficulties of students can actually interfere with their learning how to write compositions (Graham, 1990).
- ❑ The inventive spelling approach dramatically reduces the possibility that students will learn writing mechanics in such a way that this knowledge will transfer to their other school subjects.
- ❑ Shifting away from teaching writing mechanics is apt to produce long-term deficits in the knowledge of how to write successfully.
- ❑ This approach assumes that writing mechanics and learning to spell correctly will take care of themselves as the students write more compositions. However, no research exists to support this notion (Stein, Dixson, and Isaacson, 1994).
- ❑ Because practice makes permanent, the more frequently students use inventive spelling to write words incorrectly, the more likely they are to store the incorrect spelling in memory, thereby making it more difficult later to learn the correct spelling (Sousa, 2001).

All teachers need to emphasize that writing is more than *hand*writing. The notion of transferring thoughts and ideas from inside the brain to an outside device—paper or computer—requires teaching how to organize thoughts, analyze material, and sort out material differently, depending on whether students plan to relate an incident or persuade another person. To write an initial draft requires instruction in penmanship and learning the rules of written language including spelling, capitalization, punctuation, and sentence structure. Unfortunately, complex rules in the English language are loaded with exceptions and require substantial practice for mastery. Even after the initial draft is written, students need to learn how to edit and revise their material for clarity.

> *Because practice makes permanent, the more frequently students use inventive spelling to write words incorrectly, the more likely they are to store the incorrect spelling in memory, thereby making it more difficult later to learn the correct spelling.*

The point here is that students who demonstrate difficulty with writing need a full assessment to determine whether their obstacles are environmental or systemic. Teachers should look first at the learner's background knowledge of writing and assess the type and degree of writing instruction that has been provided in the past. Simply by providing more and sustained practice of writing skills and written language rules, teachers can help many students to eventually overcome their writing difficulties.

Neurological Causes

Given that such a complex order of operations involving several neural systems is necessary for accurate writing, difficulties can arise anywhere along the way. Because writing is so dependent on the brain's parietal lobes, for instance, problems (e.g., lesions or stroke) in this area are especially significant. On the other hand, research on brain functioning has not found much evidence to support the notion of a visual basis for most writing difficulties, even though conventional wisdom has pointed in that direction.

Whatever the neurological cause of writing difficulties, some children struggle because so much time is spent on the *process* that they often lose track of the *content* they are working on. The persistent condition of not being able to put thoughts into writing or accomplish other parts of the writing process (such as letter formation) is known as *dysgraphia*.

Dysgraphia

This is a spectrum disorder describing major difficulties in mastering the sequence of movements necessary to write letters and numbers. The disorder exists in varying degrees and is seldom found in isolation without symptoms of other learning problems.

Many students have difficulty with writing as they progress through the upper elementary grades. But those with dysgraphia

> **Dysgraphia**
>
> Symptoms:
> - Inconsistencies in letter formation; mixture of upper and lower cases, of print and cursive letters
> - Unfinished words or letters
> - Generally illegible writing (despite time given to the task)
> - Talking to self while writing
> - Watching hand while writing
> - Inconsistent position on page with respect to margins and lines
> - Slow copying or writing
> - Omitted words in writing
> - Inconsistent spaces between letters and words
> - Struggle to use writing as a communications tool
> - Cramped or unusual grip on pencil
> - Unusual body, wrist, or paper position

are inefficient at *handwriting* more than anything else, and this inefficiency establishes a barrier to learning. Their handwriting is usually characterized by slow copying, inconsistencies in letter formation, mixtures of different letters and styles, and poor legibility. Specific symptoms of the disorder are shown in the box titled *Dysgraphia*. Teachers must realize that dysgraphia is a disorder and is *not* the result of laziness, not caring, not trying, or just carelessness in writing.

What Causes Dysgraphia?

Dysgraphia is a neurological disorder that can stem from several causes. Figure 6.2 illustrates the numerous cerebral systems and stages involved in handwriting. Problems can occur almost anywhere. McCarthy and Warrington (1990) have suggested that a deficit in the phoneme-to-grapheme conversion is one of the main causes of handwriting disorders. This can lead to poorly legible written text with severely abnormal spelling, also referred to as dyslexic dysgraphia.

Problems with muscles controlling motor output to the hands, wrists, and fingers lead to a motor clumsiness that also produces poorly legible handwriting and copying, but with mostly correct spelling. Sometimes, deficits in the spatial processing functions of the brain's right hemisphere cause poorly legible text, but with accurate spelling (Deuel, 1994). Table 6.1 summarizes these three types of dysgraphia. Determining which type of writing disorder a child has requires the assessment of various factors, such as fine motor coordination, writing speed, organization, knowledge and use of vocabulary, spelling, and the degree of attention and concentration.

Table 6.1 Different Types of Dysgraphia

Type	Symptoms	Possible Cause
Dyslexic Dysgraphia	Spontaneously written text is poorly legible with severely abnormal spelling. Copying of text is satisfactory.	Deficits in phoneme-to-grapheme conversion
Motor Clumsiness Dysgraphia	Spontaneously written text is poorly legible but spelling is satisfactory. Copying of text is poorly legible.	Deficits in muscle control of motor output to fingers, wrist, and hand
Spatial Dysgraphia	Spontaneously written text is poorly legible but spelling is satisfactory. Copying of text is satisfactory.	Deficits in spatial processing systems of the brain's right hemisphere

We now know that the centers for processing spoken language and written language are separated in the brain. Teachers should not assume, therefore, that a student with symptoms of dysgraphia will have other language problems as well. In fact, students with dysgraphia but who are otherwise linguistically talented find enormous frustration when trying to convert their thoughts into written expression. Their frustration can eventually turn them away from writing. Teachers sometimes misinterpret this behavior as laziness, carelessness, or poor motivation. Administering assessment instruments will be useful in determining whether the cause of poor writing is of neurological or some other origin.

Associating Dysgraphia With Other Disorders

Sequencing Problems. Some individuals have a cerebral deficit that makes it difficult for them to process sequential and rational information. Students with this difficulty will have problems with the sequence of letters, numbers, and words as they write. Usually they slow down their writing to focus on the mechanics of spelling, punctuation, and word order. As a result, they may get so bogged down with the details of writing that they lose the thoughts they are trying to express.

Attention-Deficit Hyperactivity Disorder (ADHD). Students with ADHD (Chapter 3) often have difficulty with writing in general and with handwriting in particular. They are processing information at a very rapid rate and don't possess the fine motor skills needed to write down their thoughts legibly.

Auditory Processing Disorders. Students who have language disorders (Chapter 5) as a result of auditory processing deficits will usually have difficulty with writing. Those with expressive language disorder are particularly weak at writing because it is the most difficult form of expressive language.

Visual Processing Disorders. Most students with dysgraphia do not have visual processing problems. However, the small percentage of students who *do* will have difficulty with writing speed and legibility simply because they are not able to fully process the visual information as they are transferring it to paper.

> *Students with dysgraphia have problems with the writing process. They are often frustrated and are not necessarily lazy or unmotivated.*

What Do Educators Need to Consider?

One of the main goals of writing is to help individuals express their knowledge and ideas. Students with dysgraphia have writing problems that lead to excessively rapid or slow writing, messy and illegible papers, and frustration. It is wrong to label them as lazy or unmotivated. Rather, educators should look for ways to help these students cope with their writing difficulties.

Regina Richards (1998) and Susan Jones (2000) suggest that educators develop three types of strategies for helping students with dysgraphia: accommodation (also called compensation) strategies, modification strategies, and remediation strategies. Accommodations bypass the problem by avoiding the difficulty and by reducing the impact that writing has on learning. Modification looks to change the types and the expectations of assignments. Remediation strategies focus on reteaching the concept or skill or providing additional structural practice that more closely matches the student's needs and learning style.

To help students, educators must first determine the point at which a student begins to struggle. Does the problem occur as the student begins to write or does it appear later in the writing process? Is there a problem with organization of thoughts? Is the struggle more evident when the student changes from just copying material to generating complex ideas and trying to commit those to writing? Is the struggle because of confusion over printed and cursive letters, over grammar, or because of punctuation? Once the struggle area is identified, then it becomes a matter of selecting the appropriate combination of accommodation, modification, and remedial techniques for the student.

Impact on Learning

- Because technology allows writing to be done on computers, students need to have reasons for learning, practicing, and improving their handwriting.
- Writing difficulties can be so frustrating that the student avoids all learning.
- Because practice makes perfect, practicing inventive spellings for too long will lead to the permanent storage of misspellings, which will be difficult to change later.

Strategies to Consider

Suggestions to Build Confidence in Students With Writing Disorders

Lack of confidence is one of the major difficulties of students with writing disorders. Here are a few suggestions to give to students with dysgraphia to help them regain confidence and overcome the frustrations they often experience when writing.

✓ **Organize Your Thoughts.** First try to get your major ideas down on paper. Then go back and fill in the details.

✓ **Use a Tape Recorder.** If you are feeling frustrated with your writing, stop and dictate what you want to write into a tape recorder. Listen to the tape later and write down your major ideas.

✓ **Use the Computer.** Even if you are not great at the beginning, it is important to practice your keyboarding skills. You will get better and faster at it once you have learned the pattern of the keys. Computers can help you organize your thoughts, put them in the proper sequence, and even check your spelling. In the long run, it will be faster and clearer than handwriting.

✓ **Continue to Practice Handwriting.** No matter how frustrating handwriting is, you will need to be able to write things down in the future. Like any other skill, your handwriting will get better with continued practice.

✓ **Talk While Writing.** Talk to yourself while writing. This auditory feedback is a valuable tool to help you monitor what and how you write.

✓ **Use Visual Aids.** Drawing a picture or diagram can help you organize your thoughts. Some computer programs also have the capability of producing your graphic organizers.

Strategies to Consider

Accommodation Strategies for Students With Writing Disorders

Accommodation strategies help bypass writing difficulties and reduce the impact that writing has on the learning process so that students can focus more completely on the content of their writing. The accommodations can adjust the rate and volume of writing, the complexity of the task, and the tools used to create the final product. Here are some accommodating strategies to consider in each of these areas (Richards, 1998; Jones, 2000).

Accommodating the Rate of Work Produced

- **Allow more time** for students to complete written tasks, such as note-taking, written tests, and copying. Also, allow these students to begin written projects earlier than others. Consider including time in the student's schedule for acting as an aide, and then have the student use that time for making up or starting new written work.

- **Encourage developing keyboarding skills and using the computer.** Students can begin to learn keyboarding in first grade. Encourage them to use various word processing programs. Teaching handwriting is still important, but students may be more likely to produce longer and more complex writing with the computer.

- **Have students prepare worksheets in advance,** complete with the required headings, such as name, date, and topic. Provide a standard template for them with this information already on it.

– Continued –

Accommodation Strategies—Continued

Accommodating the Volume of Work Produced

- **Provide partially completed outlines** and ask students to fill in the missing details. This is a valuable, but not burdensome, exercise in note taking.

- **Allow students to dictate to another student.** One student (scribe) writes down what another student says verbatim and then allows the dictating student to make changes without help from the scribe.

- **Correct poor spelling in first drafts,** but do not lower the grade because of it. However, make clear to the students that spelling does eventually count, especially in assignments completed over time.

- **Reduce copying of printed work.** Avoid having students copy over something already printed in a text, like entire mathematics problems. Provide a worksheet with the text material already on it or have the students just write down their original answers or work.

- **Allow students to use abbreviations** in some writing, such as b/4 for before, b/c for because, and w/ for with. These are also helpful shortcuts during note taking.

Accommodating the Complexity of the Work Produced

- **Allow students to use print or cursive writing.** Many students with dysgraphia are more comfortable with print (manuscript) letters.

Accommodation Strategies—Continued

- **Teach students the stages of writing,** such as brainstorming, drafting, editing, and proofreading.

- **Encourage students to use a spell checker.** Using the spell checker decreases the demands on the writing process, lowering frustration and diverting more energy to thought production. For students who also have reading difficulties, concurrently using a computer reading program also decreases the demands on the writer.

- **Have students proofread after a delay** when they are more likely to catch writing errors. This way, they will see what they *actually* wrote rather than what they *thought* they wrote.

Accommodating the Tools of Work Production

- **Allow students to use lined and graph paper.** Lined paper helps students keep their writing level across the page. Have younger students use graph paper for mathematics calculations to keep columns and rows straight. Older students can turned lined paper sideways for column control.

- **Allow students to use different writing instruments.** Students should use the writing instrument they find most comfortable. Some students have difficulty writing with ballpoint pens, preferring thin-line marker pens that have more friction with the paper. Others prefer mechanical pencils.

- **Have pencil grips available** in all styles. Even high school students enjoy these fun grips and some like the big pencils usually associated with primary school.

- **Allow some students to use speech recognition programs.** For students with very difficult writing problems, using a speech recognition program within a word processing program allows them to dictate their thoughts rather than type them. However, this is not a substitute for learning handwriting.

Strategies to Consider

Modification Strategies for Students With Writing Disorders

For some students, accommodation strategies will not remove the barriers that their writing difficulties pose. Teachers may need to make modifications in these students' assignments. Here are some suggested modifications in the volume, complexity, and format of written work.

Modifying the Volume of Work Produced

- ❑ **Limit the amount of copying that students do.** For example, to copy definitions, have the students rewrite and shorten them without affecting the meaning. Another option is to have them use drawings or diagrams to answer questions.

- ❑ **Reduce the length** of written assignments. Emphasize quality over quantity.

Modifying the Complexity of Work Produced

- ❑ **Prioritization of tasks.** Stress or de-emphasize certain tasks for a complex activity. For example, students could focus on complex sentences in one activity and on using descriptive words in another. Evaluate the assignment based on the prioritized tasks.

Modification Strategies—Continued

- ❏ **Encourage graphic organizers.** Preorganization strategies such as the use of graphic organizers will help students get their main ideas in line before tackling the writing process.

- ❏ **Use cooperative learning groups** to give students a chance to play different roles, such as brainstormer, encourager, organizer of information, etc.

- ❏ **Provide intermittent deadlines** for long-term assignments. Work with other teachers when setting due dates, especially those involving writing assignments. Parents may also be able to monitor the student's work at home so that it can comply with deadlines.

Modifying the Format of the Work Produced

- ❏ **Allow students to submit alternative projects,** such as an oral report or visual project. Ask for a short written report to explain or expand on the oral or visual work. However, these alternatives should not replace all writing assignments.

Strategies to Consider

Remediation Strategies for Students With Writing Disorders

Students should not be allowed to avoid the process of writing, no matter how severe their dysgraphia. Writing is an important skill that they will eventually use to sign documents, write checks, fill out forms, take messages, or make a grocery list. Thus, they need to learn to write even if they can do so for just a short time.

Remediation strategies focus on reteaching information or a particular skill to help students acquire mastery and fluency. Substantial modeling of all strategies is essential for the students to be successful. Here are some suggested areas for remediation (Richards, 1998; Jones, 2000).

★ **Teaching Handwriting Continuously.** Many students would like to have better handwriting. Build handwriting instruction into the students' schedule. Provide opportunities to teach them this, keeping in mind the age, aptitude, and attitude of each student.

★ **Helping With Spelling.** Spelling difficulties are common for students with dysgraphia, especially if sequencing is a major problem. The students with dysgraphia who also have dyslexia need structured and specific instruction in learning to spell phonetically. This skill can help them use technical tools that rely on phonetic spelling to find a word.

★ **Correcting the Pencil Grip.** Young children should be encouraged to use a proper pencil grip from the beginning of their writing experience. Descriptive research indicates that, for the best results, the grip should be consistently between 3/4 inch to 1 inch from the pencil tip. Moderate pressure should be applied and the angle of the pencil to the paper should be about 45 degrees and slanted toward the student's writing arm. Accomplishing the proper slant will be difficult for left handed writers.

Remediation Strategies—Continued

A poor pencil grip can be changed to the appropriate form by using plastic pencil grips, which are commercially available. Obviously, it is easier to encourage the correct grip as soon as the student begins writing; older students with poor grip posture find it very difficult to make changes. The teacher needs to consider whether it is worth the time and effort to get the student to change the grip to be more efficient. If not, identify compensatory strategies that are available for the student.

★ **Writing a Paragraph.** Students can be taught this eight-step process for writing a paragraph. The eight steps can be easily remembered by using the acronym, **POWER**.

1. Plan the paper by thinking about the ideas that you want to include in it.
2. Organize the idea by using a graphic organizer or mind map. This places the main idea in the center and supporting facts are written on lines coming out from the center, much like the spokes of a wheel. Other visual formats can be used depending on the paragraph's topic.

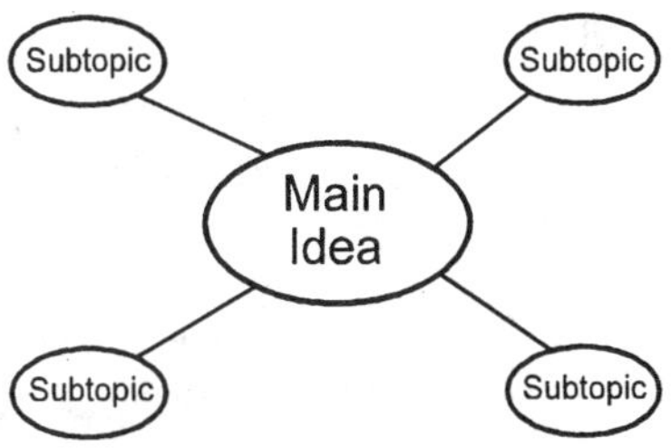

3. Analyze the graphic organizer to ensure that all your ideas have been included. Check your spelling.
4. Write a draft of the paragraph, focusing on the main ideas.
5. Edit your work for punctuation, capitalization, grammar, and spelling.
6. Use the corrections made in step 5 to revise the paragraph.
7. Proofread again, editing and revising as needed.
8. Develop a final product in written or typed form.

P...... Plan the paper (Step 1)
O...... Organize your thoughts and ideas (Steps 2 and 3)
W...... Write the draft (Step 4)
E...... Edit your work (Steps 5, 6, and 7)
R...... Revise your work and produce a final copy (Step 8)

– Continued–

Remediation Strategies—Continued

★ **Increasing the Speed of Writing.** Many students with dysgraphia write very slowly. To identify the appropriate remediation strategy, teachers need to determine the cause of the slowness.

- Is it the actual formation of the letters? If so, the students need more practice on this skill, perhaps by saying the letters aloud while writing. Air writing can be helpful because it uses many more muscles to form the letters. Also, have the students write large letters on a big surface, such as a chalkboard or dry-erase board.
- Is it in the organization of ideas? If so, provide the students with graphic organizers to help them sort and prioritize their thoughts and facts.

★ **Dealing With Fatigue.** Poor motor sequencing or an incorrect pencil grip can lead to fatigue with the writing process. The following can help students relieve the stress of writing and relax the writing hand.

- Take writing breaks at regular intervals. Students should realize that it is permissible to stop occasionally and relax the muscles of the hand. This break also gives them a chance to review what has been written and to continue to organize their thoughts.
- Shake the hands quickly to relax the muscles. This increases blood flow to the finger and hand muscles.
- Rub the hands on some texture, like the carpet or clothes.
- Rub the hands together and focus on the feeling of warmth. The rubbing also helps to restore blood flow to the area.

★ **Giving Praise, Being Patient, and Encouraging Patience.** Genuinely praise the positive aspects of students' work. Be patient with their efforts and problems, and encourage them to have patience with themselves.

Strategies to Consider

Expressive Writing for Students With Learning Disabilities

One of the goals of teaching writing is to help students express their thoughts and ideas in personal narratives and persuasive essays. Students whose learning disabilities include problems with writing often have great difficulty with this. Finding ways of helping these students has been the subject of considerable research.

A recent analysis studied the effectiveness of research-based instructional approaches for teaching expressive writing to students with learning disabilities. The following three components of instruction consistently led to improving student success in learning expressive writing (Gersten, Baker, and Edwards, 1999):

1. Adhering to a basic framework of planning, writing, and revision

Most of the successful interventions used a basic framework of planning, writing, and revision. Each step was taught explicitly, followed by multiple examples and the use of memory devices, such as prompt cards or mnemonics.

Planning. Advance planning results in better first drafts. One way of helping students develop a plan of action is to provide a planning think sheet that uses structured and sequential prompts. It specifies the topic and poses questions to guide the student's thought processes. See the sample sheet at the right.

Planning Think Sheet

TOPIC:____________________

Who am I writing for?

Why am I writing this?

What do I already know about this?

How can I group my ideas?

How will I organize my ideas?

– Continued –

Expressive Writing—Continued

Creating a First Draft. The planning think sheet helps students create first drafts by serving as a guide through the writing process. The guide also gives the student and teacher a common language for an ongoing discussion about the assignment. This student-teacher interaction emphasizes cooperative work rather than the recent method of writing mainly in isolation.

Revising and Editing. The skills of revising and editing are critical to successful writing. Some researchers found a peer editing approach to be particularly effective (Gersten and Baker, 1999). Here's how it worked:

- Pairs of students alternated their roles as student-writer and student-critic.
- The student-critic identified ambiguities and asked the writer for clarification. The writer then made revisions, with the teacher's help if needed.
- Once the clarifications were made, the student pair then moved on to correct capitalization, punctuation, and spelling.
- Throughout the process, the student writers had to explain the intent of their writings and continue revising their essays to reflect their intent accurately. These clarifying dialogues helped the student pairs to understand each other's perspective.

2. Teaching explicitly the critical steps in the writing process

Because different types of writing (e.g., personal narrative or persuasive essay) are based on different structures, explicitly teaching text structures provides the students with a specific guide to complete their writing task. For example, writing a persuasive essay requires a thesis and supporting arguments. Narrative writing focuses on character development and a story climax. Teach these structures, using explicit models of each text type.

Expressive Writing—Continued

3. Providing feedback guided by the information explicitly taught

The researchers found that successful interventions always included frequent feedback to the students on the quality of their overall writing, strengths, and missing elements (Gersten and Baker, 1999). Combining feedback with instruction strengthens the dialogue between student and teacher, thereby helping students to develop a sensitivity to their own writing style. This sensitivity may lead students to reflect on, realize, and correct writing problems as well as perceive their ideas from another's perspective. The research studies also showed that student gains were more likely to occur when the teachers and other students provided feedback mainly in the areas of organization, originality, and interpretation.

Researchers found that frequent feedback was a powerful tool for improving students' writing.

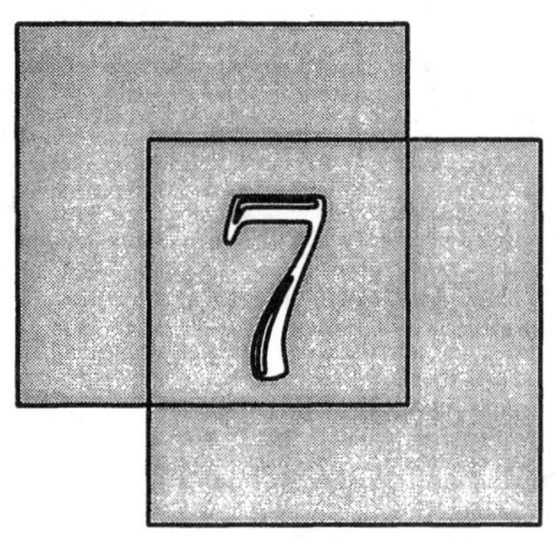

MATHEMATICAL DISABILITIES

Learning to Calculate

How and when the young brain begins to deal with number logic and arithmetic calculations are unknown. However, mounting evidence shows that toddlers have a sense of numbers and can already deal with limited arithmetic operations (e.g., simple adding and subtracting) before the age of one year (Diamond and Hopson, 1998). This early ability makes sense in terms of our past development as a species. In primitive societies, a youngster going for a stroll out of the cave needed to determine quickly if the number of animals in an approaching pack might spell danger or just an opportunity for play. Young hunters had to determine how *many* individuals would be needed to take down a large animal. Recognizing that three apples provide more nourishment than one was also a valuable survival asset. Numeration, then, persisted in the genetic code.

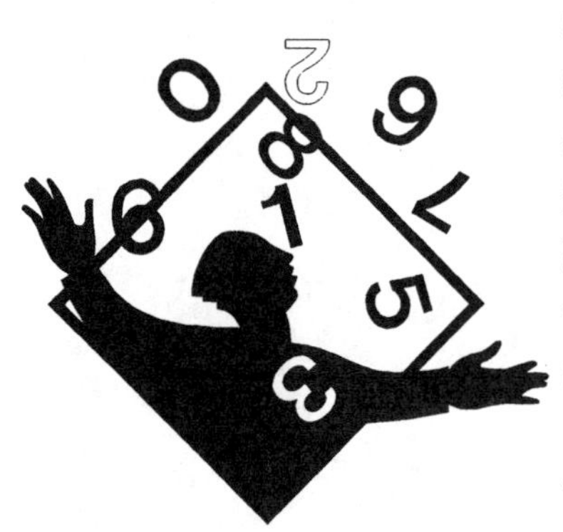

For many years, educators recognized that some children were very adept in mathematical calculations while others struggled despite much effort and motivation. But the percentage of school-age children who experience difficulties in learning mathematics has been steadily growing in the last three decades. Why is that? Is the brain's ability to perform arithmetic calculations declining? If so, why? Does the brain get less arithmetic practice because technology has shifted computation from brain cells to inexpensive electronic calculators?

It is only in the past few years that brain scanning studies have revealed clues about how the brain performs mathematical operations. Functional MRI scans indicate that the parietal and

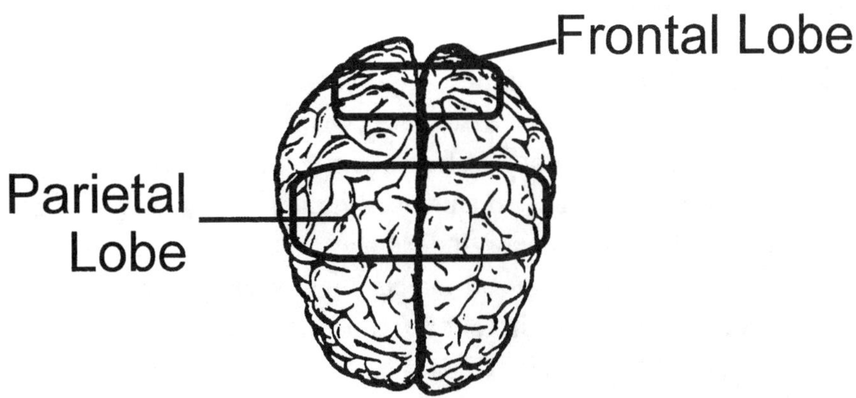

Figure 7.1 *Mathematical calculations primarily activate the brain's frontal and parietal lobes. Other areas may be activated as the calculations become more complex.*

frontal lobes (Figure 7.1) are primarily involved in basic mental mathematics (e.g., counting forward or doing serial calculations). However, other areas of the brain are recruited into action when dealing with more complex calculations (Rueckert, Lange, Partiot, Appollonio, Litvan, LeBihan, and Grafman, 1996).

Mathematical Disabilities

In previous chapters, we have referred to the considerable amount of research that has been conducted in an effort to understand how the human brain learns. As a result, we also have a greater understanding of the diagnosis and remediation of learning disorders, especially in areas of language, reading, and writing. In addition, a few researchers have been studying why students have problems with learning early mathematics, despite normal intelligence and adequate instruction.

About 6 percent of school-age children have some form of difficulty with processing mathematics. This is about the same number as children who have reading problems. However, because of the strong emphasis that our society places on the need to learn reading, many more research studies have focused on problems in this area than on mathematics. Nonetheless, the growing number of students who are having problems with mathematics has renewed research interest in how the brain does calculations and the possible causes of mathematical disorders. The condition that causes persistent problems with processing numerical calculations is often referred to as *dyscalculia*.

Environmental Causes

Even individuals with normal abilities in processing numerical operations can display mathematical disorders. Because they have no inherent mathematical deficits, their difficulties most likely arise from environmental causes. In modern American society, reading and writing have become the main measures of a good student. Mathematics ability is regarded more as a specialized function rather than as a general indicator of intelligence. Consequently, the stigma of not being able to do mathematics is reduced and becomes socially acceptable. Just hearing their parents say "I wasn't very good at math" allows children to embrace the social attitudes that regard mathematics failure as acceptable and routine. A recent Harris poll revealed that although more than 90 percent of parents expect their children to go to college and almost 90 percent of kids want to go to college, fully half of those kids want to drop mathematics as soon as they can (USDE, 1998). To help these students, educators and parents must recognize the importance of more study in this field.

Fear of Mathematics. Some children develop a fear (or phobia) of mathematics because of negative experiences in their past or a simple lack of self-confidence with numbers. No doubt, mathematics phobia can be as challenging as any learning disability, but it is important to remember that these students have neurological systems for computation that are normal. They need help primarily in replacing the memory of failure with the possibility of success. Students with mathematical disorders, on the other hand, have a neurological deficit that results in persistent difficulty in processing numbers.

Quality of Teaching. One critical factor in how well students learn mathematics is the quality of the teaching. Recent studies show that student achievement in mathematics is strongly linked to the teacher's expertise in mathematics. Students of an expert teacher perform up to 40 percent better on achievement tests compared to students of a teacher with limited training in mathematics. The average K-8 teacher has taken only three or fewer mathematics or mathematics education classes in college. Partly because of the current teacher shortage, less than half of eighth grade mathematics teachers have taken a single class on how to teach mathematics, and 28 percent of high school mathematics teachers do not have a major or minor in mathematics (USDE, 1998).

Neurological and Other Causes

Because the parietal lobe is heavily involved with number operations, damage to this area can result in difficulties. Studies of individuals with Gerstmann syndrome—the result of damage to the parietal lobe—showed that they had serious problems with mathematical calculations as well as right-left disorientation, but no problems with oral language skills (Suresh and Sebastian, 2000).

Individuals with visual processing weaknesses almost always display difficulties with mathematics. This is probably because success in mathematics requires one to visualize numbers and mathematical situations, especially in algebra and geometry. Students with sequencing difficulties also may have dyscalculia because they cannot remember the order of mathematical operations nor the specific formulas needed to complete a set of computations.

Genetic factors also seem to play a role. For example, studies of identical twins reveal close mathematics scores. Children from families with a history of mathematical giftedness or retardation show common aptitudes with other family members. Girls born with Turner syndrome—a condition caused by the partial or complete absence of one of the two X chromosomes normally found in women—usually display dyscalculia, among other learning problems (Mazzocco, 1998).

Mathematical Disorders

General Symptoms:

- Inconsistent results with addition, subtraction, multiplication, and division
- Inability to remember mathematical formulas, rules, or concepts
- Difficulty with abstract concepts of time and direction
- Consistent errors when recalling numbers including transpositions, omissions, and reversals
- Difficulty remembering how to keep score during games

Types of Mathematical Disorders

The complexity of mathematics makes the study of mathematical disorders particularly challenging for researchers. Learning deficits can include difficulties in mastering basic number concepts, counting skills, and processing arithmetic operations as well as procedural, retrieval, and visual-spatial deficits (Geary, 2000). As with any learning disability, each of these deficits can range from mild to severe.

Number Concept Difficulties. As mentioned before, the understanding of small numbers and quantity appears to be present at birth. The understanding of larger numbers and place value, however, seems to develop during the preschool and early elementary years. Studies show that most children with mathematical disorders nevertheless have their basic number competencies intact (Geary, 2000).

Counting Skill Deficits. Studies of children with mathematical disorders show that they have deficits in counting knowledge and counting accuracy. Some may also have problems keeping numerical information in working memory while counting, resulting in counting errors.

Difficulties With Arithmetic Skills. Children with mathematical disorders have difficulties solving simple and complex arithmetic problems. Their difficulties stem mainly from deficits in both numerical procedures (solving 6+5 or 4 x 4) and working memory. Moreover, deficits in visual-spatial skills can lead to problems with arithmetic because of misalignment of numerals in multicolumn addition. Although procedural, memory, and visual-spatial deficits can occur separately, they are often interconnected.

Procedural Disorders. Students displaying this disorder

- use arithmetic procedures (algorithms) that are developmentally immature,
- have problems sequencing the steps of multi-step procedures,
- have difficulty understanding the concepts associated with procedures, and
- make frequent mistakes when using procedures.

The cause of this disorder is unknown. However, researchers suspect a dysfunction in the left hemisphere, which specializes in procedural tasks.

Memory Disorders. Students displaying this disorder

- have difficulty retrieving arithmetic facts,
- have a high error rate when they do retrieve arithmetic facts, and
- retrieve incorrect facts that are associated with the correct facts.

Here again, a dysfunction of the left hemisphere is suspected, mainly because these individuals frequently have reading disorders as well. This association further suggests that memory deficits may be inheritable.

Visual-Spatial Deficits. Students with this disorder

- have difficulties in the spatial arrangement of their work, such as aligning the columns in multicolumn addition;
- often misread numerical signs, rotate and transpose numbers, or both;
- misinterpret spatial placement of numerals, resulting in place value errors; and,
- have difficulty with problems involving space in areas, as required in algebra and geometry.

This disorder is more closely associated with deficits in the right hemisphere, which specializes in visual-spatial tasks. Some studies suggest that the left parietal lobe also may be implicated.

Many students eventually overcome procedural disorders as they mature and learn to rely on sequence diagrams and other tools to remember the steps of mathematical procedures. Those with visual-spatial disorders also improve when they discover the benefits of graph paper and learn to solve certain algebra and geometry problems with logic rather than through spatial analysis alone. However, memory deficits do not seem to improve with maturity. Studies indicate that individuals with this problem will continue to have difficulties retrieving basic arithmetic facts throughout life. This finding may suggest that the memory problem exists not just for mathematical operations, but may signal a more general deficit in retrieving information from memory.

> *Children often outgrow procedural and visual-spatial difficulties, but memory problems may continue throughout life.*

What Is the Future of Research in Mathematics Disorders?

Many questions remain unanswered regarding the environmental and innate causes of mathematical disorders. For example, we now believe that infants are born with an innate sense of number logic and the ability to perform simple arithmetic operations. Some researchers believe that toddlers can even communicate with each other about their counting through a form of "toddler arithmetic" (Diamond and Hopson, 1998). How do they do that? By learning more about exactly how infants' brains process arithmetic calculations, we can build on this foundation when exposing children to more complex mathematics. Likewise, researchers need to determine which types of mathematical disorders are simply delays in development and which may represent more fundamental problems.

Other questions for research include the following: What genetic factors affect the neural networks and cognitive skills that support mathematical operations? What types of mathematical disorders are related to reading disorders, and why?

The ultimate goal of research is to develop remedies to help individuals deal with their problems. Remediation becomes difficult when a disorder is not well understood. Nonetheless, enough is now known to suggest some strategies that are likely to help those challenged by mathematical processing. Further research can only improve on this situation.

What Do Educators Need to Consider?

Determining the Source of the Problem. The first task facing educators who deal with children with mathematics disorders is to determine the nature of the problem. Obviously, environmental causes require different interventions than developmental causes. Low performance on a mathematics test *may* indicate that a problem exists, but tests do not provide information on the exact source of the poor performance. Standardized tests, such as the *Brigance Comprehensive Inventory of Basic Skills—Revised,* are available that provide more precise information on whether the problems stem from deficits in counting, number facts, or procedures.

*Seven prerequisite skills can help **all** students learn mathematics more successfully.*

Prerequisite Skills. Examining the nature of mathematics curriculum and instruction may reveal clues about how the school system approaches teaching these topics. A good frame of reference is the recognition that students need to have mastered a certain number of skills before they can understand and apply the principles of more complex mathematical operations. Mahesh Sharma (1989) and other mathematics educators have suggested that the following seven skills are prerequisites to successfully learning mathematics. They are the ability to

1. Follow sequential directions.
2. Recognize patterns.
3. Estimate by forming a reasonable guess about quantity, size, magnitude, and amount.
4. Visualize pictures in one's mind and manipulate them.
5. Have a good sense of spatial orientation and space organization, including telling left from right, compass directions, horizontal and vertical directions, etc.
6. Do deductive reasoning, that is, reason from a general principle to a particular instance, or from a stated premise to a logical conclusion.
7. Do inductive reasoning, that is, come to a natural understanding that is not the result of conscious attention or reasoning, easily detecting the patterns in different situations and the interrelationships between procedures and concepts.

Sharma notes, for example, that those who are unable to follow sequential directions will have great difficulty understanding the concept of long division, which requires retention of several different processes performed in a particular sequence. First one estimates, then multiplies, then compares, then subtracts, then brings down a number, and the cycle repeats. Those with directional difficulties will be unsure which number goes inside the division sign or on top of the fraction. Moving through the division problem also presents other directional difficulties: One reads to the right, then records a number up, then multiplies the numbers diagonally, then records the product down below while watching for place value, then brings a number down, and so on.

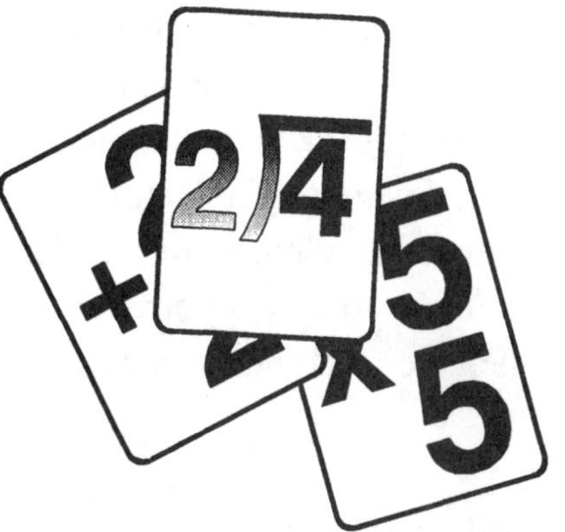

Less Is More. Another lesson that research has taught us is that students with special needs are likely to be more successful if taught fewer concepts in more time. The notion that "less is more" can apply to all students, and is particularly important for those with learning problems. Studies of mathematics (as well as science) courses in the United States and other countries show that spending more time on fewer key concepts leads to greater student achievement in the long run. Yet, our mathematics curriculum does not challenge students to study topics in depth. We tend to present a large number of ideas but develop very few of them (National Center for Education Statistics, 1996). Students with special needs should focus on mastering a few important ideas and learn to apply them accurately.

Use of Manipulatives. Students with special needs who use manipulatives in their mathematics classes outperform similar students who do not. Manipulatives support the tactile and spatial reinforcement of mathematical concepts, maintain focus, and help students develop the cognitive structures necessary for understanding arithmetic relationships. In addition to physical manipulatives (e.g., Cuisenaire rods and tokens), computers and software also help these learners make connections between various types of knowledge. For example, computer software can construct and dynamically connect pictured objects to symbolic representations (such as cubes to a numeral) and thus help learners generalize and draw abstract concepts from the manipulatives.

Search for Patterns. One of the more surprising research findings is that many children with learning disabilities—including those with mathematical disorders—can learn basic arithmetic concepts. What is needed for these children is an approach that relies less on intensive drill and practice and more on searching for, finding, and using patterns in learning the basic number combinations and arithmetic strategies.

Build on Students' Strengths. As obvious as this statement seems, teachers can often turn a student's failure into success if they build on what the student already knows how to do. Too often teachers get so focused on looking for ways to improve an area of weakness that they unintentionally overlook an individual's learning strengths. Yet many years of research into learning styles has demonstrated effective ways of recruiting style strengths to build up weaknesses.

Most people learn mathematics best in the context of real-world problems. School systems will increase all their students' chances for learning mathematics successfully if they plan curriculum content and instructional strategies that enhance prerequisite skills while developing knowledge and application of mathematical concepts and operations. Students are more comfortable with mathematics when they perceive it as a practical tool and not as an end unto itself. Integrated curriculum units provide opportunities for mathematics to be threaded through diverse and relevant topics. Finally, if the notion that babies are born with a sense of number logic continues to be supported by further research, then educators will need to reconsider how and when we teach mathematics in schools.

Mathematics for Students Studying English as a Second Language

Little attention or research has been devoted to studying the problems of learning mathematics for students with learning disabilities who are also studying English as a second language (ESL). Yet, mathematics is one of the first subjects where these students are mainstreamed. One explanation for this lack is the perception that mathematics is a universal language and, thus, should transcend the language barriers posed by other subjects.

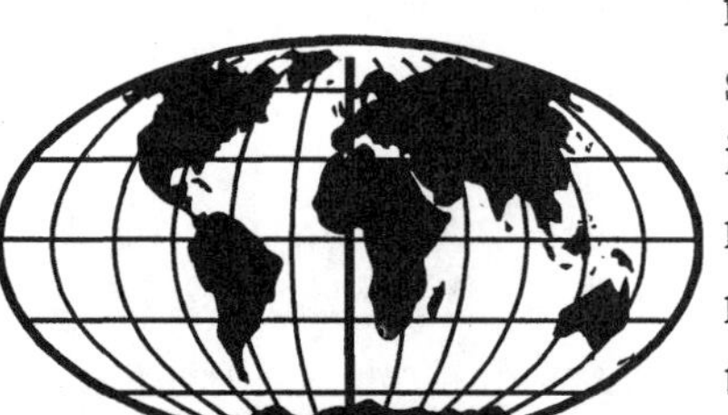

The few studies that have investigated this situation have indicated that language factors are indeed a concern. Although the language of mathematics is precise, it is not always translated accurately by ESL students. Those who also have learning disabilities already have problems understanding mathematical concepts in their native language. When faced with mathematical statements in English, these difficulties are compounded. The students have to cope with applying the rules of vocabulary, syntax, and grammar to both the English language *and* to mathematics. Consequently, they may have problems distinguishing differences in mathematical relationships, such as size, time, speed, and space.

Cultural differences also play a role, especially in the interpretation of story problems. The values, mores, and customs of different cultures can vary significantly from those represented in American textbooks. One study found that problems written for American children often contained biases of values and gender that caused confusion in children from other cultures (Fellows, Koblitz, and Koblitz, 1994).

> *The algorithms that an ESL student uses to make calculations may be misinterpreted as a mathematics disorder.*

Differences in algorithms—the procedures used to find the solution to a mathematical problem—also pose difficulties for ESL students. Asian and South American students, for example, learn algorithms that are different in sequence from those taught in American schools. The algorithms that an ESL student uses to make calculations may be misinterpreted as a mathematics disorder. Rather than being concerned about differing algorithms, teachers should determine whether the student can explain the procedure and arrive at the correct answer. See the Strategies to Consider at the end of this chapter for more suggestions on helping ESL students.

Impact on Learning

- Students with difficulties in mathematics are likely to focus when the mathematics instruction forms patterns and has meaning.
- Mathematics will be very difficult to master if certain prerequisite skills are not in place.
- Some students can learn successfully if they process mathematics more as a language than as a collection of formulas and theorems.
- ESL students can have difficulties because of language problems and cultural differences.

Strategies to Consider

General Guidelines for Teaching Mathematics to Students With Special Needs

What we have learned about how students in general education learn mathematics can apply as well, with appropriate modifications, to students with mathematical disorders. Here are some recommendations gleaned from the research (Clements, 2000).

- ❑ **Help students develop conceptual understanding and skills.** These students need time to look at concrete models, understand them, and link them to abstract numerical representations. Allow them more time for mathematics study and for completing assignments.

- ❑ **Consider giving more oral and fewer written tests.** The stress of written tests increases the mental burden on these students who often are better at telling you what they know than writing it.

- ❑ **Develop meaningful (relevant) practice exercises.** No one questions the value of practice—it makes permanent! But extensive practice that has little meaning for students is perceived as boring and may actually be harmful to special needs students (Baroody, 1999). Practice solving problems that are purposeful and meaningful.

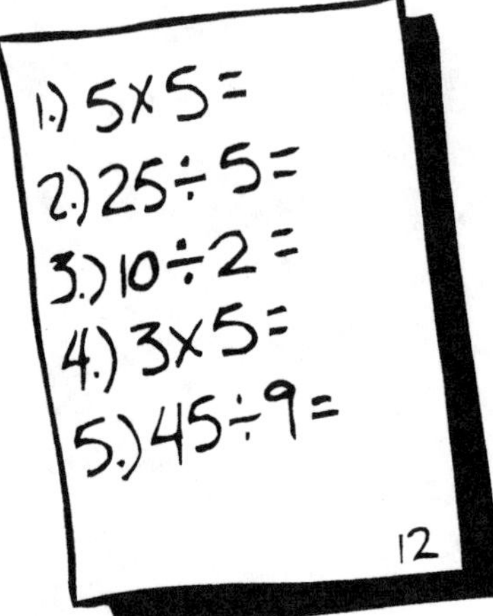

- ❑ **Maintain reasonable expectations.** If we really want all students to have basic competencies in mathematics, then we must establish expectations that are reasonable. This should include problem-based learning, solving authentic problems, and showing the applications of mathematics to other

General Guidelines for Teaching Mathematics—Continued

subject areas, such as science. Similarly, setting expectations that are too low—explicitly or implicitly—increases the burden that children with all types of special needs may need to carry as adults.

- ❑ **Build on children's strengths.** In all areas of learning, teachers can often turn a student's failure into success if they build on what the student already knows how to do. Many years of research into learning styles has demonstrated effective ways of recruiting style strengths to build up weaknesses.

- ❑ **Use manipulatives appropriately.** Manipulatives can be valuable tools if students are able to connect what they are handling with what they are thinking. Have students explain aloud the connections they are making and make sure they refer to the mathematical concepts and skills they are learning.

- ❑ **Help students make connections.** Students perceive meaning when they are able to connect what they are learning to prior knowledge or to future usefulness. Help students connect symbols to verbal descriptions. Find ways to link social situations to solving practical mathematical problems (e.g., splitting a restaurant check, determining an appropriate tip).

- ❑ **Determine and build on a student's informal learning strategies.** All learners develop informal strategies for dealing with their world. Determine what strategies the student is using and build on them to develop concepts and procedures.

- ❑ **Accommodate individual learning styles as much as practicable.** Use as many multisensory approaches as possible. Include modeling, role-playing, demonstrations, simulations, and cooperative learning groups to provide variety and maintain student interest. Use mnemonic devices and games to help students remember number combinations and other important facts. Limit direct instruction (i.e., teacher talk) and use more interactive teaching strategies.

– Continued –

General Guidelines for Teaching Mathematics—Continued

- ❑ **Use technology appropriately.** All students should have access to electronic tools. They can use them to understand mathematical concepts as well as how to benefit their adult lives. Using computer software that includes speech recognition and three-dimensional design, for instance, can be very helpful for students with special needs.

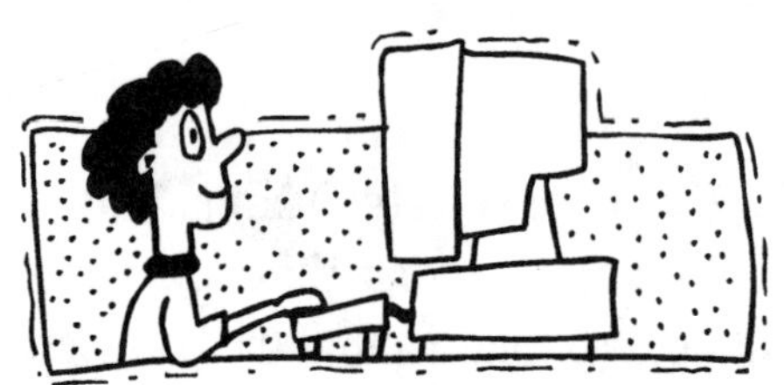

Strategies to Consider

Diagnostic Tools for Assessing Learning Difficulties in Mathematics

Research studies over the last 15 years suggest that five critical factors affect the learning of mathematics. Each factor can serve as a diagnostic tool for assessing the nature of any learning difficulties students may experience with mathematical processing.

1. **Level of Cognitive Awareness.** Students come to a learning situation with varying levels of cognitive awareness about that learning. The levels can range from no cognitive awareness to high levels of cognitive functioning (Sharma, 1989). The teacher's first task is to determine the students' level of cognitive awareness and the strategies each brings to the mathematics task. This is not easy, but it can be accomplished if the teacher does the following:
   - Interviews the students individually and observes how each one approaches a mathematical problem that needs to be solved.
   - Asks "What is the student thinking?" and "What formal and informal strategies is the student using?"
   - Determines what prerequisite skills are in place and which are poor or missing.
   - Determines if a mathematics answer is correct or incorrect and asks students to explain how they arrived at the answer.

   Knowing the levels of the students' cognitive awareness and prerequisite skills will give the teacher valuable information for selecting and introducing new concepts and skills.

– Continued –

Diagnostic Tools—Continued

2. **Mathematics Learning Profile.** Researchers agree that each person processes mathematics differently and that these differences run along a continuum from primarily quantitative to primarily qualitative (Sharma, 1989; Marolda and Davidson, 1994).

Quantitative learners:

- Prefer to deal with entities that have definite values such as length, time, volume, and size.
- Prefer procedural approaches to problem-solving and tend to be very methodical and sequential in all they do.
- Approach mathematics as though following a recipe.
- Prefer to break down problems into their parts, solve them, and then reassemble the components to deal with larger problems.
- Are better at deductive reasoning, that is, reasoning from the general principle to a particular instance.
- Learn best when mathematics is presented as a highly structured subject and with a continuous linear focus.
- Prefer hands-on materials with a counting basis, such as base-10 blocks and number lines.
- Stick with one standardized way of solving problems because alternative solutions are often perceived as uncomfortable and distracting.

Qualitative learners:

- Approach mathematics tasks holistically and intuitively.
- Describe mathematical elements in terms of their qualities rather than by separate parts.
- Are social learners who reason by talking through questions, associations, and examples.
- Learn by seeing relationships between concepts and procedures.
- Draw associations and parallels between familiar situations and the current task.
- Focus on visual-spatial aspects of mathematical information.

Diagnostic Tools—Continued

- Have difficulty with sequences, algorithms, elementary mathematics, and precise calculations.
- In their work, tend to invent shortcuts, bypass steps, and consolidate procedures with intuitive reasoning.
- Often do not practice enough to attain levels of automaticity.

Because both types of learning styles are present in mathematics classes, teachers need to incorporate multiple instructional strategies. Teaching to one style alone leaves out students with the other style, many of whom may do poorly in mathematics as a result. In fact, some may even exhibit the symptoms of mathematics disorders.

3. **Language of Mathematics.** Mathematical disorders often arise when students fail to understand the language of mathematics, which has its own symbolic representations, syntax, and terminology. Solving word problems requires the ability to translate the language of English into the language of mathematics. The translation is likely to be successful if the student recognizes English language equivalents for each mathematical statement. For example, if the teacher asks the class to solve the problem "76 take away 8," the students will correctly write the expression in the exact order stated, "76 - 8." But if the teacher says, "Subtract 8 from 76," a student following the language order could mistakenly write, "8 - 76." Learning to identify and correctly translate mathematical syntax becomes critical to student success in problem solving.

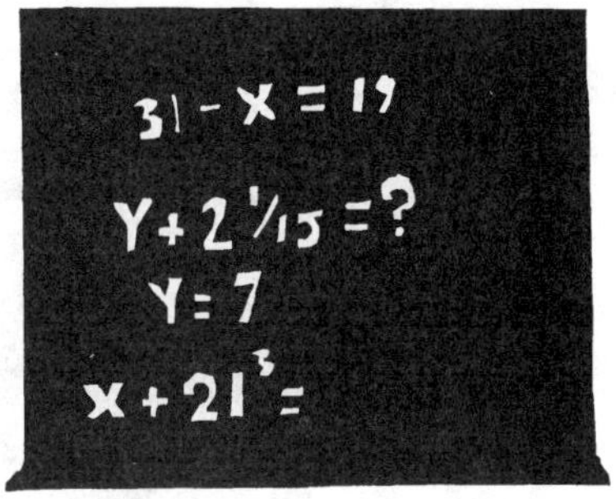

   Language can be an obstacle in other ways. Students may learn a limited vocabulary for performing basic arithmetic operations, such as "add" and "multiply," only to run into difficulties when they encounter expressions asking for the "sum" or "product" of numbers. Teachers can avoid this problem by introducing synonyms for every function: "Let us *multiply* 6 and 5. We are finding the *product* of 6 and 5. The product of 6 *times* 5 is 30."

– Continued –

Diagnostic Tools—Continued

4. **Prerequisite Skills.** The seven prerequisite skills necessary to learn mathematics successfully are non-mathematical in nature. However, they must be mastered before even the most basic understandings of number concepts and arithmetic operations can be learned. Teachers need to assess the extent to which these seven skills are present in each student.

   Teachers might consider using this simple profile diagram to assist in their assessment. After assessing the student's level on each skill, analyze the results and decide on a plan of action that will address any areas needing improvement.

Prerequisite Skills Profile for Mathematics

Student's Name:____________________ Date:___________

Directions: On a scale of 1 (lowest) to 5 (highest), circle the number that indicates the degree to which the student displays mastery of each skill. Connect the circles to see the profile.

Skill					
Follows sequential directions	5	4	3	2	1
Recognizes patterns	5	4	3	2	1
Can estimate quantities	5	4	3	2	1
Can visualize and manipulate mental pictures	5	4	3	2	1
Sense of spatial orientation and organization	5	4	3	2	1
Ability to do deductive reasoning	5	4	3	2	1
Ability to do inductive reasoning	5	4	3	2	1

Action Plan: As a result of this profile, we will work together to____

by doing____

Diagnostic Tools—Continued

Students with four or more scores in the 1 to 2 range will have significant problems learning the basic concepts of mathematics. They will need instruction and practice in mastering these skills before they can be expected to master mathematical content.

5. **Levels of Learning Mastery.** How does a teacher decide when a student has mastered a mathematical concept? Certainly, written tests of problem solving are one of the major devices for evaluating learning. However, they are useful tools only to the extent that they actually measure mastery rather than rote memory of formulas and procedures. Cognitive research suggests that a person must move through six levels of mastery to truly learn and retain mathematical concepts. For mastery, the student

   - Level One. Connects new knowledge to existing knowledge and experiences.
   - Level Two. Searches for concrete material to construct a model or show a manifestation of the concept.
   - Level Three. Illustrates the concept by drawing a diagram to connect the concrete example to a symbolic picture or representation.
   - Level Four. Translates the concept into mathematical notation using number symbols, operational signs, formulas, and equations.
   - Level Five. Applies the concept correctly to real world situations, projects, and story problems.
   - Level Six. Can teach the concept successfully to others, or can communicate it on a test.

Too often, paper-and-pencil tests assess only level 6. Thus, when the student's results are poor, the teacher may not know where learning difficulties lie. By designing separate assessments for each level, teachers will be in a much better position to determine what kind of remedial work will help each student.

Strategies to Consider

Teaching Strategies in Mathematics for Different Learning Styles

Cognitive researchers are suggesting that students approach the study of mathematics with different learning styles that run the gamut from primarily quantitative to primarily qualitative (Sharma, 1989; Marolda and Davidson, 1994). The implication of this research is that students are more likely to be successful in learning mathematics if teachers use instructional strategies that are compatible with the students' cognitive styles. Tables 7.1 and 7.2 illustrate teaching strategies that are appropriate for the mathematical behaviors exhibited by quantitative and qualitative learners, respectively. Table 7.3 suggests a sequence for using inductive and deductive approaches when introducing a new mathematical concept.

Table 7.1 Teaching Strategies for Learners With Quantitative Style

Mathematical Behaviors	Teaching Strategies to Consider
Approaches situations using recipes	Emphasize the meaning of each concept or procedure in verbal terms.
Approaches mathematics in a mechanical, routine-like fashion	Highlight the concept and overall goal of the learning.
Emphasizes component parts rather than larger mathematical constructs	Encourage explicit description of the overall conceptual framework. Look for ways to link parts to the whole.
Prefers numerical approach rather than concrete models	Use a step-by-step approach to connect the model to the numerical procedure.
Prefers the linear approach to arithmetic concept	Start with the larger framework and use different approaches to reach the same concept.
Has difficulty in situations requiring multistep tasks	Separate multiple tasks into smaller units and explain the connections between the units.

Teaching Strategies for Different Learning Styles—Continued

Table 7.2 Teaching Strategies for Learners With Qualitative Style	
Mathematical Behaviors	Teaching Strategies to Consider
Prefers concepts to algorithms (procedures for problem solving)	Connect models first to the concept, and then to procedures before introducing algorithms.
Perceives overall shape of geometric structures at expense of missing the individual components	Emphasize how the individual components contribute to the overall design of the geometric figure.
Difficulties with precise calculations and in explaining procedure for finding the correct solution.	Encourage explicit description of each step used.
Can offer a variety of approaches or answers to a single problem.	Use simulations and real word problems to show application of concept to different situations.
Prefers to set up problems but can not always follow through to a solution	Provide opportunities for the student to work in cooperative learning groups. To ensure full participation, give the student one grade for problem approach and set-up and one grade for exact solution.
Benefits from manipulatives and enjoys topics related to geometry	Provide a variety of manipulatives and models (e.g., Cuisenaire rods, tokens, or blocks) to support numerical operations. Look for geometric links to new concepts.

Tables 7.1 and 7.2 are meant to help teachers address specific mathematical behaviors that they identify in individual students. Such strategies target specific needs and, with practice, can strengthen a student's weakness. It is perhaps unrealistic, however, to expect teachers to identify and select individual strategies for problems encountered by all their students during a single learning episode.

– Continued –

Teaching Strategies for Different Learning Styles—Continued

Table 7.3 suggests an instructional sequence for introducing a new mathematical concept. The order first accommodates qualitative learners and then moves to techniques for quantitative learners (Sharma, 1989).

Table 7.3 Inductive to Deductive Approach for Introducing a New Concept

Steps of the Inductive Approach for Qualitative Learners	■ Explain the linguistic aspects of the concept. ■ Introduce the general principle or law that supports the concept. ■ Provide students opportunities to use concrete materials to investigate and discover proof of the connection between the principle and the concept. ■ Give many specific examples of the concept's validity using concrete materials. ■ Allow students to discuss with each other what they discovered about how the concept works. ■ Demonstrate how these individual experiences can be integrated into a general principle or rule that applies equally to each example.
Steps for the Deductive Approach for Quantitative Learners	■ Reemphasize the general principle or law that the concept relates to. ■ Demonstrate how several specific examples obey the general principle or law. ■ Allow students to state the principle and suggest specific examples that follow it. ■ Ask students to explain the linguistic elements of the concept.

By understanding the different approaches to the learning of mathematics, teachers are more likely to select instructional strategies that will result in successful learning for all students.

Strategies to Consider

Mathematics for ESL Students With Learning Disabilities

Researchers in the area of mathematics education offer the following recommendations for teachers of students with learning disabilities who are also studying English as a second language (ESL)(Raborn, 1995).

- **Appraising Abilities in Mathematics.** ESL students may have high abilities in mathematics but have problems expressing these because of difficulties with the English language. To appraise mathematics ability, teachers need to use measurement and assessment instruments that can distinguish mathematics competency and cognitive ability separately from the student's proficiency in English or from any language-based learning disability. Measurement is designed to compare the performance of one individual to others, generally through norm-referenced instruments. Assessments are used to highlight the student's strengths and weaknesses in mathematical content so that school officials can make a decision on appropriate class placement. Subsequent diagnostic procedures will help focus on patterns of performance in specific areas.

- **Selecting the Language of Instruction.** Educators should determine proficiency in *all* languages to which the student has been exposed. Although bilingual education regulations vary from state to state, if the student is stronger in his or her native language than in English, then mathematics instruction should start in the native language. This allows students to learn developmentally appropriate mathematical content without requiring English language proficiency. That is, students who are stronger in mathematics content than in English competency should be taught at their level of mathematics ability, not at their level of English proficiency.

– Continued –

Mathematics for ESL Students—Continued

- **Moving From Concrete Experiences to Abstract Concepts.** Tying concrete models with verbal descriptions (in English) to mathematical concepts is a valuable way of helping ESL students bypass language barriers. This verbal labeling can demonstrate the language sense of a mathematical concept through context. Ask students to practice using English to explain the concrete concept and to demonstrate with manipulatives where appropriate. Finally, remove the manipulatives and ask students to imagine the concept while explaining it aloud.

- **Using Strategies for Concept Development.** The strategy of concept attainment has proven very effective for ESL students. Students compare and contrast examples that *do* contain the concept's attributes (positive exemplars) with examples that *do not* contain the attributes (negative exemplars). In this way, the students must determine for themselves the attributes of the concept or category. Concept attainment is appropriate for any age level and is most effective if the following steps are employed (adjusted, of course, for student age):
  - Begin by presenting a category that includes the concept. For example, if the concept is that of rectangles, then perhaps start with the category of "shape."
  - Present information in the form of words, concrete materials, or diagrams that introduce an approximately equal number of positive and negative exemplars. Separate the exemplars into "yes" and "no" categories and ask students to examine them. Students will need to determine what the positive exemplars have in common and show how they differ from the negative exemplars.
  - Ask the students to develop a hypothesis and explain how they got it. Following this discussion, the students must name the concept that was presented.
  - When the concept has been correctly identified and named, the students offer their own exemplars as a check of their understanding. In a further test, the teacher can offer an exemplar and ask the students to place it in the "yes" or "no" category.

Mathematics for ESL Students—Continued

- **Using Mathematics to Develop Language.** The language of mathematics offers students the opportunity to deal with precise vocabulary, sequence, and syntax that can be helpful in acquiring both their native and a second language. Mathematics teaches predictable patterns and can develop proficiency in social and academic language skills. Give students the opportunity to talk to their peers and to adults so they can validate their ideas in mathematics while also practicing native and secondary language skills.

- **Using Students' Strengths.** Teacher observations and testing often reveal students' strengths as well as their weaknesses. Strengths should be pointed out to students and used in planning a variety of instructional techniques. Address visual and kinesthetic learning strengths by incorporating visual materials, manipulatives, and opportunities for movement in the classroom throughout each lesson. Demonstrations, models, and simulations are also helpful, although they are more appropriate for learning mathematics skills than mathematical concepts. They also aid in maintaining interest and student motivation. Cooperative learning groups have been shown to be particularly effective for ESL students because the group structure helps students attain intellectual and social goals. Further, the group format affords students an opportunity to take responsibility for cooperative roles and obligations.

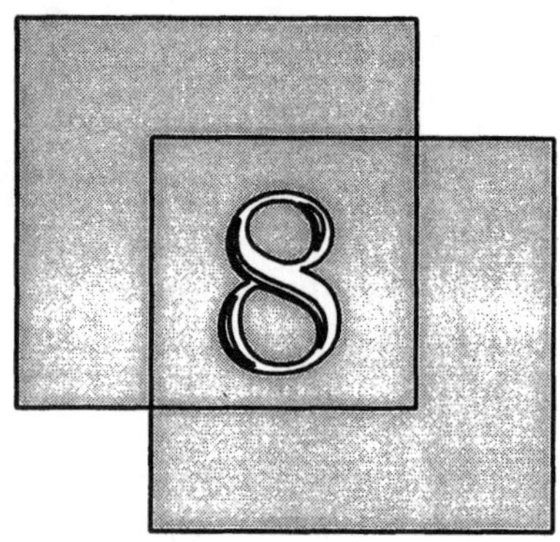

Sleep Disorders

The idea that the amount of sleep an individual gets each night can have an impact on learning is not shocking, yet it has probably been the most overlooked factor affecting student performance in school. Lack of sleep has become a national affliction and fiscal estimates of how much toll it takes on productivity range in the billions of dollars per year. Apart from these losses, researchers are just beginning to understand the negative repercussions that lack of sleep has on the learning process. Before we get into the problems of sleep deprivation, we need a brief review of the biology of sleep.

What Is Sleep?

How Does Sleep Occur?

Before the advent of brain imaging technology, most scientists thought of sleep as the time when the brain was quiet, dormant, and passive. We now know that our brains are very active during sleep, and we are just beginning to understand the ways that sleep affects our daily functioning and our mental and physical health.

Sleep is controlled by a biological clock that resides deep within the brain. Called the *suprachiasmatic nucleus* (SCN), it is a pair of pinhead-sized structures containing about 20,000 neurons. It actually rests near the *hypothalamus*, just above the point where the *optic nerves* cross. Light from the eye's *retina* creates signals that travel along the optic nerve and are monitored by the SCN (Figure 8.1). When darkness falls, the light signals decrease and the SCN prompts the *pineal gland* to produce the hormone *melatonin*. As the amount of melatonin in the blood

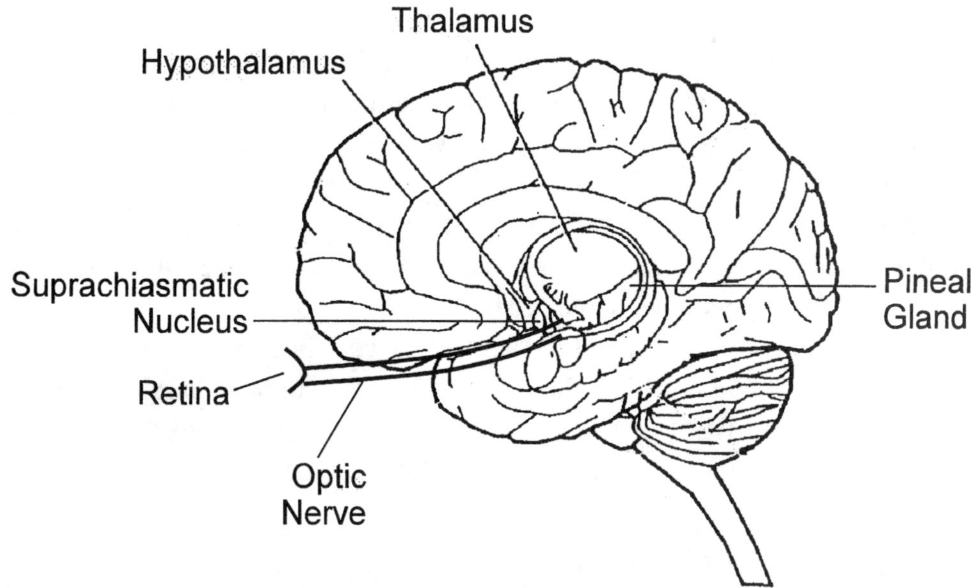

Figure 8.1 *Light signals traveling from the retina along the optic nerves are monitored by the suprachiasmatic nucleus (SCN). When the light signals decrease, the SCN prompts the pineal gland to release melatonin into the blood, beginning the sleep cycle.*

increases, we feel drowsy. Meanwhile, the SCN is altering and synchronizing other body functions, such as blood pressure, body temperature, and urine production, in preparation for sleep. In the morning, the melatonin concentration drops and the waking phase begins. This sleep-wake cycle is one of our daily rhythms, called a *circadian* (from Latin, about a day) rhythm.

Because sleep and wakefulness are regulated by different neurotransmitter signals in the brain, foods and medicines can alter the balance of these signals and affect our sleep patterns. For example, caffeinated products (e.g., coffee, soda, diet pills, and decongestants) stimulate parts of the brain that can interfere with sleep. Antidepressant drugs can also prevent deep sleep. Heavy smokers tend to wake up several times during the night because of nicotine withdrawal. Some people try to improve their sleep by drinking alcohol just before bedtime. Although alcohol does help people fall into light

A Word About Melatonin

Some people with chronic sleep problems (or jet lag) rely on melatonin supplements to improve their sleep. Because of the high dosage of melatonin in these pills, the long-term use of this supplement may create new problems. Because the potential side effects of long-term melatonin usage are unknown, medical experts do not recommend their use by the general public. See the Strategies to Consider at the end of this chapter for suggestions on how to deal with sleep problems.

sleep, it also robs them of the restorative value of deep sleep. Instead, it keeps them in the light sleep stages where they can be easily awakened.

Stages of Sleep. Sleep has five successive phases, called stages 1, 2, 3, 4, and REM. We progress through the five stages and the cycle repeats itself several times during the night. The Stage 1 is a transitional period where we are easily awakened. Stage 2 is light sleep. In stages 3 and 4, we move into deeper sleep. The last stage is called REM, for Rapid Eye Movement. Although brain and body activity increase during REM, this is the restorative stage in which neurons are repaired, dreaming occurs, and memories are consolidated and stored. Table 8.1 shows the five stages of sleep and the characteristics of each stage.

Most people spend about 50 percent of their total sleep time in stage 2, about 20 percent in REM, and the remaining 30 percent in the other stages. By contrast, infants spend about 50 percent of their sleep time in REM. This may be because infants fall into deeper sleep faster, allowing more REM time for the consolidation of rapidly growing neural networks.

Table 8.1 Five Stages of Sleep and Their Characteristics

Stage	Characteristics
Stage 1 (Transitional sleep) 15 to 20 minutes	• Eyes move very slowly • Muscle activity slows • Drift in and out of sleep • Easily awakened • When awakened, can remember pieces of visual images
Stage 2 (Light sleep) 10 to 15 minutes	• Eye movements stop • Brain waves slow down
Stage 3 (Deep sleep) 15 to 20 minutes	• Very slow brain waves (called delta waves) appear with occasional faster waves • No muscle activity or eye movement
Stage 4 (Deepest sleep) 15 to 20 minutes	• Almost exclusively delta waves • No muscle activity or eye movement • Very difficult to awaken • When awakened, feel groggy and disoriented
REM (Rapid eye movement) 4 to 5 REM cycles per night, varying 10 to 40 minutes per cycle	• Breathing becomes more rapid, irregular, and shallow • Eyes jerk rapidly in various directions • Limb muscles become temporarily paralyzed • Heart rate and blood pressure increase • When awakened, can describe dreams • Long-term memory consolidation occurs for storage

How Much Sleep Do We Need?

Age is one of the more important factors determining the amount of sleep a person needs. Infants need about 16 hours a day. Between the ages of 1 to 3 years, the sleep requirement drops to 10 to 12 hours a night. From then until the preteen years, 9 to 10 hours is normal. Teenagers need 8 to 9 hours. For these pre-adult age groups, we are talking about *sleep time*, not *bedtime*.

Most adults do well with between 7 and 8 hours a night, although the range is about 5 to 10 hours. The length of sleep needed does not correlate with intelligence or personality, despite the often-cited fact that Thomas Edison slept very little. Albert Einstein, on the other hand, was notorious for sleeping long hours (Restak, 2000).

If we do not get enough sleep, our bodies begin to create a sleep debt. Eventually, the body will demand that the debt be paid. If we continue to get less sleep than we need, our judgment, reaction time, and other functions become impaired.

What Happens If We Don't Get Enough Sleep?

Adequate sleep is so important to normal body maintenance that undesirable repercussions appear if we do not get enough sleep. Yet, many school-age children and adults are sleep deprived. Recent research studies have highlighted the dangers of sleep deprivation. For example, tests of driving skills in a simulator and monitored eye-hand coordination tasks of people who were sleep deprived showed that they performed as bad as or worse than those who were intoxicated with alcohol. Moreover, sleep deprivation intensifies alcohol's affect on the body, so a fatigued person who drinks will likely become much more impaired than someone who is well rested (NINDS, 2000).

Why Do We Need Sleep?

The best evidence that sleep is an important and necessary biological function is what happens if we don't get enough of it. For instance, sleep-deprived rats die at the age of five weeks (rather than two to three years) and develop sores on their bodies, probably because their immune systems are impaired.

Hence, sleep must be necessary for the health of our nervous system. When we get too little sleep, we have difficulty concentrating, physical performance declines, and our memory is impaired. If sleep deprivation continues, hallucinations and severe mood swings may develop. These symptoms lead researchers to believe that sleep allows the neurons (used while we are awake) the time to shut down and repair themselves. Without sleep, the neurons become depleted of energy and so polluted with the byproducts of cellular metabolism that they begin to malfunction. Some research evidence strongly suggests that sleep also gives the brain a chance to exercise important neural connections that might otherwise deteriorate from inactivity (Schacter, 1996).

In children and young adults, deep sleep coincides with the release of growth hormones. Deep sleep is also the time when cell production increases and protein breakdown decreases. Because proteins are the building blocks of cells, this fact may indicate that the body is repairing cellular damage resulting from the day's activities and other harmful factors, such as stress and ultraviolet rays. Further, the parts of the brain that control decision making, emotions, and social interactions are much quieter during this time, suggesting that deep sleep helps us maintain our emotional and social balance when awake.

Recent brain imaging studies reveal that the parts of the brain used for learning are very active during REM sleep. One study found that REM sleep affects the learning of certain mental skills. People taught a skill and then deprived of non-REM sleep still remembered the skill, but people deprived of REM sleep could not (Restak, 2000). We spend more time in REM sleep while we are learning new things. Apparently, REM sleep is a time to consolidate memories already in the system. Consequently, students who are sleep deprived may be memory deprived as well.

Sleep Deprivation

As with most disorders, the problems associated with sleep can have environmental or neurological origins. Both types affect school-age children, although environmental causes affect far more students. The primary environmental cause of problems with sleep is just not getting enough of it each night.

Preteens

We know that preteens need about 9 to 10 hours of sleep, that is, of *sleep*, not of *time in bed*. Too many preteens with televisions in their bedrooms stay awake watching TV for hours, robbing them of needed sleep. Some children lose sleep because of family situations, such as parents coming home late at night, or other household disturbances. As a result of not enough sleep, children often doze off in school.

Sleep Deprivation

Symptoms:

- Difficulty waking in the morning
- Falling asleep spontaneously during the day
- Irritability later in the day
- Sleeping for extra long periods on weekends

If children are sleep deprived, they can become distracted, aggressive, oppositional, and easily frustrated. Some evidence indicates that long-term sleep deprivation can even lead to permanent learning disabilities, although this is rare. There should be no need for the problem to get to this stage, however, because sleep deprivation is easily corrected with adequate sleep.

Adolescents

Malls, computers, television, homework, and changing family patterns all contribute to rob adolescents of their nightly sleep, and continued sleep deprivation can lead to tragic consequences. For example, the sudden increase in traffic accidents caused by adolescents and young adults falling asleep at the wheel recently brought national attention to this problem. In 1997, the National Institutes of Health convened a scientific working group to examine the issue of adolescent sleepiness. Much of the research gathered by that group and others was published in 2000 by the National Sleep Foundation (NSF) in a report titled *Adolescent Sleep Needs and Patterns*.

Amount and Patterns of Sleep. The NSF report noted research studies showing the average sleep time for 13-year-olds during the school week was 7 hours, 42 minutes, dropping to just over 7 hours for 19-year-olds. Only 15 percent of adolescents reported sleeping 8.5 hours or more on school nights, and 26 percent reported sleeping 6.5 hours or less each school night.

Weekend sleep schedules were very different from weekday schedules. The adolescents in the studies slept about 1.5 to 2 hours longer on weekends with over 90 percent of them going to bed after 11:00 p.m. Such irregular patterns of weekday to weekend sleep schedules combined with inadequate sleep can shift the adolescent body clock to a later sleep and wake cycle (circadian rhythm) than for the average adult or preadolescent (Wolfson and Carskadon, 1998).

> *Many adolescents come to school every day with sleep deprivation.*

Delayed Sleep Phase Disorder. With their body clocks shifted to a later time for going to sleep (around midnight), adolescents need to sleep until 9:00 a.m. to get their full complement of 9 hours sleep. But on weekdays, they have to wake up around 6:00 a.m. because the school buses come by at 7:00 a.m. Consequently, many high school students get up after only 6.5 to 7 hours of sleep and with their bodies still loaded with melatonin. Figure 8.2 shows the concentration of melatonin (measured in saliva) in adolescents with a strict 10:00 p.m. sleep and 8:00 a.m. wake cycle, and what this probably would be in adolescents whose sleep-wake cycle has shifted to roughly an hour later (NSF, 2000).

When students arrive at school, they are often drowsy and fall asleep in class at the first opportunity. The mismatch between the shift of adolescents' sleep phase and the time we ask them

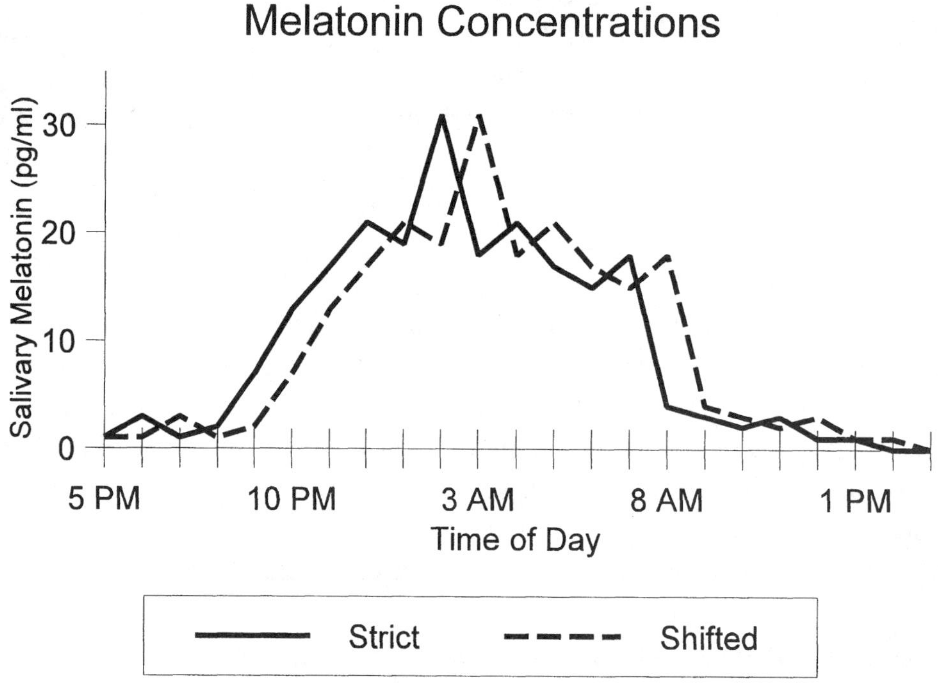

Melatonin Concentrations

Salivary Melatonin (pg/ml)
30
20
10
0
5 PM
10 PM
3 AM
8 AM
1 PM
Time of Day
Strict
Shifted

Figure 8.2 *The solid line shows the concentration of melatonin in saliva in an adolescent with a strict sleep/wake cycle (10 p.m. to 8 a.m.). The dotted line shows what the concentrations are likely to be in an adolescent whose sleep/wake cycle has shifted to a later cycle of 11 p.m. to 9 a.m. (NSF, 2000)*

to start high school has led to a chronic condition known as Delayed Sleep Phase Disorder (DSPD). The name is a bit misleading because it implies a permanent systemic or organic condition that can be treated, but not cured. However, DSPD is a temporary condition and can be easily remedied with adequate sleep.

Nonetheless, this disorder can have serious detrimental effects. That is,

- Drowsiness and fatigue can lead to accidents, especially motor vehicle collisions.
- Sleep loss reduces one's ability to control emotional responses, leading to more arguments, emotional outbursts, and depression.
- More high school students with academic problems and with average or lower grades report that they are sleep deprived than do students with better grades.
- Sleep deprivation can produce symptoms similar to attention-deficit hyperactivity disorder (ADHD).
- Lack of sleep increases the likelihood of the use of stimulants such as caffeine, nicotine, and alcohol.

Sleep Disorders

Several sleep disorders exist that are not the direct result of sleep deprivation, but may cause it. The most common ones are insomnia, sleep apnea, restless legs syndrome, and narcolepsy. These conditions require medical attention and professional intervention.

Insomnia

Most people suffer occasional insomnia, which can be relieved by practicing good sleep habits (see the Strategies to Consider for tips on sleep). Some people have chronic insomnia, which robs them of sleep every night and sets the stage for other medical problems to arise. Chronic insomnia tends to increase with age and may also be a symptom of some underlying medical disorder. For chronic insomnia, researchers are experimenting with light therapy and other ways to alter the body's sleep-wake cycle.

Sleep Apnea

Rarely found in children, this is a condition that interrupts breathing during sleep. It can be caused by the loss of muscle tone with ageing, or by the malfunction of neurons that control breathing during sleep. The individual's effort to inhale causes the windpipe (trachea) to collapse during sleep, reducing the supply of oxygen to the body. When the blood oxygen level falls too low, the brain awakens the individual enough to open the windpipe. As the person falls back asleep, the windpipe closes again. This cycle can be repeated hundreds of times a night, leaving the person feeling groggy and irritable in the morning. Sleep apnea can be treated through weight loss, sleeping on one's side, or surgery.

Restless Legs Syndrome

Another condition of ageing, but also found in young children, restless legs syndrome is a genetic disorder that causes tingling or prickling sensations in the legs and feet and an urge to move them to get relief. This constant leg movement leads to insomnia at night. The disorder is treated with drugs that affect the neurotransmitter dopamine, which suggests that dopamine abnormalities may be the underlying cause of the syndrome.

Narcolepsy

Narcolepsy affects an estimated 250,000 Americans. It is characterized by frequent and overwhelming urges to sleep at various times during the day, even if the person has had a normal night's sleep. The sleep sessions can last from several seconds to 30 minutes. The disorder often begins in adolescence but is difficult to identify and diagnose at that age. It is usually hereditary, but can also result from head injury or neurological disease. Narcolepsy is most often treated with antidepressant and stimulant drugs.

What Is the Future of Research in Sleep Disorders?

This area has been attracting the attention of more researchers, especially as brain scanning technologies are revealing how different brain regions function during sleep. Understanding the factors that affect sleep may lead to therapies to help those with sleep deprivation and sleep disorders.

What Do Educators Need to Consider?

Educators may want to review their schedules and discuss with parents and community groups the merits of a later start time for high school students. Some results of a study of several school districts that made such a change are shown in the Strategies to Consider at the end of this chapter. In the meantime, teachers, school health providers, and parents should be educated about adolescent sleep patterns and needs, becoming alert for signs of sleep deprivation or sleep disorders.

> *Information about sleep should be part of every high school curriculum.*

Students, too, should learn about the physiology and benefits of sleep and the consequences of sleep deprivation. A sleep education unit needs to be considered as part of every high school curriculum. It could be included in biology, health, psychology, and driver education courses, for example.

Impact on Learning

- Students who come to school with Delayed Sleep Phase Disorder (DSPD) typically have a difficult time focusing and concentrating for an extended period of time.
- Sleep deprivation robs the brain of the time it needs to encode information into long-term storage sites (a process that occurs during REM sleep).
- Loss of sleep affects student performance in all areas of school life including athletics, music, and drama.
- Prolonged sleep deprivation interferes with motor coordination, so driving vehicles and operating machinery can be very hazardous.

Strategies to Consider

Starting High Schools Later

One way to address Delayed Sleep Phase Disorder in adolescents is to delay the start times for high schools. This is no easy task, given all the ramifications such a change has for bus schedules, athletic programs, employment of adolescents in the community, family schedules, and safety issues related to daylight and darkness. But some communities have dealt successfully with these ramifications. A recent study of the effects of later start times on these high schools and their students has yielded such positive results that more communities nationwide are considering doing the same. Here is a part of what that study found (Wahlstrom, Wrobel, and Kubow, 1998).

1. What Is the Desirable Start Time for High Schools? The study asked nearly 3,000 high school teachers to suggest the optimal high school start time. Figure 8.3 shows the summary of their responses. Note that nearly 80 percent of the teachers preferred a start time of 8:00 a.m. or later, and 35 percent preferred 8:30 a.m. or later.

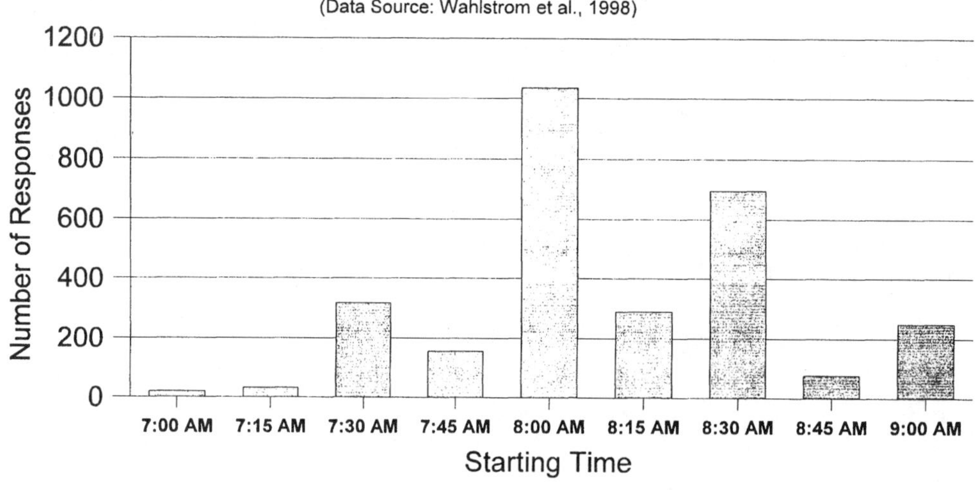

Figure 8.3 *This chart shows the responses of nearly 3,000 secondary teachers who were asked the optimal start time for the first high school class.*

Starting High School Later—Continued

2. What Did Teachers Observe? In schools with later start times, 335 teachers were asked whether students seemed more alert and attentive during the first two periods of the day. Figure 8.4 shows the percentage of teachers who agreed or disagreed with this question, or had no opinion. Note that over 57 percent of the teachers agreed or strongly agreed that students were more alert during the early part of the school day.

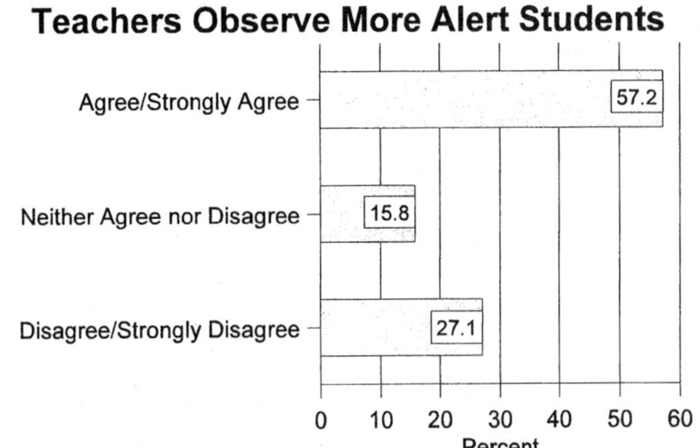

Figure 8.4 *This graph shows the degree to which teachers agreed that students were more alert in the first two class periods. (Wahlstrom et al., 1998)*

3. Does Student Performance Improve With More Sleep? The study examined how the amount of sleep that students got on school nights compared to the grades they received. Figure 8.5 compares the amount of average school-night sleep time to the students' self-reported average grades. No causal relationship is implied, here. That is, the researchers cannot say that longer school-night sleep time was the *cause* of the better grades. Nonetheless, this finding has been observed in all of the few studies of later high school start times to date.

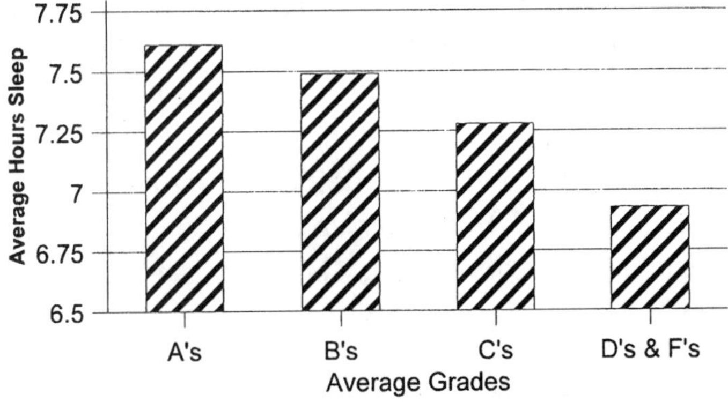

Figure 8.5 *This is a comparison of the average hours of sleep that students had on school nights to their self-reported average grades. (Wahlstrom et al., 1998)*

– Continued –

Starting High School Later—Continued

4. Parents' Response to Later Start Times. Parents in the Edina, MN, schools were surveyed and asked if they were pleased with the later high school start time. Table 8.2 shows the results of that survey. Over 93 percent of all the parents surveyed said they were pleased with the change in start time (Wahlstrom et al., 1998).

Table 8.2 Parent Responses to "Are You Pleased With the Later High School Start Time?"

Parents of:	Percent "Yes"	Percent "No"	Percent "Not Sure"
Sophomores	90.6	5.6	3.8
Juniors	94.4	4.5	1.1
Seniors	96.0	4.0	0
Totals	93.1	4.9	2.0

5. Other Considerations. The study also reported the following findings (NSF, 2000):

- Overall student attendance increased and tardiness decreased.
- Some students reported eating breakfast more frequently.
- Teachers noticed better student behavior; the hallways were quieter between periods and there was less misbehavior in the lunchroom.
- Suburban teachers did not report any noticeable decrease in student participation in extracurricular activities. However, urban teachers did notice a decrease in extracurricular participation along with some problems for students who worked after school.

Strategies to Consider

Tips for Teachers on Dealing With Sleep

1. **Learn about sleep.** Get educated about the sleep needs and patterns of children and adolescents. Students with excessive sleepiness during the day may have some other underlying biological disorder that needs attention.

2. **Teach about sleep.** Tell your students (with age-appropriate language) about the importance of sleep. Remind them that deep sleep is necessary for the brain to store the information and skills they are learning into their long-term memory sites.

3. **Keep the lights on.** One effective way to reduce the amount of melatonin in the blood is with bright light. Taking students for a quick walk in the sun will also help. Resist the temptation to turn the lights off when using an overhead projector or television, especially in the early morning. Better to have some glare on the screen and most students awake than to have a beautiful picture and students half asleep.

4. **Help students assess their sleepiness.** High school students are often unaware of how sleepy they are during their day and evening. Ask them to assess their sleepiness (especially during school days) for at least one school week by using a five-point rating scale to record how tired they are at different times (see sample at right). Review the overall class results with them. Explain that recording a 3 or greater when they should be feeling alert is an indication of sleep deprivation.

Rating the Degree of Sleepiness

Rating Scale:

1. Feeling alert and wide awake
2. Functioning okay, but not at peak
3. Somewhat groggy, tough to concentrate
4. Groggy, losing interest, sluggish
5. Fighting sleep, want to lie down

Name of Student:________________ Date:__________

Time of Day	Rating	Time of Day	Rating
8:00 AM		3:00 PM	
9:00 AM		4:00 PM	
10:00 AM		5:00 PM	
11:00 AM		6:00 PM	
12:00 PM		7:00 PM	
1:00 PM		8:00 PM	
2:00 PM		9:00 PM	

– Continued –

Tips for Teachers on Dealing With Sleep—Continued

5. **Talk to parents.** When talking with parents, emphasize the importance of their children getting adequate sleep. Cite any specific evidence you have of sleepiness that you have noticed in their children.

6. **Look for opportunities to accommodate the school to adolescent sleep needs.** Talk with other educators about the appropriateness of a later start time for high school. Incorporate some physical activity into those early morning lessons.

7. **Use more interactive strategies.** Cooperative learning groups, simulations, demonstrations, and role-playing activities are more likely to keep students alert, especially during the early hours.

8. **Get enough sleep.** It is difficult to be alert and to encourage others to get adequate sleep if you yourself are sleep deprived. Getting adequate sleep makes you a good role model for the class and for your own children.

Strategies to Consider

Tips for Parents About Sleep

When talking to parents about sleep, consider sharing some helpful tips (NSF, 2000). Say to parents the following:

- Learn about the sleep needs and patterns of your children at the various stages of their development.

- Consider whether your children should have television sets in their bedrooms. This is seldom a good idea because watching television interferes with reading, homework, and hobbies. Further, it isolates children from the family and may rob them of their sleep.

- Enforce regular sleep schedules for all your children. Adjust the schedules as they grow older. Remember that it is normal for the sleep-wake cycle of adolescents to be different from that of younger children.

- Look for signs of sleep deprivation in your children. They are not always easy to spot but may include irritability during the day, unusual sleepiness at times when they should be alert, sleeping much longer on weekends, and persistent difficulty in waking up in the morning. Don't allow a drowsy teenager to drive to school or anywhere else.

- Talk to your children about their sleep habits. Does after-school employment or extracurricular activities interfere with their sleep? Make adjustments as needed.

- Encourage your children to keep track of their sleep and wake schedule. This information will be helpful in determining whether their sleep schedules need to be revised or can be used by professionals should you seek outside help for your children's sleepiness.

- Be a good role model and practice good sleep habits.

Strategies to Consider

Tips for Teens About Sleep

When talking to teenage students about sleep, consider sharing some of these tips (NSF, 2000). Encourage them to

- ❑ Get enough sleep. Your brain needs it to store information and your body needs it to repair itself. Even mild sleep deprivation can hurt your academic and athletic performance.

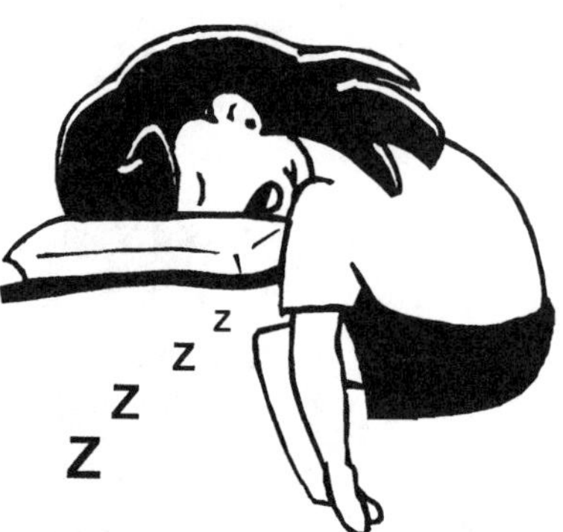

- ❑ Keep a regular sleep schedule. You need between 8 to 9 hours a night. Plan your homework time and other activities carefully to allow enough time for sleep.

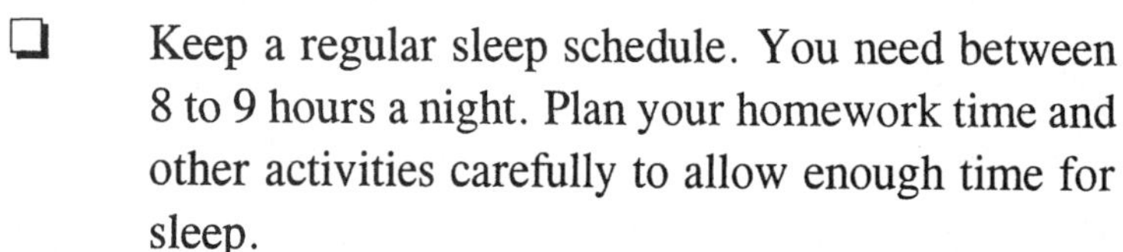

- ❑ Get some bright light as soon as possible in the morning. Bright light helps to awaken the brain. Avoid bright light in the evening so that the sleep cycle can begin normally.

- ❑ Get to know your own body clock. Try to get involved in stimulating activities during that groggy period. Avoid driving if you feel sleepy.

- ❑ Later in the day, stay away from substances that can interfere with your sleep, such as coffee, sodas containing caffeine, and nicotine. Alcohol also disrupts sleep.

- ❑ Start relaxing about one hour before bedtime. Avoid heavy reading or computer games during this time. Don't fall asleep watching television because the flickering light and sound can inhibit deep sleep, which is important for complete rest.

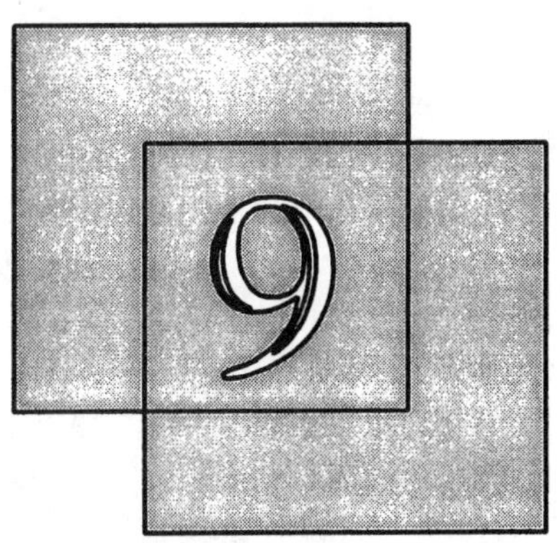

Emotional and Behavioral Disorders

It has been only in recent years that researchers have really begun to recognize the contribution that the emotions make to the development of the human brain and the impact they have on the learning process. Although these contributions are not always considered to be positive, understanding their impact can help parents and educators make appropriate decisions to meet the emotional needs of children and adolescents.

Emotions, Behavior, and Learning

The brain is genetically programmed to gather information and to develop skills that are likely to keep its owner alive. Among other things, human survival depends on the family unit, where emotional bonds increase the chances of producing children and raising them to be productive adults. Consequently, the human brain has learned over thousands of years that survival and emotional messages must have first priority when filtering through all the incoming signals from the body's senses.

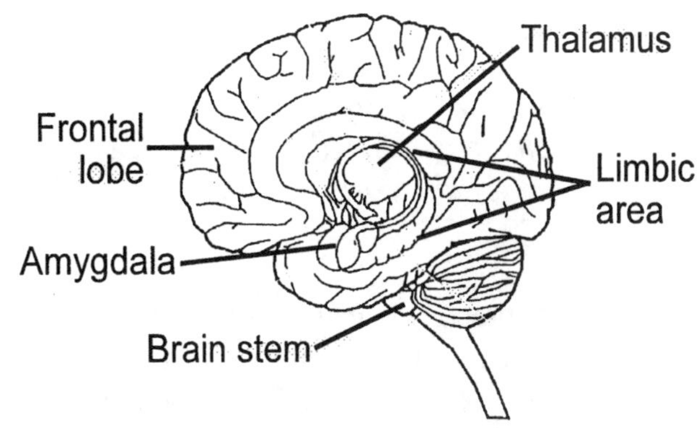

Figure 9.1 *Survival functions are controlled from the brainstem. Emotional signals are processed and interpreted by the limbic area and frontal lobe.*

The brainstem monitors and regulates survival functions such as body temperature, respiratory rate, and blood pressure (Chapter 1). Emotional messages are carried through and interpreted in the limbic area, usually with the help of the frontal lobe (Figure 9.1). These survival and emotional messages guide the individual's behavior, including directing its attention to a learning situation. Specifically, emotion drives attention and attention drives learning.

But even more important to understand is that emotional attention comes before cognitive recognition. You see a letter from a former lover in the mail and within a few seconds your palms are sweating, your breathing is labored, and your blood pressure rises—all this before you even know what is written in the letter. Joseph LeDoux (1996) has done extensive research on emotions and, as a result of using brain imaging, concludes that the amygdala is the part of the limbic system responsible for emotional responses, and that it can act without input from the cognitive parts of the brain (usually the frontal lobe in the cerebrum). This is an intriguing finding because it suggests that the brain can respond emotionally to a situation without the benefit of cognitive functions, such as thinking, reasoning, and consciousness. Of course, we have already sensed the truth of this from our past experiences.

Pathways of Emotional Signals

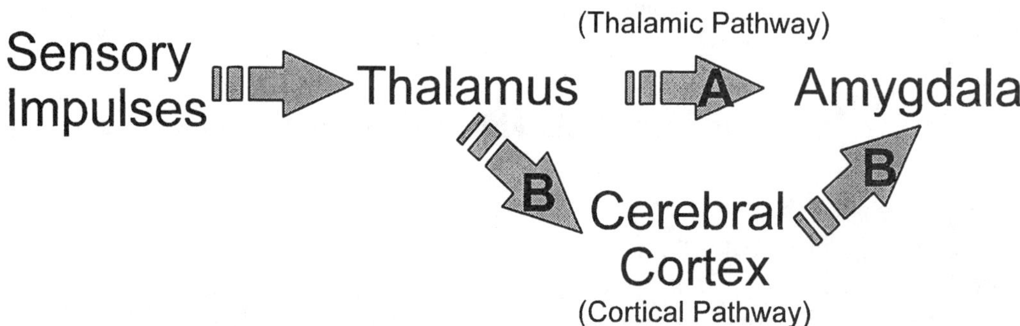

Figure 9.2 *Sensory information travels to the thalamus where it can be routed directly to the amygdala (thalamic pathway, A) or first to the cerebrum and then to the amygdala (cortical pathway, B). (See also Figure 1.2)*

In Chapter 1, we learned that the thalamus receives all incoming sensory impulses (except smell) and directs them to other parts of the brain for further processing. As a result of his research, LeDoux is convinced that incoming sensory information to the thalamus can take two different routes to the amygdala. The quick route (called the thalamic pathway) sends the signals directly from the thalamus to the amygdala (pathway A in Figure 9.2). The second possibility (called the cortical pathway) is for the thalamus to direct the signals first to the cerebral cortex (in the cerebrum) for cognitive processing and then to the amygdala (pathway B).

The time it takes for signals to travel along the two pathways is different. For example, it takes sound signals about 12 milliseconds (a millisecond is 1/1,000th of a second) to travel pathway A and about twice as long to travel pathway B. Which pathway the signals take could mean the difference between life and death. If the sound from a car blasting its horn travels along pathway A, it will probably be fast enough to get you to jump out of the way even though you are not sure what is coming. Only later does your cerebral cortex provide the explanation of what happened. Survival is the first priority, an explanation second.

Disturbances in this dual pathway system can explain some abnormal behaviors. Anxiety disorders, for example, can result whenever a certain action, such as walking into a crowd, is associated with fear. If this activity always takes pathway A, then a phobia develops that cannot be easily moderated through rational discussion. This probably explains why psychotherapy alone is rarely successful in treating phobias and anxiety disorders (Restak, 2000).

Different Brain Areas for Different Emotions

Although the amygdala is the center of emotional response, neuroscientists now believe that different areas of the brain interpret specific emotions. The frontal cortex of the left hemisphere deals with positive emotions; the right frontal cortex is concerned with negative emotions. Damage to the front of the left hemisphere results in feelings of hopelessness and bouts of depression. However, if the front right side is damaged, the individual often expresses inappropriate cheerfulness, even denying the injury.

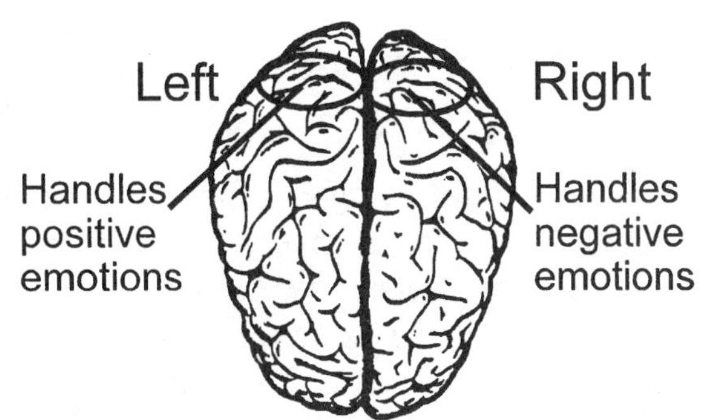

***Figure 9.3** The left hemisphere's frontal cortex is concerned with positive emotions. The right hemisphere's frontal cortex deals with negative emotions and nuance.*

People who normally have right hemisphere preference (Sousa, 2001) tend to have basically anxious and fearful approaches to life. Those with left hemisphere preference exhibit a more confident approach. The preference is probably caused by a number of factors including genetics, experience, and the way an individual's brain is organized.

The Nature of Anxiety. Anxiety serves a useful purpose in that it signals us that something needs to be corrected in our environment. The anxious feelings you got when seeing the letter from a former lover were soon tempered when cognitive reflection reminded you that a wedding was coming soon, and this was most likely an invitation to it. This return to emotional stability is the result of the interactions between the emotion-generating amygdala and the emotion-inhibiting left frontal cortex. Both the amygdala and left frontal cortex need to be functioning properly for this balance to be maintained and, thus, for good mental health. If either one is malfunctioning, then the person's behavior will be abnormal.

First Survival and Emotions, Then the Textbook

The human brain is programmed to deal first with its owner's survival and emotional needs. Therefore, the brain is unlikely to attend to any other task until it is assured that these needs have been met and that the environment poses no threat. If we transfer this notion to schools, it means that students are not going to care about the curriculum unless they feel physically safe and emotionally secure.

> *Students must feel physically safe and emotionally secure before they can focus on the curriculum.*

Physical Safety. For students to feel physically safe, schools must be free of weapons and violence. A student will have trouble concentrating on the lesson if a nearby student displays a weapon or threatens physical harm. Physical safety also refers to the safe condition of the student's body. Has the student had enough sleep and an adequate breakfast? Rest and fuel are important requirements for attention and learning.

Emotional Security. Emotional security refers to the degree to which a student feels accepted as a valued member of a group. In my opinion, the emotional needs of children can be met in just three places:

- in the home (and those entities to which the family belongs, such as religious or community groups)
- in school, through the formal organization of educators and school groups
- outside the school, from an informal organization of peers

Until recently, the emotional needs of children and adolescents were met at home. The family dined together nightly, spending quality time to strengthen emotional bonds through reassurances, caring, and love. In today's fast-paced lifestyle, many families dine together only once or twice a week. Hectic family schedules mean that parents and children have less time together. When the children *are* at home, they spend more time in their own bedrooms—playing computer games and watching television—than with their parents. A recent survey showed that children 10 to 17 years of age spend an average of 13.4 hours a week watching televison and using computers, but only 47 minutes a week of quality time talking with their parents. These children are spending about 17 times more time connecting to their outside world than to their inside world.

> *A recent survey showed that children 10 to 17 years of age spend an average of 13.4 hours a week watching televison and using computers, but only 47 minutes a week of quality time talking with their parents.*

Because the amount of quality time at home is so small, many students are not getting their emotional needs met. They come to school looking for emotional support from the formal organization through teachers and other professionals in the school environment. Finding emotional support in the primary grades is easier because those teachers are trained to provide it. But it is an entirely different matter in secondary schools. High school teachers are trained to deliver curriculum efficiently and effectively. Few have had training in how to deal with the emotional needs of students, and even fewer ever believed that such training would be necessary. However, more high school teachers are now recognizing that they must meet the emotional needs of their students before they can be successful at presenting the curriculum.

If the students' emotional needs are not met in the home or in school, then some students resort to the third alternative—joining an informal organization of peers, usually called a gang. These are family-like units that have a name, a set of values, and a system of rewards and punishments. Regrettably, their behavior is too often directed toward deviant, rather than socially acceptable, goals.

Emotional and Behavioral Disorders

Because emotions and behavior affect each other and are so closely intertwined, disorders of these areas are usually discussed together. Although a few of these disorders can appear in early adulthood or later, many appear in childhood and adolescence. Some are more common than others, and conditions can range from mild to severe. Often, a person has more than one disorder.

The causes of all the types of disorders can be biological, environmental, or a mixture of both. Biological factors include genetics, chemical imbalances in the body, and damage to the central nervous system, such as a head injury. Environmental causes can include exposure to violence, extreme stress, or the loss of an important person, such as by death or divorce.

A discussion of all the major types of emotional and behavioral disorders that afflict humans is beyond the scope of this book. Rather, the following represents those emotional and behavioral disorders that are most common among children and adolescents and that educators are likely to encounter in almost any school.

Anxiety Disorders

Most people experience feelings of anxiety before an important event, such as a business presentation, big test, or first date. But people with anxiety disorders have anxiety and fears that are chronic and unrelenting, and that can grow progressively worse. Sometimes, their anxieties are so bad that people become housebound.

Anxiety Disorders

- Phobias
- Generalized anxiety disorder
- Panic disorder
- Obsessive-compulsive disorder
- Post-traumatic stress disorder

Anxiety disorders are the most common of childhood disorders, affecting an estimated 8 percent of the child and adolescent population. These young people experience excessive worry, fear, or uneasiness that interferes with daily routines. Anxiety disorders include the following:

- **Phobias** – Two major types are social phobia and specific phobia. Children with social phobia have an overwhelming fear of scrutiny, embarrassment, or humiliation when with their peers. Specific phobia is an unrealistic and overwhelming fear of some situation or object that leads to avoiding the situation or object.
- **Generalized anxiety disorder** – A pattern of unrealistic and excessive worry not attributable to any recent experience, but disruptive to routine life and events. Those with the disorder almost always anticipate the worst even though there is little reason to expect it. It usually strikes in childhood or adolescence.
- **Panic disorder** – Repeated episodes of terrifying attacks of panic that strike without warning. They include physical symptoms such as rapid heartbeat, chest pain, abdominal distress, and dizziness.
- **Obsessive-compulsive disorder** – A pattern of repeated thoughts and behaviors (e.g., hand washing or counting) that are impossible to control or stop. Although rare in young children, the occurrence of the disorder increases slightly in adolescents.
- **Post-traumatic stress disorder** – A pattern of flashbacks and other symptoms that occurs in children who have experienced a psychologically distressing event (e.g., physical and sexual abuse, being a witness or victim of violence, or exposure to some other traumatic event, such as a hurricane or bombing). Nightmares, numbing of emotions, and feeling angry or irritable are common symptoms.

What Causes Anxiety Disorders? Normal emotional behavior relies on the integrating balance between the emotions initiated by the amygdala and the mediating effect of our thoughts. If either one of these components malfunctions, problems arise. Brain imaging has helped neuroscientists gain a greater understanding of the source of these problems and, thus, the causes of anxiety disorders. For example, if a malfunction causes nonthreatening sensory signals to always take the thalamic pathway (Figure 9.2), panic attacks result because the signals are not benefitting from the mediating effect of cognitive thought. Here is an example: To most of us, the sound of a car backfiring is annoying but we usually would not mistake it for a gunshot. However, to an adolescent brought up in a neighborhood where gunfire has killed a friend or family member, that backfiring could activate a full-fledged stress response. This post-traumatic stress response might send the adolescent diving for cover and in full panic. Apparently, the sounds of the backfiring went directly to the amygdala (thalamic pathway), triggering the panic behavior. No input from the cerebral cortex was present to curtail the post-traumatic response.

For many years, psychiatrists thought that obsessive-compulsive disorder had psychological roots and attempted to treat it with psychoanalysis. Recent brain scans, however, suggest that obsessive-compulsive behavior is the result of hyperactivity in a circuit of the brain that connects the frontal lobe to a part of the limbic area called the caudate nucleus. Activity in this circuit decreases between obsessive-compulsive episodes and after treatment. The disorder responds to a combination of drugs that increases the action of the neurotransmitter serotonin, followed by psychotherapy that addresses the specific nature of the behavior. It is common for anxiety disorder to accompany depression, eating disorders, substance abuse, or another anxiety disorder. These conditions can also coexist with physical disorders.

Depressive Disorders

Children and adolescents with learning disabilities are susceptible to chronic depression. Although much of the scientific research on depression has focused on adults, recent studies have revealed that an unexpectedly large number of today's youth suffer from some type of depressive disorder. A study by the National Institute of Mental Health estimates that about 6 percent of 9- to 17-year-olds have major depression. In addition, the study indicated that the onset of depressive disorders is occurring earlier in life today than ever before (NIMH, 2000). The depressive disorders, including major depressive disorder (unipolar depression) and bipolar disorder (manic-depression), can have far-reaching effects on the functioning and adjustment of young people. Children and adolescents with depressive disorders are at an increased risk for illness and interpersonal and social difficulties. These adolescents also have an increased risk for substance abuse and suicidal behavior.

Unfortunately, depressive disorders in adolescents often go unrecognized because their signs are interpreted as normal mood swings typical of this age group. For example, instead of communicating how bad they feel, they may act out and be irritable toward others, which may be interpreted simply as misbehavior or disobedience. Research has

Depressive Disorders

Depression: Symptoms common to all ages

- Persistent sad or irritable mood
- Loss of interest in activities once enjoyed
- Significant change in appetite or body weight
- Difficulty sleeping or sleeping too much
- Psychomotor agitation or retardation
- Loss of energy
- Feelings of worthlessness or inappropriate guilt
- Difficulty concentrating
- Recurrent thoughts of death or suicide

Bipolar Disorder: Symptoms for pre-teens and older

- Severe changes in mood
- Overly-inflated self-esteem
- Increased energy
- Able to go without much sleep
- Talks too fast and too much, cannot be interrupted
- Excessive involvement in risk behaviors

found that parents are even less likely to identify major depression in their adolescents than are the adolescents themselves.

Symptoms. The symptoms of major depressive disorders are common to children, adolescents, and adults. Five or more of these symptoms must persist for an extended period of time before a diagnosis of depression is indicated. Because of the difficulty in diagnosing younger people using just the common symptoms, clinicians often look for other signs that are usually associated with the disorder.

Bipolar disorder, or manic-depression, in children and adolescents is marked by exaggerated mood swings between extreme lows (depression) and highs (excitedness or manic behavior). Periods of quiet may occur in between. The mood swings may recur throughout life.

Causes of Depressive Disorders. Below-normal concentrations of one or more neurotransmitters were often cited as the underlying cause of depression. Support for this notion came from the apparent relief that drugs targeting neurotransmitters gave to depressed patients. Drugs that increased the levels of neurotransmitters (e.g., dopamine, norepinephrine, and serotonin) exerted an antidepressant effect; drugs that depleted their levels made the depression worse.

Neuroscientists today realize that depression is far more complicated than previously thought. It seems that depression can result from the imbalance of any one of many neurotransmitters. Another contributing factor seems to be a problem that causes neurons in the limbic area to overproduce a hormone called corticotropin releasing factor, or CRF. Several studies of patients with chronic depression showed they had about twice the normal level of CRF in their bodies. Apparently, elevated CRF makes one vulnerable to depressive disorders. This finding is leading to the development of drugs that inhibit CRF production in the hope that reducing CRF will reduce the incidence of chronic depression (Restak, 2000).

Depressive Disorders

Signs associated with depressive disorders in children and adolescents

- Frequent, nonspecific complaints of headaches, tiredness, and stomach and muscle aches
- Frequent absences from school or poor performance in school
- Talking about running away from home
- Outbursts of crying, shouting, and complaining
- Being bored
- Lack of interest in playing with friends
- Alcohol or substance abuse
- Social isolation, poor communication
- Fear of death
- Extreme sensitivity to rejection or failure
- Increased hostility and irritability
- Reckless behavior
- Difficulty with relationships

Treatment. Treatment for depressive disorders in children and adolescents often involves short-term psychotherapy, medication, or the combination of both plus targeted interventions involving the home and school environment. Recent research shows that certain types of short-term psychotherapy, particularly cognitive-behavioral therapy (CBT), can help relieve depression in children and adolescents. CBT is based on the premise that people with depression have cognitive distortions in their views of themselves, the world, and the future. CBT, designed to be a time-limited therapy, focuses on changing these distortions. A study supported by the National Institutes of Mental Health that compared different types of psychotherapy for major depression in adolescents found that CBT led to remission in nearly 65 percent of cases, a higher rate than either supportive therapy or family therapy. CBT also resulted in a more rapid treatment response time (NIMH, 2000).

Research clearly demonstrates that antidepressant medications, especially when combined with psychotherapy, can be very effective treatments for depressive disorders in adults. Using medication to treat mental illness in children and adolescents, nevertheless, has caused controversy. Many doctors have been understandably reluctant to treat young people with psychotropic medications because, until fairly recently, little evidence was available about the safety and efficacy of these drugs in youth. In the last few years, however, researchers have been able to conduct studies with children and adolescents showing that the newer antidepressant medications, specifically the selective serotonin reuptake inhibitors (SSRIs), are safe and effective for the short-term treatment of severe and persistent depression in young people.

Treatment of children and adolescents diagnosed with bipolar disorder has been based mainly on experience with adults because so far there is limited data on the safety and effectiveness of mood stabilizing medications in youth. Researchers currently are evaluating both pharmacological and social interventions for bipolar disorder in young people.

Other Emotional and Behavioral Disorders

A number of other emotional and behavioral disorders are found in the school population, such as the following:

Attention-Deficit Hyperactivity Disorder (ADHD). This disorder has received much attention from the media and from researchers. ADHD is discussed more fully in Chapter 3.

Oppositional-Defiant Disorder. All children are occasionally oppositional by arguing, talking back, or defying their parents, teachers and other adults. However, persistent and openly hostile behavior that interferes with a child's daily functioning is called Oppositional-Defiant Disorder. It is characterized by deliberate attempts to annoy others, excessive arguing with adults, frequent temper tantrums, and refusal to comply with adult requests. The cause is unknown, but treatment centers around psychotherapy. If the child does not respond to treatment, the behavior may worsen and become a general conduct disorder.

Conduct Disorder. This disorder usually begins with the appearance of hostile and defiant behavior during the preschool years, known as oppositional-defiant disorder. As the child gets older, conduct disorder may appear which causes children and adolescents to act out their feelings or impulses toward others in destructive ways. Young people with conduct disorder consistently violate the general rules of society and basic rights of others. The offenses they commit get more serious over time and include lying, aggression, theft, truancy, setting fires, and vandalism. However, most young people with conduct disorder do not have lifelong patterns of conduct problems or antisocial behavior.

Conduct Disorder

Symptoms
- Shows aggressive behavior that harms or threatens to harm other people or animals
- Damages or destroys property
- Lying or theft
- Truancy or other violation of rules

Conduct Disorder is one of the most difficult behavior disorders to treat. Even so, progress can be made with family therapy, parent training, and the use of community support services. A recent study of children and adolescents with conduct disorder showed that their aggressive behavior also responded to treatment with lithium carbonate. Further studies are planned because although lithium may be safe for short-term treatment, there is concern over its adverse side effects if used for extended periods (Malone, Delaney, Luebbert, Cater, and Campbell, 2000).

Eating Disorders. Anorexia nervosa (the compulsive need to continually lose weight) and bulimia nervosa (the compulsion to eat large amounts of food and to take subsequent radical measures to eliminate it) can be life threatening disorders. No generally accepted view of the causes of these disorders exists at present, although most experts believe the problem to be psychologically based.

Adolescents displaying the symptoms of these disorders need immediate medical attention. Various forms of treatment are available, such as psychotherapy (individual, group, or family), counseling, self-help groups, and medication.

Autism. Autism is a spectrum disorder that usually appears before the child's third birthday. Children with autism have difficulty communicating with others and display inappropriate and repeated behaviors over long periods of time. Autism is discussed more fully in Chapter 10.

Impact on Learning

- All students need to be in schools where the learning environment is physically safe and emotionally secure before they can focus on the curriculum.
- With appropriately trained teachers, students with emotional and behavioral problems sometimes can have their needs met in the context of what they are learning in the classroom.
- Teachers can take *ad hoc* opportunities in class to teach students how to handle their emotions, to delay gratification, to control impulses, and to conduct themselves in personal relationships.
- Any positive emotional experience—such as praise and other positive reinforcement techniques—will enhance learning.

Strategies to Consider

Establishing a Positive Emotional Climate in the Classroom

All students—especially those with emotional and behavioral disorders—need to be in an emotionally secure setting before they can be expected to give attention to curriculum. The classroom climate is set by the teachers and the school climate is set by the administration. Teachers and administrators need to recognize that many more students than ever come to school wanting to get at least some of their emotional needs met. Working together, faculty and staff should take **purposeful** steps to ensure that a positive emotional climate is established and maintained in the school and in all classrooms. Some ways to set a positive emotional climate are as follows:

- ❑ **Use humor, but not sarcasm.** Humor is a very effective device for getting attention and for establishing a warm climate. Laughter is common to us all and it helps diverse people bond and feel good about being with each other. Sarcasm, on the other hand, is destructive. It hurts, no matter how familiar a teacher is with students. Occasionally, a teacher has said, "Oh, he knows I was only kidding." In fact, we don't know that, and we need to wonder whether the student's sly grin means the brain is laughing or plotting revenge. Besides, there is so much good humor available that there should be no need for sarcasm.

- ❑ **Insist on respect among students.** Not only is it important for teachers to respect students, and vice versa, but teachers must also ensure that students show respect for each other. This includes
  - listening to each other's class contributions (as opposed to just waiting for their turn to speak),
  - respecting different and opposing opinions,
  - acknowledging other students' comments,
  - complimenting and helping each other when appropriate,
  - asking others for their opinions, and
  - refraining from sarcasm.

Establishing a Positive Emotional Climate—Continued

- ❑ **Have just a few rules that all teachers enforce.** Students with emotional problems are likely to get upset when they believe that they are not being treated fairly. Studies on school discipline show that schools with few discipline problems tend to be those with just a few rules (five to seven) that all teachers enforce uniformly. Keep in mind that secondary students usually see six to eight teachers during the school day. Perhaps one teacher allows gum chewing, but it drives the next period's teacher to distraction. An absent-minded, gum-chewing student going from the first to the second teacher's class may be headed for trouble.

- ❑ **Get training in how to handle emotional situations.** Most secondary teachers were not trained to deal with the emotional scenarios that appear in today's classrooms, mainly because emotional needs of adolescents are expected to be addressed in the family. But the reality is that more students are turning to the school setting for emotional fulfillment, and teachers must be trained to cope effectively with this situation.

- ❑ **Look for opportunities to teach students how to handle their emotions.** With training, teachers can use classroom and school opportunities to teach students how to handle their emotions. Look for ways to help them delay gratification, control impulses, express their feelings, and conduct themselves in their in-school relationships.

- ❑ **Use genuine praise.** Students with emotional problems often have low self-esteem. Genuinely praising their efforts can go a long way in helping them improve their self-image. Use "you" statements rather than "I" statements. For example, "You should be proud of the work you accomplished" is more effective for building self-esteem than, "I am pleased with what you accomplished."

Strategies to Consider

Interventions for Students With Behavioral Problems

Research on programs designed to help students with behavioral problems covers a wide variety of students, situations, and settings. As a result, there is a broad range of possible approaches that teachers and schools can take to make a difference in students' behavior. Here are some suggestions from that research.

- **Identifying the cause of the misbehavior.** Problem behavior is obvious, but the reasons for it might not be. Schools need to investigate **why** the student is exhibiting undesirable behavior. As more is known about the cause, appropriate interventions can be identified and implemented.

- **Selecting classroom management and teaching strategies.** Walker, Colvin, and Ramsey (1995) note that blaming, punishing, and threatening students works only in the short term. They found that effective teachers rely instead, on proactive strategies, such as reinforcing social behavior and teaching social problem solving. For difficult students, they use point or token systems, time-out, contingent reinforcement, and response cost.

- **Adapting curriculum and instruction.** Disruptive behavior is sometimes the result of inappropriate curriculum and ineffective teaching. When investigating the cause of student misbehavior, check whether curricular and instruction modifications have been made to accommodate these students (Deschenes, Ebeling, and Sprague, 1994).

- **Teaching social problem solving.** Effective programs for preventing discipline problems include the direct teaching of social problem solving. Although the interventions vary, they usually teach thinking skills that students can use to avoid and resolve interpersonal conflicts, resist peer pressure, and cope with their emotions and stress. The most effective programs also include a broad range of social competency skills taught over a long period of time.

Interventions for Students With Behavior Problems—Continued

- **Schoolwide and districtwide programs.** School and district policies should make clear that appropriate behavior is a precondition to learning. Rules of behavior should be clear and communicated to staff, parents, and students. It is important that they be consistently enforced so students perceive the system as fair. The staff should also be trained to teach alternatives to vandalism and disruptive behavior.

- **Parental involvement.** Effective programs to control behavior almost always have a parental component. Kazdin (1994) found that parental management training and family therapy are two promising approaches for controlling student behavior. Parental management training teaches techniques such as strategic use of time-out, rewards, praise, and contingency contracting. Parents have ongoing opportunities to discuss, practice, and review these techniques. Family therapy is designed to empower parents with the skills and resources to solve their own family problems. Although parental management training and family therapy are very effective approaches, less intensive parental training should suffice for most children and adolescents.

- **Some cautions.** A study by Gottfredson (1997) examined various approaches to dealing with disruptive students. She found that some programs are not effective in controlling disruptive and antisocial behavior in the long run. These ineffective programs included individual counseling, peer counseling and peer-led information groups, and programs designed to arouse students' fears and appeal to their sense of right and wrong. Schools considering these types of programs may wish to rethink their decision or do further investigation before investing their resources.

Strategies to Consider

Reducing the Risk of Antisocial Behavior

Behavior is the result of the interaction of environmental influences and genetic predispositions. Schools can do nothing to alter the genetic coding. But recent research seems to indicate that genes affecting personality traits are either activated or repressed by the individual's environment. Consequently, if schools undertake comprehensive efforts to provide supportive structures and reduce risk factors, then fewer children may fall victim to emotional and behavioral problems that can seriously interfere with their schooling and life. These efforts that will encourage prevention of problem behaviors fall into the broad areas of school organization and effectiveness, student achievement and early intervention, parent and community involvement, and professional development for staff (Appalachia Educational Laboratory, 1996).

School Organization and Effectiveness

The school should

- Have high expectations for learning and behavior for all students and help all children achieve them
- Clearly communicate expectations for learning and behavior to all students
- Include staff, students, parents, and community members in the decision-making process
- Promote student engagement and attachment
- Have a consistent system of reinforcement and recognition to shape student behavior
- Provide alternatives to suspension and expulsion
- Conduct risk assessment as part of safe schools improvement plans

Student Achievement and Early Intervention

The school should

- Intervene early to identify and assist students who fail to meet expectations for learning and behavior
- Evaluate students' social, emotional, and adaptive functions, as well as cognitive function
- Include special education students in regular classrooms
- Not disproportionately discipline students with disabilities

Reducing the Risk of Antisocial Behavior—Continued

Parent and Community Involvement	The school should ▸ Work with parents and community groups to educate and care for children ▸ Involve parents and community groups in developing the safe schools improvement plan ▸ Provide information to parents about how to help their children learn and behave appropriately in school ▸ Collaborate with other agencies to meet family and community needs
Professional Development for Staff	The school should ▸ Train teachers to use a variety of instructional and classroom management strategies to prevent academic failure and problem behavior for all students ▸ Encourage preservice programs in teacher-training institutions to provide this training ▸ Encourage state departments of education to include this training in their inservice programs

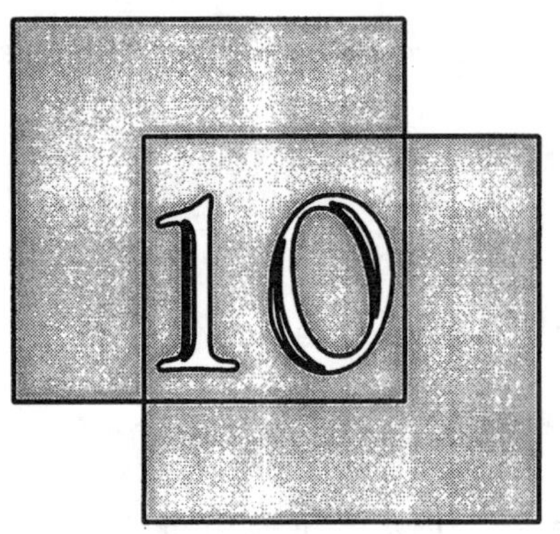

AUTISM

In previous chapters we have discovered how the brain acquires language, learns to read and write, calculates, and generates the emotions to interact and communicate with other human beings. Different neural networks must work in harmony to carry out these activities successfully. When several networks malfunction early in a child's life, developmental disorders appear. Describing and categorizing these disorders are not easy. Nonetheless, the Diagnostic and Statistical Manual of Mental Disorders (DSM-IV) calls this category Pervasive Developmental Disorder, which includes five disorders: Autistic Disorder, Asperger's Disorder, Rett's Disorder, Childhood Disintegrative Disorder, and Pervasive Developmental Disorder Not Otherwise Specified.

In Autistic Disorder (or autism), neurological problems develop that make it difficult for a person to communicate and form relationships with others. It is a spectrum disorder that runs the gamut from mild to severe. Some people with autism are relatively high functioning (called high-functioning autism), while others are mentally retarded or have serious language delays.

Autism affects one person in 500, and four out of five of those affected are males. The prevalence of autism has probably been underestimated in the past.

Autism affects about one person in 500, and four out of five of those affected are males. Although it may appear that the incidence of autism is increasing in American children, the medical community believes it is more likely that the prevalence of autism has been underestimated in the past.

The symptoms of autism usually appear before the age of three. Children with autism do not interact and may avoid eye contact. They may resist attention and affection, and they rarely seem upset when a parent leaves or show pleasure when the parent returns. Understanding the cues of others—such as a smile, wink, or grimace—is difficult for them as well. Some children with autism also tend to be physically aggressive at times, particularly when they are in a strange or overwhelming environment. At times they will break things, attack others, or harm themselves.

Areas Affected by Autism

Autism can cause language difficulties, repetitive and obsessive behaviors, sensory overload, and problems with memory and recall (NIMH, 1997).

Language difficulties. About one-half of the children diagnosed with autism remain mute throughout their lives. Others will only parrot what they hear (a condition known as *echolalia*). Those who do speak tend to confuse pronouns like "I," "my," and "you," and may use the same phrase, such as "milk and cookies," in many different situations.

It is very difficult to understand the body language of people with autism. Most of us smile when we talk or shrug our shoulders when we cannot answer a question. But the facial expressions and movements of children with autism rarely match what they are saying. In addition, their tone of voice does not usually reflect their feelings. Without meaningful gestures or the language to ask for things, these children are at a loss to communicate their needs. Consequently, they may simply scream or grab what they want.

Repetitive and obsessive behaviors. Most children with autism appear physically normal and have good muscle control. But some exhibit repetitive actions, such as flicking their fingers, rocking back and forth, or running from room to room tuning lights on and off. Others demand consistency in their environment and develop fixations with certain objects, such as eating the same foods at the same time and sitting in the same place every day. Does this repetitive-obsessive behavior have the same underlying neurological cause as obsessive-compulsive disorder? It is possible but not likely. Researchers seem to favor the explanation that the demand for consistency is an attempt to bring stability in a world of sensory confusion and to block out painful stimuli.

> *Children with autism demand consistency in order to bring stability to a world of sensory confusion.*

Sensory symptoms. Many children with autism are highly attuned to the input from their senses but have difficulty sorting the input into a coherent whole. As a result, their sensory world can be confusing and lead to overwhelming sensitivity. For example, the feel of their clothes can be very disturbing. Some children will cover their ears and shout at a ringing telephone or vacuum cleaner. For some, the senses are scrambled in that they experience certain sounds as color, make audible sounds when someone touches their skin, or gag when feeling a texture.

Memory and recall. A few studies have looked at how well children with autism learn information, encode it accurately, and retrieve it correctly. This ability is known as "recall readiness." The results showed that most children with autism had greater difficulty in recall readiness compared to those without autism (Farrant, Blades, and Boucher, 1999). The study did not include any of the rare population of "savants" who can remember enormous amounts of information.

Diagnosis

To date, there are no medical tests that reliably detect autism. No two children display the disorder in exactly the same way. Further, some children can exhibit autistic-like symptoms that may indicate other disorders and not autism. These possibilities also need to be investigated.

Specialists use a variety of methods to identify the disorder. They evaluate language and social behavior, talk with parents about the child's developmental milestones, and may test for certain genetic and neurological problems. They may consider other conditions that exhibit the same behaviors and similar symptoms to autism, such as Rett's Disorder or Asperger's syndrome. Rett's Disorder is a progressive brain disease that affects only girls and can lead to loss of language and social skills. Asperger's syndrome is explained later in this chapter.

The diagnosis of autism will be made only if there is clear evidence of

- poor or limited social relationships
- underdeveloped communication skills
- repetitive behaviors, interests, and activities.

The diagnostic criteria also require that these symptoms appear by the age of 3 years. Children with fewer or milder symptoms are often diagnosed as having Pervasive Developmental Disorder.

What Causes Autism?

No one knows for sure, but it is not the result of poor parenting. Researchers in the past 15 years have made great strides in understanding the impaired abilities of people with autism and have used this understanding to develop theories about its cause. One of the prevailing theories is that people with autism fail to construe the mental states of others—a deficit in what has been called the "theory of mind." This theory refers to the everyday ability to infer what others are thinking or believing in order to explain and predict their behavior. That is, children with autism have difficulty viewing situations from another person's perspective. This may explain why they have such difficulty with simple behaviors such as attending to a situation and playing games with others.

Another notion is that autism is caused by deficits in the frontal lobe's ability to carry out its executive functions, such as controlling behavior, especially in new circumstances. The deficit reflects frontal lobe abnormalities and may explain the repetitive and obsessive behavior in autism (Russell, 1998).

> **Theory of Mind**
>
> In one of the first studies to focus on this notion, researchers quizzed children on the following scenario: Sally puts a marble into a covered basket and leaves the room. While Sally is out, her friend Anne moves the marble from the basket to a nearby covered box. When asked where Sally would later look for the marble, children without autism said she would look in the basket because that is where she *thinks* it is. By contrast, the children with autism (including some quite bright adolescents) said that Sally will look in the box, where the ball really is. This failure to interpret Sally's belief has been taken as evidence of impaired theory of mind in autism (Baron-Cohen, Tager-Flusberg, and Cohen, 1993).

More recent studies of brain structures in people with autism have led neuroscientists to look for a biological basis. Reviewing first the inheritance factor, examinations of siblings of people with autism have shown a 3 to 8 percent chance of the sibling being diagnosed with the same disorder. Although this is greater than the 0.2 percent chance (1 in 500) in the general population, it is far less than the 50 percent chance that would indicate a single dominant gene or the 25 percent chance of a single recessive gene. When an identical twin has autism, the chances of the other twin (who has the identical genes) being diagnosed with the disorder is only 60 percent. These data favor the conclusion that autism is the result of the variance of several genes contributing to the outcome, and that this situation may be modified by environmental factors. The search for the cause of autism is complicated because researchers do not know how the various factors combine to make some people display the disorder while others escape it (Rodier, 2000).

Although deficits in language, planning, and social cues are associated with the frontal lobe, other symptoms, such as lack of facial expression, hypersensitivity to sound and touch, and sleep disturbances, are more closely associated with the cerebellum and the brain stem (see Chapter 1). One consistent finding is that people with autism tend to have a proportionally smaller cerebellum than normal. A recent study found that certain parts of the brain stem were also smaller or missing in a brain with autism, a condition that probably originated between the 20th and 24th day after conception as a result of coding by a variant gene known as HOXA1. Researchers have identified at least three genes that could be responsible for autism and they are searching for more.

It is possible, so the theory goes, that the causes of this baffling disorder may lie in changes in the brain stem during early embryonic developments as a result of malfunctioning genes (Rodier, 2000). The theory is further supported by a study showing that blood samples taken at birth from children who eventually developed autism had high levels of four proteins involved in

Vaccines and Autism

Newspapers and television have reported an alleged connection between the MMR (measles/mumps/rubella) vaccination and autism. The report was based on a study of 12 patients in England that suggested the MMR vaccine may have caused bowel problems leading to decreased absorption of essential nutrients, triggering autistic behavior.

The results of that study have not been supported by subsequent tests. Further, the current theories of the causes of autism rule out vaccinations as a potential cause. More information is available at the Center for Disease Control and Prevention website: www.cdc.gov.

brain development. The finding suggests that some abnormal processes were already underway at birth (NAAR, 2000).

Tracking down all of the genes associated with autism will not be easy, and it is possible that the genetic variants will not explain all the causes of the disorder. The genetic component may just represent a predisposition to the disorder that is triggered by some other nongenetic factor. But every risk factor that is identified takes away some of the mystery and, in time, may help alleviate the suffering caused by this disorder.

Treatment. At present, there is no cure for autism, nor do children outgrow it. Nonetheless, more than ever before, people with autism can be helped. A combination of early intervention, special education support, and medication is helping children and adolescents with autism lead more normal lives. Medications can alleviate some of the symptoms and therapy can help a child to learn, communicate, and interact with others in productive ways.

Unusual Abilities

About 10 percent of people with autism display remarkable abilities and skills. At a time when other children are drawing lines or scribbling, some children with autism can draw detailed, realistic pictures with proper dimensional perspective. Some begin to read before they speak or play musical instruments without being taught. Others can memorize enormous amounts of information, such as pages from a phone book, many years of sport scores, or entire television shows. Such abilities are known as *savant skills*, and the extreme forms are rare.

About 10 percent of people with autism display remarkable abilities and skills.

Researchers have been trying to explain why certain people with autism possess savant skills. The current theory is that one characteristic of autism may provide both advantages and disadvantages. This characteristic is called *central convergence* and refers to the ability of the brain to process incoming information in its context, that is, to put parts together into a meaningful whole. Because this ability is weak in people with autism, it may explain why they focus on details and parts at the expense of global meaning. It may also explain why they have difficulties in social situations and why their piecemeal processing of faces could hamper their recognition of emotions in others (Happé, 1997).

The notion that children with autism show weak central convergence has been supported by a growing number of studies. For example, several studies have shown that children with autism are less likely to be tricked by optical illusions and are better at finding objects imbedded in pictures than children without autism. This superior ability may be due to disembedding skills in which they can perceive parts of the object independent of the surrounding context (Figure 10.1).

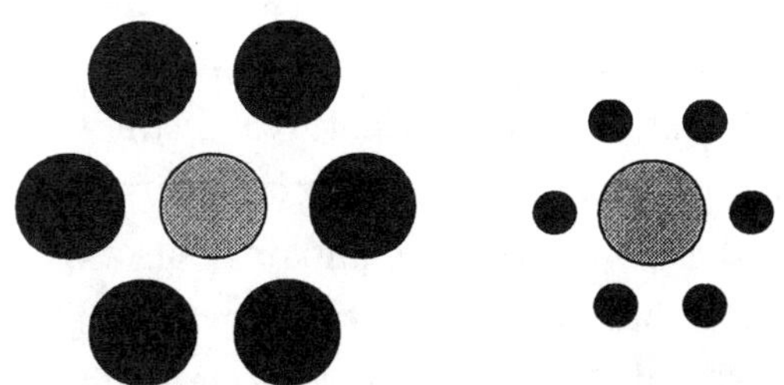

Figure 10.1 *The presence of the outside circles causes most people to believe that the inner circle on the right is larger than the inner circle on the left (The inner circles are the same size). People with autism perceive these figures in a less unified way and are less likely to succumb to the illusion.*

People with autism do appear to integrate the properties of a single object (e.g., its color and shape), and to process the meaning of individual words. The difficulty seems to be in connecting the objects and words to form larger contexts and a convergent whole.

Central convergence, then, may explain some of the assets, as well as deficits, of people with autism. Studies show that children with autism are better at learning the names of musical notes and at retaining absolute pitch later. They also do better at drawings that have details and lines of perspective. Both of these findings can be explained by a mental bias toward processing and remembering detail. A question currently under investigation is whether central convergence is an aspect of autism that is transmitted genetically (Happé, 1997).

Asperger's Syndrome

Identified in 1944 by Austrian physician Hans Asperger, this syndrome is a developmental disorder with many of the same symptoms of autism. It is usually referred to as a mild form of autism because people with Asperger's syndrome generally have higher mental functioning than those with typical autism. Like autism, Asperger's syndrome is a lifelong condition. However, the DSM-IV classifies Asperger's as a separate disorder and controversy exists as to whether Asperger's is a distinct syndrome or a form of autism. Some professionals believe that the definition of autism should include Asperger's because no biological tests have been yet identified for either disorder.

How do Asperger's and autism differ? Although many of the symptoms of the two disorders are similar, there are important differences. Because of these differences, some argue that Asperger's should carry a distinct diagnosis, which paves the way for more appropriate education and treatment. Both Asperger's and autism are classified as Pervasive Developmental Disorders, which means impairments exist in social interaction, communication, and the range of interests and activities. Differences in the two conditions are found primarily in the *degree* of impairment. For example, although an individual with autism may experience a delay in speech, an individual with Asperger's does not possess a clinically significant delay in language. However, an individual with Asperger's may have difficulty understanding abstract forms of spoken language, such as humor or irony (APA, 2000).

Cognitive ability is another distinction between the two disorders made in the DSM-IV. Persons with autism experience mental retardation, but the criteria for Asperger's state that the individual cannot possess a clinically significant cognitive delay. Of course, some people with autism do not have mental retardation, but a person with Asperger's must possess an average to above average intelligence (APA, 2000).

Professionals working with these disorders add that, compared to people with autism, those with Asperger's syndrome have a need for high stimulation, have an overdeveloped use of imagination, tend to be more social, have fewer language deficits, and are more willful in their behavior. As a result of these differences, young children with Asperger's syndrome often go undiagnosed through their early elementary years because their strengths mask their deficits.

What Is the Future of Research on Autism?

Research continues to look for genetic variants associated with autism in the hope that this may provide a more accurate diagnostic tool for the future, at least in terms of estimating the chances that the children of siblings of a person with autism may inherit the disorder. Attention is also being directed to the role that neurotransmitters, especially serotonin, play in negating the disruptive behavior associated with the disorder. The effectiveness of selective serotonin reuptake inhibitors (SSRIs) in improving some of the behaviors in autism may also lead to new insights into biochemical mechanisms (Piven, 1997).

A Word About Secretin

In 1997, television and newspaper stories publicized the claims of several families that injections of the human hormone secretin had caused noticeable improvement in the behavior of their children who had been diagnosed with autism. To date, research has not been able to affirm that secretin has any therapeutic benefit for the treatment of autism, although the clinical trials continue. One major study found no benefit from a single secretin injection (Sandler, Sutton, DeWeese, Girardi, Sheppard, and Bodfish, 1999).

> *Brain imaging is revealing variations in the brains of children with autism that may lead to the discovery of underlying physiological mechanisms of the disorder.*

Although preliminary results are inconclusive, toxic substances ingested by the mother during pregnancy as well as drugs used to induce labor continue to be investigated as possible causes of autism. Brain imaging studies are revealing variations in the brains of children with autism that may lead to the discovery of underlying physiological mechanisms of the disorder. Of particular interest is the observation that people with autism often have enlarged brains. Other studies are examining whether the normal process of synaptic pruning and programmed cell death (apoptosis) in early childhood proceeds normally in children with autism. Failure of either of these processes could lead to an enlarged brain. As researchers learn more about the development of the human brain, they will be better able to unlock the genetic, biochemical, psychological, and physiological mysteries of autism.

What Do Educators Need to Consider?

Autism is a neurological disorder that affects children's overall ability to communicate and interact socially. Their behavior may be difficult to control at times. Teachers need to be adequately trained to use interventions that will preserve a positive educational climate in the classroom for these students and their peers.

Adolescents diagnosed with autism have to bear both the burden of coping with the teenage years as well as the recognition that they are different from their peers. They typically lack friends and neither date nor plan for the future. Awareness of this often drives them to learn new and unacceptable behaviors. Success in school for students with autism should be measured not so much by whether they pass algebra, but by whether they acquire the knowledge and skills that will make them more self-sufficient as adults.

Impact on Learning

Much of what we have gleaned about how people with autism learn comes not just from professional observation but also from those with autism who have written about their world (Grandin, 1996). Children diagnosed with autism may display

- Behavioral issues that often detract from learning
- A learning style biased toward piecemeal processing
- A reluctance to communicate making it difficult to assess what they have learned
- A savant skill that can be tapped
- Ability to think more in pictures than in words
- A difficulty with long sentences or strings of verbal information
- Attention to only one sensory channel at a time
- A difficulty with generalizing.

Strategies to Consider

Enhancing Learning in Students With Autism

Children and adolescents diagnosed with autism will have an Individualized Educational Program (IEP) developed for them when enrolled in public schools. The plan serves as an agreement between the school and the family about the student's educational goals.

The items listed here are for consideration by any educator responsible for helping these students successfully cope with their situation and become self-sufficient adults (Quill, 1995).

- **Different learning style.** Students with autism learn differently in that they have difficulty understanding the perceptions of others, experience sensory overload, and use intellect instead of emotion to guide their social interactions.

- **Need for structure.** These students need structure. Their activities should
  - organize their materials,
  - give clear instructions,
  - provide stability,
  - establish patterns,
  - provide consistency and predictability, and
  - increase independence.

- **Social interaction.** These students need to learn ways to interact socially with their peers and adults. When teaching them about social interaction, use
  - a predictable sequence of interactions (no surprises),
  - a planned set of conversational scripts,
  - lots of repetition,
  - messages linked to what the student is doing,
  - speech and visual cues simultaneously, and
  - messages mixed with ongoing activities.

Strategies to Consider

Helping Students With Asperger's Syndrome

Children and adolescents diagnosed with Asperger's syndrome usually have average or above average cognitive abilities. They tend to have excellent rote memory skills and often exhibit a precocious vocabulary. However, they have problems with abstract thinking. They frequently do not understand the logic of classroom instruction and discussion and are easily distracted. Educational structure and classroom management strategies become important. Here are a few points to consider that could help students diagnosed with Asperger's syndrome to succeed in the classroom.

✓ **Educational Structure and Classroom Management.**

- Provide a predictable environment and routine and prepare students for any upcoming changes
- Ensure that each student is seated in a position of least distraction and close to the teacher or other source of information to which the student must respond
- Be consistent and do not ask for an option if there is none
- Do not do for the students what they can do for themselves
- Give clear, precise, concrete instructions, and don't assume that mere repetition means that the student has understood
- Find ways to tie new situations to old ones that students have experienced
- State expectations clearly and allow each student time to process the information
- Concentrate on changing unacceptable behaviors and do not worry about those which are simply odd
- Break tasks up into manageable segments and plan a completion schedule with the student
- Do not rely on emotional appeals by assuming students want to please you

Helping Students With Asperger's Syndrome—Continued

✓ **Instructional Approaches.**

- Support verbal information with visual aids
- Model the action you want students to use, and maintain the behavior with visual cues
- Use cooperative learning groups, but teach appropriate social responses to use in this activity
- Minimize assigned written work because these students do not understand the logic of repeating activities
- Assign enrichment activities related to the students' interests, as they will be more satisfied and productive gathering facts about a subject they like
- Avoid abstract language (e.g., metaphors and irony), and fully explain any constructions that you do use

✓ **Support and Discipline Strategies.**

- Have a strategy ready in case the students cannot cope due to overstimulation or confusion
- Have a time-out area for discipline when needed, and make sure the time-out is not more appealing than the curricular activity
- Explicitly teach the rules of social conduct
- Inform parents on a regular basis of the students' successes and failures and ask for parental advice when appropriate
- Give students some space and avoid cornering or trapping them
- Use an unemotional tone of voice when telling them what they need to do, and give sincere praise when they do it correctly
- Try not to confuse lack of tact with rudeness
- Protect them from teasing and bullying
- Teach them how to meet someone, how to recognize when someone will not talk to them, and how to tell when someone is teasing them

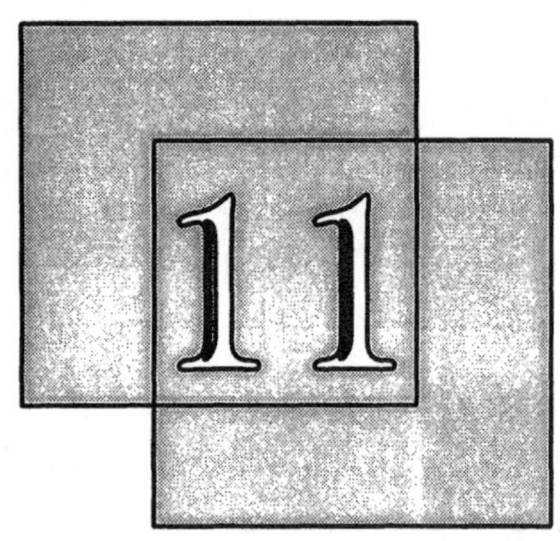

PUTTING IT ALL TOGETHER

The preceding chapters have described some of the recent research on the human brain that may shed light on problems affecting learning. Some of the problems may result from genetic mutations, fetal brain injury during gestation, or environmental impact. Whatever the cause, teachers represent the essential link between the students with learning problems and the strategies and services selected to help them.

> *Students with learning problems **can** learn when teachers find the appropriate ways to teach these students.*

It is important to remember that students with learning problems *can* learn when teachers spend the time and use their expertise to find the appropriate ways to teach these students. To that end, here are some suggestions to consider that can be adapted to most grade levels.

1. **Learn about learning.** Educators in all areas need to update their knowledge base about what neuroscience is revealing about how the brain learns. These discoveries and insights can help explain problems and improve classroom skills. Teachers should draw on the knowledge of special educators and researchers to address specific problems.

2. **Look for the warning signs.** Very often, the regular classroom teacher is the first to recognize a potential learning problem. Although many students encounter learning problems at one time or another, these problems are usually temporary and quickly overcome. For others, the problems persist

and result in a lag in academic achievement compared to their learning potential. These students need help.

3. **Assess the situation.** The question now is whether the learning problem can be addressed in the regular classroom. Asking students to take an inventory similar to the one below will help you and them learn from their perceptions of how well they perform certain tasks. Working with a student on the comments section can provide useful insights on instructional approaches to consider.

Assessment Inventory			
Area	**Strengths**	**Challenges**	**Comments**
Attention			
Speaking			
Reading			
Writing			
Calculating			
Memory			

4. **Look for abilities, not just disabilities.** Sometimes we get so concerned about the students' problems that we miss the opportunity to capitalize on their strengths. Many studies indicate that using an individual's strengths to mitigate areas of weakness often results in improved performance and a well-needed boost to that person's self-esteem.

5. **Design a learning profile for each student with learning problems.** For students with learning problems, keep a simple record of their
   - reasoning ability,
   - learning style,
   - classroom participation,
   - comprehension,
   - work level, and
   - progress.

   Design the profile to spot trends in each area. Use this information to build on students' existing strengths and identify areas needing improvement.

6. **Use technology.** Computers and other forms of advanced technology are useful tools for helping students with learning problems. Word processing programs with voice recognition are just one example of hardware and software components that can capitalize on students strengths and minimize their weaknesses.

7. **Modify the learning environment.** Just a few changes in the learning environment can sometimes make a significant difference in student achievement. Consider which students might benefit if you
   - Seat student in an areas free of distractions.
   - Consider using study carrels.
   - Keep the student's work area free of unnecessary materials.
   - Use a checklist to help get the student organized.
   - Stand near the student when giving directions.
   - Provide organizational strategies such as charts and timelines.
   - Assist in organizing the student's notebook.
   - Use materials that address the students' learning styles.
   - Provide opportunities for movement.

8. **Modify instructional strategies.** Consider modifying instructional strategies to meet the various learning styles and abilities of students with learning problems. Here are some strategies to consider:
   - Allow students to audiotape lectures.
   - Break assignment into shorter tasks.
   - Adjust the reading level of the classroom material.
   - Teach the concrete before the abstract.
   - Relate the new learning to students' experiences.
   - Reduce the number of concepts presented at one time.
   - Give an overview of the lesson before beginning.
   - Check the student's comprehension of the language used for instruction.
   - Monitor the rate at which you present material.
   - Require verbal responses from the student to check for comprehension.
   - Provide clear and concise directions for homework assignments.
   - Allow typewritten or word processed assignments.
   - Consider the oral administration of tests and open book tests.
   - Provide practice test questions for study.

- Allow use of dictionary or calculator during test.
- Provide extra time to finish a written test.

9. **Modify the curriculum materials.** Modifications to curriculum materials will vary depending on the nature of the student's learning problem. For those with **spoken language** difficulties, you can
   - Paraphrase complex information.
   - Slow the rate of presentation.
   - Provide written directions to supplement verbal directions.
   - Keep sentence structures simple.
   - Avoid the use of abstract language such as puns, idioms, and metaphors.
   - Get the student's attention before expressing key points.
   - Use visual aids such as charts and graphs.
   - Call student by name before asking questions.

   For those with **written language** difficulties,
   - Allow student to use cursive or manuscript writing.
   - Permit student to type, record, or give oral answers instead of writing.
   - Provide copies of class notes.
   - Avoid the pressure of speed and accuracy.
   - Reduce the amount of copying from the textbook or board.
   - Establish realistic standards for neatness.
   - Accept key word responses instead of complete sentences.

   For those with **organizational problems**,
   - Establish clear rules and consistently enforce them.
   - Provide an established daily routine.
   - Consider making contracts with students and use rewards when the contract is completed.
   - Ensure that due dates are clearly understood.
   - Provide a specific place for turning in assignments.

10. **Get the reluctant starter going.** Some students have difficulty getting started and need the teacher's guidance to move forward. For them,
    - Give a personal cue to begin work.
    - Check progress often, especially after the first few minutes of work.

- Provide immediate feedback and reinforcers.
- Divide work into smaller units.
- Suggest time periods for each task.
- Ensure that the student understands the instructions.
- Present the assignment in sequential steps.
- Provide a checklist for multitask assignments.

11. **Maintain attention.** Because some students with learning problems can be easily distracted, look for ways to maintain attention during the lesson.
    - Seat the students close to you.
    - Provide praise for correct answers.
    - Relate new learning to students' experiences.
    - Give an advance warning when a transition is going to occur.
    - Use physical proximity and appropriate touch to help student refocus.

12. **Use group instruction and peers.** Although some students with learning problems do not always work well in groups, persistence and guidance can often result in a productive experience.
    - Assign a peer tutor to record material dictated by the student.
    - Use cooperative learning strategies when appropriate.
    - Assign a peer helper to read important directions and information to the student and to check for understanding.

13. **Adjust time demands.** Meeting timelines and deadlines is not always easy for some students with learning problems. Some get involved in minute details, while others dart from one idea to another and lose track of time.
    - Increase time allowed for the completion of tests or assignments.
    - Reduce the amount of work or length of tests.
    - Introduce short breaks or change of tasks.
    - Follow a specific routine and be consistent.
    - Alternate active and quiet tasks.
    - Help students prioritize the steps needed to complete an assignment.
    - Set time limits for completing specific tasks.

14. **Deal with inappropriate behavior.** Inappropriate behavior is not acceptable. But keep in mind that the misbehavior may not have been intentional.
    - Provide clear and concise classroom expectations and consequences

- Enforce rules consistently.
- Avoid confrontational techniques; they often escalate the situation.
- Provide the student with alternatives.
- Avoid power struggles.
- Designate a cooling-off location in the classroom.
- Ignore attention-getting behavior for a short time (extinction).
- Assign activities which require some movement.
- Deal with the behavior and avoid criticizing the student.
- Speak privately to the student about inappropriate behavior.
- Check for levels of tolerance and be aware of signs of frustration.

15. **Modify homework assignments.** Homework can be a valuable learning tool for students with learning problems if it is relevant and not excessive.
    - Consider allowing student to work on homework in school.
    - Give frequent reminders about due dates.
    - Give short assignments.
    - Allow for extra credit assignments.
    - Develop an award system for in-school work and homework completed.

16. **Communicate with parents.** Frequent communication with parents is important so that you are all working together to assist the student in meeting expectations.
    - Develop a daily and weekly journal and share it with the parents.
    - Schedule periodic parent-teacher meetings.
    - Provide parents and students with a duplicate set of textbooks that they can use at home during the school year.
    - Provide weekly progress reports to parents.
    - Mail the parents a schedule of class and homework assignments.

Not all of these recommendations apply to every student, and individual strategies should be developed to address the needs of individual students with learning problems. Implementing accommodations such as those listed here can improve the academic achievement of students with learning disabilities. In mainstreamed classrooms, take care to balance these accommodations so as not to appear unfair to the students who are not in need of these strategies.

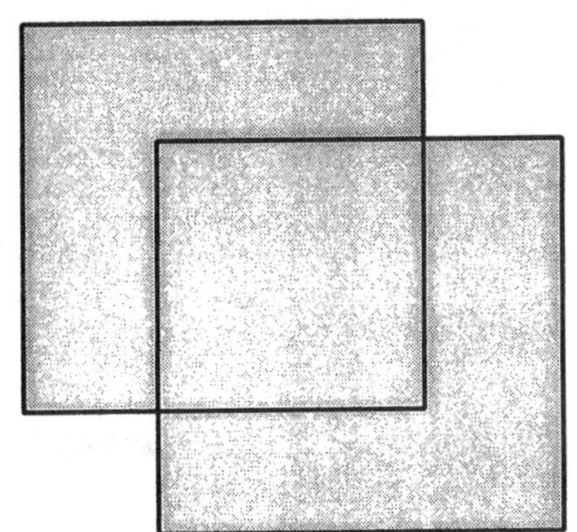

GLOSSARY

Alphabetic principle. The notion that written words are composed of letters of the alphabet that intentionally and systematically represent segments of spoken words.

Amygdala. The almond-shaped structure in the brain's limbic system that encodes emotional messages to long-term storage.

Aphasia. The loss of language function.

Apoptosis. The genetically programmed process in which unneeded or unhealthy brain cells are destroyed.

Attention deficit hyperactivity disorder (ADHD). A syndrome that interferes with an individual's capacity to regulate activity level, inhibit behavior, and attend to tasks in developmentally appropriate ways.

Autism. A spectrum disorder that affects an individual's ability to communicate, form relationships with others, and relate appropriately to the environment.

Brain stem. One of the major parts of the brain, it receives sensory input and monitors vital functions such as heartbeat, body temperature, and digestion.

Broca's area. A region in the left frontal lobe of the brain believed responsible for generating the vocabulary and syntax of an individual's native language.

Cerebellum. One of the major parts of the brain, it coordinates muscle movement.

Cerebrum. The largest of the major parts of the brain, it controls sensory interpretation, thinking, and memory.

Circadian rhythm. The daily cycle of numerous body functions, such as breathing and body temperature.

Computerized tomography (CT, formerly CAT) scanner. An instrument that uses X-rays and computer processing to produce a detailed cross-section of brain structure.

Corpus callosum. The bridge of nerve fibers that connects the left and right cerebral hemispheres and allows communication between them.

Cortex. The thin but tough layer of cells covering the cerebrum that contains all the neurons used for cognitive and motor processing.

Delayed sleep phase disorder. A chronic condition caused mainly by a shift in an adolescent's sleep cycle that results in difficulty falling asleep at night and waking up in the morning.

Dendrite. The branched extension from the cell body of a neuron that receives impulses from nearby neurons through synaptic contacts.

Dopamine. A neurotransmitter believed to control mood, behavior, and muscle coordination.

Dyscalculia. A condition that causes persistent problems with processing numerical calculations.

Dysgraphia. A spectrum disorder characterized by difficulty in mastering the sequence of movements necessary to write letters and numbers.

Dyslexia. A learning disorder characterized by problems in expressing or receiving oral or written language.

Frontal lobe. The front part of the brain that monitors higher-order thinking, directs problem solving, and regulates the excesses of the emotional (limbic) system.

Functional magnetic resonance imaging (fMRI). An instrument that measures blood flow to the brain to record areas of high and low neuronal activity.

Glial cells. Special "glue" cells in the brain that surround each neuron providing support, protection, and nourishment.

Gray matter. The thin but tough covering of the brain's cerebrum also known as the cerebral cortex.

Hippocampus. A brain structure that compares new learning to past learning and encodes information from working memory to long-term storage.

Limbic system. The structures at the base of the cerebrum that control emotions.

Magnetic resonance imaging (MRI). An instrument that uses radio waves to disturb the alignment of the body's atoms in a magnetic field to produce computer-processed, high-contrast images of internal structures.

Melatonin. A hormone that helps regulate the body's sleep-wake cycle.

Mnemonic. A word or phrase used as a device for remembering unrelated information, patterns, or rules.

Motor cortex. The narrow band across the top of the brain from ear to ear that controls movement.

Myelin. A fatty substance that surrounds and insulates a neuron's axon.

Neuron. The basic cell making up the brain and nervous system, consisting of a globular cell body, a long fiber called an axon which transmits impulses, and many shorter fibers called dendrites which receive them.

Neurotransmitter. One of nearly 100 chemicals stored in axon sacs that transmit impulses from neuron to neuron across the synaptic gap.

Orthography. The written system for a language.

Phonemes. The minimal units of sound in a language that combine to make syllables.

Phonemic awareness. The ability to deal explicitly and segmentally with sound units smaller than the syllable (i.e., the phoneme).

Phonological alexia. The inability to retain words in memory long enough to establish meaning.

Phonological awareness. The ability to recognize the production and interpretation of the sound patterns (rather than the meaning) of language.

Positron emission tomography (PET) scanner. An instrument that traces the metabolism of radioactively tagged sugar in brain tissue producing a color image of cell activity.

Prosody. The rhythm, cadence, accent patterns, and pitch of a language.

Rehearsal. The reprocessing of information in working memory.

Retention. The preservation of a learning in long-term storage in such a way that it can be identified and recalled quickly and accurately.

Reticular activating system (RAS). The dense formation of neurons in the brain stem that controls major body functions and maintains the brain's alertness.

Suprachiasmatic nucleus. A pair of small clusters of neurons within the immediate vicinity of the optic nerve that regulate the body's circadian sleep-wake cycle.

Synapse. The microscopic gap between the axon of one neuron and the dendrite of another.

Thalamus. A part of the limbic system that receives all incoming sensory information, except smell, and shunts it to other areas of the cortex for additional processing.

Transfer. The influence that past learning has on new learning, and the degree to which the new learning will be useful in the learner's future.

Visual magnocellular-deficit. A disorder of the visual processing system that leads to poor detection of visual motion, causing letters to bunch up or overlap during reading.

Wernicke's area. A section in the left temporal lobe of the brain believed responsible for generating sense and meaning in an individual's native language.

White matter. The support tissue that lies beneath the cerebrum's gray matter (cortex).

Windows of opportunity. Important periods in which the young brain responds to certain types of input to create or consolidate neural networks.

Working memory. The temporary memory wherein information is processed consciously.

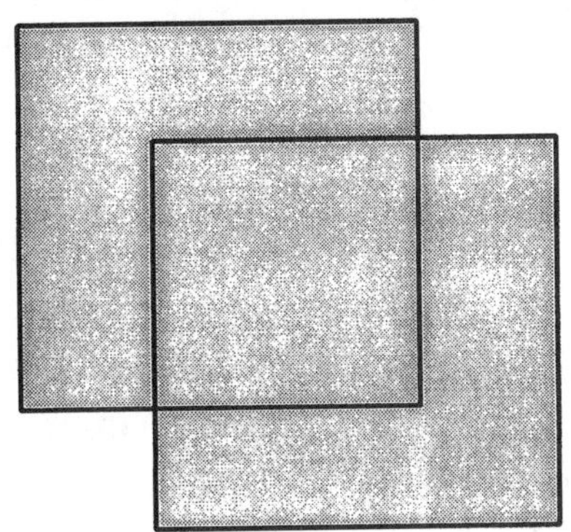

REFERENCES

American Psychiatric Association (APA). (2000). *Diagnostic and Statistical Manual of Mental Disorders*, Fourth Edition, Text Revision (DSM-IV). Washington, DC: American Psychiatric Publishing Group.

Appalachia Educational Laboratory. (1996). *Preventing antisocial behavior in disabled and at-risk students*. Charleston, WV: Author.

Barkley, R.A. (1998, September). Attention-deficit hyperactivity disorder. *Scientific American,* 66-71.

Barkley, R.A. (1998). *Attention-deficit hyperactivity disorder: A handbook for diagnosis and treatment*. New York: Guilford Press.

Baron-Cohen, S., Tager-Flusberg, H, and Cohen, D. J. (Eds.). (1993). *Understanding other minds: Perspectives from autism.* New York: Oxford University Press.

Baroody, A. J. (1999). The development of basic counting, number, and arithmetic knowledge among children classified as mentally handicapped. In L. M. Glidden (Ed.), *International review of research in mental retardation* (Vol. 22, pp. 51-103). New York: Academic Press.

Baum, S. (1994). Meeting the needs of gifted/learning disabled students. *The Journal of Secondary Gifted Education, 5*, 6-16.

Baynes, K., Eliassen, J. C., Lutsep, H. L., and Gazzaniga, M. S. (1998, May 8). Modular organization of cognitive systems masked by interhemispheric integration. *Science, 280*, 902-905.

Beatty, J. (2001). *The human brain: Essentials of behavioral neuroscience*. Thousand Oaks, CA: Sage Publications.

Borkowski, J. G., Estrada, M., Milstead, M., and Hale, C. (1989). General problem-solving skills: Relations between metacognition and strategic processing. *Learning Disabilities Quarterly, 12*, 57-70.

Brody, L. E., and Mills, C. J. (1997, May/June). Gifted children with learning disabilities: A review of the issues. *Journal of Learning Disabilities, 30*, 282-286.

Buckner, R. L., Kelley, W. M., & Petersen, S. E. (1999, April). Frontal cortex contributions to human memory formation. *Nature Neuroscience, 2*, 311–314.

Byrne, B. (1991). Experimental analysis of the child's discovery of the alphabetic principle. In L. Riehen and C. Perfetti (Eds.), *Learning to read: Basic research and its implications* (pp. 75-84). Hillsdale, NJ: Erlbaum.

Chard, D.J., and Dickson, S.V. (1999, May). Phonological awareness: Instructional and assessment guidelines. *Intervention in School and Clinic, 34*, 261-270.

Chard, D.J., and Osborn, J. (1998). *Suggestions for examining phonics and decoding instruction in supplementary reading programs*. Austin, TX: Texas Education Agency.

Cheour, M., Ceponiene, R., Lehtokoski, A., Luuk, A., Allik, J., Alho, K., and Näätänen, R. (1998, September). Development of language-specific phoneme representations in the infant brain. *Nature Neuroscience, 1*, 351-353.

Clements, D. H. (2000, Summer). Translating lessons from research into mathematics classrooms: Mathematics and special needs students. *International Dyslexia Association: Perspectives, 26*, 31-33.

Cole, P.G., and Mengler, E.D. (1994). Phonemic processing of children with language deficits: Which tasks best discriminate children with learning disabilities from average readers? *Reading Psychology, 15*, 223-243.

Coles, G. (2000). *Misreading reading: The bad science that hurts children*. Portsmouth, NH: Heinemann.

Dale, P. S., Simonoff, E., Bishop, D.V.M., Eley, T. C., Oliver, B., Price, T. S., Purcell, S., Stevenson, J., and Plomin, R. (1998, August). Genetic influence on language delay in two-year-old children. *Nature Neuroscience, 1*, 324–328.

DeGrandpre, R.J. and Hinshaw, S.P. (2000, Summer). ADHD: Serious psychiatric problem or all-American copout? *Cerebrum: The Dana Forum on Brain Science*, 12-38.

Deschenes, C., Ebeling, D. G., and Sprague, J. (1994). *Adapting curriculum and instruction in inclusive classrooms: A teacher's desk reference*. Bloomington, IN: Institute for the Study of Developmental Disabilities.

Deshler, D.D., Ellis, E.S., and Lenz, B.K. (1996). *Teaching adolescents with learning disabilities: Strategies and methods*. Denver, CO: Love Publishing.

Deshler, D.D., Shumaker, J.B., Alley, G.R., Clark, F.L., and Warner, M.M. (1981). Paraphrasing strategy. University of Kansas, Institute for Research in Learning Disabilities. Washington, DC: Bureau of Education for the Handicapped.

Deuel, R. K. (1994). Developmental dysgraphia and motor skill disorders. *Journal of Child Neurology, 10*, 6-8.

Diamond, M., and Hopson, J. (1998). *Magic trees of the mind: How to nurture your child's intelligence, creativity, and healthy emotions from birth through adolescence.* New York: Dutton.

Dinklage, K. T. (1971). Inability to learn a foreign language. In G. Blaine, and C. MacArthur (Eds.), *Emotional problems of the student.* New York: Appleton-Century-Crofts.

Edelen-Smith, P.J. (1998). How now brown cow: Phoneme awareness activities for collaborative classrooms. *Intervention in School and Clinic, 33*, 103-111.

Elkonin, D.B. (1973). In J. Downing (Ed.), *Comparative reading: Cross-national studies of behavior and processes in reading and writing* (pp. 551-559). New York: Macmillan.

Ellis, E.S., Deshler, D.D., Lenz, B.K., Schumaker, J.B., and Clark, F.L. (1991). An instructional model for teaching learning strategies. *Focus on Exceptional Children, 23*, 1-24.

Fagerheim, T., Raeymaekers, P., Tønnessen, F.E., Pedersen, M., Tranebjaerg, L., and Lubs, H.A. (1999, September). A new gene (DYX3) for dyslexia is located on chromosome 2. *Journal of Medical Genetics, 36*, 664-669.

Farrant, A., Blades, M., and Boucher, J. (1999, October). Recall readiness in children with autism. *Journal of Autism Developmental Disorders, 29,* 359-366.

Fellows, M., Koblitz, A. H., and Koblitz, N. (1994). Cultural aspects of mathematics education reform. *Notices of the American Mathematical Society, 41*, 5-9.

Foorman, B.R., Francis, D.J., Fletcher, J.M., Schatschneider, C., and Mehta, P. (1998). The role of instruction in learning to read: Preventing reading failure in at-risk children. *Journal of Educational Psychology, 90*, 1-15.

Fowler, M. (1994, October). Attention-deficit/hyperactivity disorder. *National Information Center for Children and Youth with Disabilities Briefing Paper*, 1-16.

Fulk, B. (2000, January). Twenty ways to make instruction more memorable. *Intervention in School and Clinic, 35*, 183-184.

Ganschow, L., and Sparks, R. (1995). Effects of direct instruction in Spanish phonology on native language skills and foreign language aptitude of at-risk foreign language learners. *Journal of Learning Disabilities, 28*, 107-120.

Geary, D. C. (2000, Summer). Mathematical disorders: An overview for educators. *International Dyslexia Association: Perspectives, 26*, 6-9.

Gersten, R., and Baker, S. (1999). *Teaching expressive writing to students with learning disabilities: A meta-analysis.* Eugene, OR: University of Oregon.

Gersten, R., Baker, S., and Edwards, L. (1999, December). Teaching expressive writing to students with learning disabilities. *ERIC/OSEP Digest, E590.*

Goswami, U. (1994). Phonological skills, analogies, and reading development. *Reading Behaviour*, 32-37.

Gottfredson, D. (1997). School-based crime prevention. In L. W. Sherman et al. (Eds.), *Preventing crime: What works, what doesn't, what's promising: A report to the United States Congress*. Washington, DC: U.S. Department of Justice, Office of Justice Programs.

Graham, S. (1990). The role of production factors in learning disabled students' compositions. *Journal of Educational Psychology, 80*, 356-361.

Grandin, T. (1996). *Thinking in pictures: And other reports from my life with autism.* New York: Vintage Books.

Happé, F. G. E. (1997). Central coherence and the theory of mind in autism: Reading homographs in context. *British Journal of Developmental Psychology, 15*, 1-12.

Idol, L. (1987). Group story mapping: A comprehension strategy for both skilled and unskilled readers. *Journal of Learning Disabilities,20*, 196-205.

Johnson, D.W., and Johnson, R.T. (1989). Cooperative learning: What special educators need to know. *The Pointer, 33*, 5-10.

Johnson, S. (1999, May). *Strangers in our homes: TV and our children's minds*. Paper presented at the Waldorf School, San Francisco.

Jones, S. (2000). Accommodations and modifications for students with handwriting problems and/or dysgraphia. *LDOnline* [Online]. Available at http://www.ldonline.org/ld_indepth/writing/dysgraphia.

Kazdin, A. (1994). Interventions for aggressive and antisocial children. In L. D. Eron, J. H. Gentry, and P. Schlegel (Eds.), *Reason to hope: A psychosocial perspective on violence and youth* (pp. 341-382). Washington, DC: American Psychological Association.

Klingner, J.K., Vaughn, S., and Schumm, J.S. (1998). Collaborative strategic reading during social studies in heterogeneous fourth grade classrooms. *Elementary School Journal, 99*, 3-22.

Learning Disabilities Association of America (LDA). (2000). Speech and language milestones chart. *LDOnline* [Online]. Available at http://www.ldonline.org/ld_indepth/speech-language/lda_milestones.html.

LeDoux, J. (1996). *The emotional brain: The mysterious underpinnings of emotional life*. New York: Simon and Schuster.

Lenhoff, H. M., Wang, P. P., Greenberg, F., and Bellugi, U. (1997, December). Williams syndrome and the brain. *Scientific American, 280*, 68-73.

Lenz, B. K., Ellis, E. S., and Scanlon, D. (1996). *Teaching learning strategies to adolescents and adults with learning disabilities*. Austin, TX: PRO-ED.

Leonard, L. B. (1998). *Children with specific language impairment*. Cambridge, MA: MIT Press.

Malone, R. P., Delaney, M. A., Luebbert, J. F., Cater, J., and Campbell, M. (2000, July). A double-blind placebo-controlled study of lithium in hospitalized aggressive children and adolescents with conduct disorder. *Archives of General Psychiatry, 7*, 649-654.

Marolda, M. R., and Davidson, P. S. (1994). Assessing mathematical abilities and learning approaches, in *Windows of opportunity*. Reston, VA: National Council of Teachers of Mathematics.

Mazzocco, M. M. (1998, August). A process approach to describing mathematical difficulties in girls with Turner syndrome. *Pediatrics, 102*, 492-496.

McCarthy, R. A., and Warrington, E. K. (1990). *Cognitive neuropsychology: A clinical introduction*. San Diego: Academic Press.

Merzenich, M.M., Jenkins, W.M., Johnston, P., Schreiner, C., Miller, S.L., and Tallal, P. (1996, January 5). Temporal processing deficits of language-learning impaired children ameliorated by training. *Science, 271*, 77-81.

Moats, L.C. (2000, October). *Whole language lives on: The illusion of "balanced" reading instruction*. Washington, DC: Thomas B. Fordham Foundation.

Montgomery, J. W. (2000, April). Verbal working memory and sentence comprehension in children with specific language impairment. *Journal of Speech, Language, and Hearing Research, 43*, 293-308.

National Alliance for Autism Research (NAAR) (2000, Summer). Autism in the blood: Can proteins in a newborn's blood predict autism, or lead us to new therapeutic opportunities? *Naarative, 6*, 1, 18-23.

National Center for Education Statistics. (1996). Pursuing excellence: Initial findings from the Third International Mathematics and Science Study, NCES 97-198. Washington, DC: Author.

National Information Center for Children and Youth with Disabilities (NICHCY). (1997, August). Interventions for students with learning disabilities. *NICHCY News Digest, 25*, 2-12.

National Institute of Mental Health (NIMH). (1995). *Learning disabilities*. Bethesda, MD: Author.

National Institute of Mental Health (NIMH). (1997). *Autism*. Bethesda, MD: Author.

National Institute of Mental Health (NIMH). (2000, August). *Depression in children and adolescents: A fact sheet for physicians.* Bethesda, MD: Author.

National Institute of Neurological Disorders and Stroke (NINDS). (2000, June). *Brain basics: Understanding sleep.* Bethesda, MD: Author.

National Institute on Deafness and Other Communication Disorders (NIDCD). (2000, April). *Speech and language: Developmental milestones.* Bethesda, MD: Author.

National Sleep Foundation (NSF). (2000). *Adolescent sleep needs and patterns.* Washington, DC: Author.

Patterson, K., and Lambon Ralph, M.A. (1999). Selective disorders of reading? *Current Opinion in Neurobiology, 9*, 235-239.

Piven, J. (1997). The biological basis of autism. *Current Opinion in Neurobiology, 7*, 708-712.

Posner, M.I., and Raichle, M.E. (1994). *Images of mind.* New York: Scientific American Library.

Pressley, M., Symons, S., Snyder, B. L., and Cariglia-Bull, T. (1989). Strategy instruction research comes of age. *Learning Disabilities Quarterly, 12*, 16-30.

Quill, K. (1995). *Teaching children with autism: Strategies to enhance communication and socialization.* Albany, NY: Delmar Publishing.

Raborn, D. T. (1995, Summer). Mathematics for students with learning disabilities from language-minority backgrounds: Recommendations for teaching. *New York State Association for Bilingual Education Journal, 10*, 25-33.

Restak, R. (2000). *Mysteries of the mind.* Washington, DC: National Geographic Society.

Richards, R. G. (1998). *The writing dilemma: Understanding dysgraphia.* Riverside, CA: RET Center Press.

Rief, S.F. (1998). *The ADD/ADHD Checklist: An Easy Reference for Parents and Teachers.* New York: Prentice Hall.

Rodier, P. (2000, February). The early origins of autism. *Scientific American, 282*, 56-63.

Rueckert, L., Lange, N., Partiot, A., Appollonio, I., Litvan, I., LeBihan, D., and Grafman, J. (1996, April). Visualizing cortical activation during mental calculation with functional MRI. *Neuroimage, 3*, 97-103.

Rumsey, J.M., Horwitz, B., Donohue, B.C., Nace, K.L., Maisog, J.M., and Andreason, P. (1999, November). A functional lesion in developmental dyslexia: Left angular gyral blood flow predicts severity. *Brain and Language, 70*, 187-204.

Russell, J. (Ed.). (1998). *Autism as an executive disorder.* New York: Oxford University Press.

Sandler, A. D., Sutton, K. A., DeWeese, J., Girardi, M. A., Sheppard, V., and Bodfish, J. W. (1999, December). Lack of benefit of a single dose of synthetic human secretin in the treatment of autism and pervasive developmental disorder. *New England Journal of Medicine, 341*, 1801-1806.

Schacter, D. (1996). *Searching for memory: The brain, mind, and the past*. New York: Basic Books.

Shankweiler, D., Crain, S., Katz, L., Fowler, A.E., Liberman, A.E., Brady, S.A., Thornton, R., Lunquist, E., Dreyer, L., Fletcher, J.M., Steubing, K.K., Shaywitz, S.E., and Shaywitz, B.A. (1995). Cognitive profiles of reading-disabled children: Comparison of language skills in phonology, morphology, and syntax. *Psychological Science, 6*, 149-156.

Shannon, T.R., and Polloway, E.A. (1993). Promoting error monitoring in middle school students with LD. *Intervention in School and Clinic, 28*, 160-164.

Sharma, M. (1989). *How children learn mathematics: Professor Mahesh Sharma, in an interview with Bill Domoney*. London: Oxford Polytechnic, School of Education, Education Methods Unit. Videocassette.

Shaywitz, S.E. (1996, November). Dyslexia. *Scientific American*, 98-104.

Shaywitz, S.E., Shaywitz, B.A., Pugh, K.R., Fulbright, R.K., Constable, R.T., Mencl, W.E., Shankweiler, D.P., Liberman, A.M., Skudlarski, P., Fletcher, J.M., Katz, L., Marchione, K.E., Lacadie, C., Gatenby, C., and Gore, J.C. (1998, March 3). Functional disruption in the organization of the brain for reading in dyslexia. *Neurobiology, 5*, 2636–2641.

Snow, C. E., Burns, M. S., and Griffin, P. (Eds.). (1998). *Preventing reading difficulties in young children*. Washington, DC: National Academy Press.

Sousa, D. A. (2001). *How the Brain Learns*, (2nd ed.). Thousand Oaks, CA: Corwin Press.

Sousa, D. A. (1997). Sensory preferences of New Jersey students, grades 3 to 12. Unpublished data collected by graduate students at Seton Hall University, 1994-1997.

Sowell, E. R., Thompson, P. M., Holmes, C. J., Jernigan, T. L., and Toga, A. W. (1999). In-vivo evidence for post-adolescent brain maturation in frontal and striatal regions. *Nature: Neuroscience, 2*, 859–861.

Sparks, R., and Ganschow, L. (1993). Searching for the cognitive locus of foreign language learning difficulties: Linking first and second language learning. *Modern Language Journal, 77*, 289-302.

Stein, J., Richardson, A., and Fowler, M. (2000). Monocular occlusion can improve binocular control and reading in dyslexics. *Brain, 123*, 164-170.

Stein, J., Talcott, J., and Walsh, V. (2000). Controversy about the visual magnocellular deficit in developmental dyslexics. *Trends in Cognitive Sciences, 4*, 209-211.

Stein, M., Dixon, R. C., and Isaacson, S. (1994). Effective writing instruction for diverse learners. *School Psychology Review, 23*, 392-405.

Sturomski, N. (1997, July). Teaching students with learning disabilities to use learning strategies. *NICHCY News Digest, 25*, 2-12.

Suresh, P. A., and Sebastian, S. (2000). Developmental Gerstmann's syndrome: A distinct clinical entity of leaning disabilities. *Pediatric Neurology, 22*, 267-278.

Swanson, J., Castellanos, F. X., Murias, M., LaHoste, G., and Kennedy, J. (1998). Cognitive neuroscience of attention deficit hyperactivity disorder and hyperkinetic disorder. *Current Opinion in Neurobiology, 8*, 263-271.

Swanson, L. J. (1995, July). *Learning styles: A review of the literature*. ERIC Document No. ED 387 067.

Tallal, P., Miller, S. L., Bedi, G., Byma, G., Wang, X., Nagarajan, S., Schreiner, C., Jenkins, W. M., and Merzenich, M. M. (1996, January 5). Fast-element enhanced speech improves language comprehension in language-learning impaired children. *Science, 271*, 81-84.

Tomblin, J. B., and Buckwalter, P. (1998). The heritability of poor language achievement among twins. *Journal of Speech, Language, and Hearing Research, 41*, 188-199.

United States Department of Education (USDE). (1998, January 9). *The state of mathematics education: Building a strong foundation for the 21st century*. [Online]. Available at http://www.ed/gov/inits.html#2. Washington, DC: U. S. Government Printing Office.

United States Department of Education (USDE). (1999, August). *Annual report to Congress on the implementation of the Individuals with Disabilities Education Act*. Washington, DC: U.S. Government Printing Office.

United States Department of Education (USDE). (2000). *The condition of education 1999*. Washington, DC: U.S. Government Printing Office.

Van Petten, C., and Bloom, P. (1999, February). Speech boundaries, syntax, and the brain. *Nature Neuroscience, 2*, 103-104.

Viadero, D. (2001, January). Soft science. *Teacher Magazine, 12*.

Wagner, A. D., Schacter, D. L., Rotte, M., Koutstaal, W., Maril, A., Dale, A. M., Rosen, B. R., & Buckner, R. L. (1998, August 21). Building memories: Remembering and forgetting of verbal experiences as predicted by brain activity. *Science, 281*, 1188–1191.

Wahlstrom, K., Wrobel, G., and Kubow, P. (1998). *Minneapolis Public Schools Start Time Study*. Center for Applied Research and Educational Improvement, University of Minnesota.

Walker, H. M., Colvin, G., and Ramsey, E. (1995). *Antisocial behavior in school: Strategies and best practices*. Pacific Grove, CA: Brooks/Cole.

Weismer, S. E., Evans, J., and Hesketh, L. J. (1999, October). An examination of verbal working memory capacity in children with specific language impairment. *Journal of Speech, Language, and Hearing Research, 42*, 1249-1260.

Williams, D., Stott, C. M., Goodyer, I. M., and Sahakian, B. J. (2000, June). Specific language impairment with or without hyperactivity: Neuropsychological evidence for frontostriatal dysfunction. *Developmental Medical Child Neurology, 42*, 368-375.

Wing, A. M. (2000). Mechanisms of motor equivalence in handwriting. *Current Biology, 10*, R245-R248.

Wolfson, A. R., and Carskadon, M. A. (1998). Sleep schedules and daytime functioning in adolescents. *Child Development, 69*, 875-887.

Wong, B. Y. L., and Jones, W. (1982). Increasing metacomprehension in learning disabled and normally achieving students through self-questioning training. *Learning Disability Quarterly, 5*, 409-414.

Wood, D., Rosenburg, M., and Carran, D. (1993). The effects of tape-recorded self-instruction cues on the mathematics performance of students with learning disabilities. *Journal of Learning Disabilities, 26*, 250-258, 269.

Wood, K. D., and Jones, J. (1998, Fall). Flexible grouping and group retellings include struggling learners in classroom communities. *Preventing School Failure, 43*, 37-38.

Wright, B. A., Bowen, R. W., and Zecker, S. G. (2000). Nonlinguistic perceptual deficits associated with reading and language disorders. *Current Opinion in Neurobiology, 10*, 482-486.

Zametkin, A., Mordahl, T. E., Gross, M., King, A. C., Semple, W. E., Rumsey, J., Hamburger, S., and Cohen, R. M. (1990). Cerebral glucose metabolism in adults with hyperactivity of childhood onset. *New England Journal of Medicine, 2*, 1361-1366.

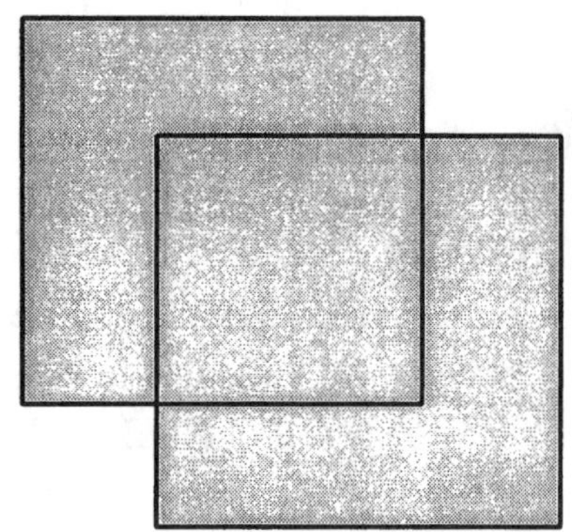

Resources

TEXTS

Cavey, D.W. (2000). *Dysgraphia: Why Johnny can't write.* Austin, TX: Pro-Ed.

Diamond, M., and Hopson, J. (1998). *Magic trees of the mind: How to nurture your child's intelligence, creativity, and healthy emotions from birth through adolescence.* New York: Dutton.

Grandin, T. (1996). *Thinking in pictures: And other reports from my life with autism.* New York: Vintage Books.

Fowler, M. (1999). *Maybe you know my kid: A parent's guide to identifying, understanding, and helping your child with ADHD* (3rd ed.). New York: Birch Lane Press.

Nadeau, K. (1998). *Help4ADD@high school.* New York: Advantage Press.

Quill, K. (1995). *Teaching children with autism: Strategies to enhance communication and socialization.* Albany, NY: Delmar Publishing.

Richards, R. G. (1998). *The writing dilemma: Understanding dysgraphia.* Riverside, CA: RET Center Press.

Rief, S. F. (1998). *The ADD/ADHD Checklist: An Easy Reference for Parents and Teachers.* New York: Prentice Hall.

Silver, L. (1998). *The misunderstood child: Understanding and coping with your child's learning disabilities* (3rd ed.). New York: Time Books.

Sousa, D. A. (2001). *How the brain learns* (2nd ed.). Thousand Oaks, CA: Corwin Press.

ORGANIZATIONS

American Speech-Language Hearing Association (ASHA)
10801 Rockville Pike
Rockville, MD 20852
(800) 638-8255
E-mail: webmaster@asha.org Web: www.asha.org

Asperger Syndrome Coalition of the U.S.
P.O. Box 49267
Jacksonville Beach, FL 32240
E-mail: info@asc-us.org Web: www.asperger.org

Autism Society of America, Inc.
7910 Woodmont Avenue
Suite 650
Bethesda, MD 20814
(800) 3-AUTISM
Web: www.autism-society.org

Children and Adults with Attention Deficit Hyperactivity Disorder (CH.A.D.D.)
8181 Professional Place, Suite 201
Landover, MD 20785
(800) 233-4050
E-mail: national@chadd.org Web: www.chadd.org

Council for Exceptional Children
1920 Association Drive
Reston, VA 20191-1589
(800) 641-7824
Web: www.cec.sped.org

Council for Learning Disabilities (CLD)
P.O. Box 40303
Overland Park, KS 66204
Web: www.cldinternational.org

International Dyslexia Association
Chester Building, Suite 382
8600 LaSalle Road
Baltimore, MD 21286-2044
(800) 222-3123
E-mail: info@interdys.org Web: www.interdys.org

International Reading Association (IRA)
800 Barkdale Road
P.O. Box 8139
Newark, DE 19714-8139
(800) 336-READ
Web: www.reading.org

Learning Disabilities Association of America (LDA)
4156 Liberty Road
Pittsburgh, PA 15234
(888) 300-6710
E-mail: ldanatl@usaor.net Web: www.ldanatl.org

National Alliance for Autism Research
414 Wall Street, Research Park
Princeton, NJ 08540
(888) 777-NAAR
E-mail: naar@naar.org Web: www.naar.org

National Attention Deficit Disorder Association
P.O. Box 1303
Northbrook, IL 60065-1303
E-mail: mail@add.org Web: www.add.org

National Center for Learning Disabilities
381 Park Avenue, Suite 1401
New York, NY 10016
(888) 575-7373
Web: www.ncld.org

National Sleep Foundation
1522 K Street, NW
Suite 500
Washington, DC 20005
Web: www.sleepfoundation.org

National Information Center for Children and Youth with Disabilities (NICHCY)
P.O. Box 1492
Washington, DC 20013-1492
(800) 695-0285
E-mail: nichcy@aed.org   Web: www.nichcy.org

National Institute on Deafness and Other Communication Disorders
31 Center Drive, MSC 2320
Bethesda, MD 20892-2320
(800) 241-1044
Web: www.nidcd.nih.gov

National Institute of Mental Health
6001 Executive Boulevard, Room 8184, MSC 9663
Bethesda, MD 20892-9663
(301) 443-4513
E-mail: nimhinfo@nih.gov   Web: www.nimh.nih.gov

U.S. Department of Education
600 Maryland Avenue SW
Washington, DC 20202
(800) USA-LEARN (872-5327)
Web: www.ed.gov

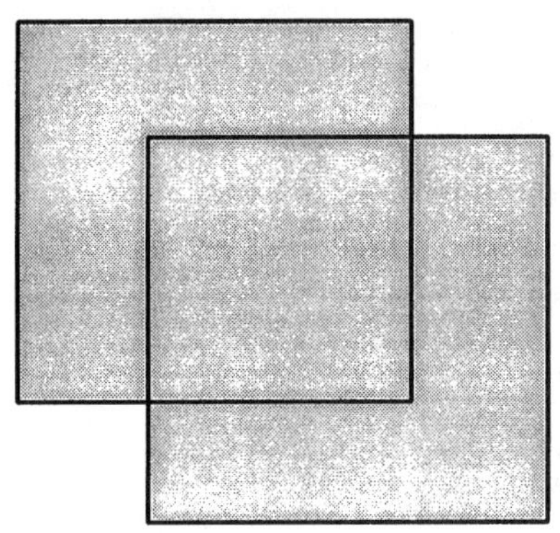

INDEX

Page numbers in **boldface** are **Strategies to Consider**.

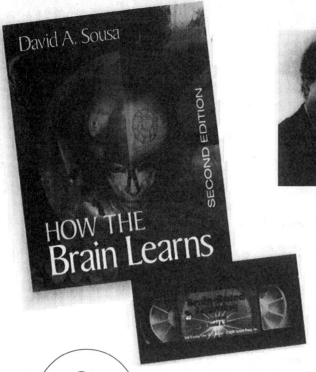

HOW THE Gifted Brain Learns

Use what talent you possess:
the woods would be very silent
if no birds sang
except those that sang best.

— Henry Van Dyke

HOW THE Gifted Brain Learns

David A. Sousa

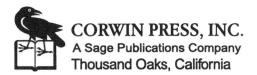

CORWIN PRESS, INC.
A Sage Publications Company
Thousand Oaks, California

For information:

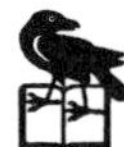

Corwin Press, Inc.
A Sage Publications Company
2455 Teller Road
Thousand Oaks, California 91320
www.corwinpress.com

Sage Publications Ltd.
6 Bonhill Street
London EC2A 4PU
United Kingdom

Sage Publications India Pvt. Ltd.
M-32 Market
Greater Kailash I
New Delhi 110 048 India

Printed in the United States of America

Library of Congress Cataloging-in-Publication Data

Sousa, David A.
How the gifted brain learns / David A. Sousa.
p. cm.
Includes bibliographical references (p.) and index.
ISBN 0-7619-3828-1 (pbk. :alk. paper)—ISBN 0-7619-3829-X (cloth : alk. paper)
1. Gifted children—Education—United States. 2. Gifted children—United States—Identification. 3. Brain—Localization of functions. I. Title.

LC3993.9 .S68 2002

2002031375

This book is printed on acid-free paper.

03 04 05 06 07 6 5 4 3 2

Acquiring Editor: Kylee Liegl
Cover Designer: Tracy E. Miller

Contents

LIST OF APPLICATIONS

About the Author

David A. Sousa, Ed.D., is an international educational consultant. He has made presentations at national conventions of educational organizations and has conducted workshops on brain research and science education in hundreds of school districts and at several colleges and universities across the United States, Canada, Europe, and Asia.

Dr. Sousa has a bachelor's degree in chemistry from Massachusetts State College at Bridgewater, a master of arts in teaching degree in science from Harvard University, and a doctorate from Rutgers University. His teaching experience covers all levels. He has taught junior and senior high school science, served as a K–12 director of science, and was Supervisor of Instruction for the West Orange, New Jersey, schools. He then became superintendent of the New Providence, New Jersey, public schools. He has been an adjunct professor of education at Seton Hall University, and a visiting lecturer at Rutgers University. He was president of the National Staff Development Council in 1992.

Dr. Sousa has edited science books and published numerous articles in leading educational journals on staff development, science education, and brain research. He is listed in *Who's Who in the East* and *Who's Who in American Education* and has received awards from professional associations and school districts for his commitment and contributions to research, staff development, and science education.

He has been interviewed on the NBC *Today* show and on National Public Radio about his work with schools using brain research. He makes his home in Florida.

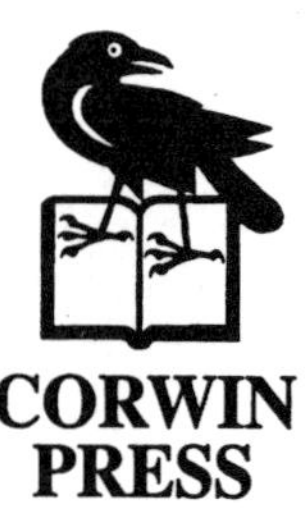
CORWIN
PRESS

Introduction

This book was inevitable. My first book, *How the Brain Learns* (Second Edition), was intended to explore the nature of teaching and learning for the majority of mainstream students. The second book, *How the Special Needs Brain Learns*, was written to help parents and educators understand what we are discovering about students who have learning difficulties. This book is designed to examine the needs of gifted and talented students, to uncover what—if anything—we are learning about the gifted brain, and to suggest strategies and programs that can help our best and brightest students achieve their full potential.

Classroom teachers, education specialists, school and district administrators, college instructors, and parents should all find items of interest in *How the Gifted Brain Learns*. Although many books have been written about the gifted, this book focuses primarily on insights to be gained about the gifted brain from the current explosion of research in neuroscience. It also reviews research information about the gifted learner for prospective and current teachers and administrators so that they may consider alternative instructional approaches.

WHAT DO WE MEAN BY *GIFTED AND TALENTED*? ■

Many terms are used to describe the student who demonstrates exceptional talent, and sometimes these terms themselves become a challenge to understand. *Gifted* is the most commonly used word, but it has hundreds of definitions, from legal to jargon. *Talented* usually describes an individual with a performance skill that has been refined through practice, such as music or dance. *Precocious* and *prodigy* are most commonly used to describe young children who display a high level of skill in a particular endeavor at a very early age.

In earlier times, *genius* was widely used, but it is now limited to the phenomenally gifted. *Superior* has recently come into vogue. Being a comparative term, it tempts one to ask superior to whom or to what, and to what degree. The vagueness of the term limits its usefulness in helping educators design an educational program for an individual student. *Exceptional* is an appropriate term when referring to a gifted child as being different from the regular school population, although it is also used to describe children with learning difficulties.

During the 1970s, the combined term *gifted and talented* came into common use. Although *gifted* and *talented* are often used interchangeably, Gagne (1985) differentiated between the two terms. For Gagne, *giftedness* is above-average aptitude (as measured by IQ tests) in creative and intellectual abilities, and *talent* is above-average performance in an area of human activity, such as music, mathematics, or literature.

In recent years, most researchers have moved away from defining *giftedness* solely in terms of IQ tests and have broadened its usage to include the characteristics of giftedness, such as creativity and motivation. Some definitions also consider the person's contributions to culture and society. People from diverse cultural and ethnic backgrounds may display their gifts and talents in ways that are recognized and valued by their own culture, but these individuals may not be recognized or valued by other cultures. A review of the literature on the characteristics of gifted and talented children from across different ethnic groups found some common indicators (e.g., problem-solving ability, intense interest, and motivation) but also found that each ethnicity had distinct and unique behavioral attributes (Frasier and Passow, 1994). As a result, one of the greater concerns in the field of gifted education is the realization that gifted children from diverse cultural backgrounds, or who have some type of learning disability, will not be recognized as gifted in our schools.

Given the various interpretations of the terminology used to describe students of high ability, I had to decide on a working definition that would be meaningful for all readers. For the purposes of this book, then, I use the term *gifted* to be an inclusive one in that it comprises high intellectual ability in academic areas as well as high levels of ability in areas of performance, such as music, theater, and dance. My simple definition is that a gifted person demonstrates (or has the potential for demonstrating) an exceptionally high level of performance in one or more areas of human endeavor. Not all readers may agree with this definition, and some may object that using it as an inclusive term de-emphasizes the importance of talent. That is certainly not my intent, which I think will become clear as one reads the book. However, to avoid any misinterpretation, and because

For the purposes of this book, a gifted person is defined as one who demonstrates an exceptionally high level of performance in one or more areas of human endeavor.

the combined term is so widespread, many references to *gifted and talented* will be found in the text.

Myths and Realities About Giftedness

Myths abound about the nature of giftedness, largely because public schools have not really had the resources to fully and accurately identify the gifted and to understand their needs. A prevailing notion for many years in public education has been that these students can take care of themselves and learn a great deal on their own. Consequently, schools have concentrated on providing a broad curriculum for mainstream students and then devoting a significant portion of remaining resources to students with learning difficulties. Little has been left over to identify or support the gifted, despite federal and state mandates to do so.

We are slowly gaining a greater understanding of the idiosyncracies of gifted children and the implications for parenting and teaching them. But to be successful at this, we must dispel the myths and look to credible research about the realities of being gifted and talented. The following list (Winner, 1996; Gentry and Kettle, 1998) summarizes some myths and realities regarding gifted children. Several of the topics are discussed in greater detail throughout the book.

Myth #1: Little is really known about how we learn. So how can we know about the gifted brain?	**Reality:** Research is providing a deeper understanding of how the human brain learns, including insights into the phenomenally gifted brain. See Chapters 1 and 2.
Myth #2: Academically gifted students have general intellectual power that makes them gifted in all areas.	**Reality:** Giftedness tends to be specific to a given domain of learning. Children can be gifted in one area and learning disabled in another. See Chapter 8.
Myth #3: *Gifted* refers just to academic ability, but *talented* refers to high ability in music and the arts.	**Reality:** There is no justification for this distinction. The domains of excellence are merely different, and in many cases the words can be used interchangeably. See Chapter 2.

Myth #4: Gifted students have lower self-esteem than nongifted students.	**Reality:** The majority of studies indicate that gifted students have a somewhat higher level of self-esteem than nongifted. However, they are at risk for isolation and loneliness, and they can become arrogant. See Chapters 2 and 7.
Myth #5: Giftedness in any domain requires a high IQ.	**Reality:** There is little evidence that giftedness in music or art requires an exceptional IQ. Moreover, IQ tests measure a narrow range of ability. See Chapters 2 and 6.
Myth #6: Acceleration options, such as grade skipping, early entrance, and early exit, tend to be harmful for gifted students.	**Reality:** Although it is important to consider the social and psychological adjustment of every student, there is little evidence that acceleration options are in any way detrimental. See Chapter 3.
Myth #7: Cooperative learning in heterogeneous groups provides academic benefits to gifted students and can be effectively substituted for specialized programs for academically talented students.	**Reality:** Recent studies show that gifted students receive greater academic benefit from being grouped with other gifted students, and that cooperative learning is not an effective replacement for specialized programs for academically talented students, such as new courses or acceleration options. See Chapter 3.
Myth #8: Giftedness is inborn, or giftedness is entirely the result of hard work.	**Reality:** True giftedness results from both genetic predispositions *and* hard work. See Chapter 2.
Myth #9: Creativity tests are effective means of identifying artistically gifted and talented students.	**Reality:** Creativity tests measure problem-solving and divergent thinking skills, but have not proved valid in predicting the success of students with high abilities in the visual arts. See Chapters 2, 6, and 9.

Myth #10: Pushy parents who drive their children to overachieve create gifted children.	**Reality:** Gifted children are usually pushing their parents, who are trying to accommodate and nurture them. However, some parents do try to live vicariously through their children and lose sight of the child's emotional well-being. See Chapters 3 and 7.
Myth #11: Early reading and writing skills should keep pace with each other.	**Reality:** Although this is a commonly held belief, there is no relationship between reading and writing skills in the development of young talented children. See Chapters 4 and 8.
Myth #12: All children are gifted, and there is no special group of children that needs enriched or accelerated education.	**Reality:** Although all children have strengths and weaknesses, some have extreme strengths in one or more areas. Extreme giftedness creates a special education need the same way that a learning disability does. See Chapters 3 and 8.
Myth #13: Highly gifted children go on to become eminent and creative adults.	**Reality:** Many gifted children, even prodigies, do not become eminent in adulthood, and many eminent adults were not prodigies. See Chapters 3, 5, 6, and 8.

GIFTED AND TALENTED PROGRAMS IN TODAY'S SCHOOLS ■

Because some parents and educators believe that truly gifted children will remain gifted and fulfill their educational needs on their own, schools have historically done little to identify and encourage the gifted. As a result, potentially gifted students have gone through school without their gifts ever being recognized. This has been a long-standing problem as history will attest. Sir Isaac Newton was considered a poor student in grammar school; he left at age 14, was sent back at 19 because he read so much, and graduated at Cambridge without any distinction whatsoever. The poet Shelley was expelled from Oxford; James Whistler and Edgar Allen Poe were both expelled from West Point. Charles Darwin dropped out of medical school, and Edward Gibbon, the noted British historian, considered his education a waste of time.

Gregor Mendel, founder of the science of genetics, flunked his teacher's examination four times in a row and finally gave up trying. Thomas Edison's mother withdrew him from school after 3 months in the 1st grade because his teacher said he was "unable to perform." Winston Churchill ended up last in his class at the Harrow School. Albert Einstein found grammar school boring. It was his uncle, showing the boy tricks with numbers, who stimulated his interest in mathematics. For a long time and in many places, traditional academic programs have often been poorly suited to humans of extraordinary potential. One is left to wonder how many Edisons did not survive their educational experiences.

Our society has not given the same attention to the education of the gifted as it has given to other special groups. For example, we spend millions every year for the mentally handicapped. But, too often, children of superior intellect spend their time in a commonplace school, assimilating a curricular diet far below their potential. Thus, gifted children pose one of our greatest present-day problems, beginning in the home and ultimately becoming a concern of the school. Teachers at all grade levels bear the responsibility to recognize and plan for the needs of the gifted.

Our society has not given the same attention to the education of the gifted as it has given to other special groups.

Currently, the process of identifying gifted students and the programs designed to address their needs vary greatly by grade level and school district. Gifted students who are not identified and served by these programs are not likely to ever have their needs fully met while in school. The loss of such potential is a serious blow to society as well as to the student and teacher. The student never feels fulfilled, loses self-esteem, and lacks direction. The teacher, meanwhile, is faced with student boredom, underachievement, and a litany of discipline problems that could have been avoided. One purpose of this book is to examine the current state of programs for the gifted and to suggest what we might do to make them better serve the gifts and talents of all students.

Programs in Elementary and Middle Schools

Identification and Teacher Bias

Identification of gifted students begins in elementary school. Students who get high scores (usually the 95th percentile or greater) on standardized achievement tests are referred by teachers as potential candidates for the gifted program. Acceptance into the program is typically made on the basis of several factors, but teacher recommendations tend to carry a lot of weight during final selections. Much debate has occurred about whether classroom teachers are qualified to identify gifted students. Some researchers argue that teacher biases related to differences in performance between male and female students, and other stereotypic beliefs, undermine the reliability and objectivity of their judgments.

A recent study to test the nature of teacher bias found that gender stereotypes and other biases still exist (Powell and Siegle, 2000). For example, classroom teachers rated males who were avid readers higher than similar females. Even males who were not interested in reading were rated higher than non-interested females. Introverted, absent-minded females were nominated with less confidence than males who also had these characteristics.

A recent study found that gender stereotypes and other biases still exist in teachers.

The study also found that students who were interested in topics unusual for their age, such as airplane design and flying, were more likely to be nominated than students interested in dinosaurs, a topic of interest for most elementary students. Meanwhile, gifted and talented specialists tended to rate students higher than did classroom teachers because, as the researchers suggested, these specialists tend to focus more on student strengths. Classroom teachers, on the other hand, often have to diagnose and prescribe and this, according to the researchers, may cause them to be more sensitive to student weaknesses. In any event, a major implication of this study is that classroom teachers probably need more training to recognize any stereotypical beliefs they may hold about the nature of gifted and talented students.

The Pull-Out Format

Elementary and middle school programs for gifted students usually follow a pull-out format in which these students meet once or twice a week to engage in problem-based learning activities or other similar experiences. Rarely is there any planned scope or sequence to the curricular activities, and little or nothing is shared when the students return to their regular classes. Research studies reveal that gifted students gain little to modest benefit from these types of classes, and that they would probably gain the same benefits if they carried out these activities in their regular classes. Undoubtedly, the pull-out format results in missed opportunities for gifted students as well as for the remaining students in the class. This book suggests some other ways to configure programs and design curriculum for gifted students at these grade levels that can result in greater achievement.

Programs in High Schools

The common belief in high schools is that honors and advanced placement-type courses are sufficient to meet the needs of gifted and talented students. Some schools also offer mentoring programs or have dual enrollment agreements with local colleges. A recent study from the National Research Center on the Gifted and Talented (NRC/GT) reported on the nature of programs for gifted high school students. Surveys were mailed to nearly 8,000 randomly selected high schools in all 50 states. Of that sample, 546 high schools responded. The following are some of the survey's findings:

- Nearly 66 percent of the respondents said they had a gifted education program at their high school and 34 percent reported that no such program existed. However, the surveys revealed that there was a great deal of overlap between what was offered in the schools claiming they *did not* have a gifted program and in the schools claiming they *did* have one. Apparently, there was a lack of understanding about what kind of program constituted gifted education at the high school level.
- About 50 percent of the schools reported having opportunities beyond academic courses for gifted students, e.g., internships/mentorships, early college programs, independent study, and academic clubs or competitions.
- Nearly all respondents offered advanced placement courses; the most common were English, calculus AB, biology, and US history.
- Approximately 50 percent of the schools had a consultant or coordinator associated with these programs, some serving only in a part-time capacity.

More attention needs to be given to clarifying what constitutes a comprehensive and effective gifted program at the high school level and to what other steps high schools can take to ensure a broad and rich variety of educational experiences for their most gifted students.

■ ORGANIZATION OF THIS BOOK

Basic brain structures and their functions are the main topics in Chapter 1. This information serves as a useful resource for identifying brain regions that are referenced in other chapters. Learning, the stages and types of memory, and retention are also reviewed.

Chapter 2 looks at various conceptual schemes (e.g., psychological, socio-emotional) that attempt to define the nature of intelligence and giftedness. Of particular interest is the discussion over the long-standing debate about whether nature (i.e., genetic programming) or nurture (i.e., environment and upbringing) has greater impact on talent development. Gender differences in cognitive styles are discussed along with some differences in brain structure and brain chemistry.

In Chapter 3, we examine specific suggestions for designing curricular and instructional strategies that are more likely to challenge the gifted brain. Because many teachers are faced with addressing the needs of gifted students within the context of the inclusive classroom, this chapter focuses on the concept of differentiated curriculum. Also discussed are acceleration, curriculum compacting, grouping formats, and other techniques that have been successful in developing the talents of gifted students.

Chapters 4, 5, and 6 deal with attempts to understand the nature of giftedness in three specific areas: language, mathematics, and music, respectively. As scientific evidence accumulated over the last few decades suggesting that the human brain is hard-wired for language, mathematics, and music, research resources were directed toward investigating the cerebral nature of these activities. Consequently, we include these areas because they currently have the largest base of research studies among all the school disciplines. Furthermore, there is little evidence at this time to indicate that the brain is specifically wired for science, economics, or history. According to current thinking, it is more likely that high ability in these areas results from high ability in one or more of the hard-wired areas (e.g., mathematics for science, and language for history) coupled with intense personal interest in, say, scientific phenomena or historical events.

Chapter 7 investigates the various symptoms, causes, and types of underachievement in gifted students. A somewhat overlooked area of gifted education, this chapter presents ways of identifying these students and suggests strategies for reversing underachievement. Particular attention is paid to the growing number of underachieving minority students and to ways for addressing their needs.

Although the notion that a person can be both gifted and learning disabled may seem strange, Chapter 8 examines the twice-exceptional student. Some of the more common combinations of giftedness and learning disabilities are discussed—gifted children with attention-deficit hyperactivity disorder, for example—as well as rare phenomena, such as savant syndrome.

Finally, Chapter 9 suggests some ways of identifying gifted children and setting up a learning environment where gifted students, along with their classmates, can excel in the inclusive classroom. The effectiveness of current programs to aid gifted students in elementary and secondary schools is also discussed.

Other Features of the Book

At the end of most chapters, a section called **Applications** includes activities reflecting my interpretation of how research might translate into effective classroom strategies. Obviously, some of the strategies are appropriate for all learners; however, the suggestions have been written specifically to address the needs of gifted students. Even though this book does not present every strategy for teaching gifted students, those that best match the research information in the corresponding chapters are mentioned. Readers are invited to critically review my suggestions and rationale to determine if these ideas have any value for their work.

The book will help answer the following questions:

- How different are the brains of gifted students?
- What kinds of strategies are particularly effective for students with specific gifts?
- What progress is brain research making in discovering the nature of intelligence and giftedness?
- Will brain research help us identify potentially gifted students sooner and more accurately?
- Are schools adequately challenging gifted students today? If not, what can we do about it?
- How can improving programs for the gifted and talented benefit other students?
- What insights are we gaining about students who are gifted in language, mathematics, and music?
- What can we do to identify and help gifted students who are underachievers?
- How can we identify students who are both gifted and learning disabled, and how can we help them?

Some of the information and suggestions you will find here came from advocacy organizations including the National Association for Gifted Children and the National Research Center on the Gifted and Talented (see **Resources**). Where possible, I have sought out original medical research reports, which are noted in the **References**. A few of the strategies are derived or adapted from the second edition of my book, *How the Brain Learns* (2001).

As we gain a greater understanding of the human brain, we may discover ways to identify gifted students sooner and more accurately.

As we gain a greater understanding of the human brain, we may discover ways to identify gifted students more quickly and more accurately. This means that schools can begin to provide for student needs earlier and with greater effectiveness. Sometimes, these students are attempting to learn in environments that are designed to help but instead inadvertently frustrate their efforts. By looking for ways to differentiate the curriculum and by changing some of our instructional approaches, we may be able to move gifted students to exceptional levels of performance. My hope is that this book will encourage all school professionals and parents to learn more about how the brain learns so that they can work together for the benefit of all students.

A WORD ABOUT ELITISM

Some parents, educators, and politicians object to any special programs for gifted children on the grounds of elitism. This word has acquired the negative connotations of snobbishness, selectivity, and unfair special attention at a time, critics say, when we should be emphasizing egalitarianism. The reality is that gifted students are elite in the sense that they possess skills to a higher degree than most people in their class. The same is true for professional athletes, musical soloists, inventors, or physicians. Parents and schools must provide children with equal opportunity, not equal treatment. Treating all students as though they learned exactly the same way is folly. Therefore, schools have a responsibility to challenge gifted students to their fullest potential while, at the same time, challenging those who cry elitism to rethink the true meaning of the word and the real purpose of education.

1

Brain Structure and Learning

No other known entity in the universe is as complicated and as fascinating as the human brain. This three-pound mass of hundreds of billions of nerve cells is intricately organized to control our feelings, behavior, and thoughts. It collects and sorts information, learns complex skills, masters spoken language, stores the memories of a lifetime, and contains the secret of ourselves. For centuries, scientists have been attempting to understand exactly how the brain grows and develops into this amazing organ.

Until recently, their efforts where thwarted by the reality that the brain could be examined only in autopsy. Microscopic and macroscopic sections of brain tissue gave clues about structure but not function. Today, however, brain imaging technologies have given neuroscientists powerful new tools to look at brain structure *and* function in living persons. Computerized tomography (CT scans, also called CAT scans), positron-emission tomography (PET scans), and magnetic resonance imaging (MRI) are especially helpful in deciphering the complex cerebral processes involved in language acquisition and reading.

In addition to the imaging techniques, advanced systems monitor and record the electrical signals (electroencephalography, or EEG) as well as the magnetic fields (magneto-encephalography, or MEG) that are produced when electrical impulses travel within the neurons. These recordings are valuable in localizing the source of signals originating in brain regions as small as one cubic millimeter of cerebral cortex and in timing any changes to the nearest thousandth of a second.

Imaging techniques offer different views of brain structure and function. Already, more advanced imaging technologies are providing innovative ways of studying the brain. Table 1.1 and Table 1.2 show the major imaging technologies and other techniques that allow us to examine the inner workings of the human brain (Beatty, 2001).

Table 1.1 Imaging Technologies for Examining Brain Structure and Function

Name	How It Works
Computerized Tomography (CT)	First introduced in 1973, CT is an enhancement of X-rays that reconstructs an image of a horizontal slice of tissue. A large number of X-ray beams pass through the tissue at a variety of angles, and the amount of radiation absorbed is measured. This allows a computer to determine the density of tissue at each point and produce the image. CT scans show *structure*.
Positron Emission Tomography (PET)	Introduced in the early 1980s, this technology indicates brain *function* and tells us what the brain is doing rather than how it looks. To accomplish this, the patient is injected with glucose containing a radioactive nucleus that emits positrons. More active portions of the brain will metabolize more glucose and thereby concentrate more radioactivity than the less active areas. The radioactivity is detected by the scanner and an image is produced by a computer.
Magnetic Resonance Imaging (MRI)	Like CT, MRI provides images of *structure*; but, unlike CT, it does not use X-rays. MRI is non-invasive and is safe to use repeatedly on the same patient. The procedure uses a strong magnetic field and radio frequency energy to generate signals from atoms (usually hydrogen) within tissue. Images are compiled that have a much greater resolution than CT and that can be taken from any angle.
functional Magnetic Resonance Imaging (fMRI)	By detecting the minute changes in the magnetic properties of blood hemoglobin and oxygen, the fMRI can measure *function* as well as *structure*. Active neurons need more blood and so generate a signal in an fMRI scan. Unlike the PET, it is non-invasive and is thus used to measure brain function in healthy subjects.

Table 1.2 Other Technologies for Examining Brain Structure and Function

Name	How It Works
Electroencephalography (EEG)	This technique dates back to the 1920s and involves measuring the electrical activity of neurons by attaching electrodes to the scalp. Because it is very difficult to determine which part of the brain is generating the signals, EEG is used mainly for examining general brain activity as in the sleep-wake cycle and during epileptic seizures.
Magnetoencephalography (MEG)	In a fashion similar to EEG, MEG measures the small magnetic fields generated by the electrical activity in neurons, but it can be more useful in localizing the source of the signals.
Brain Lesion Analysis	This procedure involves examining human brain tissue for lesions and determining whether a deficiency can be associated with the lesion. Researchers can also intentionally introduce lesions in the brains of laboratory animals and interpret the resulting behavioral changes.

BASIC BRAIN STRUCTURES ■

To understand the complexity of the human brain, we will first look at the major parts of the outside of the brain (Figure 1.1). Three major structures are visible: the cerebral hemispheres, the cerebellum, and the brain stem.

The Cerebral Hemispheres

The cerebral hemispheres comprise the largest part of the brain (about 85 percent by weight), called the *cerebrum*, and their surface is highly convoluted. The ridges of these convolutions are called *gyri* (singular is *gyrus*). This convoluted surface is covered with a laminated sheet of six layers of cells approximately two millimeters (about one-tenth of an inch) in thickness. The convolutions allow a great deal more of this laminated sheet (called the *cerebral cortex*) to be packed into the confines of the human skull. Although the minor wrinkles are unique in each brain, several major folds are common to all brains. In the largest part of the brain is a set of four lobes, each of which specializes in performing certain functions.

Four Cerebral Lobes

Frontal Lobe. Often referred to as the executive control center, the frontal lobe contains almost 50 percent of the volume of each cerebral hemisphere. It controls movement through a narrow strip across the top of the hemispheres called the *motor cortex*. The area at the very front of this lobe (i.e., just behind the forehead) is called the *prefrontal cortex*, which is believed to be the site of our personality, curiosity, decision making, and reflecting on the consequences of our actions. Curbing the excesses of our emotions is another of the prefrontal cortex's important functions. Because emotions drive attention, the efficiency of this area is linked to the limbic centers.

Most of the working memory is located in the frontal lobe, so this is the area where focus occurs. The frontal lobe, however, matures slowly. MRI studies of postadolescents reveal that the frontal lobe continues to mature into early adulthood. Thus, the emotional regulation capability of the frontal lobe is not fully operational during adolescence (Sowell, Thompson, Holmes, Jernigan, and Toga,

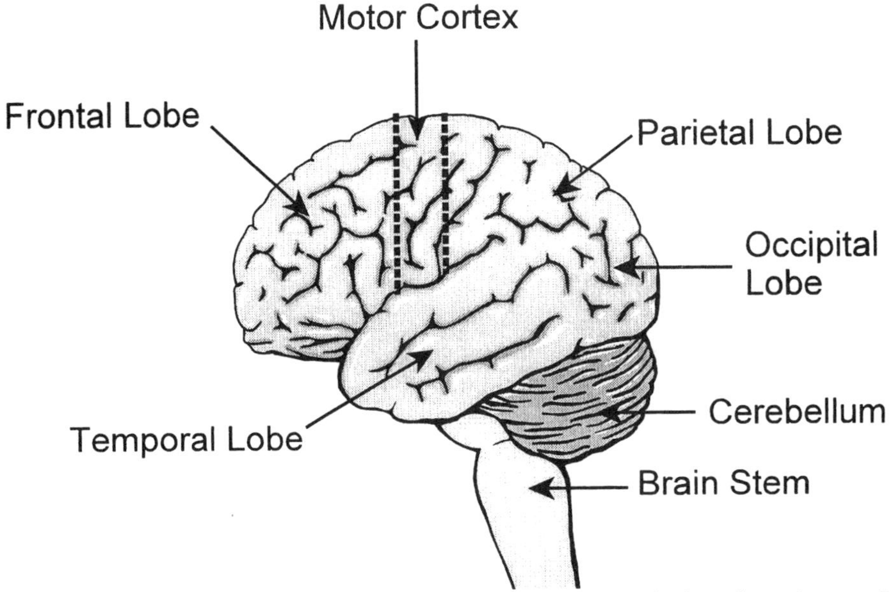

Figure 1.1 This diagram shows the four major lobes of the brain (cerebrum) as well as the motor cortex, the brain stem, and the cerebellum.

1999). This is one reason why adolescents are more likely than adults to submit to their emotions and resort to high-risk behavior.

Temporal Lobe. The temporal lobe is the speech center. It is involved in the interpretation of sound, speech (primarily on the left side), and some aspects of long-term and visual memory.

Occipital Lobe. Visual processing is the main function of the occipital lobe.

Parietal Lobe. The parietal lobe is primarily concerned with attending to stimuli, sensory integration, and orientation.

The Cerebellum

The cerebellum (Latin for "little brain") coordinates every movement. Because the cerebellum monitors impulses from nerve endings in the muscles, it is important in the learning, performance, and timing of complex motor tasks including speaking. The cerebellum may also store the memory of rote movements, such as touch-typing and tying a shoelace. A person whose cerebellum is damaged cannot coordinate movement, has difficulty with speech, and may display the symptoms of autism.

The Brain Stem

The oldest and deepest area of the brain, often referred to as the reptilian brain, the brain stem resembles the entire brain of a reptile. Here is where vital body functions (e.g., respiration, body temperature, blood pressure, and digestion) are monitored and controlled. The brain stem also houses the reticular activating system (RAS), which plays an active role in sleep, waking, and attention.

Next, we will look at the inside of the brain and at some of its major structures (see Figure 1.2). These include the limbic area and the cerebrum.

The Limbic Area

Above the brain stem lies the limbic area, most of whose structures are duplicated in each hemisphere of the brain. This area regulates fear conditioning and other aspects of emotional memory. Some parts of the limbic area process and interpret specific sensory information, but the three parts of the limbic area important to learning and memory are the following:

Thalamus. This structure is the brain's switching station. All incoming sensory information (except smell) goes first to the thalamus for preliminary

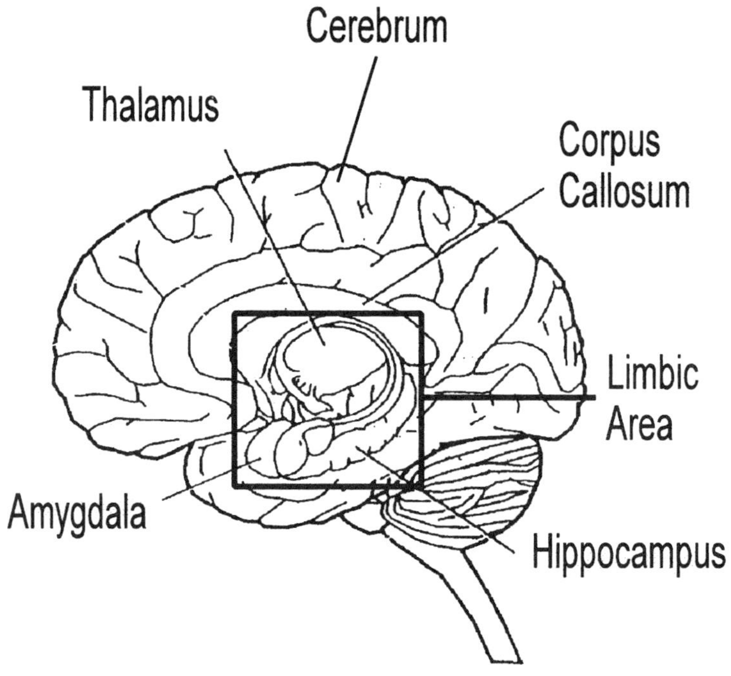

Figure 1.2 A cross section of the human brain.

processing and integration. From here it is directed to other parts of the brain for additional processing.

Hippocampus. Derived from the Greek word for a sea monster resembling a seahorse, because of its shape, the hippocampus hugs the inside of the temporal lobe. It plays a major role in consolidating learning and in converting information from working memory via electronic signals to the long-term storage regions, a process that may take from days to months. This brain area constantly checks information relayed to working memory and compares it to stored experiences. This process is essential for the creation of meaning.

Amygdala. Attached to the end of the hippocampus, the amygdala (Greek for "almond") plays an important role in emotional behavior, especially the fear response. It regulates those interactions that are necessary for the organism's survival, such as whether to fight or flee, to eat or not eat, and when to mate. Because of its proximity to the hippocampus and its activity on PET scans, researchers believe that the amygdala encodes an emotional message, if one is present, whenever an experience is destined for long-term storage. Apparently, these memories can even be established unconsciously (LeDoux, 2002). This explains why we tend to remember vividly the best and the worst things that happen to us.

The Cerebrum

The cerebrum encompasses the four lobes of the brain. For some still unexplained reason, the nerves from the left side of the body cross over to the right hemisphere, and those from the right side of the body cross over to the left hemisphere. The two hemispheres are connected by a thick cable, called the *corpus callosum*, composed of over 250 million nerve fibers. The hemispheres use this bridge to communicate with each other and to coordinate activities.

Brain Cells

The activities of the brain are carried out by signals traveling along brain cells. The brain is composed of a trillion cells of at least two known types: nerve cells and their support cells. Nerve cells are called *neurons* and represent about one tenth of the total number of cells—roughly 100 billion. Most of the cells are support cells, called *glial* (Greek for "glue") cells, that hold the neurons together and act as filters to keep harmful substances out of the neurons.

With few exceptions, all of the neurons in the human brain are produced before birth from a small number of precursor cells. During gestation, neurons are multiplying at an astonishing rate, reaching about 250,000 per minute at peak production (Restak, 2001). Neurons are the functioning core for the brain and the entire nervous system. They come in different sizes, but it takes about 30,000 brain neurons to fit on the head of a pin. Unlike other cells, the neuron (Figure 1.3) has

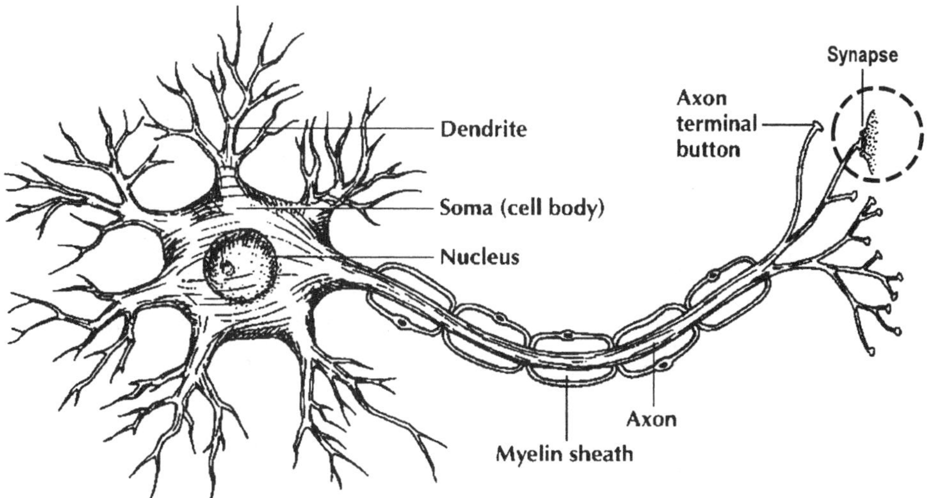

Figure 1.3 Neurons transmit impulses along an axon and across the synapse (in dotted circle) to the dendrites of a neighboring cell.

tens of thousands of branches or *dendrites* (from Greek for "tree") emerging from its center. The dendrites receive electrical impulses from other neurons and transmit them along a long fiber, called the *axon* (Greek for "axis"). Each neuron has a cell body (called the *soma*) and only one axon. Some axons are only a few millimeters in length and affect just nearby neurons. Other axons stretch over to the other side of the brain and influence neurons a considerable distance away.

Neurons have no direct contact with each other. Between each dendrite and axon is a small gap of about a millionth of an inch called a *synapse* (from Greek for "to join together"). This system allows for maximum flexibility. Because the neurons are not physically tied to each other, neuron-to-neuron interactions can form, reform, and dissolve from one moment to the next. This flexibility accounts for the brain's *plasticity* and explains why learning occurs during our entire lifetime.

Signals generated within neurons are electrical, but communication between neurons is chemical. A typical neuron collects signals from others through the dendrites. The neuron sends out spikes of electrical activity (impulses) through the axon to the synapse where the activity releases chemicals stored in sacs (called *synaptic vesicles*) at the end of the axon. The chemicals, called *neurotransmitters*, travel across the *synaptic gap* to a *receptor site* and either excite or inhibit the neighboring neuron (see Figure 1.4). Nearly 100 different neurotransmitters have been discovered so far. Some of the more common neurotransmitters are dopamine, glutamate, acetylcholine, epinephrine, and serotonin. Some neurotransmitters, such as glutamate, are found everywhere in the brain but others, like dopamine, are restricted to certain regions.

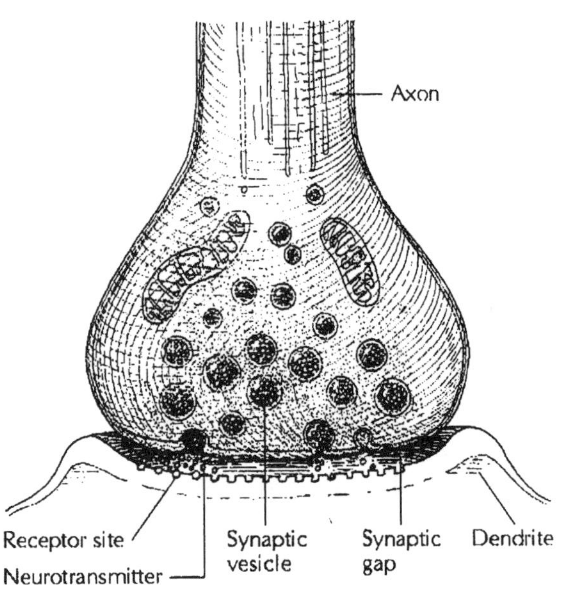

Figure 1.4 The neural impulse is carried across the synapse by chemicals called neurotransmitters that lie within the synaptic vesicles.

Electrical transmission can be exceedingly slow in brain cells. During early brain development, a layer called the *myelin* (related to the Greek word for marrow) *sheath* surrounds each axon. As the amount of electrical activity through a neuron increases, more myelin is produced, so the thickness of the sheath increases—a process called *myelination*. MRI scans confirm that myelination is carried out at a staggering rate during childhood (Blanton, Levitt, Thompson, Narr,

Capetillo-Cunliffe, Nobel, Singerman, McCracken, and Toga, 2001). The sheath insulates the axon from other cells and increases the speed of impulse transmission. The impulse travels along the neurons through an electrochemical process and can move the entire length of a 6-foot adult in two tenths of a second. A neuron can transmit between 250 and 2,500 impulses per second.

The presence or absence of myelin around neurons may be the main determinant of their fate during early brain development. Newborns have many more neurons than they need, and after the first 3 years or so after birth, the brain begins to eliminate those neurons that have little myelination, thus indicating little use. This pruning process—called *apoptosis*—ensures that the remaining neural networks can function more efficiently.

Brain Size and Intelligence

The idea that a relationship exists between brain or head size and intelligence has long been the subject of controversy. Popular in the 19th century, the concept seemed to make sense: the more brain, the more intelligence. Although early 20th-century biologists ridiculed the idea, modern brain imaging studies show a small positive correlation between brain volume and intelligence. A more specific study was carried out by Paul Thompson and his colleagues (Thompson, et al., 2001). Using MRI, they scanned the brains of 20 pairs of identical and fraternal twins. The researchers gave the subjects intelligence tests and found that intelligence as measured by these tests was significantly linked with the amount of brain matter in the frontal lobes.

Recent studies show a link between intelligence and the size of some regions of the brain.

Thompson was surprised by this result, finding it hard to believe that something as simple as frontal lobe brain volume could affect something as complex as intelligence. Nonetheless, it could be that the larger the brain cell mass, the greater the number of cell-to-cell connections. What still remains a mystery is whether the larger cell volume was the cause of higher intelligence or the other way around—people with strong motivation might use their brains more and thus develop a higher density of neurons. The researchers cautioned, however, that because this study involved collective data, the size of brain volume in the frontal lobes cannot be used to measure the intelligence of an individual.

LEARNING AND MEMORY

Learning is the process by which we *acquire* new knowledge and skills; memory is the process by which we *retain* knowledge and skills for the future. At the cellular level, learning occurs when the synapses make physical and chemical changes so that the influence of one neuron on another also changes. Investigations into the neural mechanisms required for different types of learning are revealing more about the interactions between learning new information, memory, and changes in brain structure. Just as muscles improve with exercise, the brain seems to improve with use. Although learning does not increase the number of brain cells, it does increase their size, their branches, and their ability to form more complex networks.

Learning does not always result in long-term retention.

Learning and memory also occur in different ways. Learning involves the brain, the nervous system, and the environment as well as the process by which their interplay acquires information and skills. Whether this learning becomes a memory is something else. Sometimes, we need information for just a short period of time, like the telephone number for a pizza delivery, and then the information decays after a few seconds. Thus, learning does not always result in long-term retention.

Neural Efficiency

The brain goes through physical and chemical changes when it stores new information as the result of learning. For instance, a set of neurons "learns" to fire together. Repeated firings make successive firings easier and, eventually, automatic under certain conditions. Thus, a memory is formed. Storing the memory gives rise to new neural pathways and strengthens existing pathways. Over time, these small networks of memories begin to form larger associations. Hence, every time we learn something, our long-term storage areas undergo anatomical changes that, together with our unique genetic makeup, constitute the expression of our individuality.

As the repetition of stimuli causes neural circuits to become more associated and efficient, the threshold for forming new circuits lowers. Consequently, subsequent learning may form strong neural circuits with less repetition, thereby increasing the speed of learning. This process describes *neural efficiency*. If an important aspect of intelligence is speed of learning, then it is likely that individuals born with a predisposition for developing neural circuitry rapidly are destined to be gifted in some way. Further, this trait is likely to appear during the early years in a child's development when neuron circuit building is at its peak. And so, the child genius appears.

If an important aspect of intelligence is speed of learning, then it is likely that individuals born with a predisposition for developing neural circuitry rapidly are destined to be gifted in some way.

Genetic composition is likely to be a strong determinant in an individual's predisposition for neural efficiency. But there is substantial evidence that environmental influences can also provide opportunities for improving the speed with which new learning takes place (Buckner, Kelley, and Petersen, 1999). One teaching strategy that is particularly successful in this area is rehearsal, which is discussed later in this chapter.

STAGES AND TYPES OF MEMORY ■

Trying to explain the components and mechanisms associated with human memory has confounded scientists for centuries. However, during the last 20 years, most researchers have adopted a general memory model that distinguishes between *how long* something is stored (the stages of memory) from *what* is being stored (the types of memory)(see Figure 1.5).

1. Stages of Memory

The stages of memory deal with the temporal nature of memory. They describe the length of time a memory can be present to influence behavior or thought. Neuroscientists generally agree that there are three types of temporal memory: *immediate memory* and *working memory* for temporary interactions and *long-term memory* for permanent storage.

Immediate Memory

Immediate memory is the ability to hold on to items, from a few seconds up to about a minute, to accomplish a particular task. Repeating a short list of items or remembering a telephone number just long enough to dial it are examples of using immediate memory. The task is often completed subconsciously and the memory of it quickly fades. Thus, items that have been just in immediate memory

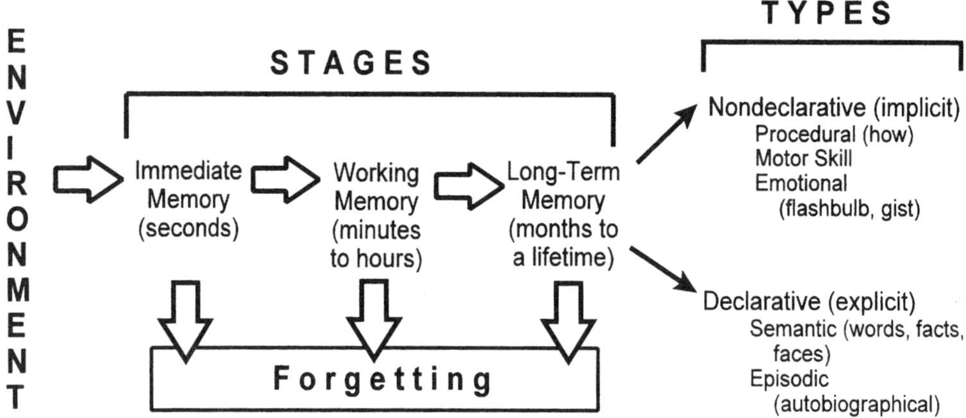

Figure 1.5 The stages and types of memory.

cannot be recalled. However, if you recite the list or dial the phone number repeatedly, there is a high probability that the information will move to the conscious processor—working memory.

Working Memory

Working memory is the ability to hold items long enough to consciously process and reflect on them and to carry out related activities during that processing, which can take from minutes to hours. If, for example, the route you normally drive from home to work were blocked by an accident, working memory and frontal lobe processing would be recruited to assess the situation and help determine an alternate route.

Studies of working memory indicate that it has a limited capacity of about six to seven verbal items for most people. This capacity (called the *phonologic loop*) is likely to be greater for highly talented individuals and less for those with learning problems. Working memory capacity seems to be closely related to the amount of attention one gives to situations requiring problem solving. Individuals with higher working memory capacity give more controlled attention to problem solving tasks and are less likely to be diverted by other distractions. Working memory also shows a strong connection to general intelligence, probably because working memory's connections within the frontal lobes keep the representation active for further processing (Engle, Laughlin, Tuholski, and Conway, 1999; Tuholski, Engle, and Baylis, 2001).

Another component of working memory is the *visuospatial sketchpad*, which holds visual and spatial information in a similar loop (Beatty, 2001). To date, only a few studies have sought to examine this facet of working memory. As might be expected, one EEG study found that high IQ individuals performed better than their lower IQ peers on tasks requiring the rehearsal of spatial information in working memory. One surprising finding, however, was that when the memory load of the task increased, areas in the rear of the brain were activated, but only in the high IQ subjects. The researchers speculated that a characteristic of high intelligence may be the ability of the frontal lobes to store and rehearse spatial information in working memory and in the posterior areas (occipital lobe) of the brain (Van Rooy, Stough, Pipingas, Hocking, and Silberstein, 2001).

A characteristic of high intelligence may be the ability of the frontal lobes to store and rehearse spatial information in working memory and in the posterior areas (occipital lobe) of the brain.

Long-Term Memory

Long-term memory is the ability to store information in a permanent form for months, years, and even for a lifetime. Storing occurs when the hippocampus encodes information and sends it to one or more long-term storage areas. The encoding process takes time and usually occurs during deep sleep, resulting in permanent physical changes and an increase in the efficiency of transmission in the synaptic areas associated with the memory. This physical embodiment of the memory is called an *engram*. Note that forgetting can occur in all stages of memory.

An important question is what factors increase the probability that information in working memory will be encoded into long-term storage sites for future recall? That is how can teachers help students to retain the learning objective for future use. This is an important matter because we cannot recall what we have not stored.

Information that has survival value is quickly stored. You don't want to have to learn every day that walking in front of a moving bus or touching a hot stove can injure you. As already mentioned, the amygdala ensures that emotional experiences also have a high likelihood of being permanently stored. But, in classrooms—where the survival and emotional elements may be minimal or absent—other factors need to come into play if the learner is ever to recall information. In this situation, it seems that permanent storage is most likely to occur when the learning makes sense and has meaning. *Sense* refers to whether the learner can understand the item on the basis of past experiences. On the other hand, *meaning* refers to whether the item is *relevant* to the learner. For what purpose should the learner remember it? Meaning, of course, is a personal thing and is greatly influenced by that person's prior experiences. The same item can have great meaning for one student and none for another. When a student asks "Why do I have to know this?" or "When will I ever use this?", it indicates that the student has not, for whatever reason, accepted this learning as relevant.

Whenever the learner's working memory decides that an item does not make sense or have meaning, the probability of it being stored is extremely low. If either sense or meaning is present, the probability of storage increases significantly (assuming, you remember, no survival or emotional component). If both sense *and* meaning are present, the likelihood of long-term storage is very high. For more on sense and meaning and how they affect retention, see Sousa (2001a).

Effect of Past Experiences on Memory

Past experiences always influence new learning. What we already know acts as a filter, helping us attend to those things that have meaning (i.e., relevancy) and discard those that don't. Meaning, therefore, has a great impact on whether information and skills will be learned and stored. If students have not found meaning by the end of a learning episode, there is little likelihood that much will be remembered.

Teachers spend about 90 percent of their planning time devising lessons so that students will *understand* the learning objective (i.e., make sense of it). But to convince a learner's brain to persist with that objective, teachers need to be more mindful of helping students establish *meaning*. We should remember that what was meaningful for us as children may not necessarily be meaningful for children today.

Curriculum Implications

If we expect students to find meaning, we need to be certain that the curriculum contains connections to *their* past experiences, not just ours. Further, the enormous size and the strict compartmentalization of secondary curriculum areas do little to help students find the time to make relevant connections between and among subjects. Helping students to link subject areas by integrating the curriculum increases meaning and retention, especially when students recognize a future use for the new learning.

Students who are gifted in acquiring information and skills often have an extensive knowledge base that allows them to make meaningful connections to new learning quickly. They are then ready to move on to other challenges.

Students gifted in acquiring information and skills have an extensive knowledge base that allows them to make meaningful connections to new learning quickly.

Rehearsal

Attaching sense and meaning to new learning can occur only if the learner has adequate time to process and reprocess it. This continuing reprocessing is called *rehearsal* and is a critical component in the transference of information from working memory to long-term storage. Two major factors should be considered in evaluating rehearsal: the amount of time devoted to it, which determines whether there is both initial and secondary rehearsal, and the type of rehearsal carried out, which can be rote or elaborative.

Time for Initial and Secondary Rehearsal

Time is a critical component of rehearsal. Initial rehearsal occurs when the information first enters working memory. If the learner cannot attach sense or meaning, and if there is no time for further processing, the new information is likely to be lost. Providing sufficient time to go beyond initial processing to secondary rehearsal allows the learner to review the information, to make sense of it, to elaborate on the details, and to assign value and relevance, thus increasing significantly the chance of long-term storage.

Scanning studies of the brain indicate that the frontal lobe is very much involved during the rehearsal process and, ultimately, in long-term memory formation. This makes sense because working memory is also located in the frontal lobe. Several studies using fMRI scans of human subjects showed that, during longer rehearsals, the amount of activity in the frontal lobe determined whether items were stored or forgotten (Wagner, Schacter, Rotte, Koutstaal, Maril, Dale, Rosen, and Buckner, 1998; Buckner, et al., 1999).

Students carry out initial and secondary rehearsal at different rates of speed and in different ways, depending on the type of information in the new learning and on their learning styles. As the learning task changes, learners automatically shift to different patterns of rehearsal. An individual's neural efficiency will most likely play a role in this process as well.

Rote and Elaborative Rehearsal

Rote Rehearsal. This rehearsal is used when learners need to remember and store information exactly as it is entered into working memory. This involves a simple strategy necessary to learn information or a skill in a specific form or sequence. We employ rote rehearsal to remember a poem, the lyrics and melody of a song, multiplication tables, telephone numbers, and steps in a procedure.

Elaborative Rehearsal. By contrast, elaborative rehearsal is used when it is unnecessary to store information exactly as learned, and when it is important to associate new learnings with prior learnings to detect relationships. This is a complex thinking process, in which the learners reprocess the information several times to make connections to previous learnings and assign meaning. For example, students use rote rehearsal to memorize a poem, but elaborative rehearsal to interpret its message. Elaborative rehearsal is also likely to enhance neural efficiency as larger associative networks are being made. When students get very little time for, or training in, elaborative rehearsal, they resort more frequently to rote rehearsal. Consequently, they fail to make the associations or discover the relationships that only elaborative rehearsal can provide. Also, they continue to believe that the value of learning is merely the recalling of information as learned rather than the generating of new ideas, concepts, and solutions.

There is almost no long-term retention without rehearsal.

When deciding how to use rehearsal in a lesson, teachers need to consider the time available as well as the type of rehearsal appropriate for the specific learning objective. Keep in mind that rehearsal only contributes to, but does not guarantee, information transfer into long-term storage. However, there is almost no long-term retention in the classroom *without* rehearsal.

2. Types of Memory

Some stimuli that are processed in the immediate and working memories are eventually transferred to long-term memory sites, where they actually change the structure of the neurons so they can last a lifetime. Although neuroscientists are not in total agreement as to all of the characteristics of long-term memory, there is considerable agreement on some of their types, and their description is important to understand before setting out to design learning activities accordingly. Long-term memory can be divided into two categories, *nondeclarative memory* and *declarative memory* (Figure 1.5).

Nondeclarative Memory

Nondeclarative memory (sometimes called *implicit* memory) exists in several different forms including procedural memory, motor skill memory, and emotional memory.

Procedural Memory. Procedural memory refers to remembering *how* to do something, like riding a bicycle, driving a car, swinging a tennis racket, and tying a shoelace. As practice of the skills continues, these memories become more efficient and can be performed with little conscious thought or recall. The brain process shifts from *reflective* to *reflexive*. For example, you may remember the first time you drove an automobile by yourself. No doubt you gave a lot of conscious attention to your speed, maneuvering the vehicle, putting your foot on the correct pedal, and observing surrounding traffic (reflective thought). However, as you continued to practice this routine, the skills were stored in procedural memory and became more automatic (reflexive activity). Now, it is possible to focus on abstract thoughts while taking that familiar and mundane drive between home and work, giving no conscious thought to the motor skills required to operate the automobile. Procedural memory drives the car while working memory plans your day.

Procedural memory helps us to learn things that don't require conscious attention and to habituate ourselves to the environment. Thus, we can become accustomed to the clothes we wear, the daily noisy traffic outside the school, a ticking clock in the den, or the sounds of construction. This adjustment to the environment allows the brain to screen out unimportant stimuli so it can focus on those that matter.

We also learn *perceptual skills*, such as reading, discriminating colors, and identifying tones in music, and *cognitive skills*, such as figuring out a *procedure* for solving a problem. Cognitive skills are different from cognitive concept building in that cognitive skills are performed automatically and rely on procedural memory rather than declarative memory. Acquiring perceptual and cognitive skills involves brain processes and memory sites that are different from those used in learning cognitive concepts. If they are learned differently, should they be taught differently?

Motor Skill Memory. Much of what we do during the course of a day involves the performance of skills. We go through the morning grooming and breakfast rituals, read the newspaper, get to work, and shake the hand of a new acquaintance. We do all of these tasks without realizing that we have learned them and without being aware that we are using our memory. Although learning a new skill involves conscious attention, skill performance later becomes unconscious and relies essentially on nondeclarative memory.

Emotional Memory. Emotions can positively or negatively affect the acquisition of new learning. Emotions associated with a learning become part of the nondeclarative memory system. These emotions can return and change how students *feel* about what they learned. This unconscious response can turn them toward or away from a similar learning experience.

A powerful emotional experience can cause an instantaneous and long-lasting memory of an event, called a *flashbulb memory*. An example is remembering where you were and what you were doing when the Challenger space shuttle exploded or during the terrorist attacks on New York City and Washington. Although these memories are not always accurate, they do attest to the brain's ability to record emotionally significant experiences. This ability most likely results from the stimulation of the amygdala and the release throughout the body of emotion-arousing substances, such as adrenaline.

Sometimes, an experience is stored merely as an emotional *gist* or summary of the event, that is, we remember whether we liked it or not. A year after seeing a movie, for example, we might be able to recall only bits of the storyline and perhaps its mood. Students often can remember whether they liked a particular topic, but cannot recall many details about it.

Declarative Memory

Declarative memory (also called *conscious* or *explicit* memory) describes the remembering of names, facts, music, and objects (e.g., where you live and the kind of car you own) and is processed by the hippocampus and cerebrum. Items in declarative memory are readily available through consciousness and thus can be expressed through language—that is, declared. Think for a moment about a person who is now important in your life. Try to recall that person's image, voice, and mannerisms. Then think of an important event you both attended, one with an emotional connection, such as a concert, wedding, or funeral. Once you have the context in mind, note how easily other components of the memory come together. This is declarative memory in its most common form—conscious and almost effortless recall. It should be noted, however, that the emotional memory you just recalled is a separate component that may be stored in declarative memory but kept as a declarative fact. The emotional memory is mediated by the amygdala and operates independently of conscious awareness (LeDoux, 2002).

Declarative memory can be further divided into episodic memory and semantic memory. *Episodic memory* refers to the memory of events in one's own life history. It helps a person identify the time and place when an event happened. *Semantic memory* is knowledge of facts and data that may not be related to any event. A veteran knowing that there was a Vietnam War in the 1970s is using semantic memory; remembering his experiences in that war—including emotional memories—is episodic memory.

It seems that procedural and declarative memories are stored differently. Studies of brain- damaged and amnesia victims show that they may still be perfectly capable of riding a bicycle (procedural) without remembering the word *bicycle* or when they learned to ride (declarative). Procedural and declarative memory seem to be stored in different regions of the brain, and declarative memory can be lost even though procedural is spared.

RETENTION

Retention is the process whereby long-term memory preserves a learning in such a way that the memory can be located, identified, and retrieved accurately in the future. This is an inexact process influenced by many factors, including the degree of student focus, the length and type of rehearsal that occurred, the critical attributes that may have been identified, the student's learning style, any learning disabilities, and, of course, the inescapable influence of prior learning. For all practical purposes, the capacity of the brain to store information is unlimited. That is, with about 100 billion neurons, each with thousands of dendrites, the number of potential neural pathways is incomprehensible. The healthy brain will never run out of space to store all that an individual learns in a lifetime.

Different parts of a memory are stored in various sites which reassemble when the memory is recalled.

Memories are not stored as a whole in one place. Different parts of a memory are stored in various sites, and they reassemble when the memory is recalled. These virtual assembly sites are sometimes referred to as *convergence zones*. Researchers believe that long-term memory is a dynamic, interactive system that activates storage areas distributed across the brain to retrieve and reconstruct memories (Squire and Kandel, 1999; Schacter, 2001).

Effects of Emotions on Memory and Retention

Any input from a person's environment that stimulates the limbic area will get high priority for processing. Highest priority goes to any situation interpreted as posing a threat to the survival of the individual. For example, data related to a burning odor, a snarling dog, or someone threatening bodily injury are processed immediately. Upon receiving the stimuli, the brain stem sends a rush of adrenaline throughout the brain, shutting down all unnecessary activity and directing the brain's attention to the source of the stimulus.

Emotional data also take high priority. When an individual responds emotionally to a situation, the older limbic system (stimulated by the amygdala) takes a major role and the complex cerebral processes are suspended. We have all had experiences when anger or fear of the unknown quickly overcame our rational thoughts. The resulting overriding of conscious thought can be strong enough to cause a temporary inability to talk ("I was dumbfounded") or move ("I froze"). This fear response occurs because the hippocampus is susceptible to stress hormones, which can inhibit cognitive functioning and long-term memory.

Under certain conditions, however, emotions can enhance memory by causing the release of hormones that stimulate the amygdala to signal brain regions to strengthen memory. Strong emotions can shut down conscious processing during the event while enhancing our memory of it. Emotion is a powerful and misunderstood force in learning and memory.

Implications for Teaching

How the learner processes new information presented in school has a great impact on the quality of what is learned and is a major factor in determining whether and how it will be retained. Memories, of course, are more than just information. They represent fluctuating patterns of associations and connections across the brain, from which the individual extracts order and meaning. Teachers with a greater understanding of the types of memory and how they form can select strategies that are more likely to improve the retention and retrieval of learning.

A good portion of the teaching done in schools centers on delivering facts and information to build concepts that explain a body of knowledge. We teach numbers, arithmetic operations, ratios, and theorems to explain mathematics. We teach about atoms, momentum, gravity, and cells to explain science. We talk about countries and famous leaders and discuss their trials and battles to explain history, and so on. Students may hold on to this information in working memory (a temporary memory) just long enough to take a test, after which the knowledge readily decays and is lost. Retention, however, requires that the learner not only give conscious attention but also build conceptual frameworks that have sense and meaning for eventual consolidation into long-term storage networks.

2

What Is a Gifted Brain?

Asking 50 people what is meant by giftedness is likely to produce 50 different definitions. Nonetheless, some common elements will emerge from most of the descriptions. These might include describing a person's aptitude in a specific subject area or a talent in the visual or performing arts, or in sports. Also mentioned might be creativity, inventiveness, or just plain "intelligent in everything." Descriptions of giftedness also vary from one culture to another. For example, in a culture with no formal schooling, a skilled hunter might be the gifted one. Gifted abilities are also more likely to emerge when the individual's talents coincide with what is valued by the culture. Chess prodigies, for example, appear in cultures where such talent is valued and nurtured. So it can be said that giftedness is what others in a society perceive to be higher or lower on some culturally embedded scale.

> **From one perspective, giftedness is what people in a society perceive to be higher or lower on some culturally embedded scale.**

THEORIES OF INTELLIGENCE AND GIFTEDNESS ■

In the 1950s, researchers and psychologists described giftedness mainly in terms of intelligence: high IQ was the same as gifted. Creativity and motivation were soon added as other characteristics of gifted performers. Consequently, as the push in schools for special programs for gifted students got underway, IQ tests became the primary screening vehicle for program selection. But IQ tests had their own problems. They assessed analytical and verbal skills but failed to measure practical knowledge and creativity, components critical to problem solving and success in life. Furthermore, the predictive abilities of IQ tests deteriorated once situations or populations changed. For example, research studies found that IQ tests predicted leadership skills when the tests were given under low-stress conditions. Under high-stress conditions, however, IQ was negatively related to leadership. In other words, it predicted the opposite.

It eventually became apparent that IQ tests were not a satisfactory measure of giftedness and that people could be gifted in different ways (e.g., academic areas, sports, performing arts, or in business ventures). Very few people are gifted in all areas. Paradoxically, some people can be gifted in some aspects of learning while displaying learning disorders in others (see Chapter 8). Clearly, relying on only one quantitative criterion (the IQ score) and maybe two qualitative criteria (creativity and motivation) was not adequate in the process of describing the collective and varied characteristics of gifted (and talented) people.

Revising the Definition of Giftedness

In an effort to challenge the notion that *giftedness* meant demonstrating high performance in nearly all areas of intellectual and artistic pursuit, Joseph Renzulli (1978) proposed his own definition. He suggested that it resulted from the interaction of three traits: general or specific abilities that were above average, commitment to task, and creativity. Later, he distinguished two types of gifted performance (Renzulli, 1986):

- Schoolhouse giftedness, which is characterized by the ease of acquiring knowledge and taking tests as demonstrated through high grades and high test scores, and
- Creative-productive giftedness, which involves creating new products and ideas designed to have an impact on a specific audience or field.

Renzulli's work stimulated school districts to include more opportunities for creative expression in their programs for gifted students.

Multiple Intelligences

During the 1980s, psychologists unleashed new and different models to describe intelligence. Harvard researcher Howard Gardner (1983) published a significant book suggesting that intelligence is not a unitary concept, that humans possess at least seven intelligences (recently, he added an eighth), and that an individual is predisposed to developing each of the intelligences to different levels of competence (Table 2.1). For Gardner, the intelligences represented ways of processing information and of thinking. He also suggested that the intelligences are the product of the interaction between genetic predisposition and the environment, a sort of nature-nurture combination that is not a question of either–or, but both–and. He selected an intelligence if it met the following eight criteria:

- Potential isolation by brain damage
- Existence of idiots savants, prodigies, and other exceptional individuals
- An identifiable core operation or set of core operations
- A distinctive developmental history, along with a definable set of expert "end-state" performances
- An evolutionary history and evolutionary plausibility
- Support from experimental psychological tasks
- Support from psychometric findings
- Susceptibility to encoding in a symbol system

According to Gardner, the intelligences are not the same as thinking style, which tends to remain consistent and independent of the type of information being processed. Rather, individuals at any given time use those intelligences which will allow them to solve specific problems, generate new problems, or create products or services of value to their particular culture. As the information and tasks change, other intelligences are called into action. One of Gardner's legacies is the oft-quoted aphorism, "Ask not how smart is the child, but how is the child smart?" Nevertheless, in this schema, *giftedness* can be defined as a child being exceptionally competent in one or more of Gardner's intelligences.

Table 2.1 Howard Gardner's Eight Intelligences

- **Bodily/Kinesthetic** - The capacity to use one's body to solve a problem, make something, or put on a production.
- **Naturalist** - The ability to discriminate among living things and sensitivity to other features of the natural world.
- **Logical/Mathematical** - The ability to understand logical systems and to manipulate numbers and quantities.
- **Musical/Rhythmic** - The capacity to think in music and to hear, remember, recognize, and manipulate patterns.
- **Verbal/Linguistic** - The capacity to use one's language (and other languages) to express oneself and understand others.
- **Visual/Spatial** - The ability to represent the spatial world internally in one's mind.
- **Interpersonal** - The ability to understand other people.
- **Intrapersonal** - The capacity to understand oneself.

Using Multiple Intelligences Theory With the Gifted

In the past two decades, the multiple intelligences (MI) theory has been used to promote all sorts of curricular and instructional changes in school systems across North America. Several curricular programs are almost exclusively based on MI. In his writings, Gardner (1983) has suggested that traditional measures for identifying gifted students rely too heavily on IQ tests that focus on linguistic and logical/mathematical skills. Consequently, schools are increasingly resorting to MI as an alternative means of identifying gifted students. However, the problem with this approach is deciding how to develop instruments that can measure each of the intelligences with reliability and validity. Some new instruments, such as those developed, by Udall and Passe (1993), show internal consistency with some student groups but not with others.

A few critics (Delisle, 1996) of using MI theory to identify gifted students point out that MI's appeal is its simplicity, convenience, and egalitarian theme. It focuses toward developing every learner's intelligence rather than the exceptionalities of the gifted. Consequently, MI has spawned "talent developers," who disregard the emotional element as well as important concepts, such as compassion, self-knowledge, and respect for others.

Other critics (White and Breen, 1998) caution that although MI may be appropriate for accommodating those children who are multiply gifted, it does not help them decide what to do and when to do it. It is their ability to reason and evaluate that allows them to make these decisions, not MI. White and Breen also question whether MI are intelligences or maybe talents or abilities, and if they remain constant during one's lifetime. Even though they lament that the use of the common word *intelligences* to describe all the abilities conceals some of the important differences among them, they commend MI theory for raising educators' awareness to the multiple talents of gifted children. Just the same, they continue, some education programs based on MI look more like entertainment and serve only to dilute the teaching of fundamental skills.

Educators need to be wary of the fad-like nature of some of the MI programs and recognize that, without further research support, they cannot depend on MI as a panacea for gifted education.

Although MI may be theoretically useful in identifying gifted and talented children, especially those from culturally diverse backgrounds, more empirical data are needed to help develop reliable measures for the identification process. Educators need to be wary of the fad-like nature of some of the MI programs and recognize that, without further research support, they cannot depend on MI as a panacea for gifted education.

Emotional Intelligence

No discussion of the different intelligences would be complete without mentioning Daniel Goleman's (1995) concept of emotional intelligence. His book summarized the breakthroughs in understanding the strong influence that emotions have as we grow and learn. Emotions interact with reason to determine how we view the world and to support or inhibit learning. According to Goleman, an individual who can use emotions effectively is likely to become a more successful and productive citizen.

Sternberg's Theories

The Triarchic Theory

Two years after Gardner's work appeared, Robert Sternberg (1985) at Yale proposed a theory that distinguishes three types of intelligence: analytical, creative, and practical. People with analytical intelligence (the analyzers) have abilities in analyzing, critiquing, and evaluating. Those who are creatively intelligent (the creators) are particularly good at discovering, inventing, and creating. By contrast, the practically intelligent (the practitioners) excel at applying, utilizing, and implementing. In this model, *intelligence* is defined by these three types of behavior, and *giftedness* results from the ability to perform the skills in one or more of these areas with exceptional accuracy and efficiency. According to Sternberg, various combinations of these three areas produce different patterns of giftedness (Figure 2.1). This concept was tested in several studies conducted by Sternberg and his colleagues. Students were assessed for their memory as well as their analytical, creative, and practical achievement. The results showed that those students who were taught in ways that best matched their achievement patterns outperformed those whose method of instruction was not a good fit for their pattern of abilities (Sternberg, Ferrari, Clinkenbeard, and Grigorenko, 1996; Sternberg, Griorenko, Jarvin, Clinkenbeard, Ferrari, and Torfi, 2000).

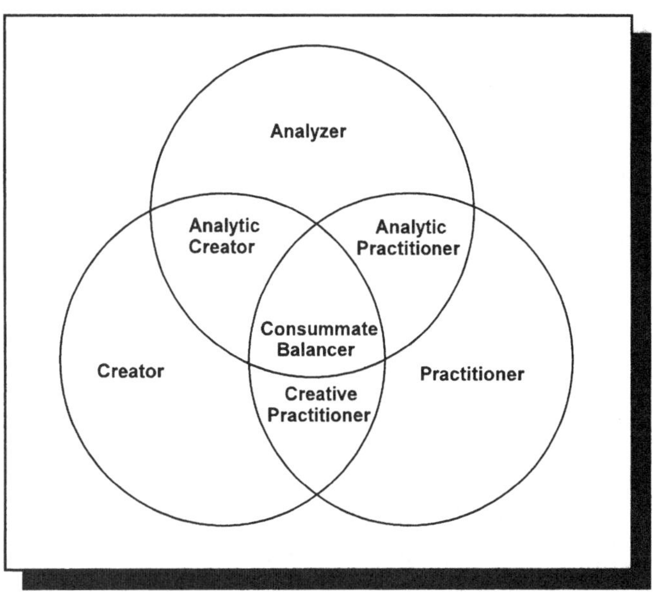

Figure 2.1 In Sternberg's model, the combinations of the three types of intelligence produce different patterns of giftedness.

The Pentagonal Implicit Theory of Giftedness

More recently, Sternberg (1995) has introduced another theory that describes a gifted person as one who meets the following five criteria:

Excellence. The individual is superior in some dimension or set of dimensions relative to peers.

- Rarity. The individual possesses a skill or attribute that is rare among peers.
- Productivity. The individual must produce something in the area of giftedness.
- Demonstrability. The skill or aptitude of giftedness must be demonstrable through one or more valid assessments.
- Value. The individual shows superior performance in a dimension that is valued by that person's society.

Sternberg's theory helps provide a basis for understanding why we call some people gifted and others not. He cautions, however, that although this theory can be helpful in identifying gifted individuals, it should be used in conjunction with other generally accepted assessment measures.

Even with all these theories, the definition of *giftedness* remains elusive. Yet, most of us recognize a gifted or talented person when we see one in action. We might wonder whether the person was born with those abilities, or whether their skills are the result of hard work, or both. As the trend toward moving away from using IQ measures to understand gifted individuals gained momentum, the question remained: What characteristics of a person should be measured instead? The many research studies designed to address this question can be categorized in various ways. One useful method, suggested by Robinson and Clinkenbeard (1998), sorts the studies into those looking either for psychological characteristics or social and emotional characteristics.

■ PSYCHOLOGICAL CHARACTERISTICS OF GIFTEDNESS

Thinking About Problems and About Thinking

Most of the research on the psychological characteristics of giftedness has focused on cognition and metacognition. In these studies, researchers observed how students identified as gifted thought through a given problem or situation (cognition), and how they reflected on their thinking throughout the problem-solving experience (metacognition).

Cognitive Strategies

Not surprisingly, the studies showed that gifted students acquired information and solved problems faster, better, or at earlier stages than other students. Some studies showed that higher IQ individuals had more efficient memories, more information- processing strategies, larger and more elaborately organized knowledge bases, and a better ability to solve mathematical problems by employing their own symbolic encoding (Robinson and Clinkenbeard, 1998).

Sternberg has also investigated how different thinking styles in gifted students affect their academic performance (Grigorenko and Sternberg, 1997). The study found that there were no differences in thinking styles among groups of students at different ability levels, and that certain thinking styles contributed significantly to prediction of academic performance. For example, the style that involved analyzing, grading, or comparing things had the highest predictive value. Further, this contribution was independent of the type of instruction the students were given. One other finding of interest was that the gifted students performed best on assessment procedures that closely matched their thinking style. (This last finding corroborates the results of decades of earlier research on different types of student learning styles.)

Metacognitive Strategies

Research studies in metacognition (i.e., thinking about one's own thinking) have focused around three aspects:

- What do students know about thinking strategies?
- Can they use the strategies?
- Can they monitor their own cognitive processing?

Gifted students may know more about metacognitive strategies but, surprisingly, do not use a wider variety of them. Nor do they monitor their strategies any more than other students.

Compared to other students, the studies showed that gifted students knew more about metacognitive strategies and could use them more easily in new contexts. However, a significant finding was that, contrary to popular beliefs, the gifted students did not use a wider variety of metacognitive strategies than other students, nor did they monitor their strategies any more than the other students (Alexander and Schwanenflugel, 1995; Carr, Alexander, and Schwanenflugel, 1996). Several researchers in this area caution that motivation and creativity may influence the results of studies on metacognition.

Neuroscientists—or more specifically, cognitive neuroscientists—also think about thinking. In recent years, they have explored what differences in the structure and functions of the gifted brain may allow it to achieve remarkable levels of performance. These researchers use many tools in their investigations, such as advanced imaging techniques, EEG, and MEG, to reveal similarities and differences in the function of high-performing brains compared with the brains of students showing no signs of the same kinds of giftedness. Here are some of their findings.

The Cortex

Any attempt to examine giftedness through the lens of neuroscience needs to begin with an understanding of the complexity and functional diversity of the brain. Of particular importance is the cortex, considered the brain's most advanced structure. In the history of our species, the cortex was the most recent part of the human brain to evolve, eventually developing two abilities that seem unique to humans: spoken language and cognitive thought. The cortex, you will recall, is the six-layer covering of the cerebrum that is divided into two hemispheres, each consisting of the frontal, temporal, parietal, and occipital lobes. Although the neurons in the cortex are heavily interconnected, certain regions in each lobe and hemisphere are organized into units that perform specific functions.

The Cerebral Hemispheres

Since the work of Roger Sperry in the 1960s (Sousa, 2001a), neuroscientists have accepted the notion that the two cerebral hemispheres are not mirror images of each other. That is, they differ structurally, biochemically, and functionally. In most people, for example, the right frontal lobe protrudes over, and is wider than, the left frontal lobe. The left occipital lobe (at the back of the brain) protrudes over, and is wider than, the right occipital lobe. The neurotransmitter norepinephrine is more prevalent in the right hemisphere, while dopamine is more prevalent in the left hemisphere. Estrogen receptors are more prevalent in the right hemisphere than in the left hemisphere.

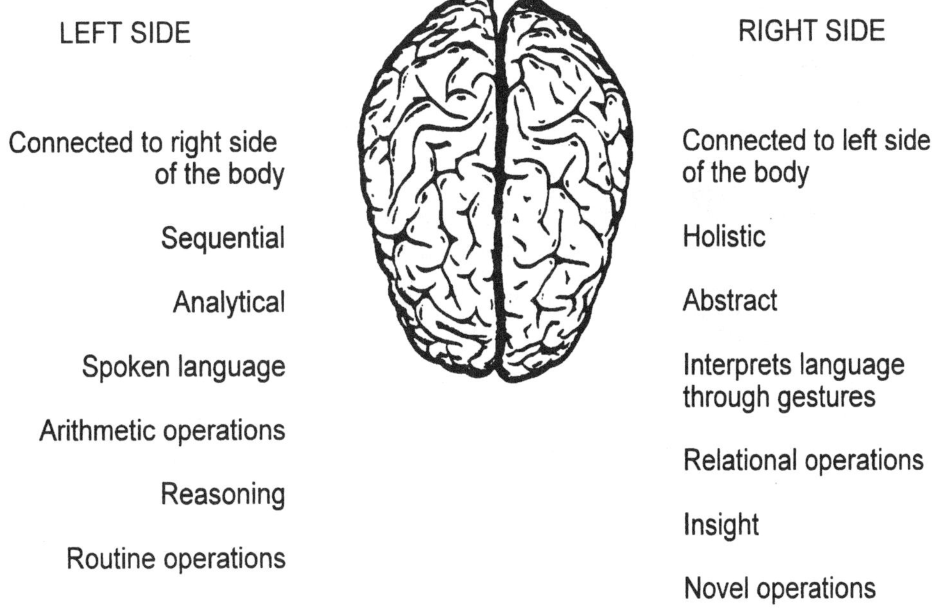

Figure 2.2 The left and right hemispheres of the human brain are specialized and process information differently.

As for brain functions, more evidence is accumulating that the brain has a much greater degree of specialization than was previously thought. Even so, because of advancements in neuroimaging, the earlier idea that the brain is a set of modular units carrying out specific tasks is giving way to a new model, which holds that moving across the cortical surface results in a gradual transition from one cognitive function to another. Goldberg (2001) refers to this as the "gradiental" view of brain organization. This view does not necessarily discard the notion that specific areas of the brain perform specific functions. Rather, it uses recent evidence from neurological studies to suggest a pattern of organization whereby the boundaries between the specific areas are fluid, not fixed. The ability of certain areas of the brain to perform unique functions is known as *lateralization* or *specialization* (Sousa, 2001a). Brain imaging scans and other studies reveal remarkable consistency in the way the two hemispheres store and process information (Figure 2.2).

Specialization and Learning

The two hemispheres of the brain communicate with each other through a tight bundle of about 200 million nerve cells called the *corpus callosum* (see Figure 1.2). Researchers have been particularly interested in how the specialized functions of each hemisphere affect new learning, and the degree to which they communicate

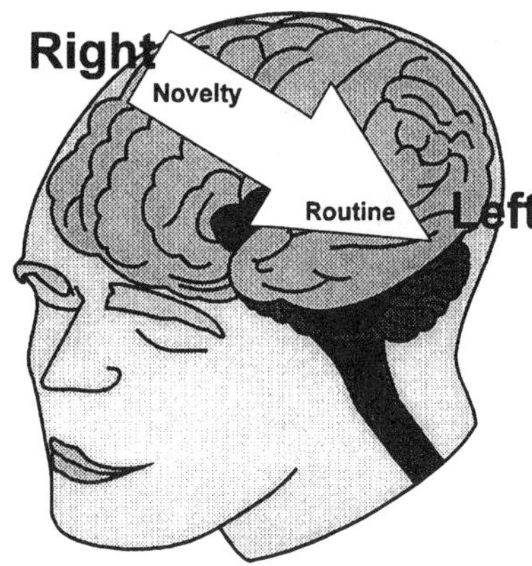

Figure 2.3 With repeated exposures, novel experiences become routine and their cortical processing areas shift from the right hemisphere to the left hemisphere.

with each other during that process. Early theories held that new learning occurs in the hemisphere mainly responsible for the functions associated with that learning. Thus, the left hemisphere would be largely involved in spoken language acquisition and sequential procedures, and the right side would support the learning of visual images and spatial relationships. These theories were based mainly on the results of tests done with patients who had damage to specific areas of the brain.

More recent research, however, lends credence to an alternative explanation. Goldberg (2001), for example, proposes that hemispheric specialization may center around the differences between novelty and routine. Closer examination of brain-damaged patients shows that those with severe right hemisphere problems experience difficulty in facing new learning situations, but can perform routine, practiced tasks (e.g., language) normally. Conversely, patients with severe left hemisphere damage can create new drawings and think abstractly, but have difficulty with routine operations.

Goldberg's notion gives us a different way of looking at how the brain learns. It suggests that upon encountering a novel situation for which the individual has no coping strategy, the right hemisphere is primarily involved and attempts to deal with the situation. With repeated exposure to similar situations, coping strategies eventually emerge and learning occurs because it results in a change of behavior. In time, and after sufficient repetition, the responses become routine and shift via the corpus callosum to the left hemisphere (Figure 2.3). The amount of time and the number of situational exposures needed to accomplish this right-to-left hemisphere transition vary widely from one person to the next. But it may be that one component of giftedness is the ability of that person's brain to make the transition in less time and with fewer exposures than average.

It may be that one component of giftedness is the brain's ability to make the transition from novelty to routine in less time and with fewer exposures than average.

Studies using neuroimaging provide evidence to support Goldberg's theory. In one study, researchers used PET scans to measure the changes in brain flow patterns when subjects were asked to learn various types of information. Changes in blood flow levels indicate the degree of neural activation. When the information was novel, regions in the right temporal lobe were highly activated. After the information had been presented several times to the subjects, activity in the right temporal lobe decreased dramatically (Figure 2.4). In both instances, however, the level of activation in the left temporal lobe remained constant (Martin, Wiggs, and Weisberg, 1997).

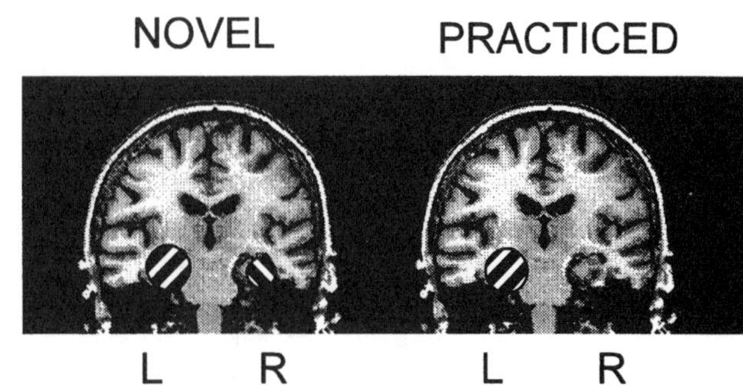

Figure 2.4 A representation of PET scans showing the changes in regional blood flow for novel and practiced tasks. The highlighted circles show areas of high activation in the left and right temporal lobes for novel tasks, but only in the left temporal lobe for practiced tasks.

Similar results were reported from other studies involving a variety of learning tasks, such as recognizing faces and symbols (Henson, Shallice, and Dolan, 2000), learning a complex motor skill (Shadmehr and Holcomb, 1997), and learning and relearning different systems of rules (Berns, Cohen, and Mintun, 1997). The same shifts were detected no matter what type of information was presented to the subjects. In other words, says Goldberg, the association of the right hemisphere with novelty and the left hemisphere with routine appears to be independent of the nature of the information being learned.

Language Functions in the Hemispheres

Although speech seems to be centered in regions of the left hemisphere, studies involving patients with brain lesions indicate that language functions are distributed across the brain. Damage to the rear part of the temporal lobe nearest to the occipital lobe causes the loss of nouns naming objects. On the other hand, damage to the frontal lobe can cause the loss of verbs. These observations suggest that words are closely associated in the brain with the objects or actions they represent, lending further support for the gradiental and not the modular pattern of organization of the cerebral cortex.

The Prefrontal Cortex

Cognitive thought and related activities are located in the foremost part of the frontal lobes, called the *prefrontal cortex*. This area comprises about 29 percent of the total cortex and is interconnected to every distinct functional region (Figure

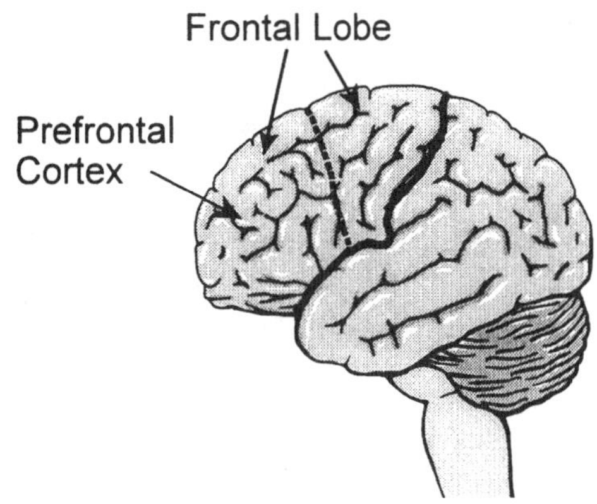

Figure 2.5 The entire area in front of the solid line is the frontal lobe. The area to the left of the dotted line is the general location of the prefrontal cortex.

2.5). Often called the executive control area, the prefrontal cortex is embedded in a rich network of neural pathways so that it can coordinate and integrate the functions of all areas. Like the conductor of an orchestra, the prefrontal cortex blends individual inputs from various regions of the brain into a comprehensive and comprehendible whole. Its interpretations ultimately define personality, and its decision-making abilities determine how successfully an individual copes with each day.

To accomplish this task, the prefrontal cortex must converge the inputs from within an individual with those from the outside world. The brain's organization facilitates this process. Sensory signals from the outside environment pass along the sensory nerves to the thalamus and are routed to other areas toward the back of the brain (reception). These inputs are then directed to specific sites in the parietal and temporal lobes, as well as in the limbic areas, for further analysis (integration). Finally, the frontal lobes combine this input with information from the individual's memory (interpretation) to determine what subsequent action, if any, should be taken (Figure 2.6).

The prefrontal cortex also seems to be strongly interested in task novelty. Several PET studies show that when processing new information, cerebral blood flow levels in the frontal lobes reached their highest levels. But when the subject became familiar with the task, frontal lobe involvement—as measured by blood flow—dropped significantly (Goldberg, 2001). If a somewhat different task was introduced, frontal lobe activation picked up once again. We noted before that the right hemisphere was more associated with novelty than the left. These findings infer that the frontal lobes are more closely aligned with the right hemisphere when dealing with novel learning situations.

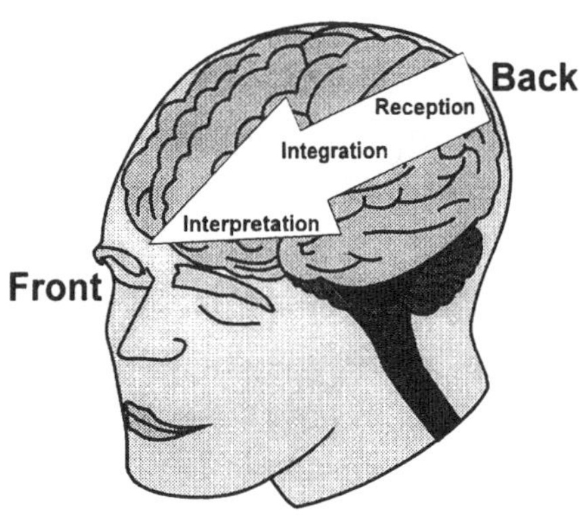

Figure 2.6 Stimuli from the outside world are received toward the rear of the brain, integrated in the center, and interpreted by the frontal lobes.

Decision Making

The prefrontal cortex faces many decisions in the course of a day. Some involve simple concrete problems, such as the following:

"What is my doctor's telephone number?"

"How much money is left in my savings account?"

"When is my nephew's birthday?"

Each question is clear and the situations require searching for a single, indisputable answer. This process is called *veridical decision making*, or finding the single, true answer.

I may be faced with other questions as well:

"Am I sick enough to see the doctor or should I wait a few days?"

"Should I use some of my savings to buy stocks or bonds?"

"What gift should I get for my nephew's birthday?"

These questions are ambiguous and have no intrinsically unique answer. I will choose the answer for a variety of reasons. My decision to see the doctor might depend on whether my body temperature rises or falls. Buying stocks or bonds might depend on where I think the stock market may be headed in the next year. In any event, my brain is engaging in *adaptive decision making,* that is, I adapt the decision on the basis of context and my priorities at the moment. At another time and place, my decision might be different.

Veridical decision making gets us through the day. Adaptive decision making gets us through life.

No one doubts that finely tuned veridical decision-making skills are valuable in certain technical occupations. But, life in general is fraught with ambiguities, and most critical decisions—personal and occupational—often require choosing from among equally valid options. Deciding among ambiguities is one of the most important functions of the prefrontal cortex. Studies show that individuals with damage to the prefrontal cortex have difficulty dealing with adaptive decision making, while damage to other parts of the brain does not seem to affect this process (Goldberg, 2001).

To be successful, we need to be competent in both types of skills. Veridical decisions help us get through the day: What time do I need to be at work and when is my first appointment? How much gasoline is in the car? Who's picking up the kids after practice? Adaptive decisions, on the other hand, get us through life: Is this the person I should marry? Is this the right job for me? When should we start a family?

Neural Efficiency

As mentioned in Chapter 1, when the frontal lobes gain more experience at making adaptive decisions and solving complex problems, neuronal pathways responsible for these processes should become more efficient and thus require less effort. Indeed, this concept—known as neural efficiency—has long been part of most theoretical models of the gifted brain. The idea is that gifted brains can perform tasks more quickly and accurately because they contain networks comprising neurons working together in vast arrays and with such efficiency that they require less cerebral energy than unorganized networks. One way to measure the level of brain activity is to monitor the pattern of waves produced by the brain's electrical activity. Obtaining experimental evidence to support this idea would require using EEG technology to measure the activity of the brain while it was performing different functions. Even though early attempts were inconclusive, advancements in EEG techniques have spurred new interest in studying this idea experimentally.

EEG Studies

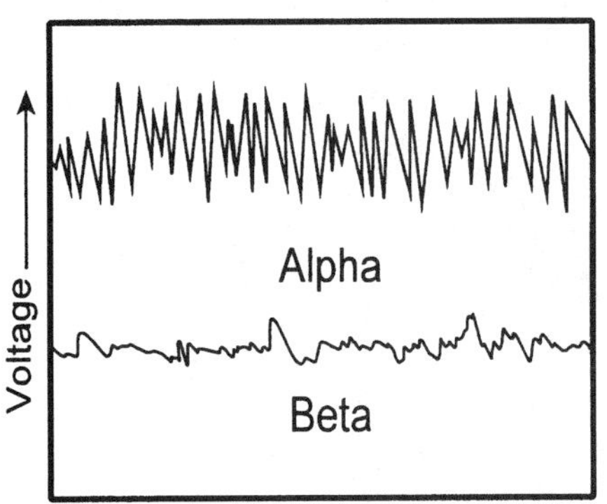

Figure 2.7 The diagram shows typical activity patterns of alpha and beta brain wave activity.

When using the EEG to detect brain functioning, two wave patterns are of particular interest: alpha waves (8-13 cycles per second) and beta waves (14-60 cycles per second). Neurobiologists theorize that alpha activity is the result of neurons firing together (in synchrony) and resting together—an indication of neural pathway efficiency. Thus, alpha activity produces high voltage, rhythmic, and sinusoidal patterns. The higher the amplitude of the alpha wave (called *alpha power*), the more efficiently the neurons are firing, resulting in less mental effort.

Beta waves, on the other hand, result from the activity of neurons that are doing different things at different times (asynchrony), producing a low voltage, irregular pattern (Figure 2.7). Beatty (2001) offers the analogy of a marching band. When the band members are marching in synchrony, their footsteps are a loud beat with silence between the steps. But as the band members disperse after the march, one hears the constant sound of many steps at random intervals.

Norbert Jausovec (2000) used EEG to study the differences in brain activity during problem solving in about 50 young adults who were separated into four groups based on their intelligence (average or high) and creativity (average or high). On the basis of their scores on various assessment measures, Jausovec placed them into the categories of intelligent, gifted, creative, and average (Figure 2.8). He then measured their alpha wave activity as they were solving closed problems (i.e., requiring convergent and logical thinking) and creative problems (i.e., requiring more adaptive decision making). His findings were threefold:

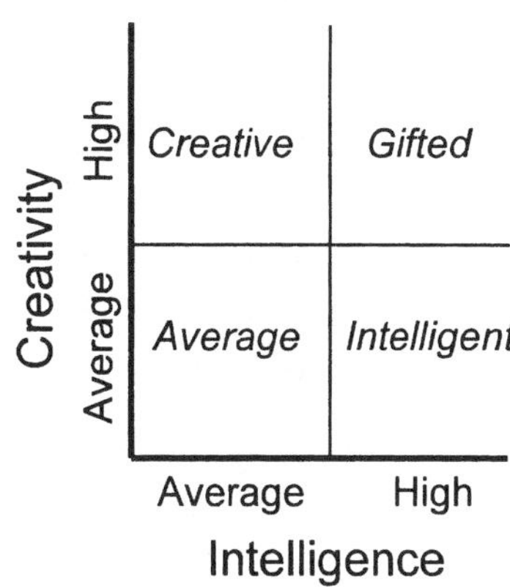

Figure 2.8 Jausovec's system for classifying subjects for the EEG study based on level of creativity and intelligence.

- Alpha wave activity showed that high IQ individuals (gifted and intelligent) used less mental effort than the average IQ individuals (creative and average) when solving closed problems.
- Alpha wave activity showed that high creative individuals (creative and gifted) used less mental effort than average creative individuals (intelligent and average) when engaged in creative problem solving.
- Creative individuals showed more cooperation among brain areas than did gifted ones, who showed greater decoupling of brain areas when solving ill-defined problems.

These results first suggest that when individuals are solving problems in their area of strength, less mental effort is needed so the alpha power is high, an indication of neural efficiency. Second, the results appear to support the concept that creativity and intelligence are different abilities that involve different areas of the cortex while solving closed or creative problems. This finding enhances the position of those who urge that creativity be considered as a separate measure of giftedness.

Creativity and intelligence are different abilities that involve different areas of the cerebral cortex while solving problems.

Implications for Schools

Far too frequently, what is taught in schools emphasizes veridical, rather than adaptive decision making. Most course work—and the resulting tests—ask students to search for the unique answers to concrete and unambiguous questions. Some students adapt to this strategy quickly and excel at veridical decision making. As a result, their test scores are high, and they may even be considered gifted. However, when faced with ambiguous problems, they often vacillate and become indecisive. Seldom do schools offer students consistent opportunities to develop adaptive decision-making skills. Instead, these are acquired individually, through trial and error.

With such emphasis on veridical decision making in schools, one wonders what happens to students who favor adaptive decision making. Do they get bored easily and act out or become withdrawn? Do they get frustrated if teachers insist they find only the unique answer? Are there areas in the curriculum where they can excel with their adaptive skills? Is it possible that those students who prefer adaptive decision making will seem different from the rest of the class? Is it also possible that a high aptitude in adaptive decision making is a characteristic of the gifted brain?

Is it possible that a high aptitude in adaptive decision making is a characteristic of the gifted brain?

Given the appropriate adjustments in curriculum, most students can be taught to improve their adaptive decision-making skills. This process involves helping students to make connections and to discover relationships between the new learning and what they already know. One valuable strategy for accomplishing this is the frequent use of elaborative rehearsal.

The Overlooked Role of Visual-Spatial Abilities

For decades, general intelligence has been measured largely by one's ability to handle verbal skills through language manipulation. Yet, there is mounting evidence that visual-spatial abilities may play just as important a role as language to indicate general intelligence. Recent studies have been able to correlate visual-spatial abilities with the brain's executive functions, which, you will recall, reside in the frontal lobes.

One major study tested 167 participants on a variety of tasks to determine their ability to solve visual-spatial problems, to temporarily store visual-spatial information, and to measure their brain's executive functioning. The study found the following:

- Participants who were good at solving complex visual-spatial problems displayed superior executive functions.
- Executive functioning had the strongest correlation with spatial visualization.
- Executive functioning had the lowest correlation with perceptual speed (the ability to match simple shapes).

In sum, participants who were better visualizers and who solved visual-spatial problems quickly had stronger executive function, even if they had slow perceptual speed. The researchers felt that these findings made sense because spatial visualization is a complex cerebral operation, requiring substantial frontal lobe resources (Miyake, Friedman, Rettinger, Shah, and Hegarty, 2001).

Implications

Because traditional IQ tests are more verbally oriented, it is easy for visual-spatial intelligence to be discounted. Individuals with strong visual-spatial abilities are often not even identified in schools as gifted. But this study highlights the relationships between visual-spatial abilities and executive functions, thereby contributing to our emerging and broader view of intelligence as multifaceted.

EFFECT OF NURTURE ON INTELLIGENCE

As mentioned earlier, psychologists long believed that an individual's intelligence was determined primarily by the genetic code. Little credence was given to the notion that the child's environment could have any major or lasting impact on overall intelligence. Today, our view of intelligence is quite different. Few cognitive neuroscientists dispute the substantial impact that environment can have on a child's intellectual development. Intellectual skills once thought to be innate seem instead to be very sensitive to a person's environment.

Intelligence can be affected by
- ★ Well-designed daycare
- ★ School attendance
- ★ Breast-feeding
- ★ Diet

Thus, IQ can be modified—up or down—by the child's environment. Well-designed day-care programs, for example, can provide the mental stimulation that young brains need during this period of rapid neural growth. Stephen Ceci (2000) has suggested that the following environmental factors can affect IQ:

- *School Attendance.* Staying in school can elevate IQ above what it would be if the student dropped out. For each year of schooling completed, there is an IQ gain of approximately 3.5 points. This indicates that other factors besides heredity are at work in shaping intelligence.
- *Breast-Feeding.* Despite skepticism over initial reports that breast-fed children grew into adults with higher IQs than siblings who were not breast-fed, more controlled studies, according to Ceci, continue to indicate a three to eight point IQ gain for breast-fed children by age 3. No one knows for sure why, however. It may be that the immune factors in mother's milk boost the infant's immune system, making it less prone to contract diseases that could affect learning. Mother's milk also contains high quantities of omega-3 fatty acids, which are used to build nerve cell membranes as well as the myelin that protects the impulses moving along the neuron.
- *Diet.* Nutritional researchers have long suspected that some of the substances added to today's food can affect brain development. Because controlled studies in this area using human children would be unethical, other types of data analysis are used. Ceci refers to one large-scale study of about 1 million students in the New York City schools, researchers found that IQ scores increased 14 percent after dyes, colorings, preservatives, and artificial flavorings were removed from the lunch food. Further, the weakest students showed the greatest improvement. Researchers also noted that the number of students who were performing two or more grade levels below average had dropped, from 120,000 before the dietary changes to 50,000 afterward.

Scientists are now starting to define the kinds of environmental stimuli that can promote (or delay) intellectual development in children.

Birth Order, Family Size, and Intelligence

The relationship between birth order, family size, and intelligence has been the subject of many research studies. Some articles have suggested that birth order and larger families expose an individual to environmental conditions that influence intellectual abilities. However, the results of a longitudinal study indicate that although low-IQ parents have been making larger families, larger families do not make low-IQ children. Further, the connection between birth order and intelligence seems to be unfounded (Rodgers, Cleveland, van den Oord, and Rowe, 2000).

SOCIAL AND EMOTIONAL CHARACTERISTICS OF GIFTEDNESS ■

Social Characteristics

Despite stories that often circulate in schools about gifted students being loners, surveys indicate that preadolescent and adolescent gifted students were at least as popular as other students their age, and most gifted students felt good about themselves and their relationships with peers. However, highly gifted students had more difficulty with the peer relationships and often developed coping strategies to deal with such circumstances (Mayseless, 1993). Swiatek (1995) found that the three most frequent coping strategies used by highly gifted students were denial of giftedness, popularity/conformity, and peer acceptance. There were no gender differences in the use of the strategies. Students more highly gifted in mathematical talents reported more peer acceptance than students who were gifted predominantly in verbal skills. It may be that verbally gifted students are more obvious to their peers and, therefore, they may feel more different.

Highly gifted adolescents
- **Often deny their giftedness**
- **Want to conform**
- **Seek popularity and peer acceptance**

A more recent study of over 220 gifted and nongifted high school freshmen found that gifted students perceived themselves as being more intimate with friends and assuming fewer family responsibilities. The gifted group also took more sports-related and danger-related risks than nongifted students. Furthermore, gifted students reported feeling that they were the same as or better than their peers in social skills, and, coincidently, their teachers agreed (Field, Harding, Yando, Gonzalez, Lasko, Bendell, and Marks, 1998).

Theory of Mind in Social Situations

Other studies also tend to show that some gifted adolescents and young adults can be very successful in social as well as intellectual situations. Is there some relationship between this capability and the brain functions of gifted individuals? One possible explanation is that a social relationship involves not only understanding how you would react in a given situation, but also forming a judgment about how the other person would think and act. In effect, you form an internal representation of that person's mental processes, what some call a "theory of mind." The more successful you are at predicting the other person's reactions and choices in a given social situation, the more likely you are to select a behavioral response that will make the interaction successful. This insight into other people's mental states is far more complicated than merely solving a puzzle, and the degree of its mastery is a reliable measure of social skills.

Emotional Characteristics

Numerous studies on the emotional, personality, and motivational characteristics of gifted students have yielded similar results. In general, the studies showed that, when compared to average students, gifted students

- Were at least as well or somewhat better adjusted
- Possessed more personality traits considered to be favorable
- Displayed personality traits similar to older students
- Had lower levels of anxiety about school
- Scored higher on measures of self-concept
- Displayed higher levels of intrinsic motivation and autonomy, especially for reading, thinking, and solitude

Some gender and age differences have been noted. For example, gifted high school girls had significantly less self-confidence, more perfectionism, and more discouragement than younger gifted girls. Gifted high school boys, however, felt less discouragement than younger boys, and there were no age differences in self-confidence and perfectionism. High school girls scored higher on discouragement than high school boys (Robinson and Clinkenbeard, 1998).

Although the studies present a useful profile, it is important to remember that some groups of gifted students will look quite different. For example, gifted students who are underachievers, and those whose talents are very far from the norm, are more likely to have difficulty fitting in socially and emotionally with their peers (see Chapter 7).

Frontal Lobe and Emotional Maturity

Why is it that many gifted students seem to be emotionally more mature than other students of the same age? Part of the answer may lie in the difference between the rate of maturation of the frontal lobes and the cerebral areas associated with emotions—the limbic area. You will recall from the previous chapter that the limbic area is located deep within the brain between the two temporal lobes where it generates, interprets, and stores emotional messages. Neurobiologists estimate that the limbic area matures (i.e., is fully functional) by the age of 10 to 12 years.

Maturity of a brain structure can be determined by measuring the amount of myelin covering the axons in the neural pathways. As structures become fully myelinated, nerve impulses can move along the pathways efficiently, making communication between various regions of the brain faster and more reliable.

Complete myelination of the frontal lobes takes a lot longer than for the limbic region, occurring for most individuals around the age of 18 to 20 years. This is because the frontal lobes have to communicate with all areas of the brain, and it takes time for the more distant pathways to be established and fully myelinated. One of the functions of the frontal lobes, you may recall, is to control the excesses of our emotions. We have all experienced situations in which our impulses could easily have got out of control if the frontal lobes had not reined them in. The approximate 8-year time lag between the full maturity of the limbic region and the frontal lobes is largely responsible for the impulsive, high-risk behavior that is typical of most adolescents. Field and her colleagues (1998) found that gifted high school students do engage in high-risk behavior. However, she suggested that this finding may be because, as gifted children, they may have had earlier psychological separation from their parents and greater intimacy with peers. Thus, as adolescents, their distance from parents, association with peers, and a self-perception of social maturity may increase their desire and need to take more risks.

For highly intelligent adolescents, it is possible that faster myelination in the frontal lobes may lead to earlier maturation of that area.

But neuroscience may provide us with another possible explanation as to why gifted students display more mature behavior and decision-making skills than other students of the same age. It may be that the greater frontal lobe volume found in more intelligent individuals (Thompson, et al., 2001) indicates that faster and more widespread myelination is occurring in those brains, thereby leading to earlier maturation of the frontal lobes. Supporting evidence for this concept may come from an EEG study that measured different alpha wave activity in 30 gifted adolescents, 30 average ability adolescents, and 30 college-age subjects. When given a series of cognitive tasks to complete, the overall alpha wave levels of the 30 gifted adolescents more closely matched that of the college-age subjects than the alpha levels of the average ability adolescents. These findings suggest that the gifted adolescents may have a more enhanced state of brain development than their average ability peers (Alexander, O'Boyle, Benbow, 1996).

GENDER DIFFERENCES

One always has to tread lightly when suggesting that males and females are different. No one disputes the obvious biological and anatomical differences that exist between the sexes. However, people often misinterpret discussions of differences in how the genders think or act to mean that one gender is inferior to another. This is not the case here. The intent is to present some valid observations from cognitive neuroscience to support the self-evident notion that males and females, in general, look at life through different lenses and approach decision making with specific gender-related preferences.

Differences in Cognitive Styles

Years of anecdotal studies, learning styles research, and real-life experiences seem to indicate that male and female brains do not think alike. Television programs, best-seller books, and even standup comedians have all tried to demonstrate and explain the different ways males and females deal with solving daily problems and arriving at important decisions. Much of the early research on male-female differences focused on veridical decision making and on the acquisition of specific skills. For instance, studies suggested that males were better at visual-spatial skills and at mathematics and that females were better at learning language. Until recently, little research was done to examine each gender's general approach to adaptive decision making and problem solving, better indicators of cognitive style.

Now, neuroscience is joining the fray by offering new evidence that male and female brains are generally different in structure, in basic biochemistry, and in cognitive style. In studies on cognitive problem solving, males tended to be more *context-dependent*, that is, they changed their choice of answer depending on how the type of question changed. Females, on the other hand, were far more *context-independent*, that is, they made their choices based on a stable set of preferences, regardless of the changes in the question type (Goldberg, 2001).

In terms of cognitive style, more males prefer a context-dependent approach and more females prefer a context-independent approach.

People who are context-dependent tend to size up the problem at hand and then tailor a response that is appropriate to the specific context. In a new situation, a different choice is made, depending again on the new context. In Goldberg's example, a context-dependent person would vary the amount put into a savings account each month, depending on that month's income. By contrast, context-independent people tend to seek solutions that can apply across a number of different situations. When the context changes, little or no change in response is usually required. Here, a context-independent individual is likely to save the same amount each month, regardless of variations in monthly income. Neither strategy works better in all situations, and few people stick entirely to just one strategy. Nonetheless, although most people can move between the two strategies at will, more males prefer context-dependence and more females prefer context-independence.

Other studies have found that, when trying to exit a virtual 3-D maze, women activated the right parietal cortex and right prefrontal cortex, but that men triggered only the left hippocampus. When viewing emotionally disturbing images, women activated the amygdala on the left side, but men activated the right side. All of these findings lead to an obvious question: Can the gender differences in decision-making strategies be explained through gender differences in brain structure and brain biochemistry?

Differences in Brain Structure and Biochemistry

The male brain is about 10 percent larger than the female brain. One major difference in brain structure between the genders relates to the thickness of the cerebral cortex covering the frontal lobes. In males, the right frontal lobe cortex is thicker than the left, and in females, the cortical thickness is about the same for both frontal lobes. The corpus callosum tends to be proportionally thicker and denser in females than in males. Biochemical differences are also found. Estrogen receptors are distributed symmetrically across the frontal lobes in females, but asymmetrically in males. Gender differences also exist in the prevalence of neurotransmitter pathways—especially dopamine and norepinephrine—in the two lobes.

Given these variances, it is highly probable that the frontal lobes of males and females function differently. It is also highly probable that the left frontal lobe is functionally different from the right frontal lobe and that these differences are greater in male brains than in female brains. This may be because the female's proportionally larger corpus callosum allows for greater integration of functions (and less differentiation) between the cortical hemispheres than in males. In other words, most female brains are better at communicating *between* hemispheres, while most male brains are better *within* hemispheres.

Several recent MRI studies found that the volume of the cerebral hemispheres in most females was symmetrical, but the volume was not symmetrical in most males. The parietal lobe was significantly larger in males than in females. On tests of cognitive performance, the females outperformed males on verbal tasks, while males did better than females on visual and spatial tasks (Gur, Turetsky, Matsui, Yan, Bilker, Hughett, and Gur, 1999; Frederikse, Lu, Aylward, Barta, and Pearlson, 1999). Although researchers in learning styles observed similar results long before the advent of MRI, these imaging studies support the idea that differences in cognitive performance are related, at least in part, to differences in brain structure.

Another area where gender differences in brain architecture seem to matter is in the processing of language. When doing phonological processing, fMRI scans showed that although both sexes carried out the task with equal speed and accuracy, males activated the left temporal lobe's speech center (Broca's area), which is involved in the processing of speech, while females activated both the left and right temporal regions (see Figure 2.9). This observation helps to explain why a left hemisphere stroke often results in speech problems in men but less so in women (Shaywitz, Shaywitz, and Gore, 1995).

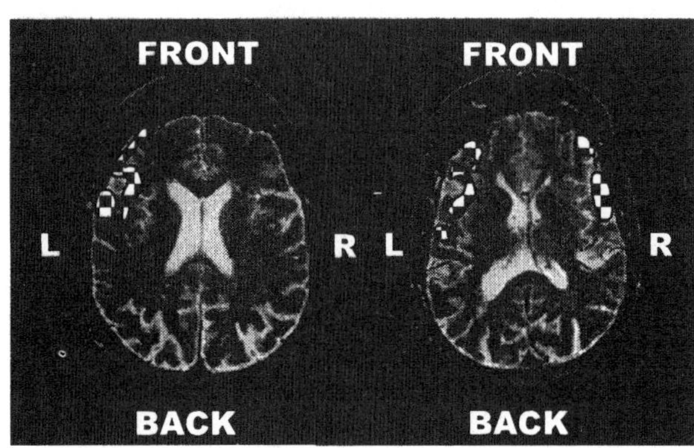

Figure 2.9 While processing phonetic language, fMRI scans show that male brains (left) use left hemisphere regions and that female brains (right) activate regions in both hemispheres (checkered areas).

■ IMPACT OF PRAISE ON GIFTED STUDENTS

Gifted children should be commended for their good grades and high test scores. However, recent research seems to indicate that excessively complimenting children for their intelligence and academic performance may lead them to believe that good test scores and high grades are more important than learning and mastering something new (Mueller and Dweck, 1998). Six studies of 412 fifth-graders compared the goals and achievement behaviors of children praised for intelligence with those praised for effort and hard work under conditions of failure as well as success. Through their studies, the psychologists demonstrated that commending children for their intelligence after good performance might backfire by making them highly performance-oriented and thus extremely vulnerable to the effects of subsequent setbacks. In contrast, children who are commended for their effort concentrate on learning goals and strategies for achievement.

The researchers also observed that children who were commended for their ability when they were successful learned to believe that intelligence is a fixed trait that cannot be developed or improved. The children who were explicitly commended after their successes were the ones who blamed poor performances on their own lack of intelligence. However, when children praised for their hard work performed poorly, they blamed their lack of success on poor effort and demonstrated a clear determination to learn strategies that would enhance subsequent performances.

Studies show that children who are praised for their intelligence learn to value performance, while children praised for their effort and hard work value opportunities to learn.

The studies demonstrated that children who are praised for their intelligence learn to value performance, while children praised for their effort and hard work value learning opportunities. Virtually all of the findings were similar not only for boys and girls but also among children from several different ethnic groups in rural and urban communities.

These findings may also explain why bright young girls who do well in grade school often perform poorly in upper grades. In their desire to bolster young girls' confidence in their abilities, educators have praised them for their intelligence which, these studies have shown, could have an undesired impact on their subsequent motivation and performance.

Labeling children as gifted or talented too soon may also have a negative impact on them. Such labeling may cause the children to become overly concerned with justifying that label and less concerned with meeting challenges that enhance their learning and mastery skills. They may begin to believe that academic setbacks indicate that they do not deserve to be labeled as gifted. The researchers advised that gifted and talented programs should emphasize how to meet challenges, apply effort, and search for new learning strategies. Furthermore, when students succeed, attention and approval should be directed at their effort and hard work rather than for the final product or their ability.

APPLICATIONS

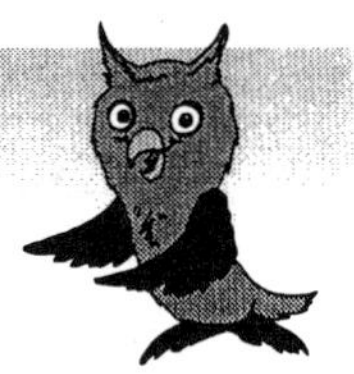

USING ELABORATIVE REHEARSAL

Rehearsal refers to the learner's reprocessing of new information in an attempt to determine sense and meaning. It occurs in two forms. Some information items have value only if they are remembered *exactly* as presented, such as the letters and sequence of the alphabet, spelling, poetry, telephone numbers, notes and lyrics of a song, and the multiplication tables. This is called *rote rehearsal.* Sense and meaning are established quickly, and the likelihood of long-term retention is high. Most of us can recall poems and telephone numbers that we learned years ago.

More complex concepts require the learner to make connections and to form associations and other relationships in order to establish sense and meaning. Thus, the information will need to be reprocessed several times as new links are found. This is called *elaborative rehearsal.* The more senses that are used in this elaborative rehearsal, the more reliable the associations. Thus, when visual, auditory, and kinesthetic activities assist the learner during rehearsal, the probability of long-term storage rises dramatically. That is why it is important for students to talk about what they are learning *while* they are learning it, and to have visual models as well.

Elaborative rehearsal can also develop adaptive decision-making skills because students will have more opportunities to make new connections and to see relationships that would otherwise not be possible through rote rehearsal.

Rehearsal is teacher-initiated and teacher-directed. Much of what students practice in schools is rote rehearsal. Recognizing the value of elaborative rehearsal as a necessary ingredient for retention of learning, teachers should consider the following when designing and presenting their lessons:

Elaborative Rehearsal Strategies

- ***Paraphrasing***. Students orally restate ideas in their own words, which then become familiar cues for later storage. Using the auditory modality helps the learner attach sense, making retention more likely.

- ***Selecting and Note Taking***. Students review texts, illustrations, and lectures, deciding which portions are critical and important. They

USING ELABORATIVE REHEARSAL— Continued

make these decisions on the basis of criteria from the teacher, authors, or other students. Students then paraphrase the idea and write it into their notes. Adding the kinesthetic exercise of writing furthers retention.

- *Predicting*. After studying a section of content, the students predict the material to follow or what questions the teacher might ask about that content. Prediction keeps students focused on the new content, adds interest, and helps them apply prior learnings to new situations, thus aiding retention.

- *Questioning*. After studying content, students generate questions about the content. To be effective, the questions should range from lower-level thinking of recall, comprehension, and application to higher-level thinking of analysis, synthesis, and evaluation. When designing questions of varying complexity, students engage in deeper cognitive processing, clarify concepts, predict meaning and associations, and examine options—all contributors to retention and to improving adaptive decision-making skills.

- *Summarizing*. Students reflect on and summarize in their heads the important material or skills learned in the lesson. This is often the last and critical stage, in which students can attach sense and meaning to the new learning.

3

Challenging the Gifted Brain

Understanding the nature of the gifted brain is one thing; deciding how to help it learn is quite another. Addressing the needs of gifted students can occur in different classroom settings, using a variety of curriculum resources and teaching strategies and having expectations of specific student products that demonstrate learning. As for classroom settings, elementary and middle school students identified as gifted might participate in a special pull-out class, and high school students can opt for advanced placement courses. But apart from these limited choices, most gifted students—except for those few with extraordinarily abilities—will get their learning opportunities in the normal school setting. Consequently, this chapter examines some considerations for selecting curriculum content, choosing teaching strategies, and deciding on the learning products of gifted students in the regular classroom.

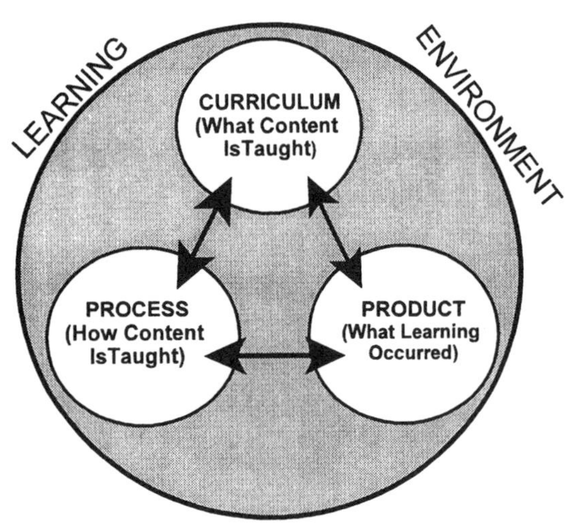

Figure 3.1 The diagram shows the relationship between the elements of curriculum, process, and product and their setting within the learning environment (dark circle).

Figure 3.1 illustrates the relationship between the elements of curriculum, process, and product and their setting within the total learning environment. Curriculum identifies *what is being taught* as well as the classroom structures and environment in which the teaching occurs. Process refers to *how the curriculum is taught*, that is, the teaching strategies and resulting learning behaviors that are used in the classroom during the teaching/learning episode. Product describes the various ways students can demonstrate *what they have learned.* Of course, there will be some overlap among the three components, and the learning environments affect all three. But the essential areas focus on what and where material is taught (curriculum), the teacher (process), and the student (product).

DIFFERENTIATED CURRICULUM AND LEARNING ■

Because most gifted students—especially in elementary and middle school—will be taught primarily in the regular classroom, teachers need to find ways to differentiate the learning experiences for these students.

- Differentiating the curriculum means moving students beyond grade-level standards or connecting what is taught to their personal interests.
- Differentiating the processes means using the learning strategies that provide depth and complexity appropriate to the students' abilities.
- The products are differentiated in that they demonstrate student learning at an advanced level, going beyond paper-and-pencil tests and allowing students to develop their talents and curiosities and to present their findings to an appropriate audience.
- Differentiating the learning environment means allowing students to work more independently on their own projects, collaborate with other students, or pursue interests outside the regular classroom (Winebrenner, 2000).

Gifted students are expected to learn the same basic concepts, facts, issues, and skills as all other students. However, they make connections faster, work well with abstractions, and generally have the deep interests found in older individuals. Consequently, they need to work with the curriculum at higher instructional levels, at a faster pace, and using a variety of materials appropriate for their learning style.

Federal regulations and those of most states require that school districts establish curriculum modifications to meet the needs of students identified as gifted. (Federal regulations on educational programs can be found on the Internet at: *http://www.ed.gov/legislation/FedRegister.*) However, the standards movement will be of little value if it does not respond to the needs of all students, including the gifted. The standards need to be flexible so that gifted students can be assured access to a stimulating, rich, and thought-provoking curriculum. Furthermore, standardized tests should not be the primary means for measuring student achievement. A wide range of assessment tools, e.g., journals, learning logs, self-evaluation questionnaires, interviews, and portfolios, are likely to yield more accurate information about how much a student has learned. To assist districts in deciding what those modifications should be, the National Association for Gifted Children (NAGC) has published standards for pre-K through grade 12 gifted programs. Specifically, the standards suggest (NAGC, 1998) that

- Curriculum for the gifted learner should be differentiated and span grades pre-K through 12.
- Regular classroom curricula must be adapted, modified, or replaced to meet the needs of the gifted.
- The pace of instruction must be flexible to allow for the accelerated learning of the gifted.
- Gifted students must be allowed to skip subjects and grades.
- Gifted learners must have opportunities that provide a variety of curriculum options, instructional approaches, and resources.

Exactly how to best address the different learning styles and needs of the gifted has been a question that schools have pondered for years. Some schools offer pull-out programs at the elementary and middle school levels, where gifted children can interact with their peers for a set time period. But for budgetary and philosophical reasons, schools in recent years have been moving away from pull-out programs and toward providing enrichment services to all students in the regular classroom environment. Some researchers in gifted education are alarmed at this trend, fearing that gifted students will not be appropriately challenged in this format.

Teachers need to establish a flexible learning environment and differentiate the curriculum so that gifted students will be challenged rather than bored.

The reality is that, as budgetary reductions take their toll on pull-out programs for the gifted, an increasing number of these elementary and middle school students will have to get their needs met in their regular classroom. To accomplish this successfully, teachers need to establish a flexible learning environment and differentiate the curriculum content so that gifted students will be challenged rather than bored.

A SUPPORTIVE LEARNING ENVIRONMENT ■

Teaching gifted students in an inclusive classroom requires a flexible and supportive learning climate that encompasses both the physical setting of the classroom and its climate. The teacher maintains a challenging environment by encouraging responsibility and autonomy, emphasizing student strengths, and addressing individual student needs.

Classroom Organization and Management

To organize the classroom for flexibility and openness, the teacher provides space for students to work independently and in small groups. Students may move around the room freely as long as they remain on task. They may also go to the computer lab, library, or other in-school location, if appropriate. In this setting, the teacher's role changes from presenting the curriculum to selecting and creating learning opportunities, guiding students, and assessing their progress. Students are given choices and allowed to schedule their activities, at least for part of the classroom time. Of course, students are still responsible for completing specific activities or periodically demonstrating what they have learned. However, they can choose how and when they will work.

Social and Emotional Climate

A positive learning environment includes the elements of safety and acceptance. Teachers create this atmosphere by modeling care and respect for all members of the classroom, emphasizing every student's strengths. All students need to recognize and appreciate their own strengths and those of others. Acceptance is a particularly important component of classroom climate because gifted learners are prone to being perfectionists and thus place great emphasis on completing a task quickly and getting the right answer. Their unusual abilities may make them outsiders among their classmates, or they may be accustomed to having a higher status than others in the classroom.

Gifted students sometimes feel insecure when presented with problem-solving activities or open-ended inquiry. They want to know the procedures that will ensure that they do it the right way. Here the teacher needs to remind these students that mistakes are an important part of the learning process and that there may be several "right" ways to solve a problem.

Not all gifted students like to display or explain their work. Some see this as redundant or as slowing them down. Teachers need to assure students that explaining how they got an answer is as important as being correct. Using a scoring guide or rubric may help these students recognize the value of the steps used to work through a problem.

CURRICULUM CONTENT INITIATIVES FOR GIFTED LEARNERS

Gifted students need to work at higher instructional levels and at a faster pace than non-gifted students. Several initiatives have emerged to enhance content within the context of the self-contained classroom as well as within the middle and high school curricular formats. Numerous studies in recent years have investigated the impact of these initiatives on student performance, the extent of which is assessed by a statistical measure known as *effect size*.

A Note About Research and Effect Sizes

One way to measure the impact of an educational strategy on student achievement is with a statistical measure known as *effect size* (ES). It is determined by dividing the standard deviation of the control group into the difference between the mean scores of the treatment and control groups.

$$\text{Effect Size} = \frac{\text{(Mean of Treatment Group)} - \text{(Mean of Control Group)}}{\text{Standard Deviation of Control Group}}$$

An effect size of 0.25 or greater is considered educationally significant. In classroom terms, an effect size of 1.00 is approximately equal to one school year. Thus, if a study found an effect size of 0.33, it would mean that the treatment group outperformed the control group by 1/3 of a school year, or about 3 grade-equivalent school months of additional achievement.

In the following sections, references are made to effect size results if they are available. (For more information on effect size, see Glass, McGaw, and Smith, 1981.)

Acceleration

Acceleration assumes that different students of the same age are at different levels of learning. This requires a diagnosis of the learning level and the introduction of curriculum at a level slightly above it. Essentially, acceleration recognizes that different students will learn different material at different rates in different subject areas and at different stages of their development. However, schools have found great difficulty in achieving the flexibility required to meet these varying student needs. No one pretends that this is easy, and several components need to be considered.

Early Entrance and Exit

One component should allow for early entrance and early exit of students who complete the curricular requirements and any grade level. Getting into high school early eliminates the slower moving middle school years. Despite the cry over standards, they do provide a clear way to determine mastery of curriculum, thus allowing students to move ahead.

Content-Based Acceleration

Another component involves content-based acceleration in all subject areas while the student remains in grade. Although schools have become more open to acceleration in mathematics, other areas of acceleration languish. Gifted learners with verbal, scientific, and artistic abilities need access to accelerated programs in these subjects as well. Some educators and parents express concern that gifted children should not accelerate more than six months to a year for fear they will get too far out of step with the curriculum or socially with their peers. Yet, there is little reliable research to support either of these fears.

Telescoping

Courses often overlap material and skills from one grade level to the next. Because gifted students learn and remember material faster, telescoping reduces the amount of time a student takes to cover the curriculum. An example is when a student completes grades 7 and 8 mathematics in one year, thus allowing the student to move on to more challenging work.

Grade-Level Advancement

Acceleration can involve advancing students who have learned all areas of a grade's curriculum, to the next grade. This step is particularly warranted for students who demonstrate more than 2 years' advancement in all school subjects. Once again, the concerns raised about the students, potential mismatch of social and emotional growth between these students and their new peers seems unfounded, especially when compared with how grade acceleration can counter the boredom and disenchantment of our most able learners. Given its powerful effect sizes (see box that follows), grade advancement should be far more common than it is.

Yet, many practitioners continue to have concerns about this practice and use it infrequently (Southern, Jones, and Stanley, 1993). However, when it does occur, skipping a grade is not always accompanied by adaptations to the curriculum to meet the needs of the advancing student (Southern, et al., 1993; Shore and Delcourt, 1996). Because grade skipping is applied to an individual student, a curriculum plan needs to be designed to ensure that appropriate curriculum experiences will occur for that student in the new placement.

Problems With Advanced Placement and International Baccalaureate Programs?

Advanced Placement (AP) and International Baccalaureate (IB) programs have recently come under scrutiny. A study in 2002 by the National Research Council criticized AP and IB mathematics and science courses as

- cramming too much material at the expense of depth of understanding
- failing to keep up-to-date with developments in the area
- not providing adequate guidance to teachers on modern methods of instruction
- lacking research on what the examinations actually measure
- lacking systematic and continuing professional development for teachers.

(Gollub, Bertenthal, Labov, and Curtis, 2002)

Advanced Study Programs

In high school, acceleration has traditionally meant enrollment in the College Board's Advanced Placement (AP) Program or the International Baccalaureate (IB) program. Both programs allow students to engage in college-level work and get the reward of college placement or credit for work done during their high school years. However, recent concerns about the integrity of both these programs have led some colleges to give credit only to students who score a five (the highest grade) on the AP exam.

Dual Enrollment

Acceleration can also mean dual enrollment at local community and 4-year colleges, where students can sample the college environment and gain the opportunities needed for early academic and socialization processes to occur.

Acceleration Through Technology

Advances in telecommunications now permit university on-line courses to reach distant rural areas. Some of these distance learning courses (e.g., the

Stanford Education Program for Gifted Youth) are tailored for younger students, and others offer the equivalent of freshman-level college courses. On-line communications also offer independent study with university faculty and opportunities to work on research projects.

Acceleration and Effect Sizes

After conducting an exhaustive search of research literature on gifted education through 1998, Rogers (1998) performed an analysis of acceleration formats and found the following effect sizes (ES):

- Early Entrance and Exit: ES = 0.49
- Content-Based Acceleration: ES = 0.57
- Telescoping: ES = 0.40
- Grade-Level Advancement: ES = 0.49 (Academic effect); 0.31 (Socialization effect)
- Advanced Study Courses: ES = 0.27
- Dual Enrollment: ES = 0.22

Curriculum Compacting

Compacting is one of the most common curriculum modifications for academically gifted students. This strategy reduces the amount of time the student spends on the regular curriculum. It allows students to demonstrate what they know, to do assignments in those areas where work is needed, and then to move on to other curricular areas. The strategy makes appropriate adjustments for students in any curriculum area and at any grade level. Essentially, the process involves defining key concepts and skills of a specific curriculum unit, determining and documenting which students have already mastered most or all of the learning objectives, and providing replacement strategies for material already mastered that result in a more challenging and productive use of the student's time (Reis, Burns, and Renzulli, 1992).

Occasionally, there will be specific areas in which the student is still developing competence. In this instance, the teacher can ask the student to rejoin the class at strategic points during the unit. The student may also need to join the class for discussions and inquiry or for problem-solving activities.

Teachers can compact basic skills as well as course content. Compacting basic skills involves determining which ones the students have mastered and eliminating the repetition or practice of those skills. For example, beginning algebra students who demonstrate mastery of some algebraic functions have little need for drill and practice in those areas and should move on to more complex course content.

Compacting is also useful for those gifted students who have not mastered the course material at the regular classroom pace but can do so at an accelerated pace. They usually have some understanding of the content but may require only minimal instructional time to reach mastery.

A teacher's fear that curriculum compacting will cause decreases in students' achievement scores is not supported by research studies.

Some elementary teachers are reluctant to use curriculum compacting for fear that doing so could cause declines in students' scores on achievement tests. However, a recent study looked at the achievement scores of a national sample of 336 high-ability students from second- through sixth-grade heterogeneous classrooms in urban, suburban, and rural settings. The teachers selected one to two students who demonstrated superior knowledge of the material prior to instruction and eliminated 40 to 50 percent of the curriculum across content areas for those students. The results of the Iowa Test of Basic Skills indicated that the achievement scores of the students whose curriculum was compacted did not differ significantly from the scores of similar students whose curriculum was not compacted (Reis, Westberg, Kulikowich, and Purcell, 1998).

In a study of language arts curriculum for advanced learners in grades 4 through 6, teachers replaced the regular readings with selections that were advanced for the grade levels in which they were introduced. The readings emphasized abstract concepts in literary analysis, such as mood, tone, theme, and

Curriculum Compacting and Effect Sizes

- Compacting: ES = 0.83, 0.26;
  11, 0.99, 1.57

Different effect sizes were found in the research literature on curriculum compacting, depending on the type of replacement activity provided. The 0.83 represents the replacement of math and science curriculum with advanced math and science at the student's true learning level and at an accelerated pace. The 0.26 represents the replacement of social studies and reading curriculum with enrichment activities in those areas (Rogers, 1998).

When regular readings in grades 4 through 6 were replaced with advanced-level readings for gifted students, the effect size of 11 represents literary analysis, the 0.99 represents writing, and the 1.57 is grammatical understanding (VanTassel-Baska, et al., 1996).

motivation. Outcome measures showed that the learners who received the advanced material outperformed students in the comparison groups in three areas: on a reading assignment that focused on literary analysis, on a persuasive writing assignment, and on an objective measure of grammatical understanding (VanTassel-Baska, Johnson, Hughes, and Boyce, 1996).

Grouping

Grouping can be an effective component in educating all students. But this technique is particularly effective with gifted students because it is an ideal medium for differentiation. Furthermore, several studies have found that gifted students benefit most from like-ability grouping because they are able to access more advanced knowledge and skills and to pursue their learning tasks in greater depth (Pallas, Entwisle, Alexander, and Stluka, 1994; Gamoran, Nystrand, Berends, and LePore, 1995). Grouping formats run the gamut from within-class ability groupings to independent grouping options, such as internships and mentor programs.

Within-Class Ability Grouping

Gifted students benefit most from like-ability grouping because they can get more deeply involved in the learning task.

This format can occur at all grade levels. In elementary schools, many classes are now heterogeneous and inclusive—settings where little challenge or differentiation is provided for the gifted learner. In secondary schools, instruction in even the honors, Advanced Placement, or International Baccalaureate programs are set for the norm. Thus, high ability students may find the instructional pace too slow and miss out on opportunities for more in-depth and challenging work. Within-class groups can be formed around term papers, for example, allowing advanced students more latitude for their work. Groups for differentiated reading assignments can have the same effect.

Pull-Out Grouping

This program is particularly popular at the elementary level and is one of the primary ways to deliver differentiated curriculum. Students identified as gifted from different classes meet as one group on a regular basis. In this setting, effective acceleration practices can be used for individual students because the content level of the class, by its very nature, needs to be more advanced.

Full-Time Ability Grouping

Also known as tracking, this format usually starts in upper elementary grades. Students are in the same group for most of the day and tend to remain in the same track throughout their school year. Tracking allows students to pursue a more advanced series of courses through middle and high school. The recent trend toward heterogenous classes has diminished tracking, especially in middle school where it all started. Where it still occurs, tracking usually provides for special grouping in mathematics and language arts, but not in science and social studies. To be truly successful, full-time grouping should apply across all subject areas, where the school size allows.

A Word About Cooperative Learning

Cooperative learning is an effective instructional strategy, especially in heterogeneous classes. However, when the range of abilities gets very wide, gifted students may not benefit from the heterogenous cooperative group. One study found that gifted students participated in higher-level discussions when grouped with other gifted students (Lando and Schneider, 1997), and that their absence from the heterogeneous group did not adversely affect the learning of other students in the group (Kenney, Archambault, and Hallmark, 1994). These findings suggest that teachers may want to use caution when using this practice with gifted students.

Cluster Grouping

Cluster grouping is different from tracking in that the group is composed of only three to six students, usually the top 5 percent of ability in the class. This format allows the gifted children to learn together while avoiding permanent grouping arrangements with students of other ability levels. If the cluster group is kept to a manageable size, teachers report a general improvement in achievement for the whole class. This is probably because teachers who learn how to provide opportunities for gifted students also modify those opportunities for the rest of the class, raising achievement for all. Cluster groups can also be formed in secondary schools in any heterogeneous classroom, especially in smaller schools, where there may not be enough students to form an advanced section in a particular subject (Winebrenner and Devlin, 2001).

Independent Work Grouping

This format offers students options for more personalized opportunities for intellectual growth. It can occur by one or two students working on a well-designed independent project, interning in a professional setting (e.g., a hospice or senior care center), or associating with an adult mentor who has expertise in an area of the student's interest. Such options require close collaboration between school and community leaders.

Grouping Formats and Effect Sizes

- Within-Class Ability Grouping: ES = 0.34
- Pull-Out Grouping: ES = 0.65, 0.44, 0.32
- Full-Time Ability Grouping: ES = 0.49, 0.33
- Cluster Grouping of Gifted Students: ES = 0.62
- Independent Work With Mentors: ES = 0.47, 0.42, 0.57

There are only a few reliable studies on pull-out groups, so the effect size numbers may be inflated. The 0.65 refers to pull-outs that are a direct extension of the regular school curriculum; the 0.44, to pull-outs that focus on thinking skills; the 0.32, to pull-outs that focus on creative skills.

For full-time ability grouping, the 0.49 represents the yearly effect for all academic areas for elementary gifted students (grades K-6); the 0.33, for secondary students (grades 7-12).

Mentor programs can advance gifted students in many ways. The 0.47 represents the socialization effect; the 0.42 is the self-esteem effect; and 0.57 is the academic effect (Rogers, 1998).

INSTRUCTIONAL PROCESSES FOR GIFTED LEARNERS ■

Processes refers to the instructional strategies that engage students during the learning episode that will help them find sense and meaning. This is more likely to happen if the instructional techniques help students see purpose to the new learning and have opportunities to probe for understanding and relevancy. Such process skills might involve higher-level thinking, creative thinking, problem solving, and independent or group research.

Higher-Level Thinking

Trying to classify levels of human thought is no easy feat. But that has not kept psychologists from trying. One model, published nearly 50 years ago by Benjamin Bloom (1956), still passes the test of time and remains useful as a starting point for understanding the complexity of human thought. I have discussed the value of Bloom's Taxonomy at great length in a previous publication (Sousa, 2001a) so my purpose here is just to present a short version to set the stage for discussing thought processes further.

Bloom's model is a hierarchy of six levels describing human thought, from the least to the most complex: knowledge, comprehension (understanding), application, analysis, synthesis, and evaluation. Although there are six levels, the hierarchy is not rigid, and an individual may move easily among the levels during extended processing. Here are brief definitions of each level:

- **Knowledge:** The mere recall of rote learning, from specific facts, to a memorized definition or complete theory. This is semantic memory and there is no presumption that the learner *understands* what has been recalled.
- **Comprehension:** This level describes the ability to make sense out of the material, goes beyond recall, and represents the lowest level of understanding. Here the material becomes available for future use to solve problems and to make decisions.
- **Application:** Application refers to the ability to use learned material in new situations with a minimum of direction. It includes the application of such things as rules, concepts, methods, and theories to solve problems. The learner activates procedural memory and uses convergent thinking to select, transfer, and apply data to complete a new task. Practice is essential at this level.
- **Analysis:** Analysis is the ability to break material into its component parts so that its structure may be understood. It includes identifying parts, examining the relationships of the parts to each other and to the whole, and recognizing the organizational principles involved. The learner must be able to organize and reorganize information into categories. The brain's frontal lobes are working hard at this level. This stage is more complex because the learner is aware of the thought process in use (metacognition) and understands both the content and structure of the material.
- **Synthesis:** Synthesis refers to the ability to put parts together to form a plan that is new to the learner. It may involve the production of a unique communication (essay or speech), a plan of operations (research proposal), or a scheme for classifying information (a taxonomy). This level stresses creativity, with major emphasis on forming *new* patterns or structures. This is the level where learners use divergent thinking to get an *Aha!* experience. Although most often associated with the arts, synthesis can occur in all areas of the curriculum.
- **Evaluation:** Evaluation describes the ability to judge the value of material on the basis of specific criteria. The learner examines

criteria from several categories and selects those that are the most relevant to the situation. Activities at this level almost always have multiple and equally acceptable solutions. This is the highest level of cognitive thought in this model because it contains elements of all the other levels, plus conscious judgments based on definite criteria. At this level, learners tend to consolidate their thinking and become more receptive to other points of view. (Note: The name of this level often creates confusion because one immediately thinks of testing. Bloom intended for *evaluation* to mean a judgment or assessment of different individual options within a group and the selection of one option supported by a defensible rationale.)

Convergent/Critical and Divergent/Creative Thinking

The first three levels of Bloom's taxonomy describe what can be called *convergent* or *critical* thinking whereby the learner recalls and focuses what is known and comprehended to solve a problem through application. While using the upper three levels, the learner often gains new insights and makes discoveries that were not part of the original information. This describes a *divergent* or *creative* thinking process.

The Important Difference Between Complexity and Difficulty

Complexity and difficulty describe completely different mental operations, but are often used synonymously (Figure 3.2). This error, resulting in the two factors being treated as one, limits the use of the taxonomy to enhance the thinking of all students. By recognizing how these concepts are different, the teacher can gain valuable insight into the connection between the taxonomy and student ability. *Complexity* describes the *thought process* that the brain uses to deal with information. In Bloom's Taxonomy, it can be described by any of the six words representing the six levels. The question, "What is the capital of Florida?" is at the knowledge level, but the question, "Can you tell me in your own words what is meant by a state

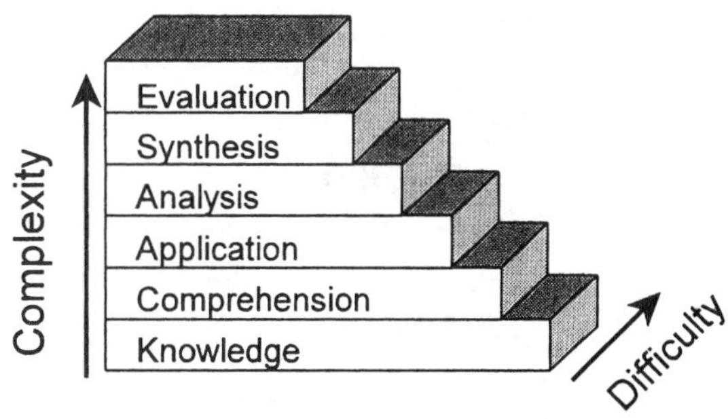

Figure 3.2 Complexity and difficulty are different. Complexity establishes the level of thought; difficulty determines the amount of effort within each level.

capital?" is at the comprehension level. The second question is more *complex* than the first because it is at a higher level in Bloom's Taxonomy.

Difficulty, on the other hand, refers to the *amount of effort* that the learner must expend *within* a level of complexity to accomplish a learning objective. It is possible for a learning activity to become increasingly difficult without becoming more complex. For example, the question, "Can you name the states of the Union?" is at the knowledge level of complexity because it involves simple recall (semantic memory) for most students. The question, "Can you name the states of the Union and their capitals?" is also at the knowledge level but is more difficult than the prior question because it involves more effort to recall more information. Similarly, the question, "Can you name the states and their capitals in order of their admission to the Union?" is still at the knowledge level, but it is considerably more *difficult* than the first two. It requires gathering more information and then sequencing it by chronological order.

Bloom's Taxonomy and Gifted Students

These are examples of how a student can exert great effort to achieve a learning task while processing at the lowest level of thinking. When seeking to challenge students, classroom teachers are more likely (perhaps unwittingly) to increase difficulty rather than complexity as the challenge mode. This may be because they do not recognize the difference between these concepts or that they believe that difficulty is the method for achieving higher-order thinking. Moreover, for all sorts of reasons including the overcrowded curriculum and the continued educational emphasis on fact acquisition, more class time is spent with instruction at the lower levels of the taxonomy. Obviously, all students benefit when teachers include activities that engage students at the upper levels of analysis, synthesis, and evaluation. Gifted students, particularly, can pass through the first three levels quickly and schools do these students a great disservice if they fail to provide opportunities for higher-level thinking.

Creative Thinking

Is creativity the result of innate abilities or of a learned set of behaviors? Psychologists and others have debated this question for decades, more often siding with the view that creativity is a gift from nature or the result of genetic heritage. Now studies in cognitive neuroscience seem to be indicating that creativity is more likely the result of a series of cognitive processes that can be developed in most individuals. Surely, genetic heritage still has some influence. But the notion that some degree of creativity can be *taught* is exciting, and strategies to accomplish this will make valuable additions to a teacher's repertoire.

In Bloom's model, synthesis is the level most closely associated with creativity, but there certainly are other ways to define creative thinking, usually in terms of the learning behaviors creativity evokes. Four behaviors often associated with creativity are

Fluency: This describes the ability to generate new ideas. This skill is required for students to explain what they know, to think of ways to solve a problem, to develop ideas for writing or speaking, and to draw diagrams or models. A question like, "In what ways can we do this?" evokes fluency.

Flexibility: This behavior requires generating a broad range of ideas, such as "How many different ways can we do this?"

Originality: This behavior refers to unusual or unique responses to a situation. Original responses usually occur at the end of an idea-seeking activity and after the more obvious ideas have been rendered. A question stem might be, "What is the most unusual way to accomplish this?"

Elaboration: Here, other ideas and details are added to the reasoning. "What else can we do here?" and "Can you tell me more?" are questions that elicit elaboration.

Mental Imagery and Creativity

At least three of these creativity behaviors—fluency, originality, and elaboration—seem to be closely associated with mental imagery. One large study of 560 high school students compared scores on tests of imaging ability with those on tests of creative thinking. The results indicated a significant correlation between imaging ability and creativity in general and that imaging ability had strong effects on fluency, originality, and elaboration (González, Campos, and Pérez, 1997). The researchers did not offer an explanation for the correlation. However, it seems reasonable to speculate that because other scanning studies have shown separately that imagery and creative activities engage the right frontal and temporal

Creativity appears to be closely associated with the ability to do mental imagery.

lobes of the brain, individuals having high imaging capabilities would also have high capabilities in creativity as well.

Creativity as Decision Making

If being creative is more a learned pattern of behavior than genetic heritage, the question arises as to what behaviors or skills are likely to develop creativity. Sternberg (2000) suggests that students can develop their creativity by learning the attitudes they will need to be successful in their work. Thus, they develop what Sternberg calls "creative giftedness" as a decision-making skill. He describes ten decisions that students can make to be more creative:

Creativity is a decision-making skill that can be developed.

1. **Redefine Problems.** Creative people take a problem and force themselves to see it differently from the way most other people see it. For example, Manet and Monet challenged artistic representations, Beethoven redefined classical music, and Einstein totally altered our views of the universe.
2. **Analyze One's Ideas.** Creative people analyze the value of their ideas, recognizing that not all of them are worthy of pursuit and that they will make mistakes. This self-skepticism prevents them from believing that they have all the answers and encourages them to admit when they are wrong.
3. **Sell One's Ideas.** Because creative ideas usually challenge existing methods, they will not be easily accepted and thus need to be sold to the public.
4. **Knowledge Is a Double-Edged Sword.** Knowledge can help people decide what new areas need to be explored, or it can entrench people so that they lose sight of other perspectives.
5. **Surmount Obstacles.** Creative people inevitably confront obstacles and must have the determination to surmount them.
6. **Take Sensible Risks.** Creative people must be willing to take reasonable risks, recognizing that they will sometimes fail and sometimes succeed.
7. **Willingness to Grow.** Creative people avoid getting stuck with one idea forever. Rather, they look for new ways to expand the idea or add new ones.
8. **Believe in Yourself.** Creative people maintain their belief in themselves even when their ideas are poorly received and when other sources of intellectual and emotional support are gone.

9. **Tolerance of Ambiguity.** Creative people often face ambiguity when trying creative things. A high tolerance for ambiguity is important if the creative venture is to succeed.
10. **Find What You Love to Do and Do It.** Creative people are at their best when they are doing what they love to do.

Sternberg proposes that anyone can make the decision to be creative. Because the ten decisions are not fixed abilities, teachers can encourage students to decide in favor of creativity and to reward those students who do.

Problem-Based Learning

Problem-based learning places students in the position of trying to solve a multifaceted problem of significant complexity. The problem resembles a real-life situation in that the students lack some of the information they need to solve the problem or are not clear on the steps they will need to take. The students critically analyze the problem from different points of view, look for alternative solutions, select a solution, and develop a plan of action for its implementation.

Students usually work in groups and are responsible for retrieving the additional information and resources they will need. In addition, students decide which group members will focus on the various parts of the problem and on how to present their findings to demonstrate what they have learned. Their presentations can be in the form of portfolios, videotapes, exhibits, or written reports (Burruss, 1999).

The teacher's role in problem-based learning is to act as a metacognitive coach by asking questions, helping students plan their work, guiding them toward the questions they need to pursue, and assessing their progress. In this format, the teacher is more of a guide than a provider of information.

The open-ended nature of problem-based learning allows for considerable differentiation of curriculum and instruction. The process calls upon the varied strengths of the learners, involves a multitude of in-school and out-of-school resources, and provides opportunities for students to pursue their interests. Sources of real problems to study may be

- Environmental: Why is the amount of mercury increasing in our drinking water?
- School: What are the implications of starting high school an hour later?
- Community: Should we adopt an evening curfew for teenagers?

- Political: Should city councilors be subject to term limits?
- Global: What can be done to stem the rise of AIDS in Africa?

The Triarchic Approach

The text in Chapter 2 explains the Triarchic Theory of Intelligence (Sternberg, 1985). To apply the theory in the classroom, teachers need to present instruction so that at different times it engages the students in analytical, creative, and practical thinking while solving problems. The problem-solving cycle involves five steps: identifying the problem, acquiring the resources for solving the problem, devising a strategy for solving the problem, and monitoring and evaluating the problem solving (see Figure 3.3). Properly implemented, the cycle promotes the three different types of thinking. For example, evaluating the problem-solving approach might involve analytical thinking. Creative thinking would help to formulate the strategy, and practical thinking would be helpful in determining and acquiring the resources for solving the problem at hand.

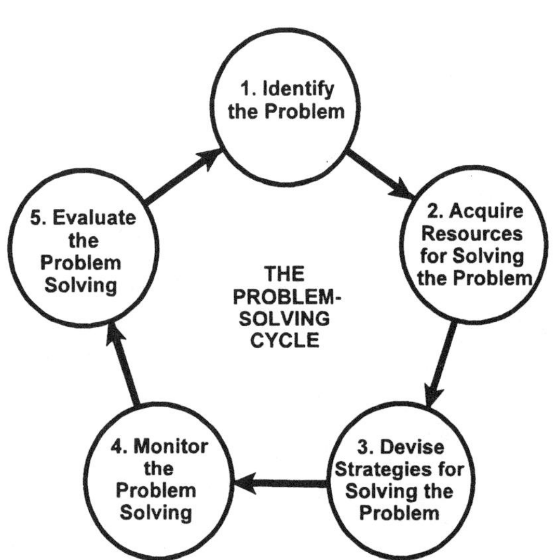

Figure 3.3 The five steps in the problem-solving cycle.

In the triarchic approach, teachers plan their lessons not only for memory but also for analytical, creative, and practical processing. Analytical thinking occurs then teachers ask students to judge, compare and contrast, evaluate, and critique. Creative thinking activities would have students suppose, invent, imagine, explore, and discover. Practical thinking is involved when students implement, use, apply, and contextualize. Classroom applications of the theory have shown positive results in terms of student achievement (Sternberg, et al., 1996; Sternberg, et al., 2000).

Independent Study

Independent study can be a useful strategy for differentiating curriculum. However, students generally need help in learning how to become independent workers. But with proper teachers' guidance, students can learn to pursue interests on their own by setting learning goals, establishing criteria for judging their work, assessing their progress, and presenting their work products to an audience. The goal of this program is to help the student move from being teacher-directed to being self-directed.

These ventures are more likely to be successful if the student has a clear focus on what material and skills are to be learned. The selected independent learning activities should help develop creative and critical thinking skills as well as time management strategies and research skills. Maintaining a learning log and a portfolio of results also is an important component of a successful independent study program. It should be noted that assessment results of the effect size of independent study are inconclusive.

Tiered Assignments

Tiered assignments provide for differentiation by allowing students at different ability levels to work on the same content. However, students seek out the answers to different questions and are assigned different activities based on their ability. One approach is to teach Bloom's Taxonomy and to ask them to design questions and activities at the different levels of complexity. The teacher then works with the students to decide which questions they will pursue and to set the criteria for evaluating their results.

Before starting on tiering, the teacher needs to identify the core elements—those components that *all* students should master. The teacher then devises separate versions of the activities so that the low-, middle-, and high-ability students are adequately challenged. The advantage of this approach is that, with a little advance planning, the teacher can keep students of differing ability levels engaged and working toward the same learning objective through differentiated tasks.

THE PRODUCTS OF GIFTED LEARNERS

Products are the vehicles through which students demonstrate what they have learned as a result of their engagement with a particular body of knowledge and skills. The products referred to in this context are culminating activities that result from a considerable amount of student time and involvement with the learning unit; they are not the worksheets or quizzes that are part of daily routine.

To be effective, the culminating products need to be able to do the following (Tomlinson, 1995):

- Offer students opportunities to extend their knowledge, stretch their abilities, and pursue authentic and challenging learning experiences.
- Evolve from advanced materials, original research, or primary documents.
- Transform information so that students are not merely repeating information but creating a new idea or product.
- Be similar to those created by professionals in that the products address real-world problems and are intended for real audiences, for example, are published in student literary magazines, displayed in public places (banks, malls, and shop windows), or prepared as oral history tapes for a library.
- Be assessed by experts associated with the field of endeavor, such as researchers, college professors, or other professionals.

Student products can be centered around tiered assignments, independent studies, the Triarchic and Multiple Intelligences models, and any complex investigations that result in the learning of a body of knowledge and skills. They can include the following:

- ☞ Written reports
- ☞ Oral reports
- ☞ Plays, skits, or pantomimes
- ☞ Songs
- ☞ Charts and graphs
- ☞ Photo essays
- ☞ Demonstrations
- ☞ Videotapes
- ☞ 3-D sculptures
- ☞ Storyboard displays
- ☞ Audiotapes
- ☞ Poems
- ☞ Oral history tapes
- ☞ Charcoal sketches
- ☞ Watercolors
- ☞ Puppet shows

GIFTED VISUAL-SPATIAL LEARNERS

The information in human brains can be organized in specialized patterns that result in different views of the world, as discussed in Chapter 2. Left-hemisphere-preferred individuals develop a highly-organized sequential system that is strong on analysis, progression from simple to complex, and specializing in linear deductive reasoning. This system seems to be greatly influenced by auditory input and language. By contrast, right-hemisphere-preferred individuals develop thinking patterns that use synthesis, have an intuitive grasp of complex systems, process concepts simultaneously, and specialize in inductive reasoning.

Visualization and spatial abilities are thought to be strongly associated with this preference. Although more males are right-hemisphere preferred and more females are left-hemisphere preferred (Sousa, 2001a, Ch. 5), it is important to remember that integration of both hemispheres is necessary for higher-level thought. All learners use both hemispheres, but not with equal fluency.

Linda Silverman (1989) was among the first researchers to identify visual-spatial learners as a result of working with children with many types of giftedness. She identified two groups of gifted visual-spatial learners. The first group scores extremely high on IQ tests because they have high ability in tasks requiring visual-spatial processing as well as those tasks requiring sequential thinking processes. The second group consists of students who are brighter than their IQ scores would indicate but do not score well because they have weaknesses in sequential processing skills. Although these students may have difficulty achieving their potential in school, they may not have a learning disability, but perhaps a teaching-style disability. That is, traditional teaching methods tend to favor strong sequential learners. Concepts are usually presented step-by-step, practiced with drill and repetition, reviewed, and then tested under timed conditions. Consequently, gifted visual-spatial learners may have greater difficulty in traditional classrooms and their talents may not be fully recognized.

Characteristics of Visual-Spatial Learners

There is no single test to determine visual-spatial giftedness. Identification is best accomplished by looking for a collection of behaviors that often indicate visual-spatial preference. For example, IQ tests generally show higher scores on nonverbal tasks compared with verbal tasks. Essentially, this type of learner enjoys constructing toys and rarely follows directions. These students are reflective and need time to think. Consequently, they may appear off task when they are really probing some inner meaning or mentally creating a new conceptual scheme. As children, they often pull toys apart, trying to determine how they work. Organizational skills are not their strong point and they have difficulty keeping to schedules and being on time. Table 3.1 lists some of the

Table 3.1 Characteristics of Visual-Spatial Learners

- Rely on vision and visualization
- Preoccupied with space at the expense of time
- Intuitive grasp of complex systems
- Prefer synthesis approach
- Simultaneous processing of concepts
- Active use of imagery
- Prefer visual directions
- Poorly organized
- Prefer puzzles, jigsaws, computer games
- Get difficult concepts, struggle with easy ones

characteristics of visual-spatial learners (Silverman, 1989b), who thrive on complex ideas, abstract concepts, holistic methods, multidisciplinary studies, inductive learning strategies, and any other activities requiring synthesis of thought.

Once visual-spatial learners create a mental image of a concept, it creates a permanent change in the students' understanding and awareness. Repetition is unnecessary and may cause difficulty because it emphasizes their weaknesses instead of their strengths.

These students are ideally suited for the kinds of activities and learning experiences associated with programs for the gifted. However, to reach their full potential, visual-spatial learners must be placed in a learning environment that is a good match between their learning style and the way they are taught.

AVOIDING THE PITFALL OF ACADEMICS VERSUS THE ARTS

Much of the research in areas related to programs for the gifted and talented focuses on the education of students with high ability in academic areas. Little research exists that suggests how to develop curriculum, teach, or assess students who are artistically gifted, probably because educators—and the communities they serve—generally place much greater emphasis on the academic areas than the arts. Furthermore, researchers and educators traditionally have used the terms *gifted* and *talented* to describe different things. *Gifted* often referred to high ability in one or more academic areas; *talented* usually meant superior abilities in the visual or performing arts. Researchers in the past often claimed that there was little direct evidence that students who were talented in the arts also exhibited high abilities in academic areas. To this day, it is not unusual to find school districts that have separate programs for the academically and artistically gifted.

Researchers today, who have worked with both types of high-ability students, argue that academically gifted students are often equally gifted in the arts, and vice versa. In a study of teenage students at a summer institute for the arts, all the participants were superior students in academic areas as well (Clark and Zimmerman, 1998). Perhaps we need to adopt a broader view of giftedness that includes all areas of both academic and artistic talents for all students who participate in gifted education programs. The theories of Renzulli, Sternberg, and Gardner discussed in Chapter 2 define a wide range of abilities that can contribute to a more inclusive description of what constitutes programs for gifted students. This multidimensional approach allows for the inclusion of students with abilities in a wide range of school subjects and from all racial, ethnic, and socioeconomic groups.

Fortunately, the growing recognition that students may have multiple abilities, such as mathematics and music, has prompted some school districts to use multiple criteria to identify students for special programs. Regrettably, this process is moving much too slowly. Given the enormous economic and technological threats facing our society, we need to accelerate and expand our efforts to identify and support all the gifts of our children, for it is their knowledge and skills that will ultimately determine the nature and quality of our lives in the future.

APPLICATIONS

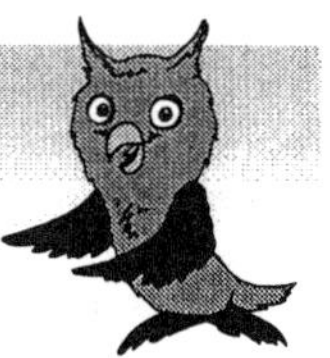

ASSESSING THE LEARNING ENVIRONMENT

The following list of questions is designed to help teachers assess the effectiveness of the learning environment for gifted students in their classroom:

- Have you helped students become more aware of their learning styles?
- Have you asked students what helps them learn effectively?
- Do you model the process of talking about *how* we learn, rather than just *what* is learned?
- Have you established an environment in which wrong answers are a productive opportunity for learning?
- Do you actively encourage creative thinking by asking open-ended questions to which there are no single right answers?
- Do you encourage students to question themselves, each other, and other adults in the classroom?
- Are students involved in self-assessment?
- Do you encourage students through challenging and interactive displays?
- Have you developed a resource collection including websites and in-school and out-of-school resource centers, and how do you know if the resources are being well used?

APPLICATIONS

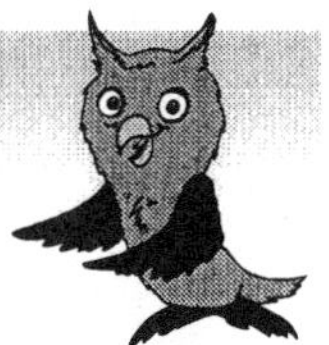

PROCEDURES FOR COMPACTING CURRICULUM

Compacting curriculum simply means determining what students already know about a particular unit of instruction, deciding what they still need to learn, and replacing it with more interesting and challenging material that they would like to learn. There are eight basic steps to the process (Reis, Burns, and Renzulli, 1992a):

Define and Assess Key Concepts and Skills	1. The first step is to identify and define the key concepts and skills for the unit to be taught. Teachers' manuals, district curriculum guides, scope-and-sequence charts, and even some textbooks list the goals and key learning objectives for each curriculum unit. 2. Examine these key objectives to decide which represent the acquisition of new learning and which review and practice material is already presented in earlier grades or courses. Comparing the scope-and-sequence charts or tables of contents of basic textbooks will often reveal new versus repeated material.
Identify and Assess Student Candidates for Compacting	3. Identify the students who have the potential for mastering the new material at a faster than normal pace. Use completed assignments, scores on previous tests, classroom participation, and standardized achievement tests as some of the measures for identifying potential candidates for compacting. 4. Develop appropriate techniques for assessing specific learning objectives. Any unit pretests can be helpful here. The analysis of the pretest results will help determine proficiency and identify instructional areas that may need additional practice.

PROCEDURES FOR COMPACTING CURRICULUM—Continued

	5. Streamline the instruction and practice activities for students who demonstrate mastery of the learning objectives. 6. Provide individualized or small group instruction for students who have not yet mastered all the objectives, but who are able to do so more quickly than their classmates.
Provide Acceleration and Enrichment Options and Keep Records	7. Offer more challenging learning alternatives based on student interests and strengths. Deciding which replacement activities to use is guided by space, time, and the availability of resource persons and materials. Resource persons can be other classroom teachers, media specialists, content area or gifted education specialists, and outside mentors. The materials can include self-directed learning activities, instructional materials that focus on developing particular thinking skills, and a variety of experiences designed to promote research and investigative skills. 8. Use a simple three-column form for maintaining a record of the compacting process and of the instructional alternatives provided. In the first column, list the objectives of a particular unit of study and data on the students' proficiency in those objectives. Use the second column specifically to detail the pretest measures and their results. In column three, record information about the acceleration and enrichment options that were used.

PROCEDURES FOR COMPACTING CURRICULUM—Continued

Guidelines. Curriculum compacting takes time and energy at first, but usually saves time once teachers and students are familiar with the process. For educators who are hesitant to try curriculum compacting, here are a few guidelines that are likely to increase your chances of success (Reis, Burns, and Renzulli, 1992b):

- Start with one or two responsible students who have a positive attitude and who are more likely to welcome the change and be successful with the replacement activities.
- Talk with these students and discuss the content with which they feel comfortable. Select the appropriate activities, but be sure to give them some options.
- Try a variety of methods to determine how much they already know about the material. Sometimes a brief conversation with the students is just as reliable as a formal pretest.
- Compact the topic rather than the time. Because the alternative activities are usually more interesting, students may take more time to complete them than you estimated.
- Define proficiency in learning the material or skills based on conversations with school staff, administrators, and parents.
- Do not hesitate to request help from other school personnel or from community volunteers to accomplish the replacement activities.

Teachers who use curriculum compacting on a regular basis report increased interest and enthusiasm among their students and thus often expand the compacting program from just one or two students to a broader segment of the class. The process can be used at any grade level and in any subject area and is not aligned with any specific curricular reform. It is adaptable and flexible to meet the needs of almost any classroom. More information on this strategy is available from the National Research Center on the Gifted and Talented (see **Resources**).

APPLICATIONS

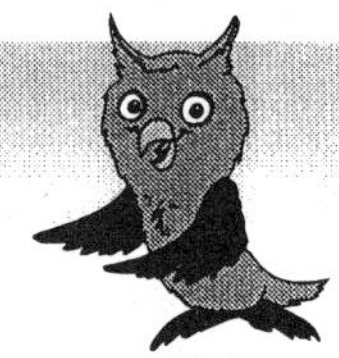

STRATEGIES FOR FLEXIBLE GROUPING

Grouping is common in the elementary school classroom. Creating small groups of gifted students to work together provides a productive learning situation. Here are some guidelines to consider when organizing these groups (Smutny, 2000).

CREATE GROUND RULES

Certain ground rules need to be established to ensure that all participants have an opportunity to participate and share ideas. Discuss these ground rules with the class. The rules should be grade- and age-appropriate, but most need to include the following:

- If you cannot agree on what to do, move on to another idea
- Listen to others in your group and respond to their comments
- Take turns sharing ideas
- Help each other
- Make your best effort
- If you don't understand something, talk it out with your group
- Seek the teacher's help when needed

PROVIDE VARIETY

Organize a variety of groups based on the learning objective. Groups can be formed around student interests, motivation, and the complexity level of the assignment.

OFFER CHOICES

When appropriate, allow students to choose their group members as well as their topic. Of course, teacher discretion may be necessary to allow for variety of groupings over time or to ensure that certain students do not always dominate a group.

STRATEGIES FOR FLEXIBLE GROUPING—Continued

ASSESS STUDENTS INDIVIDUALLY

Although some reward can be given to the group upon completion of their work, it is important to assess each student individually. Assessment measures can include checklists, portfolios, mastery tests, drawings, written compositions, and oral responses.

COMPACT THE CURRICULUM

Compress the essentials so that students can move beyond what they have already mastered. Assess their level of mastery and then allow students to choose activities of particular interest to them. Another option is to design an activity related to the current lesson that challenges their abilities. Some teachers find that signing a learning contract with a student can be effective. The contract stipulates the chosen activities or projects, the conditions for their completion, and the expected outcomes.

INCORPORATE CREATIVE THINKING

Using creative thinking activities benefits all students. The "what if" questions are always interesting to pursue and they challenge students to come up with alternative explanations. Teachers can then suggest other resources to help students with their new explorations. Brainstorming and other metacognitive strategies can stimulate discussions and add to the depth of understanding that students have about a particular subject or theme.

APPLICATIONS

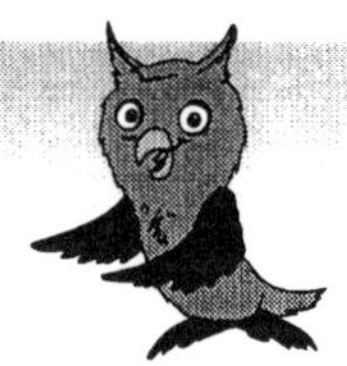

DIFFERENTIATING CONTENT

Content refers to what the student needs to know, understand, and be able to do as a result of a particular unit of study. It should be highly relevant to students, coherent, transferable through instructional techniques, and authentic. Content includes any means by which students acquire information and skills. The teacher promotes differentiation through (Tomlinson, 1999) the use of the following:

- ✓ Multiple textbooks
- ✓ Field trips
- ✓ Supplementary readings
- ✓ Videos
- ✓ Guest speakers
- ✓ Demonstrations
- ✓ Lectures
- ✓ Computer programs
- ✓ Internet
- ✓ Learning contracts
- ✓ Mentors
- ✓ Media centers
- ✓ Experiments
- ✓ Interest centers
- ✓ Audio tapes
- ✓ Internships
- ✓ Group investigations

APPLICATIONS

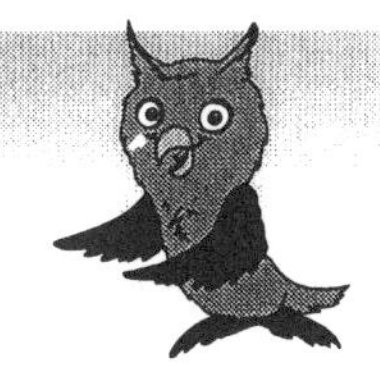

TEACHING FOR CREATIVITY

Sternberg (2000) proposes that creativity results from a set of 10 decision-making skills that can be learned. He further suggests that teachers can encourage students to be creatively gifted by doing the following:

Decision	Teacher Activity
1. Redefine Problem	• Goal: To help students see an aspect of the world in a different way from which it is usually seen. • Example: Select or have students provide a well-known phenomenon, such as seasonal differences in the northern and souther hemispheres. "Summer vacation" in the USA has to be redefined for students living in Australia.
2. Analyze One's Ideas	• Goal: To help students critique strengths and weaknesses of their ideas. • Example: Have students analyze the phenomenon they presented above. What were its strengths and weaknesses? How can they improve the idea?
3. Sell One's Ideas	• Goal: To teach students the importance of selling their ideas to others. • Example: Have students present an oral or written report in which they explain, defend, and promote an idea in which they truly believe. Remind them to defend their idea against possible criticism.
4. Knowledge Is a Double-Edged Sword	• Goal: To help students realize that theories apply only to a limited range of behavior. • Example: Lead students to study a major idea (e.g., any person born in the United States can become president). What kind of information would we need to determine if this really applies to all children? What other factors could limit this statement's validity?

TEACHING FOR CREATIVITY—Continued

Decision	Teacher Activity
5. Surmount Obstacles	• Goal: To help students realize that new ideas are not immediately accepted. • Example: Ask students to reflect on ideas they may have encountered (e.g., Darwin's Theory of Evolution, the Wright brothers' concept of flight, or the "big bang" theory of the formation of the universe) or on one of their own ideas that others had difficulty accepting. What strategies would help these ideas gain acceptance? Can we relate them to ideas people already accept?
6. Take Sensible Risks	• Goal: To help students realize that creativity involves some degree of risk. • Example: Have students write a brief essay critiquing an interpretation you (the teacher) gave in class. They must support their belief and their criticism must be constructive. Assure the students that you welcome alternative interpretations. Evaluate their essay and offer ways for them to improve their critique. Here they realize they can take a sensible risk and be rewarded.
7. Willingness to Grow	• Goal: To encourage students to grow by challenging their own beliefs. • Example: Ask students to select a belief they have about human behavior, such as why people fall in love, why they get angry, how they chose their friends, or whether capital punishment is effective (or ineffective). Have them commit to this belief in writing and then compose an essay that persuasively supports an opposite point of view. Afterwards, ask if writing this essay helped them to better understand people who disagree with them.
8. Believe in Yourself	• Goal: To show students that if they believe they can do something, they often can. • Example: Ask students to select a task they think would be very difficult to do (e.g., learning to play an instrument, losing weight, or achieving an athletic goal), and then ask them to develop a plan for accomplishing that task. In some cases, students may be encouraged to follow through on their plan and report on their progress periodically.

TEACHING FOR CREATIVITY—Continued

Decision	Teacher Activity
9. Tolerance of Ambiguity	• Goal: To help students recognize and appreciate that ambiguity is inherent in much thinking in the academic disciplines. • Example: Ask students to read a piece that seems to present a theory, analysis, or explanation persuasively. The ask them to read a critique of what they have read and to let you know if the original analysis is still convincing. Why or why not? The reading and critique can be on any set of opposing ideas, such as communism versus capitalism, the North's and South's views of the Civil War, or capital punishment versus life without parole. Students should realize that attaining understanding can be a slow process and that one must tolerate ambiguity for a long time in order to better understand the world.
10. Find What You Love to Do and Do It	• Goal: To show students how any field of endeavor can accommodate a wide variety of outside interests. • Example: Ask students to reflect on an interest they have that is outside a field of study and to relate orally or in writing this interest to the field being studied. These investigations might relate music or art to a scientific field, or compare science fiction to real science, or delve into the psychological makeup of a literary character. The point is to show that they can pursue a diversity of interests while still following a specific area of study.

APPLICATIONS

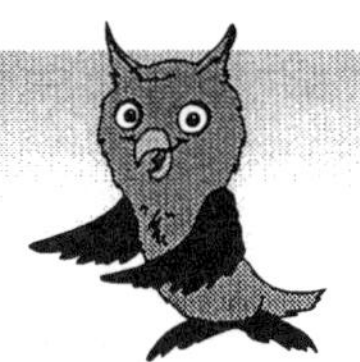

CREATIVE THINKING THROUGH QUESTIONING

Open-ended questions are effective for encouraging creative thinking because they rarely have one answer and they stimulate further inquiry. They ask for clarification, probe for assumptions, search for reasons and evidence, and look for implications and consequences. Here are a few examples of these types of questions:

What would you have done? Why do think this is the best choice?

Could this ever really happen? What might happen next?

What do you think might happen if … ? What do you think caused this?

Is what you are saying now consistent with what you said before?

How is it different from …? Can you give an example?

Where do we go next? Where could we go for help on this?

What do you mean by that expression?

Can we trust the source of this material?

In what other ways could this be done? How can you test this theory?

What might be the consequences of behaving like that?

Do you agree with this author/speaker? Why or why not?

How could you modify this? How would changing the sequence affect the outcome?

CREATIVE THINKING THROUGH QUESTIONING—Continued

The Question Spinner. Here is a tool to promote creative questioning. Make a copy of this page. Cut out the arrow. Insert a paper fastener through the white dot on the arrow and through the center of the inner circle. A student spins the arrow and answers the indicated question.

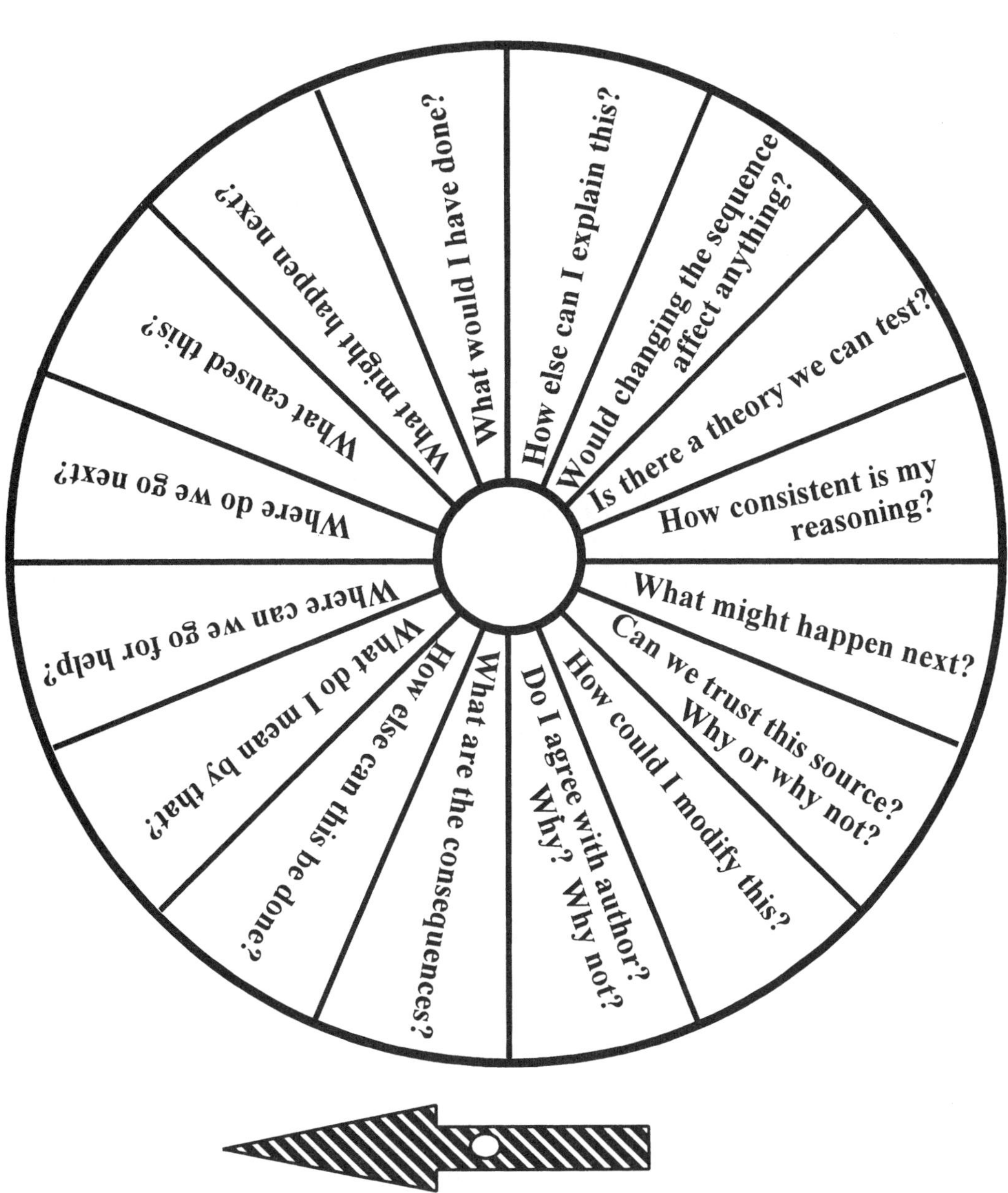

APPLICATIONS

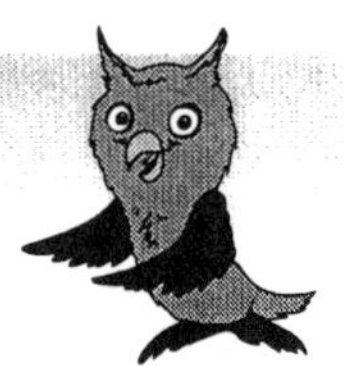

GUIDELINES FOR PROBLEM-BASED LEARNING ACTIVITIES

Problem-based learning activities are usually labor-intensive and time consuming. Before embarking on these activities, the teacher should consider working with other teachers to plan the problem that the students will undertake. Here are some guidelines to consider (Burruss, 1999):

- Identify some complex issues or problem situations. Selecting a local issue, such as environmental preservation or city planning, adds relevancy to the process. The following are examples of local issues:
    - ➨ Should a city park be sold for commercial development to increase dwindling property tax revenues?
    - ➨ What can be done to prevent or lessen the runoff of fertilizers into the community's water table?
    - ➨ What are the advantages and disadvantages of building a strip mall next to the middle school?
    - ➨ Should all smoking be banned from local restaurants?

- Examples of regional and national issues can be found in books, newspapers, magazines, and television news and documentary programs. Here are a few examples:
    - ➨ Should the elected county commissioners be subject to term limits?
    - ➨ What are the pros and cons of electing the US president by popular vote?
    - ➨ Should Americans give up some liberties in the fight against terrorism?

- State the problem in a way that is interesting for students and that puts the situation in an intriguing context. The statement should suggest avenues they can pursue but should not provide all the information and resources they need.

PROBLEM-BASED LEARNING ACTIVITIES—Continued

- Because your program may have time restrictions, be sure to align the problems with the curriculum and standards. Think about the curriculum areas involved and the skills the students will use as they pursue the problem and generate solutions.

- Carefully select the best time to discuss and present the problem in class, and make sure to allow sufficient time for students to complete their work.

- To ensure a productive start, give the students a partial list of materials and resources they may need at the onset of their work.

- If the project falters, revise the problems as needed to resume progress.

APPLICATIONS

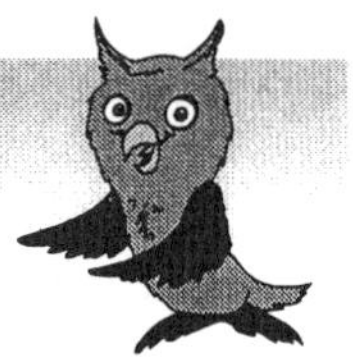

USING THE TRIARCHIC MODEL IN THE CLASSROOM

Practical applications of Sternberg's Triarchic model in the classroom require that the teacher incorporate activities that provoke analytical, creative, and practical thinking whenever students are involved in complex problem solving (Sternberg, 1985; Sternberg, et al., 2000). This approach to differentiated instruction helps all students, but is particularly beneficial for gifted students who can use their strengths for in-depth study.

General Guidelines

- Use *analytical activities* at times that encourage students to compare and contrast, analyze, evaluate, judge, and critique.

- Use *creative activities* at times that encourage students to discover, imagine, explore, invent, and create.

- Use *practical activities* at times that encourage students to use, contextualize, apply, and put into practice.

- Allow all students occasionally to capitalize on their strengths.

- More often, enable students to correct or compensate for their weaknesses.

- Use assessments that match the analytical, creative, and practical activities you are using, as well as testing for memory skills.

- Value the diversity of learning styles in all students.

USING THE TRIARCHIC MODEL IN THE CLASSROOM—Continued

Examples

Activity	Science	Language Arts	Social Studies
Analytical	• Draw the major parts of an animal cell, and explain what the parts do.	• Identify simile, analogy, and metaphor, and explain their function.	• Describe the steps necessary for a bill to become law in the state legislature.
Creative	• Write a story (or play) using characters representing the parts of an animal cell, and describe a potential conflict.	• Using unusual materials, act out simile, analogy, and metaphor in mime, and see if other students can guess them.	• Become a state senator, and use your position to help us think about the merits and problems of laws to restrict campaign financing.
Practical	• Find a system in the world around you that mimics the activities and relationships in an animal cell, and explain it.	• Demonstrate how someone would use similes, analogies, or metaphors in their work or life.	• Underage drinking is a problem here at school. Devise legislation that would address this problem.

APPLICATIONS

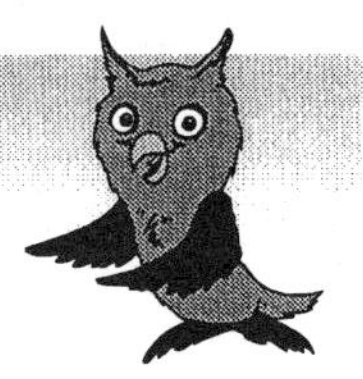

GUIDING STUDENTS FOR INDEPENDENT STUDY

Independent study is another useful strategy for differentiating curriculum and instruction, especially in the self-contained classroom. However, even gifted students often need guidance in pursuing learning objectives independently. Here are some considerations.

- Prepare options in advance for the students to select as part of the curriculum unit's work. These options should include a variety of ability levels, involve different skills, and address different learning styles.

- Encourage students to select the option they feel is most relevant to their topic. The teacher may need to help with this decision by discussing with the students how the options match their needs, strengths, and desires.

- Guide students toward appropriate resources that they can seek out independently.

- Ensure students that they can also develop other options for the curriculum unit, but that they should discuss them with the teacher before embarking on any work with the options.

- Suggest to students that they can occasionally work in small groups if necessary to accomplish their learning objectives.

- Encourage students to seek out other environments (e.g., another classroom, the media center, or computer lab) that will help them with their task.

APPLICATIONS

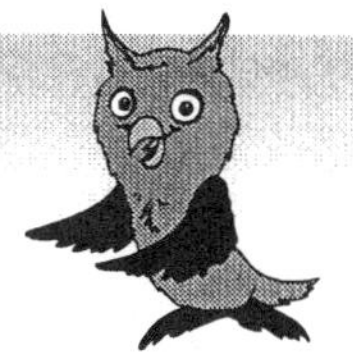

STEPS FOR DEVELOPING TIERED ACTIVITIES

In a classroom with students of mixed abilities, tiered activities offer choices for accomplishing a learning objective at different levels of complexity. The following guidelines are useful for planning tiered activities (Tomlinson, 1999).

- Decide which concepts, themes, and skills all students will be expected to learn in the instructional unit. These selections are the core fundamentals for developing an understanding of the curricular material.

- Use simple assessments to determine the range of readiness of the students who will be studying this unit. Other measures and previous experience will also allow you to determine the students' interests, talents, and learning styles as they pertain to the learning objectives.

- Select a past activity, or create a new one, that focuses students to use an important skill to understand an important idea. This activity should be interesting, relevant, and able to engage students in higher-level thought (e.g., Bloom's analysis or synthesis levels).

- Next, chart the complexity of the activity along some linear scale (Tomlinson suggests a ladder) that runs from low to high complexity. Think about the students who will be using the activity you developed in the previous step and place it on that scale. Its placement will help you determine what other versions of the activity need to be developed. For example, will the lesson challenge only the average ability students? If so, you need to develop versions for the low- and high-ability learners.

STEPS FOR DEVELOPING TIERED ACTIVITIES—Continued

- Devise the versions of the activity needed along the scale at the different degrees of complexity. These versions can be created by varying the material the students will use (from basic to very challenging), by developing a range of applications of the learning (from those that are close to the student to those that are very remote), and by allowing different products that students can use to demonstrate achievement.

- Finally, match each version of the activity to the appropriate students based on their learning profile and the requirements of the learning task. The goal is to closely match the degree of complexity to the students' readiness, but to add a measure of challenge.

APPLICATIONS

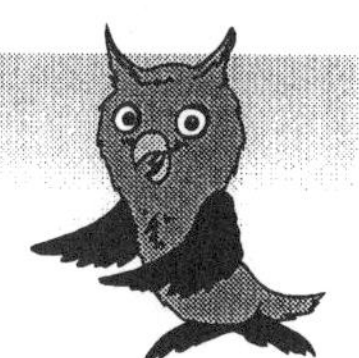

COMPONENTS OF EFFECTIVE CULMINATING PRODUCTS

A culminating product created by students at the end of a major unit of inquiry is an excellent opportunity to assess how much the students have learned. Teachers can use differentiation in their classes when they allow students to select from a broad variety of possible culminating projects. This venture is more apt to be successful if the teacher (Tomlinson, 1999)

- Makes clear to students what they should transfer, demonstrate, explain, or apply to show what they have learned and what they can do as a result of their inquiry.

- Allows students to choose from among a variety of product possibilities, such as videos, photo essays, charts and graphs, and written reports.

- Presents specific expectations about what (1) type of information, concepts, and resources constitute high-quality content; (2) steps should be used in developing the product, such as planning, editing, effective use of time, and originality; and (3) details describe the nature of the product itself, such as size, durability, format, construction, accuracy, and the anticipated audience.

- Supports student efforts by providing in-class workshops on how to use research materials, for brainstorming ideas, for discussing timelines, and for peer reviewing, critiquing, and editing.

- Provides for variations in student learning styles, interests, and learning readiness.

APPLICATIONS

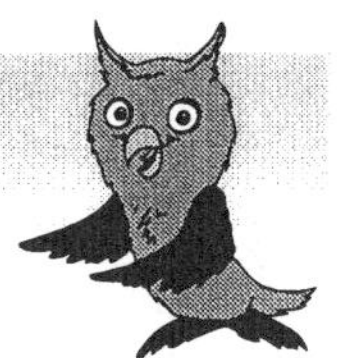

STRATEGIES FOR WORKING WITH GIFTED VISUAL-SPATIAL LEARNERS

Gifted visual-spatial learners do best with a holistic approach to learning. They prefer complex systems, abstract concepts, and inductive reasoning and problem solving. Recognizing the strengths and weaknesses of these learners, and making a few simple academic modifications, can help these students become successful and innovative leaders. Here are some strategies that have been found to be effective with visual-spatial learners (Silverman, 1989b).

- Use visual aids, such as overhead projectors, computers, diagrams, graphic organizers, and other visual imagery.
- Give them the larger scheme at the beginning of each unit and explain the major objectives so that the students understand the instructional goal.
- In spelling, use a visualization approach: Show the word, have students close their eyes and visualize it, have them spell it backward (this is visualization), then spell it forward, and then write it once.
- Find out what they have already mastered about the unit's topics before teaching them.
- Use manipulative materials for hands-on experiences.
- Avoid rote memorization. Use more conceptual and inductive approaches.
- Help students discover their own methods of problem solving. When they succeed, give them a harder problem to see if their system works.

WORKING WITH GIFTED VISUAL-SPATIAL LEARNERS—Continued

- Emphasize concepts over details. Encourage new insights, creativity, and imagination.
- Avoid drill and repetition. Instead, have them try the hardest tasks in the unit with at least 80 percent accuracy. If they accomplish this, then the students may not have to complete the rest of the assignment.
- Group gifted visual-spatial learners together for instruction. Give the group handouts if they have difficulty with dictation.
- Allow them to accelerate in school.
- Give them abstract, complex material at a faster pace.
- Use real-life scenarios and service-oriented projects whenever possible.
- Allow students to construct, draw, or create other visual representations of concepts.
- Have students discuss the moral, ethical, and global implications of their learning.
- For foreign language learning, total immersion is much more effective than being in the typical classroom setting for these students.
- At the end of each class or school day, ask the students to take a few deep breaths, close their eyes, and visualize what happened during the class (or day) and what they will need to do for homework.

APPLICATIONS

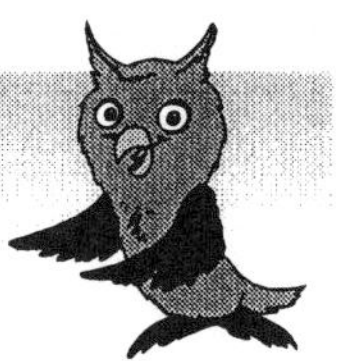

INTEGRATING ACADEMIC AND ARTS-RELATED ACTIVITIES FOR ALL GIFTED STUDENTS

Many academically talented students are also capable of being high performers in artistic endeavors. Because the artistic areas are often ignored in gifted programs, educators should incorporate the visual and performing arts into comprehensive gifted and talented programs. Here are some recommendations for accomplishing this task (Clark and Zimmerman, 1998).

- The arts should be included as an integral part of all comprehensive gifted and talented programs. This type of program will more likely accommodate the varying needs of the wide variety of abilities represented in a comprehensive program that includes academically and artistically gifted students.

- Just as scientifically talented students need access to modern, well-equipped laboratories, artistically gifted students should have access to facilities that resemble the studios, stages, and other workplaces of artists who are trying to solve problems in the arts. The goals of programs designed to educate artistically gifted students should be carefully integrated with those for students who are academically gifted so that all students benefit from comprehensive and enriching experiences.

- Traditionally, schools often encourage academically gifted students to take advanced classes in academic subjects within the school but suggest that they pursue artistic endeavors outside the school. Teachers, administrators, and parents need to be educated about the importance of including the arts as an integral part of the gifted education program, and to encourage all students to pursue the arts within the school setting.

ACADEMIC AND ARTS-RELATED ACTIVITIES—Continued

- Educators who teach academically and artistically talented students should collaborate in planning programs that provide equity and excellence, that reinforce shared goals, and that emphasize common strengths for the benefit of their students and the entire school community. Such collaboration would inevitably benefit all students who participate in programs that develop talent.

- More work needs to be done on developing resources and teaching strategies that incorporate the arts into the comprehensive programs for gifted students. If these resources are available, teachers are more likely to include them as a regular part of their repertoire. Furthermore, these strategies need to be appropriate to the learning styles and cultural backgrounds of individual students.

Developing integrated programs should not be solely the responsibility of teachers. Local, community, and state resources should be gathered to support these efforts and to establish liaisons with out-of-school entities (e.g., organizations, government agencies, and businesses) that can contribute to the success of the comprehensive program.

4

Language Talent

One of the most extraordinary features of the human brain is its ability to acquire spoken language quickly and accurately. We are born with an innate capacity to distinguish the distinct sounds (phonemes) of all the languages on this planet. Eventually, we are able to associate those sounds with arbitrary symbols to express our thoughts and emotions to others. Ever since Paul Broca discovered evidence in 1861 that the left hemisphere of the brain was specialized for language, researchers have attempted to understand the way in which normal human beings acquire and process their native language.

SOURCES OF LANGUAGE ABILITY

In most people, the left hemisphere is home to the major components of the language processing system (Figure 4.1). Broca's area is a region of the left frontal lobe that is believed to be responsible for processing vocabulary, syntax, and rules of grammar. Wernicke's area is part of the left temporal lobe and is thought to process the sense and meaning of language. However, the emotional content of language is governed by areas in the right hemisphere.

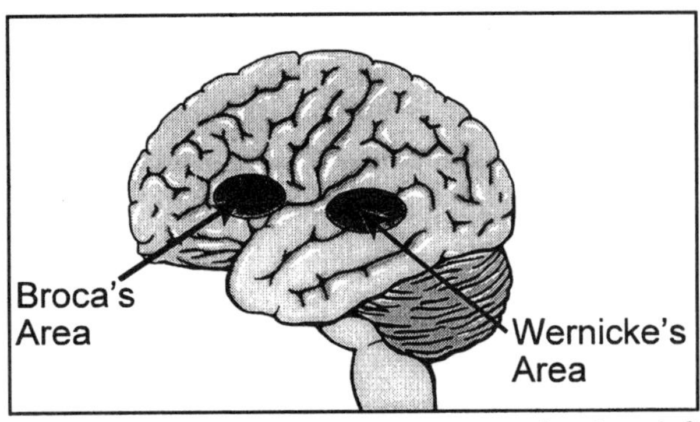

Figure 4.1 The language system in the left hemisphere is comprised mainly of Broca's area and Wernicke's area.

Brain imaging studies of infants as young as 4 months of age confirm that the brain possesses neural networks that specialize in responding to the auditory components of language. Dehaene-Lambertz (2000) used EEG recordings to measure the brain activity of sixteen 4-month-old infants as they listened to language syllables and acoustic tones. After numerous trials, the data showed that syllables and tones were processed primarily in different areas of the left hemisphere, although there was also some right hemisphere activity. For language input, various features, such as the voice and the phonetic category of a syllable, were encoded by separate neural networks into sensory memory. These remarkable findings suggest that, even at this early age, the brain is already organized into functional networks that can distinguish between language fragments and other acoustical input.

The apparent predisposition of the brain to the sounds of language explains why normal young children respond to and acquire spoken language quickly. How long the brain retains this responsiveness to the sounds of language is still open to question. However, there does seem to be general agreement among researchers that the window of opportunity for acquiring language within the language-specific areas of the brain tapers off for most people around 10 to 12 years of age. Obviously, one can still acquire a new language after that age, but it takes more effort because the new language will be spatially separated in the brain from the native language areas (Sousa, 2001a).

Structure of Language

Languages consist of distinct units of sound called *phonemes*. Although each language has its own unique set of phonemes, only about 150 phonemes comprise all the world's languages. These phonemes consist of all the speech sounds that can be made by the human voice apparatus. Around the age of 6 months or so, infants start babbling, an early sign of language acquisition. Their babbling consists of all those phonemes, even ones they have never heard. Within a few months, however, pruning of the phonemes begins, and by about one year of age, the neural networks focus on the sounds of the language being spoken in the infant's environment (Beatty, 2001).

Syntax and Semantics

With more exposure, the brain begins to recognize the hierarchy of language (Figure 4.2). Phonemes, the basic sounds, can be combined into morphemes, which are the smallest units of language that have meaning. Morphemes can then be combined into words, and words can be put together according to the rules of syntax to form phrases and sentences. Toddlers show evidence of their progression through these levels when simple statements, such as

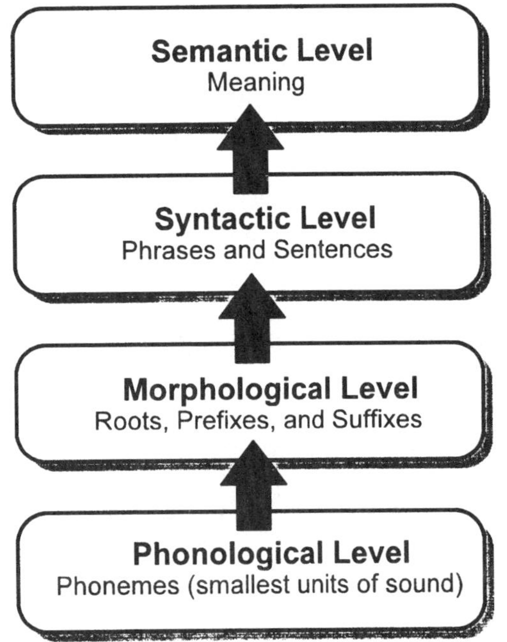

Figure 4.2 These four levels represent the hierarchical structure of language and language acquisition.

"Candy," evolve to more complex ones, "Give me candy." They also begin to recognize that shifting the words in sentences can change their meaning.

The brain's ability to recognize different meanings in sentence structure is possible because Broca's and Wernicke's areas establish linked networks that can understand the difference between "The dog chased the cat" and "The cat chased the dog." In an fMRI study, Dapretto and Bookheimer (1999) found that Broca's and Wernicke's areas work together to determine whether changes in syntax or semantics result in changes in meaning. For example, "The policeman arrested the thief" and "The thief was arrested by the policeman" have different syntax but the same meaning. The fMRI showed that Broca's area was highly activated when subjects were processing these two sentences. Wernicke's area, on the other hand, was more activated when processing sentences that were semantically—but not syntactically—different, such as "The car is in the garage" and "The automobile is in the garage."

How is it that Wernicke's area can so quickly and accurately decide that two semantically different sentences have the same meaning? The answer may lie in two other recently discovered characteristics of Wernicke's area. One is that the neurons in Wernicke's area are spaced about 20 percent further apart and are cabled together with longer interconnecting axons than the corresponding area in the right hemisphere of the brain (Galuske, Schlote, Bratzke, and Singer, 2000). The implication is that the practice of language during early human development results in longer and more intricately connected neurons in the Wernicke region.

The ability to understand language may be rooted in the brain's ability to recognize predictability.

The second recent discovery regarding Wernicke's area is its ability to recognize predictable events. An MRI study found that Wernicke's area was activated when subjects were shown differently colored symbols in various patterns, whether the individuals were aware of the pattern sequence or not (Bischoff-Grethe, Proper, Mao, Daniels, and Berns, 2000). This predictability-determining role for Wernicke's area suggests that our ability to make sense of language is rooted in our ability to recognize syntax. The researchers noted that language itself is very predicable because it is constrained by the rules of grammar and syntax.

Genes, Language, and the Environment

The production of phonemes by infants is the result of genetically determined neural programs; however, language exposure is environmental. These two components interact to produce an individual's language system and, assuming no pathologies, sufficient competence to communicate clearly with others. Scientists, of course, are interested in the exact nature of that interaction in an effort to determine how genes can be modified by the environment, and vice versa. These gene-environment relationships are called *genotype-environment correlations* (GECs). Research on GECs helps to explain the degree to which a child's genetic destiny can be modified by environmental experiences. Three types of GECs have been described: evocative, active, and passive (Scarr and McCartney, 1983).

Evocative GEC occurs when young students who are talented in language are identified by their teachers and provided with special opportunities to enhance their gifts. In other words, they evoke reactions from other individuals on the basis of their genetic predispositions. Consequently, these students will receive more verbal input and be better stimulated than students without such talents. Over time, the talented group's environment and genetics mutually influence each other, favoring the development of greater language ability.

Environmental variables in the home may not be reliable predictors of a child's language ability.

Active GEC occurs when students talented in language arts seek out environments that are rich in language experiences. For example, they may want to associate with like-talented peers or take part in poetry or essay contests. Once again, this type of GEC can enhance language skills due to the different groups that the students place themselves into over time.

Passive GEC occurs when students talented in language arts inherit both the genes from their similarly talented parents *and* the environment that promotes the development of language ability. Hence, the children passively receive a family environment that is closely correlated to their genetic predispositions.

Evocative and active GECs can occur inside or outside the family and become increasingly important as the child moves outside the family and becomes involved in other environments. Passive GEC, on the other hand, occurs only within the biological family and tends to decrease in importance as the child matures. Consequently, children who are passive GEC candidates are the most appropriate group to study when trying to determine how much various environmental factors moderate genetic traits.

To that end, a major longitudinal study of passive GEC, by Jeffrey Gilger and his colleagues, looked at language development in children from about 400 families over a 12-year period (Gilger, Ho, Whipple, and Spitz, 2001). In order to isolate the genetic propensities from the environmental influences on linguistic development, the children were selected from an almost even split of adoptive and nonadoptive families. Language-related assessment measures were administered to the subjects during the second, fourth, seventh, tenth, and twelfth years.

Evidence emerged from this study that genetic predispositions *can* dampen the influence of four environmental variables: the provision of toys and games in the home, the degree of maternal involvement in the child's language development, the number of people living in the home, and the degree of intellectual/cultural orientation in the home. Using statistical analysis, the researchers estimated the genetic contribution to these variables to range from 11 to 100 percent.

Keep in mind that passive GECs decrease in importance as the child ages because the family becomes less significant than peers and other adults in the child's environment. Two major implications arise from this study: (1) It is important to avoid drawing conclusions from family data about the impact of the environment on language-based skills, and (2) children possessed of genetic predisposition for high language ability, but raised in family environments that do not evoke the ability, can still realize their potential when they encounter teachers who recognize and nurture these talents.

Learning to Read

Speech will develop in the human brain without any specific instruction. Reading, on the other hand, is an acquired skill. To read correctly, the brain must learn to connect abstract symbols (the alphabet) to those sound bits (phonemes) it already knows. In English, the brain must first learn and remember the alphabet, and then connect those 26 letters to the 44 sounds of spoken English that the child has been using successfully for years. Thus, reading involves a recognition that speech can be broken into small sounds and that these segmented sounds can be represented by symbols in print called *graphemes*. The brain's ability to recognize that written symbols can represent sounds is known as the alphabetic principle. Unfortunately, the human brain is not born with the insight to make these sound-to-symbol connections, nor does it develop naturally without instruction. Children of literate homes may encounter this instruction before coming to school. If these children possess any type of genetic predispositions for high language ability, they are likely to learn quickly the complex process of reading earlier than other children of the same age.

Successful reading involves the coordination of three neural networks: visual processing (orthography), sound recognition (phonology), and word interpretation (semantics). In reading the word *dog*, for example, the visual processing system puts the symbols together. The decoding process alerts the auditory processing system that recognizes the alphabetic symbols to represent the sound "dawg." Other brain regions, including the frontal lobe, search long-term memory sites for meaning. If all systems work correctly, a mental image emerges of a furry animal that barks (Figure 4.3).

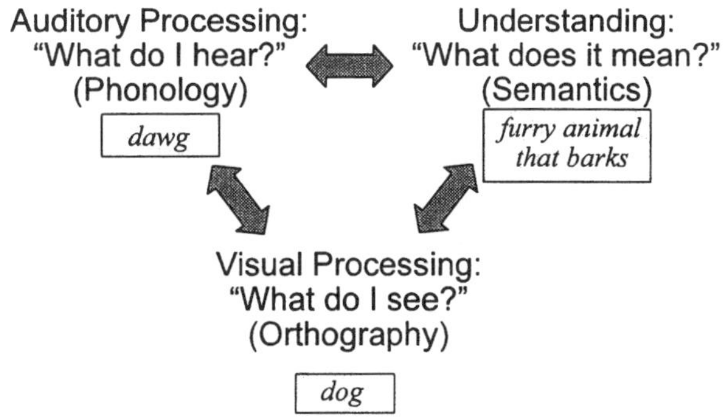

Figure 4.3 Successful reading requires the coordination of three systems: visual processing to see the word, auditory processing to hear it, and semantic processing to understand it.

Learning to read also requires good memory systems. Working memory has to keep words available so that letter sounds found at the beginning of the word can be connected to those found at the end of the word. Eventually, the learner has to be able to remember the meaning of the word if future reading is to be successful. Because so many words in English have different meanings in different contexts, the learner must also remember every word in the sentence in order for the brain to select the correct meaning and put everything together.

Some brains acquire the skills associated with reading, such as phonemic awareness and the alphabetic principle, very quickly, and reading becomes an easy task. Most neuroscientists who study how the brain reads agree that genetic predispositions likely enhance processing within various neural networks that contribute to reading. In rare cases, the predisposition is so strong that it produces a condition known as *hyperlexia*, where the child becomes a voracious reader at the expense of developing spoken language and communication skills. See Chapter 8 for more about hyperlexia.

IDENTIFYING STUDENTS GIFTED IN LANGUAGE ARTS

Students who are gifted in the language arts of reading, writing, and communication skills will demonstrate competencies in some or all of the following areas:

Awareness of language. These students understand the nature of language and show special interest in language features, such as rhyme, accent, and intonation in spoken language, and the use of grammar in written texts. They often have an interest in other languages and demonstrate an awareness of the relationship between the sounds and words of other languages.

Communication skills. These students can easily gain the attention of an audience by exploiting the humorous or dramatic components of a situation in imaginative ways. They tend to write and talk with a creative flair that is exceptional for their age, often using metaphors and poetry. They can also express ideas elegantly and succinctly, in ways that reflect the knowledge and interests of specific audiences. They will guide a group to achieve its shared goals, while being sensitive to the participation of others.

Reasoning and arguing. These students can use reasoned arguments at an abstract and hypothetical level in both spoken and written language. They can justify their opinions convincingly, and they know how to use questioning strategies to challenge the points of view of others.

DEVELOPING LANGUAGE ABILITY

Students talented in language arts will develop their abilities when they are challenged by experiences involving sophisticated language. Too often in the regular classroom, the reading materials and language activities are not sufficiently challenging for gifted students, who then become bored when their learning needs are not being adequately met. For these students to grow, they should be given language problems that are not easily solved, that are open-ended, and that force them to think, study, reread, and reformulate. Thus, a curriculum designed for these students should build upon the characteristics of the intellectually gifted. It should carefully identify which components and strategies will be used at each grade level in order to eliminate the content redundancy that plagues too many curriculum guides.

As explained earlier, teachers can have a great impact on evoking language-related talents in students. The teachers in this program should be highly intelligent, emotionally secure, comfortable interacting with gifted students, and able to demonstrate advanced knowledge of the subject matter. Evaluate the success of the program through the students' work product and not by tests of mastery of lower-level skills. This may require developing new assessment instruments because most current tests evaluate acquisition of knowledge rather than the application of knowledge in creative ways.

Some Instructional Approaches and Strategies

In an effort to address the needs of students who are gifted in language arts, teachers have devised various instructional approaches and strategies to generate exciting experiences in all aspects of language including vocabulary development, grammar, reading, and writing. Here is just a sampling of those ideas, which, of course, could be appropriate for all students. The activities are explained in greater detail in **Applications** at the end of this chapter.

Focus on the Classics (Grades 5 and Higher)

Thompson (1999) suggests that to develop verbal talent, students need go beyond the regular basal texts and be exposed to classical literature. Great books are called great because they can have different meaning for different readers. The classics stretch imaginations, challenge ideas, and open a new world of possibilities for expressing the human condition in language. Gifted students often see themselves in classic stories, whose characters can become their virtual mentors.

The classics also provide an exposure to rich vocabulary somewhat lacking, according to Thompson, from the literature anthologies used in today's classrooms. In addition to their value as sources of mentors and vocabulary, the classics expose students to a wealth of divergent and often conflicting ideas. They shock students into thought, forcing them to confront new concepts.

Author's Chair (Grades 3 and Higher)

This is an opportunity for writers to share their final compositions with an audience in order to receive positive feedback that will assist them in future writing efforts. A particular chair in the classroom is designated for this activity. In addition to the value of the feedback, this strategy also develops listening skills for students in the audience.

Student Journal Writing (Grades 3 and Higher)

Journal writing provides a natural way to integrate language through reading, writing, and discussion. Gifted students generally enjoy expressing their ideas verbally, but keeping a continuous written journal requires them to write, rephrase, and reflect on their thoughts. Different types of journals can be used for different purposes. *Dialogue journals* are conversations in print, designed to promote fluent oral and written communication. In *literary journals*, students enter their responses to works of literature that they have read. A third type is the *subject journal*, in which students record information related to specific topics (e.g., ecology, dinosaurs, and minerals).

Literature Circles (Grades 3 and Higher)

In literature circles, small groups of students discuss a literary work in depth, guided by their responses to what they have read. The circles help students engage in reflection and critical thinking, building on their understanding and ability to construct meaning with other readers.

Writer's Workshop (Grades 7 and Higher)

Writer's workshops were first used to develop the work of adult writers who were pursuing writing as a profession. However, the format can be adapted to younger individuals. Essentially, writer's workshop is a thoughtful and more sophisticated form of Author's Chair that is best suited for older middle and high school students who are gifted in language arts. As in Author's Chair, students who have read a writer's paper give feedback that identifies positive features, such as the literary forms and patterns that the author used, and offer constructive criticism as well. The comments are intended to help the author improve the paper, but the author is not obligated to follow all the suggestions. Because it is time consuming, this strategy should be used sparingly and only with students who are comfortable with feedback that includes constructive criticism.

Out-of-School Activities (High School)

Opportunities often exist in the local community and region for these students to extend and enrich their experiences with language arts.

APPLICATIONS

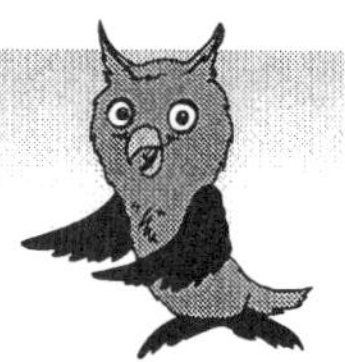

IDENTIFYING STUDENTS WITH LANGUAGE TALENT

Students with high ability in language do tend to display common characteristics, especially by the time they reach middle school where language fluency rapidly develops. Use the scale below to help decide if a particular student is gifted in language arts. If you rate the student with scores of 4 or 5 on more than half of the characteristics, then further assessment is warranted.

The student...	A little Some A lot
1. Writes or talks in imaginative and coherent ways.	1 — 2 — 3 — 4 — 5
2. Organizes text in a manner that is exceptional for the student's age.	1 — 2 — 3 — 4 — 5
3. Expresses ideas succinctly and elegantly.	1 — 2 — 3 — 4 — 5
4. Writes with a flair for metaphorical and poetic expression.	1 — 2 — 3 — 4 — 5
5. Takes the lead in helping a group reach its writing goal.	1 — 2 — 3 — 4 — 5
6. Easily grasps the essence of a writing style and adapts it for personal use.	1 — 2 — 3 — 4 — 5
7. Can capture and maintain the attention of an audience by using drama and humor in imaginative ways.	1 — 2 — 3 — 4 — 5
8. Engages creatively and seriously with social and moral issues expressed in literature.	1 — 2 — 3 — 4 — 5
9. Justifies opinions convincingly.	1 — 2 — 3 — 4 — 5
10. Shows special awareness of language features, such as intonation, rhyme, accents in spoken language, and grammatical organization in written texts.	1 — 2 — 3 — 4 — 5
11. Presents reason arguments at the hypothetical or abstract level in both spoken and written language.	1 — 2 — 3 — 4 — 5

APPLICATIONS

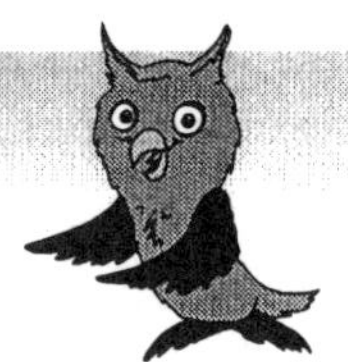

WORKING WITH GIFTED READERS

Young gifted readers are those who start to read early, read better with less drill, read longer, and read a variety of literature. Teachers promote the intellectual development of gifted readers by selecting books and materials that allow the students to (Halsted, 1990)

- Work with intellectual peers
- Build skills in productive thinking
- Have more time for processing ideas and concepts
- Share ideas in depth verbally
- Pursue ideas as far as their interests take them
- Encounter and use increasingly difficult vocabulary and concepts
- Draw generalizations and test them

Promoting Intellectual Development

Teachers can use books to promote intellectual development by requiring students to read whole books in addition to their reading in the basal series. This approach is positive for gifted students because it rewards them for something they already enjoy. To ensure quality control and choice, the teacher should prepare the reading list from which students can choose their required books. Teachers may also suggest that students keep notebooks for recording the title, author, short comments about the book, and the dates the book was read.

Librarians, teachers, and volunteers can lead discussion of the books that students have read. These group discussions should focus on main themes and ideas, encouraging students to pursue higher-level thinking, such as analysis and syntheses, rather than to give just plot summaries and statements of fact.

Books can also be a part of the educational program for individual students, provided that an adult (teacher, parent, librarian, or other mentor) offers guidance appropriate to the student's interests, reading ability, and reading background.

WORKING WITH GIFTED READERS—Continued

Nurturing Emotional Development

Gifted children may experience feelings of difference and even inferiority, isolation, and a sense of being misunderstood by others. They must constantly choose between the alternatives of using their abilities and the need to fit into their group. Choices like this make growing up more difficult for them. Consequently, teachers need to nurture the social and emotional development of gifted children, in addition to meeting their intellectual needs. Many novels written for children address these affective concerns. The adults who discuss these books with gifted young students can help them cope with the additional considerations that being gifted add to the process of maturing.

Promoting Emotional Development

Books can be used to help individuals who are facing a particular situation, such as giftedness, become better prepared through reading and discussion. This process, known as developmental bibliotherapy, includes three components: a book, a reader, and a leader who reads the same book and prepares a productive discussion on the issues raised in the book. The goal is to help the reader identify with a character in the book, experience that character's emotions, and apply the experience to the reader's own life. The leader's role is to guide this process and to develop questions that will confirm and expand on these elements. Used appropriately, developmental bibliotherapy can be an effective tool for helping young students cope successfully with their giftedness.

APPLICATIONS

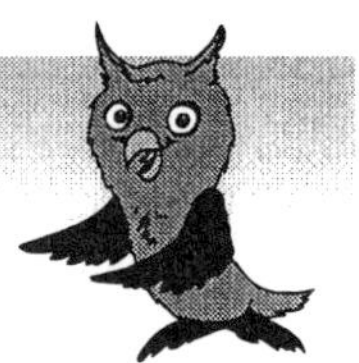

LANGUAGE ARTS STRATEGIES FOR GIFTED ELEMENTARY STUDENTS

Gifted students who have already mastered much of the required oral and written language skills for their grade level need strategies to stimulate imaginative and higher-order thinking. Although the following strategies, suggested by Smutny (2001), are appropriate for all students, they encourage gifted students to work at their own pace and level of complexity.

Exploring Poetic Language: Free Verse

Teachers can use poetry to help gifted students explore the quality of words, the power of metaphoric language, and the subtly and complexity of meaning. Without the constrictions of a rhyming scheme, free verse allows students to focus on imagery and to experiment with various writing styles.

> *Creating a group poem.* One method for demonstrating the different ways to write free verse is to have the students work as a group to create a free verse poem together. Using a picture or poster as the theme, ask the students to think about the picture's color, any feelings they get, and what the picture's components mean to them. Ask questions that will provoke their imagination: "If you were to think of the animals in this picture as colors, what colors would they be? If they were music, what sounds would you hear?" Write on the chalkboard the words and phrases that the students contribute. Read the words as a poem and talk about the images that are generated.
>
> *Creating individual poems.* All kinds of media, such as music recordings, games, pictures, posters, puzzles, films, and paintings, can be used as the basis for creating poetry. Help the students select the medium and stimulate original thinking by asking focused questions: "What is the main character in this painting staring at? What mood is he in? What else could be happening around him? What could have happened minutes later?"

LANGUAGE ARTS STRATEGIES—Continued

Exploring the Elements of Fiction

Divergent thinking. Exploring fiction becomes much more exciting if students think divergently about their stories. Divergent thinking involves pursuing the answers to open-ended questions, such as "How would you change this story, and why? Given all that has happened so far, what are some possible endings to this story? What would you have done in these circumstances, and why?"

Exploring fiction with fractured fairy tales. Altering the plot, setting, or character of a fairy tale in an unexpected way can produce a humorous twist of fiction and stimulate the imagination. For example: What if the big, bad wolf fails to blow down any of the pigs' homes, or the pigs come out and confront the wolf? What if the three bears return home while Goldilocks is still snooping around the place? After presenting a fractured fairy tale, asking some questions can help the students think through what changes have been made and what they mean: "Which events occur in the new tale that do not occur in the original? How do the changes in plot and character behavior affect the overall meaning of the story?"

A Study of Perspective: Biographical and Historical Fiction

Biographies and histories enable gifted students to conceive imaginary versions of actual events from different viewpoints. It gives them an opportunity to critically and creatively debate points in history and politics based on their own revisions of events. By writing biographical and historical fiction, they can explore new and exciting perspectives.

Researching the facts. Use books, short films, and magazines to introduce students to the work of prominent men and women. Get students to research what influenced these individuals in their youth, how they overcame difficulties or obstacles in their lives, and what were the most significant contributions they made to society. As they write down this information, they should also note any questions they have about the person's life. Then ask them to find out the answers to these questions. One of the values of this activity is that it inspires further research and analysis of issues that appear in the story.

LANGUAGE ARTS STRATEGIES—Continued

Creating a point of view. Ask students to choose a person, animal, or object in this prominent person's life and describe an event from this perspective. Students often discover how individual points of view can create quite a different focus from that of the author who wrote the biography. For historical fiction, students can create a fictional character who, for example, fought in the Civil War. They could devise a fictional biography of this character and write an anecdote of an event that could have happened to this person in this time and place. This approach helps gifted students to see history in a different light, recognizing that within each daily news story, there are many individuals who see an event with slightly different perspectives.

These types of investigations with language arts engage the analytical minds and creative talents of gifted students. The strategies allow these students to expand their experiences with literature through their own creative designing and writing, and to gain a deeper insight into the people and events that have influenced our lives and shaped our world.

APPLICATIONS

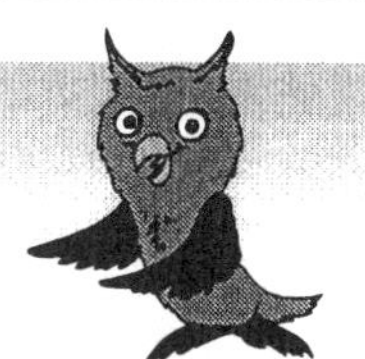

USING CLASSICAL LITERATURE TO DEVELOP LANGUAGE ABILITY

Thompson (1999) makes a strong case for using classical literature to lure students away from the basal readers and to encounter new ideas that extend their capabilities in language. Here are some of this suggestions.

- *Identifying with a character.* Encourage students to read classics, such as those found in the Junior Great Books or Great Books programs. The characters in these literary masterpieces provide a powerful source of virtual mentors. Suggest that students talk about which characters they like and explain their reasons. Describe something the character did that they would like to do. What other choices can the character make, and what are their consequences?

- *Enriching vocabulary.* Classic literature offers a rich source of vocabulary not usually found in basal readers. Ask students to select words they found particularly interesting, to define them, and to speculate why the author might have chosen those words. What other words might the author have used? Thompson has compiled a word database, which includes a number of unusual items found in common classics. Here are the first ten books on his list, followed by the number of noteworthy words each contains:

  Uncle Tom's Cabin, Harriet Beecher Stowe, 714
  Ivanhoe, Sir Walter Scott, 519
  Gulliver's Travels, Jonathan Swift, 472
  The War of the Worlds, H. G. Wells, 379
  Dracula, Bram Stoker, 345
  Tom Sawyer, Mark Twain, 293
  Robinson Crusoe, Daniel Defoe, 279
  Treasure Island, Robert Louis Stevenson, 254
  Silas Marner, George Eliot (Mary Ann Evans), 216
  To Kill a Mockingbird, Harper Lee, 208

USING CLASSICAL LITERATURE—Continued

- *Classic ideas.* Classic literature exposes students to the divergent, complex, and conflicting ideas of heroes like Mark Twain, Martin Luther King, Henry David Thoreau, and Thomas Jefferson. These voices express all kinds of humanitarian and uplifting themes: be yourself, be free, be ethical, find happiness, and protect the people.

- *Quality and quantity.* Some of these books will need to be assigned as home reading because few schools can dedicate time for the amount of reading necessary for gifted students. Two classics per semester might be reasonable for middle and high school students. Teachers should also ensure that they assign books rich in vocabulary.

- *The power of ancient words.* Teachers should encourage students with high ability in language arts to study the structure of words, thereby enriching their own vocabulary and ensuring their success in tackling examinations (e.g., the SAT) that assess vocabulary development. Just studying the Greek and Latin stems, for example, can help a student gain understanding of over 5,000 new words. Some other advantages of learning these stems are

  Power learning - Because the stems appear in many words and combinations, this approach to learning vocabulary is more powerful than learning one word at a time.

  Spelling - Thousands of English words are nothing more than several stems in a row. By learning the stems, a student learns spelling for many words at the same time.

  Standardized tests - The final few, and most difficult, questions on the SAT analogies test contain vocabulary words that are almost always stem-based. Students who have studied these stems, therefore, are likely to do better.

  Sense of history - As students study the stems of words, they realize that language was not just invented in our time, but also reflects a historic development of many voices over eons.

  Advanced vocabulary - Many stem-based words are big words used by science and technology. The names of biological species and diseases are just two examples of how

USING CLASSICAL LITERATURE—Continued

new words are continually created from Latin and Greek roots.

- *The power of stems.* Greek and Latin stems form the basis for many words in English. Middle school students gifted in language arts may find the pursuit of these stems an enjoyable project. However, it is more important to learn the stem and its definition than the word example. Here are a few common stems for starters.

  ***ante-**, antecedent, anterior, anteroom*
  ***anti-**, antibody, antitoxin, antithesis*
  ***circum-**, circumnavigate, circumspect, circumvent*
  ***con-**, contract, confine, conjunction*
  ***equi-**, equivocate, equilateral, equinox*
  ***intra-**, intramural, intravenous, intracoastal*
  ***mal-**, malapropism, malodorous, malicious*
  ***non-**, nonprofit, nonchalant, nonfeasance*
  ***pre-**, presume, precede, premature*
  ***semi-**, semifinal, semicircle, semiformal*
  ***super-**, superb, supervise, superfluous*
  ***sym-**, symbiosis, symbolic, symphony*
  ***un-**, unfit, undeniable, unconventional*

- *Pursuing grammar.* Grammar is often viewed by students as tedious and a waste of time. But students gifted in language arts may find studying grammar to be a useful method for critical thinking about language. Grammar provides a way for students to think about how they use language, how grammar can clarify or muddle, and how different authors use language in their own styles. This approach offers a deeper appreciation for literature and the enjoyment of crafting good sentences and compositions.

APPLICATIONS

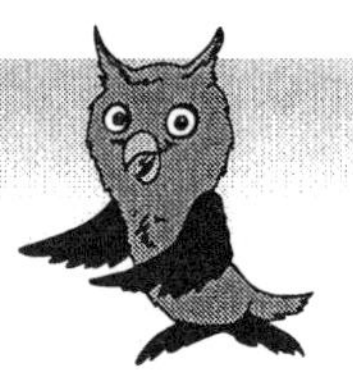

AUTHOR'S CHAIR

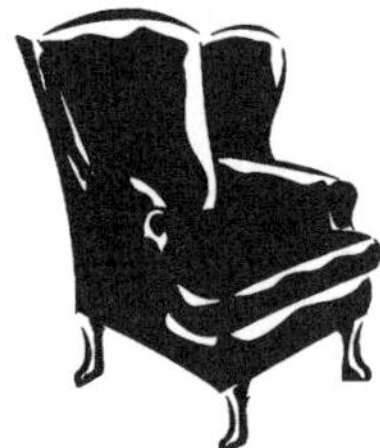

This activity gives writers an opportunity to share their writing products with an audience. A special time and chair are designated for this activity, which provides the author with valuable feedback from classmates. It is appropriate for grades 3 and higher.

Purpose

- To provide students an audience for their writings and motivation to write more in the future.
- To promote listening skills for students in the audience.
- To develop the analyzing and critical thinking skills necessary to critique someone else's work. The critical reviews benefit the writings of both the presenter and the members of the audience.

Procedure

- Select a special chair, such as an overstuffed chair or an office executive's chair, as the Author's Chair. The author orally presents the written material.
- Audience members listen carefully, mentally noting what they like and do not like about the writing.
- The teacher may wish to model the types of responses that would be appropriate from the audience. For example: "The language you used to describe the sunrise at the beach was vivid." "I could really feel the sadness in the character's words when she responded to the bad news."
- Audience members then share only what they liked about the writing, and the author responds to these comments. The author or teacher may set a limit on the number of responses from each audience member or the entire group.
- Set a time limit for the activity. For grades 3 to 5, 15 to 20 minutes is usually sufficient. Longer sessions may be appropriate for the upper grades.

APPLICATIONS

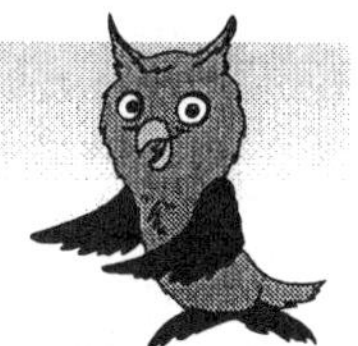

STUDENT JOURNAL WRITING

Student journals are an effective means for integrating the components of language, and they benefit all students. They are particularly effective with gifted language arts students, who usually enjoy all forms of language expression. Here are some suggestions for using this strategy effectively (Cobine, 1995).

Format

The journal writing portion of a lesson can be structured in many different ways, depending on the grade level, purpose, and type of journal. For example, the teacher can start with an oral reading of a passage from literature and follow it with journal writing about the passage (Note: *both* teacher and students write their entries). To model a critical response and to set students at ease about sharing their entries, the teacher should read his or her entry first.

In another format, the teacher initiates a 15-minute focused pre-journal writing session about the day's reading. Afterwards, the teacher separates the class into small groups, appoints a leader, and assigns a focus task or question for discussion. The groups share the results of their discussions with each other and individually write a second version that will become part of their journals.

Types of Journals

Journal writing serves several useful purposes that can be combined into one student notebook. For example, a notebook in English class might be modeled after a book, containing a preface, a body of chapters, and a glossary. These divisions suggest three different types of journal entries, designed to achieve separate goals.

Dialogue journals. Dialogue journals foster communicativeness among students and can serve as the preface for the combined notebook. These journals are personal, informal, succinct, and direct. As a preface for the notebook, students could write about their perspective and respond to questions the teacher may have written alongside their entries. Later, the teacher could write comments about the students' responses. In this way, students have a real audience who helps to enhance their reflection and rhetorical awareness.

STUDENT JOURNAL WRITING—Continued

Literary journals. The literary journal can serve as the body of chapters for the combined notebook. In this type of journal, students maintain a record of their personal responses to passages from literature. Their writings may include predictions about plot, analyses of characters, and insights about themes. Whenever the plot or actions of a character are suggestive of real-life experiences, the students can also include those personal references in their entries.

Subject journals. The subject journal serves as the glossary for the student notebook. For an English-class notebook, there are several possible uses. One section could be reserved for student responses to the author's biography or about historic events mentioned in the literary work. Another section might represent a personalized dictionary of literary and linguistic terms for further study. A third section could be a personalized stylebook of grammatical, rhetorical, and mechanical concerns about their writings. Here, the students track the progress of their language usage throughout the course.

Journal writing promotes communication, clarity of thought, and investigation into language styles. At the same time, it connects the processes of reading, writing, and discourse. The different types of journals and the diverse student participation accommodate multiple learning styles and offer exciting challenges to gifted students.

APPLICATIONS

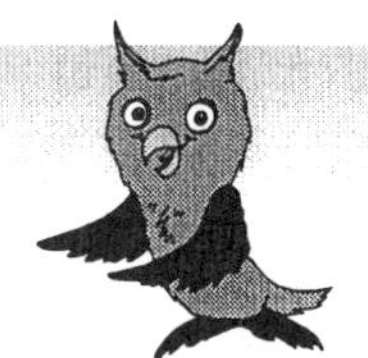

LITERATURE CIRCLES

In literature circles, small groups of students read and discuss the same book. The discussions are led by their reactions to the characters and events in the book. Collaboration is critical to the success of this activity because it forms the bridge by which students connect their understandings about the literary work with those of others in the real world.

Procedure

- Students choose their own reading material from a list provided by the teacher.
- Small temporary groups are formed, based upon the book choice of the student. Different groups read different books.
- Groups meet on a regular schedule to discuss their reading. The students use written (or sketched) notes to guide their discussions.
- Discussion topics come from the student but are cleared through the teacher.
- The group discussions should be open, so personal connections and open-ended questions are welcome.
- Students play a rotating assortment of task roles. For example, the roles and tasks might include

    Discussion director: This student develops a list of questions that the group wants to discuss about the book. The questions should focus on big ideas and stay away from small details.

    Literary presenter: This student selects a few special sections that the group would like to hear read aloud. This is to help students remember some powerful, mysterious, puzzling, humorous, or important sections of the text.

    Connector: This student looks for connections between the group's book and the real world. It may involve connecting the reading to students' lives, to happenings at school or in the community, or to similar events at other times and places.

LITERATURE CIRCLES—Continued

Illustrator: This student draws a quality picture related to the reading. Other students should comment on the picture before the illustrator explains it.

Summarizer: This student prepares a brief summary of the day's reading, which includes key points, main highlights, and the essential theme of the group's literary choice.

- The teacher serves as a facilitator, not as a group member or instructor.
- The group's work is evaluated by student self-evaluation and by teacher observation.
- When the books are finished, the groups share with each other and new groups are formed around new literary choices.

Guidelines

- Literature circles are *not* meant to be teacher- or text-centered activities.
- Groups should not be formed solely by ability. However, a group formed entirely of students who are gifted in the language arts may be appropriate.
- These circles are not the place to do skills work.
- The group's operating rules should encourage student responsibility, independence, and ownership.

APPLICATIONS

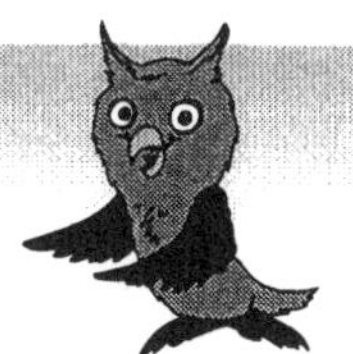

CONDUCTING A WRITER'S WORKSHOP

A writer's workshop is a sophisticated format that is particularly effective in reviewing, evaluating, and improving an author's literary descriptions and style. It was first used with adult writers who were interested in pursing writing as a career. The basic structure, however, can be modified to accommodate younger writers.

Because it is a labor- and time-intensive strategy, it should be used sparingly and only with more mature middle and high school students who are gifted in language arts, who have a strong self-image, and who can devote the required time and effort. During the workshop, a panel of peers examines the strengths and weaknesses of an author's paper, accentuating positive aspects and suggesting improvements in style and content.

Format

- A group of panel members (usually other student authors) reads the author's paper carefully before the workshop.
- In one format, the author is present but does *not* participate during most of the discussion. The author takes notes in order to respond later to the panelists' comments. (Another variation allows the written paper to be discussed by a group that includes the author, a moderator, and several reviewers who are familiar with the author's work. The author selects and reads a paragraph and expresses feelings about the selection. One or two reviewers then briefly summarize their viewpoint of the author's paper, but they should avoid debating inconsistencies between their interpretations of the work's content.)
- The panel then discusses and praises what they liked about the paper in terms of content and style.
- Following the discussion on positive aspects, the panel presents ways to improve the content and style of the paper, offering constructive suggestions on how to make the work better. The protocol is to first state the problem and then follow with a suggestion on how to solve the problem.

CONDUCTING A WRITER'S WORKSHOP—Continued

- During the discussion of both the positive aspects and the areas needing improvement, the author does not participate. Nor do the reviewers address the author directly. The reviewers should refer to the author in the third person and should not look at the author when making comments.
- After this discussion, the author may ask questions of the reviewers to clarify and better understand their comments.
- The audience thanks the author for writing the paper.

Guidelines

- The teacher's main duty during this process is to act as moderator and ensure that the students behave courteously towards each other and towards the author. People feel uneasy when being evaluated, even under the best of circumstances. The teacher needs to insist on an atmosphere that is constructive and conducive to insightful discussions, rather than allowing students to show off their intellect by attacking others.
- Panel reviewers are usually authors themselves, whose papers will also go through this process. In some situations, teachers may wish to include non-authors in the class as reviewers. Nonauthors may have good comments to contribute but may not be good writers.

APPLICATIONS

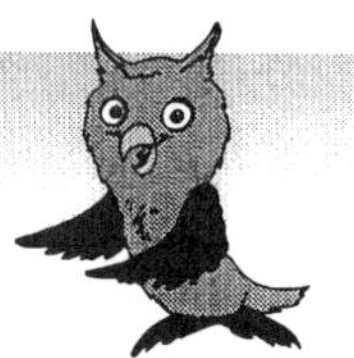

OUT-OF-SCHOOL ENRICHMENT ACTIVITIES FOR STUDENTS GIFTED IN LANGUAGE ARTS

The following activities offer students who are gifted in the language arts additional opportunities for enrichment in language and for extending their talents.

- *Local theater and drama groups.* Opportunities to participate in local theater and drama groups that include live performances can be a very enriching experience for these students. The pariticipation can be as passive as just watching rehearsals or involve being an actual member of the production.

- *Reading groups.* Exceptional readers may wish to participate in reading groups organized by older students or an interested parent. The Internet is a useful source of information about these groups and can also provide information on websites that show what students are reading in other schools and in other countries.

- *Creative writing and poetry societies.* Some communities have societies dedicated to creative writing or poetry, giving students the opportunity to write for pleasure (and for an audience) outside school.

- *Visiting the media.* Visits to the offices of radio and television stations, newspapers, and publishing companies can provide exciting insights into the world of journalism. Gifted students might even be able to contribute copy of their own.

- *Lectures and seminars.* Gifted students may be able to enroll in lectures and seminars on topics of special interest at local universities, galleries, and museums, as a way of extending the breadth and depth of their subject knowledge.

5

Mathematical Talent

Quick, how much is 37 times 489? What is the square root of 7,569? If you are like most people, you will need a few minutes along with pencil and paper to answer these questions. But people who are highly skilled at mathematics can solve these problems in a few seconds without a calculator or a pencil. How do they do it? Is it an inherited gift?

Mathematics is often viewed with such awe that those who understand and manipulate numbers with ease are usually considered gifted. Yet, studies show that infants demonstrate number sense very early in their development and begin to do addition and subtraction much earlier than previously thought. The notion that number sense is hard-wired into the brain makes sense in terms of our development as a species. Counting (e.g., determining how many animals in a pack represented a danger) and arithmetic operations (e.g., deciding how much to plant to feed the clan) were major contributors to our survival and, over time, became part of our genetic code.

Some researchers believe that number sense is hard-wired into the brain, and that human infants can do simple addition and subtraction.

Debates continue over the nature of the number sense that infants have and over whether addition and subtraction are actually innate or are arithmetic competencies that develop in the early years. Karen Wynn (1992, 1998), now at Yale University, believes that infants are genetically programmed to recognize discrete numbers of objects and to perform rudimentary addition and subtraction. Her studies also found that 8-month-old infants could reliably distinguish individual objects from collections and could discriminate among different objects within their visual field (Chiang and Wynn, 2000). Other researchers, such as Ann Wakeley at the University of California, Berkeley, believe that infants can distinguish general numbers of objects through contour and shape, but they cannot count discrete items and have weak or no innate ability to add or subtract (Wakeley, Rivera, and Langer, 2000).

Given the difficulty of carrying out these types of studies with infants and of trying to speculate on what the infants are thinking, the debate is likely to continue for some time. What is of greater importance, perhaps, is that regardless of whether mathematical abilities are innate or quickly acquired, they are important skills for success in a complex world.

MATHEMATICAL THINKING AND THE BRAIN ■

How does the brain process arithmetic and mathematical operations? Is the processing dependent on language or visual-spatial representations? What conditions affect an individual's mathematical competence? These and similar questions have been the focus of scientific investigations for decades. In the past, answers to these types of questions came from observing the behavior of mathematicians and from their own musings about what occurred in their minds while thinking about mathematics. Some mathematicians, including Albert Einstein, insisted that words and language had little or no role in their thought processes; others stressed that language played a vital role in their interpretation of symbol systems. Still others claimed that mathematical insights were opaque operations that did not emerge from conscious, explicit thought. Now brain imaging and stimulation techniques are studying cerebral activity during various types of mathematical operations and have produced some fascinating revelations.

Arithmetic Fact Retrieval and Processing

Several recent studies have focused on determining where simple arithmetic functions, such as addition and multiplication, are processed in the brain. One study showed that electrical stimulation of the cortex in the left parietal lobe (Figure 5.1) impaired performance on simple multiplication problems and disrupted the retrieval of arithmetic facts (Whalen, McCloskey, Lesser, and Gordon, 1997). This finding supported the observations of other researchers who noted that patients with left parietal lobe damage had difficulty with arithmetic operations (Hittmair-Delazer, Semenza, and Denes, 1994). However, the

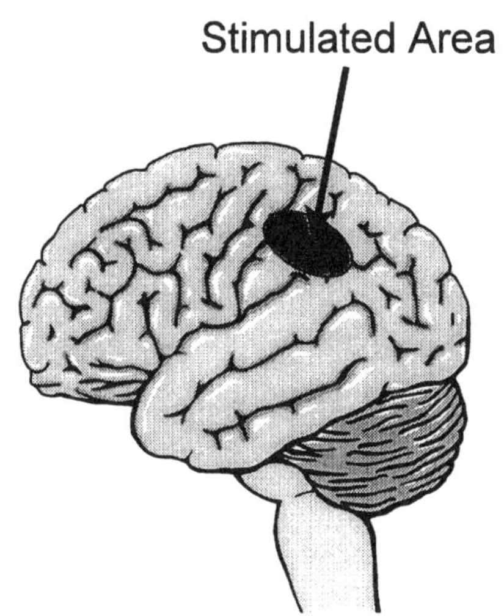

Figure 5.1 The shaded area shows the region of the left parietal lobe where arithmetic processing may occur.

results of these studies do not exclude the possibility that other regions of the brain may play a lesser role in arithmetic fact retrieval and processing.

The left parietal lobe is also the part of Albert Einstein's brain that was about 15 percent larger than normal. Because of the size of his related cortical structures, the researchers who examined Einstein's brain estimated that this extensive development of the parietal lobe probably occurred early in Einstein's lifetime, when he was already showing prowess at number manipulation and spatial abilities (Witelson, Kigar, and Harvey, 1999). The unanswered question, of course, is whether the larger parietal lobe is the cause or result of Einstein's intense work with mathematical operations.

Number Processing, Language, and Visual-Spatial Dependence

An area of considerable research interest has been the degree to which mathematical operations are dependent on other cerebral functions. If the ability to manipulate numbers is innate, as some researchers believe, then it would seem that mathematical processing would be associated with other innate human talents, such as language and visual-spatial representations.

Apparently, different brain regions are called into action when we change the way we process numbers. An fMRI study found that multiplication, subtraction, and number comparison activate different regions of the brain's left and right parietal lobes (Chocon, Cohen, van der Moortele, and Dehaene, 1999). The researchers hypothesized that although both parietal areas are involved in manipulating quantity information, only the left parietal region provides the connection between quantity information and the linguistic code stored in Broca's and Wernicke's areas.

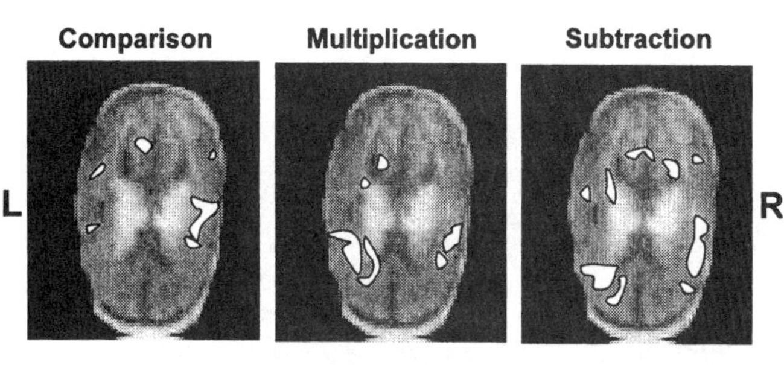

Figure 5.2 These representations of fMRI scans show that the right parietal lobe is most activated during number comparison but the left parietal lobe is most activated during multiplication. However, during subtraction, both lobes are highly activated (Chochon, et al., 1999).

Results from the study seemed to support this hypothesis. During number comparison, the right parietal region was the most activated region because comparison involves accessing the Arabic number system and does not require any linguistic translation (Figure 5.2). During multiplication, the left parietal lobe was more strongly activated because the brain monitors the results of the process through verbal computations (i.e., verbalized the results internally).

Finally, during subtraction, both the left and right parietal lobes were activated because subtraction requires both the internal numbering system and the verbal naming of the resulting quantity.

A study by Stanislas Dehaene and his colleagues of bilingual adults used fMRI techniques to examine brain activity while the subjects performed exact and approximate arithmetic calculations (Dehaene, Spelke, Pinel, Stanescu, and Tsivkin, 1999). For example, in the tasks requiring *exact* addition, subjects were asked to give the sum of two numerically close numbers shown on a card (e.g., 5+4 =?), and to identify the answer on the following card (7 or 9?). Using the same problem, the exercise was repeated and subjects were asked to find an *approximate* calculation (3 or 8?).

Exact and approximate arithmetic calculations appear to be processed in different parts of the brain.

The results of the study were quite surprising. First, with repetition, the performance of the subjects improved considerably (i.e., response times dropped about 45 percent), regardless of the language used to present the problem. However, in exact calculations, the bilingual subjects responded significantly faster when the problem was presented in the same language in which they were given the original instructions for the study, but more slowly if the problem was presented in the other language. This was true regardless of the subjects' native language. Apparently, the instructions were stored in a language-specific format that accelerated the exact arithmetic calculations when the language of the problem and instructions were the same, but hindered the exact calculations when the languages were different. In contrast, no differences were noticed because of language changes in problems involving approximate calculations, indicating that those operations were independent of language.

In the second phase of the study, a different group of bilingual adults was asked to perform more complex exact and approximate arithmetic calculations. The fMRI results showed that different areas of the brain were used for exact calculations than were used for approximate calculations. Exact arithmetic calculations activated mainly the left frontal lobe and the left angular gyrus. Both of these areas have been associated with language tasks, indicating that this network is probably using language-dependent coding to carry out verbal processes needed to perform exact arithmetic calculations. In contrast, approximation tasks activated the left and right parietal lobes and portions of the right occipital lobe. These areas are outside the language processing regions and are usually associated with visual-spatial operations, such as mental rotation and guided hand movements (Figure 5.3).

Implications for Studying Mathematics

These several studies seem to confirm that there is no one area of the brain for mathematical computation. Different cerebral regions are activated to perform different calculations, some of which require input from the language areas located in the left hemisphere. This would suggest that people who have strong neural connections between the quantity and language centers are likely to be more proficient in mathematics than individuals whose connections are weaker.

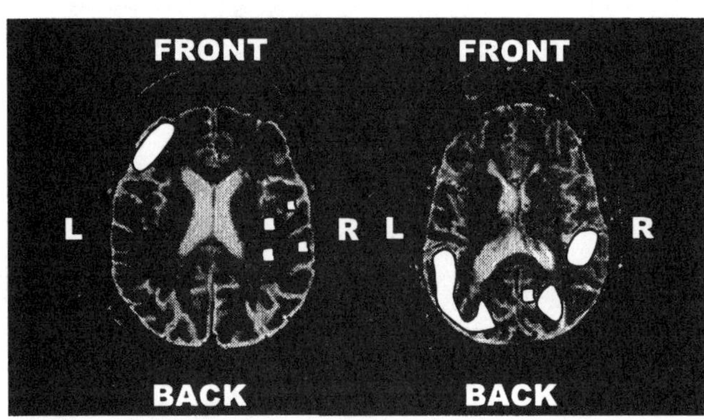

Figure 5.3 The illustration on the left is a representation of an fMRI image showing that the left frontal lobe was the area of main activation during exact calculations. The representation on the right shows that approximate calculations activated the left and right parietal lobes and portions of the occipital lobe (Dehaene, et al., 1999).

Even for simple arithmetic computations, multiple mental representations are used to perform different tasks. To some degree, they also help explain the diverse views that mathematicians have about their own thinking processes. Exact computations seem to involve language-specific operations and rely on left-hemisphere circuits in the frontal lobe to complete their work. Thus, success in learning symbolic arithmetic and calculus may depend heavily on an individual's ability to process verbal language, which may affect the recognition and processing of mathematical language. In other words, good verbal language skills mean good exact computation skills.

Approximate arithmetic, on the other hand, shows no dependence on language and seems to rely more on visual-spatial representations in the left and right parietal lobes. This may be called the Einstein area (see Chapter 2), where complex spatial portrayals are created and enriched. It is possible that this language-independent representation of quantity is associated with our evolutionary history, whereby approximating the number of animals in a herd or pack was sufficient for our survival. This tendency toward approximation allowed neural networks the freedom to focus on holistic relationships and patterns rather than to get bogged down in handling discrete numbers.

Exact computation seems related to verbal language skills, while approximate computation is related to visual-spatial skills.

Conceptual knowledge has a greater influence on procedural knowledge than the reverse.

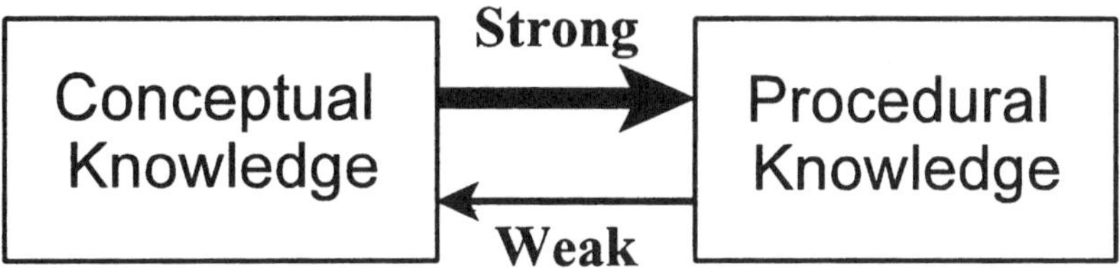

Figure 5.4 The diagram illustrates the different influences that conceptual and procedural knowledge have on each other.

Conceptual and Procedural Knowledge

Understanding mathematics, like most learning endeavors, requires acquiring the grand scheme of a topic, usually referred to as *conceptual knowledge*, as well as the steps and procedures needed to achieve a solution to a problem, known as *procedural knowledge*. Psychologists have long debated how these two components interact with each other during the acquisition of new learning, especially in the early years.

A study of 4th- and 5th-grade students examined the relationship between the students' conceptual understanding of mathematical equivalence and their procedures for solving problems involving equivalence (e.g., $4+5+7 = 4+\underline{?}$). The students were pretested on their conceptual and procedural knowledge of equivalence. They were split into two groups and taught either the concept of equivalence or the steps needed to solve problems of equivalence. Posttests were given to determine how easily they could transfer their understanding to solve problems (Rittle-Johnson, and Alibali, 1999).

Those taught with conceptual knowledge had a good conceptual understanding of equivalence and could also devise the correct procedures for solving equivalence problems. In contrast, the students taught only the procedural knowledge had some conceptual understanding but only limited transfer of the procedure to a new problem. The findings seem to indicate that there is a causal relationship between conceptual and procedural knowledge, and that conceptual knowledge has a greater influence on the acquisition of procedural knowledge than the reverse (Figure 5.4).

Experienced teachers will not be surprised by the results of the preceding study. Most of us have experienced learning situations in which we were more or less following a series of steps without really understanding why we were doing it. Beginning cooks can carefully follow a written recipe and even produce a decent product, but they have no clue about how the ingredients came together to make the dish. Moreover, they would not know how to make modifications if they lacked one of the ingredients.

Implications for the Study of Mathematics

In most lessons, teachers should ensure that they find ways to present mathematics conceptually first and check for the students' conceptual understanding before moving on to any procedural steps involved in solving problems associated with the concept.

IDENTIFYING THE MATHEMATICALLY GIFTED

Mathematically promising students are not always easy to spot. They may feel self-conscious about their abilities and may prefer to remain in the background rather than have attention brought to them. As a result, their competence may not be identified at all, or they may be encouraged to skip classes or grades in the hope that their specific needs eventually will be met.

Some Attributes of Mathematical Giftedness

Students with high mathematical ability

- Learn and understand mathematical ideas very quickly.
- Display multiple strategies for solving problems. They prefer to approach the problem from different perspectives and at varying levels of difficulty. The more layers the problem has, the more involved these students become in seeking solutions.
- Engage other students in their activities. They tend to talk to themselves or others as they walk through various approaches to the problem. They make convincing arguments about their views and try to recruit others to their position.

- Sustain their concentration and show great tenacity in pursuing solutions.
- Switch approaches easily and avoid nonproductive approaches.
- Operate easily with symbols and spatial concepts.
- Quickly recognize similarities, differences, and patterns.
- Look at problems more analytically than holistically.
- Work systematically and accurately.
- Demonstrate mathematical abilities in other subject areas by using charts, tables, and graphs to make their points and illustrate their data.

Of course, not all the students who possess these attributes are willing to work hard at mathematics, or even to be very creative. We see potential, but students may put little effort into using their mathematical capabilities. Truly gifted students not only possess these attributes but are also creative, working hard to develop their abilities. The earlier that school personnel identify these students, the better. Whether mathematical ability is innate or acquired, however, the early years are an important time for developing the cerebral areas and establishing the neural networks that perform arithmetic computation as well as create and manipulate mathematical abstractions.

TEACHING THE MATHEMATICALLY GIFTED ■

Classroom Challenges

Providing Unique Opportunities

One reason that mathematically gifted students are not identified may be that the method of teaching mathematics in the classroom does not evoke the type of thinking processes associated with high mathematical ability. Instruction that focuses mainly on memorizing rules, formulas, and procedural steps will provide few opportunities for gifted students to demonstrate their higher-level competencies. In this environment, they are more likely to be bored, withdrawn, or even act out to show their displeasure with activities that offer little or no challenge. Teachers are more likely to spot gifted students when the instruction is differentiated so that the mathematically talented can pursue interesting and thought-provoking problems.

Some teachers of mathematics are not prepared to deal with highly-gifted students. Interviews of 12 middle and high school mathematics teachers found that some harbored resentment toward their gifted students. The teachers said that their own poor training in mathematics or lack of a strong mathematical background was the main source of these feelings. They felt intimidated by the questions gifted students asked and often responded by shifting to classroom activities that replaced creativity with routine. Some teachers who tried to impress these students with their own mathematical competence found that the bright students took that as a challenge. Ironically, interviews of the students revealed that they appreciated teachers who were honest about their own mathematical abilities and who were willing to be co-learners and explore mathematics along with the students (Mingus and Grassi, 1999).

Because of their own lack of knowledge, some mathematics teachers admit to feeling intimidated by, and even resenting, mathematically gifted students.

Creating a learning environment that encourages and nurtures the talents of mathematically gifted students requires sustained effort and is no easy task. These students grasp information quickly and seek higher meaning and challenge in what they are learning. Because the mathematics curriculum in most schools today is designed for that school's average learner, the needs of students who are exceptionally talented in mathematics often go unmet. Thus, the teacher has to search for unique opportunities for gifted students, such as designing open-ended problems, setting up cooperative learning groups of high-ability students, and helping students become involved in the talent searches sponsored by nearly a dozen US universities.

Diversity in Homogeneity

Even among groups of mathematically gifted students, there can be a great deal of individual variability. Thus, engaging these students in diverse projects that allow them to use their strengths improves their achievement dramatically. Kalchman and Case (1999) conducted a study whereby the same teacher presented a curriculum unit on mathematical functions to two groups of highly motivated and gifted high school boys. For the control group, the unit centered around solving problems from the textbook plus compiling and applying definitions related to functions. The students engaged in activities that were largely procedural, such as creating tables and graphs and relating their solutions to prior problems. The sequential nature of the follow-up exercises in the textbook made individualization very difficult.

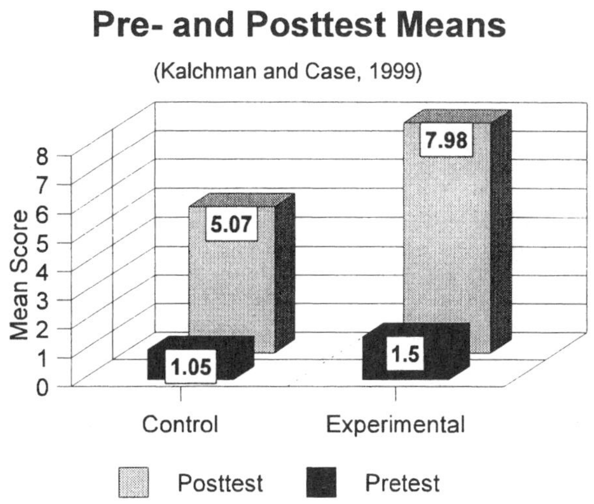

In the experimental group, however, the teacher used a technique called jigsaw learning. In this format, different groups of students acquired specialized knowledge about mathematical functions. They then reformed into new teams so that the expertise of all the group members had to be combined to solve a new problem. This approach promoted an environment whereby these high-ability students could feel part of a community of learners and could have the opportunity to display their unique talents. Although the experimental and control groups had similar scores on a pretest, the experimental group's scores on the posttest were significantly higher than the control group's scores (Figure 5.5). These findings, as in other studies, reaffirm that variations in degree of talent and ability exist in a seemingly homogeneous group of mathematically gifted students. Teachers, therefore, need to consider and recognize the individual needs and differences of gifted students, even within the same class.

Figure 5.5 This graph compares the pre- and posttest mean scores of the control and experimental groups.

Assessing Achievement in Mathematics

Assessing how well our students are doing in mathematics can be done by comparing their performances on tests to those of similar students in other countries. Started in the 1960s, the International Mathematics and Science Study was designed to do just that. In the first two mathematics studies, conducted in the mid-1960s and the early 1980s, US students did not fare well. Curriculum reform movements in the late 1980s and 1990s were supposed to improve achievement in several areas including mathematics and science. But, when the Third International Mathematics and Science Study (TIMSS) was completed, the American public was surprised to learn that in 1995, US 8th graders scored only 28th among the 41 countries whose students took the test (NCES, 1999). Four years later, the followup TIMSS report showed that in 1999, 8th graders had scored somewhat better: 19th among the 38 participating nations (NCES, 2001). (The US 8th graders' scores on the science portions of the TIMSS were only slightly better.)

Of particular concern in the 1995 study was the fact that US high school seniors in advanced mathematics classes (pre-calculus, calculus, and AP calculus) scored 15th among the 16 nations participating in this portion of the TIMSS. Coming in next to last prompted a national outcry for curriculum reform in K-12 mathematics. As a result, the 1995 report forced many districts to reexamine how secondary school teachers were delivering mathematics and science to advanced-ability students. Frances and Underhill (1996) proposed an integrated program of mathematics and science instruction on the basis of guidelines from the National Council of Teachers of Mathematics, the American Association for the Advancement of Science, and the National Research Council. The researchers' earlier studies had found that students achieved much better in classes where mathematics and science teachers had worked together to integrate their curriculum.

In practice, teachers of the gifted rarely have the resources or time to develop and implement an integrated mathematics-science curriculum, But when it does happen, studies show a significant improvement in student achievement. Here are a few examples of programs that have tried to improve mathematics instruction, especially for gifted students.

The Georgia GEMS Study

The Georgia program for Gifted Education in Math and Science (Ga-GEMS) was designed to give students with high potential in mathematics and science opportunities to study these two areas in an enriched environment (Tyler-Wood, Mortenson, Putney, and Cass, 2000). Sixty-four gifted high school students participated in a 2-year controlled study designed to determine whether a newly developed integrated mathematics and science curriculum would assist gifted students in their acquisition of higher-level mathematics and science. The students were divided into two matched groups of 32 each. During the academic year, the control group participated in their traditional tracked science and mathematics classes for high-ability

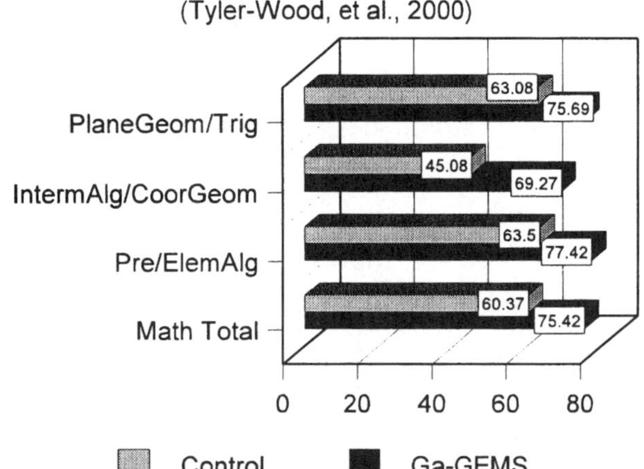

Figure 5.6 A comparison of the ACT scores of the Ga-GEMS and a control group after 2 years in the study. Each group had 32 high-ability students.

students, while the Ga-GEMS students participated in the integrated mathematics and science curriculum.

Teachers implementing the Ga-GEMS curriculum used a team-teaching approach and engaged students in hands-on experiences, extended laboratory projects, and field trips. At the end of the 2-year program, both groups were administered the science and mathematics portions of the American College Test (ACT). Students participating in the Ga-GEMS project scored significantly higher on all the ACT subtests (Figure 5.6).

The researchers in this study were also interested in comparing the frequency of seven types of classroom activities that occurred in the two groups. To do this, they videotaped each group for 45 to 55 minutes on 10 occasions. The tapes were analyzed by three different individuals and their scores were averaged. Researchers found significant differences between the frequency of activities in the Ga-GEMS group and the control groups. Compared to the Ga-GEMS classes, teachers in the control classes spent more time on lecture and seat work, less time on group work, and no time on laboratory work (Table 5.1).

Table 5.1 Percentage of Occurrences of Classroom Activities
(Tyler-Wood, et al., 2000)

Activity	Ga-GEMS %	Control %
Lecture	27	45
Lab Work	22	0
Seat Work	5	14
Question and Answer	14	17
Group Work	23	8
Teacher Giving Directions	6	9
No Structured Activities	3	7

Developing the Ga-GEMS integrated curriculum took over 1,000 hours of teacher time. Many school districts cannot afford this type of investment in time and resources. Nonetheless, this effort offered gifted students an opportunity to continue their high school experience while pursuing interests in mathematics and science. Other school districts may want to consider undertaking a similar program that may require less time but still be as effective.

The Music Spatial-Temporal (MST) Math Program

Although not designed specifically for gifted students, this program evolved from the work of Gordon Shaw, the researcher whose work in 1993 led to the so-called "Mozart Effect." After retiring from the University of California, Irvine, he established the Music Intelligence Neural Development (M.I.N.D.) Institute in 1997 to conduct research on the influence of music on spatial-temporal reasoning—the ability to form a mental image and to think ahead in space and time. Shaw, himself a theoretical physicist, believed that training primary grade students in music would build the neural structures necessary to enhance spatial-temporal reasoning, which is crucial for understanding mathematics and science. Shaw and his colleagues at the Institute developed the Music Spatial-Temporal (MST) Math Program to teach mathematics by exploiting the brain's innate ability to do spatial-temporal reasoning. This program complements the typical language-analytical methods (symbols, word problems, equations) usually begun at home during the pre-school years as well as emphasized in the primary grades. Music training is also introduced, which includes a listening component, music theory skills, and piano keyboard instruction. The students use mathematics video game software to visualize and understand difficult concepts, and to integrate them with the regular language-based mathematics curriculum.

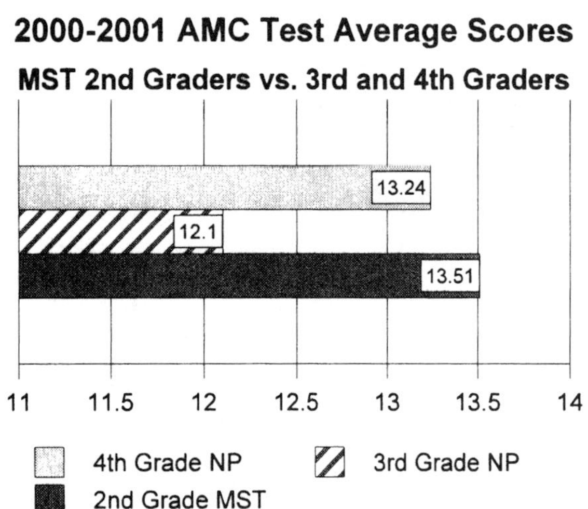

Figure 5.7 Comparison of the average scores of 2nd-grade MST Math Program students with 3rd- and 4th-grade students who were not in the program. (NP=Not in Program)

In a study designed to test the effectiveness of the MST program, nearly 1,100 2nd graders were taught difficult mathematical concepts using the video computer games. To assess their level of achievement, the MST students were first administered the 2nd-grade California standardized exams in advanced mathematics concepts (AMC). This test includes questions on fraction, proportions, symmetry, graphs, and pre-algebra. The students were then asked to answer relevant questions from the 3rd- through 5th-grade AMC tests, in which the heavily language-loaded presentations had been simplified. The 2nd-grade MST Math program students scored significantly higher than the 3rd-grade (13.51 vs. 12.1) and slightly higher than the 4th grade (13.51 vs. 13.24) students, at the same schools, who were not in the program but who had one to two years of additional mathematics training (Figure 5.7). It is also worth noting that 2nd-grade students at *all ability levels* benefitted from the MST program (M.I.N.D., 2002).

Gender Differences in Mathematics: Do They Really Exist?

Since the 1970s, gender differences in mathematics performance has been a controversial topic among educators and researchers. Statistical evidence that boys are smarter at mathematics than girls came from the Study of Mathematically Precocious Youth conducted in the early 1980s. Gifted 7th graders were administered the mathematics section of the Scholastic Aptitude Test (SAT-M). Four times as many boys scored above 600 as girls, and 13 times as many boys scored above 700 (Benbow and Stanley, 1983). Male college-bound students also displayed a mathematics advantage by consistently scoring higher on both the SAT-M and the mathematics section of the American College Test (ACT).

Gender differences in mathematics seem to be greater for high-ability students than for the general student population.

Ensuing studies found other differences between male and female performance on specific types of mathematical skills. For example, males seemed to have an advantage over females in mathematical operations involving visual-spatial ability, while females did better in mathematical computation. One possible explanation for these findings is that more male than female brains seem to have a visual-spatial preference (see Chapter 3) and would therefore perform better in solving these types of problems. In contrast, more females have analytic preferences and would tend to do better with computation problems.

Numerous other studies in the 1980s through the mid-1990s yielded conflicting results, especially with regard to the age at which the gender differences emerge. Some studies reported differences in the early elementary years, others by age 12, and still others argued that gender differences did not appear until high school. The discrepancies among these studies can be explained in part by the limited sample sizes and by the use of a select population, such as gifted or college-bound students. More recently, a major study by Leahey and Guo (2001) sought to overcome the deficiencies of previous studies by using large samples and data from the National Longitudinal Study of Youth (NLSY) and the National Educational Longitudinal Study (NELS).This approach not only reduced the bias due to small and select samples, but also allowed the researchers to examine mathematical performance from kindergarten to grade 12, rather than at one or two developmental stages. They were also able to separate out performance differences by mathematical skill and by selected student populations. Table 5.2 summarizes some of their findings.

Table 5.2 Gender Differences in Mathematics
Summary of Findings from the Study by Leahy and Guo (2001)

Major Findings (Elementary Students and NLSY data) **No. of Students: 4,126** **No. of Scores: 12,159**	**General Mathematics Skill:** Almost no gender differences in mean scores among the general population. Boys' scores did have more *variance* than girls' scores, but it was not statistically significant. **High-Scoring Students:** Boys and girls had similar overall *averages*. Ages 4-7, high-ability girls did better than high-ability boys. Ages 8-10, high-ability boys did better than high-ability girls. Ages 11-13, no significant differences. **Reasoning Skill:** Few differences in younger children; a slight advantage to female students among 11- to13-year-olds.
Major Findings (Secondary Students and NELS data) **No. of Students: 9,787** **No. of Scores: 26,253**	**General Mathematics Skill:** In 8th grade, males scored an average of 0.5 points higher than females. This difference increased to 1.32 by 12th grade. The difference was *not significant* at the 5 percent level. **High-Scoring Students:** High-ability boys did better than high-ability girls. **Reasoning Skill:** In 8th grade, no gender differences. In high school, male scores were slightly higher than female, but not statistically significant. **Geometry Skill:** In 8th grade, males held a very slight advantage, which increased to a statistically significant advantage in 12th grade.

In summary, Leahy and Guo found that there were a few and slight gender differences that did not appear until the end of high school. These differences also were greater for high-ability students than for the general population. Males seemed to have an advantage in geometry and females, in computation in the early grades. Differences in brain development and learning style preferences may account for these findings. But is it possible that there are societal and cultural factors at work as well? For example, more boys elect to take more mathematics and science courses, which could further develop their visual-spatial abilities and thereby improve their performance on certain tests, such as geometry. These skills are not really emphasized until high school, which could explain the emergence of the gender differences at that time.

Three important points need to be made at this time: First, there are gender differences in mathematics that are slight, develop late, and are subject specific. Second, the findings do *not* support the notion that males generally have a powerful innate superiority in mathematics over females. It may just be that the slight advantage they do have, especially in visual-spatial operations, are more obvious in the later high school years. Third, the fact that much of higher mathematics involves visual-spatial and abstract reasoning may explain why a large portion of top mathematicians are male.

APPLICATIONS

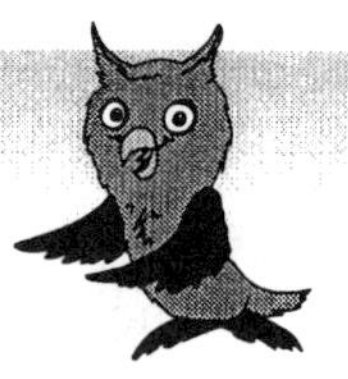

IDENTIFYING THE MATHEMATICALLY GIFTED

Students who are gifted in mathematics display certain attributes. Specific classroom activities (see the next application) can often reveal these attributes. Use the scale below to help decide if a particular student is gifted in mathematics. If you rate the student with scores of 4 or 5 on more than half of the characteristics, then further assessment is warranted.

The student....	A little Some A lot
1. Learns and understands mathematical ideas very quickly.	1 — 2 — 3 — 4 — 5
2. Displays multiple strategies for solving problems.	1 — 2 — 3 — 4 — 5
3. Engages others in problem solving.	1 — 2 — 3 — 4 — 5
4. Sustains concentration and shows great tenacity in pursuing problems.	1 — 2 — 3 — 4 — 5
5. Switches approaches easily and avoids nonproductive approaches.	1 — 2 — 3 — 4 — 5
6. Operates easily with symbols and spatial concepts.	1 — 2 — 3 — 4 — 5
7. Quickly recognizes similarities, differences, and patterns.	1 — 2 — 3 — 4 — 5
8. Looks at problems more analytically than holistically.	1 — 2 — 3 — 4 — 5
9. Works systematically and accurately.	1 — 2 — 3 — 4 — 5
10. Demonstrates mathematical abilities in other subject areas.	1 — 2 — 3 — 4 — 5
11. Prefers to present information through charts, tables, and graphs.	1 — 2 — 3 — 4 — 5

APPLICATIONS

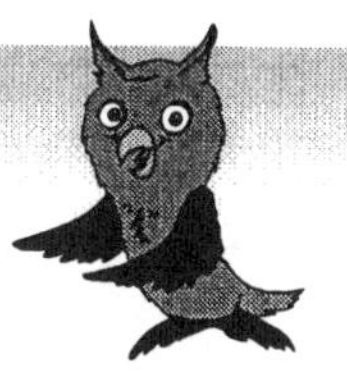

CLASSROOM ACTIVITIES TO HELP IDENTIFY MATHEMATICALLY GIFTED STUDENTS

When teaching mathematics at any grade level, offering classroom activities at varying levels of difficulty and complexity can help teachers identify mathematically gifted students. Here are a few suggestions for accomplishing this task (Hoeflinger, 1998).

- Offer open-ended problems that have an array of discrete levels and can be solved using multiple strategies. (A simple test to identify a problem of this type: If you are unsure how to proceed in order to solve the problem, then it most likely requires a multistep approach.)

- Provide thought-provoking and nonroutine problems about once a week. Look for the ways the students organize knowledge, argue their position, make conjectures, and clarify their thoughts. Are they looking for patterns and can they recognize and explain them? What type of reasoning and logic are they using? How quickly and accurately can they solve the problem? Make anecdotal notes on how students respond to specific problems, the types of strategies they use, and their progress.

- As problems are solved, raise the level of complexity for ensuing problems until the students are involved in a spirited debate about potential approaches to solutions. Be certain, however, that the students know and understand the necessary mathematics vocabulary in the event that they need to seek information from other sources.

- Mathematically gifted students often show their talents in other curriculum areas. They tend to view the world in mathematical ways and to use mathematical symbols and language in their other work.
  ➢ In writing, they often demonstrate a clarity of logic, precision, and sequencing, sometimes using tables and charts to organize information.

CLASSROOM ACTIVITIES—Continued

➢ Social Studies offers another area where they can apply their unique abilities to create models and design tables and graphs to illustrate data (e.g., population growth in an area using birth and death rates, etc.). Can they use this information to make and support predictions about future growth?

➢ Science experiments also provide many opportunities for these students to show their abilities, especially in collecting, organizing, and manipulating quantitative experimental data. Can they use the data to make predictions when other experimental variables are changed?

- Avoid giving textbooks to truly gifted students and allowing them to move at their own pace. Like other students, they also need nurturing and encouragement to move ahead faster.

- Cluster the gifted mathematics students in small cooperative groups and give them a complex problem to solve while you carry on instruction with the rest of the class. Ensure that group members have time to discuss their problem-solving strategies and to make connections to curriculum objectives.

- Look to other sources for mathematical problems, games, and ideas for these students to pursue. Those sources can include texts from higher grade levels, other teacher colleagues, journals published by the National Council of Teachers of Mathematics (NCTM), curriculum materials from the state Department of Education, local public and university libraries, and the Internet.

APPLICATIONS

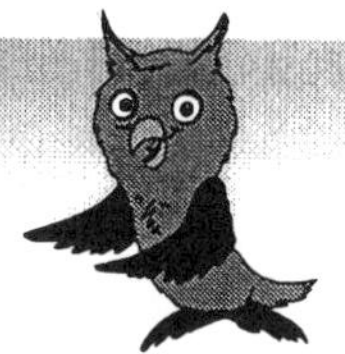

TEACHING MATHEMATICALLY GIFTED STUDENTS IN MIXED-ABILITY CLASSROOMS

After identifying students who are mathematically gifted, working with them in a mixed-ability classroom can present problems unless the teacher finds ways to differentiate instruction. Mathematically gifted students still have educational needs, but they will be better than other students at handling and organizing data, formulating problems, and expressing and transferring ideas. Here are some suggestions for differentiating instruction for the mathematically gifted (Johnson, 2000).

Assessment

- Give pre-assessments to determine which students already know the material. In the elementary grades, gifted learners still need to know the facts necessary to complete their learning objectives. Work with those students who do not know the basics, and allow the gifted students to complete more complex learning tasks.

- Develop assessments that allow for differences in creativity, understanding, and accomplishment. Give students chances to express themselves orally and in writing to show what they have learned.

Curriculum Materials

- Select textbooks that offer enriched opportunities. Too many mathematics textbooks repeat topics every year prior to algebra. Most texts are written for average students and are not appropriate for the gifted.

- Use multiple resources, such as college textbooks and research reports, because no one textbook can meet the needs of these learners.

TEACHING IN MIXED-ABILITY CLASSROOMS—Continued

- Use technology as a tool, an inspiration, or as an independent learning environment that allows gifted students the opportunity to reach the depth and breadth they need to maintain their interest. Computer programming is a special skill. Using spreadsheets, databases, and graphic and scientific calculators can lead to powerful data analysis.

- The World Wide Web is a vast source of material, contests, student and teacher resources, and information about mathematical ideas usually not found in textbooks.

Instructional Techniques

- Flexibility in pacing is important. Some students may be mastering basic skills while others are working on advanced topics.

- Use inquiry-based, discovery learning approaches that emphasize open-ended problems with multiple paths to multiple solutions. Have students design their own methods for solving complex problems or answering complicated questions. You will be surprised at what gifted students can discover.

- Ask lots of higher-level questions that encourage students to discuss and justify their approaches to problem solving.

- Differentiate assignments so that gifted students do not get just more problems of the same type. Offer choices, such as a regular assignment, a more challenging one, or one that matches the students' interests.

- Offer AP level courses in statistics, calculus, and computer science. Students should also be encouraged to take classes at local colleges if they have exhausted all the high school possibilities.

- Provide units and problems that go beyond the normal curriculum and relate to the real world. Use concrete experiences that incorporate manipulatives or hands-on activities.

TEACHING IN MIXED-ABILITY CLASSROOMS—Continued

- Ensure that students realize that you expect their learning products to be of high quality.

- Offer opportunities to participate in contests, such as the Mathematical Olympiad. Give students feedback on their performance, and use some of the contest's problems for classroom discussion.

- Allow students access to mentors who represent diverse cultural and linguistic groups. Mentors can come from within the school, the community, or be available through teleconferencing or the Internet. Use guest speakers in the classroom to talk about how mathematics has benefitted their careers.

Grouping

- Provide some activities that can be done individually or in groups, based on student choice. Grouping is productive because gifted students working alone are learning no more than they would at home. Be sure to give them guidelines on their interactions with other group members and appropriate feedback afterward.

Using differentiated instruction in regular mathematics classrooms not only benefits gifted students but also has the potential for enriching the learning experience for all students, because some may also want to try the more challenging tasks. With this approach, all students will have the chance to work at their own level of challenge.

APPLICATIONS

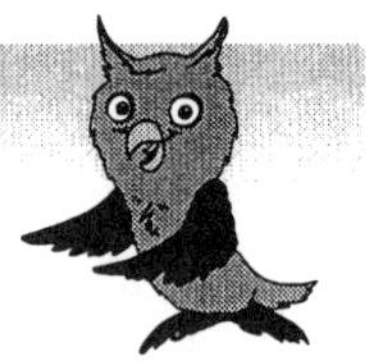

CHOOSING CONTENT FOR ELEMENTARY SCHOOL MATHEMATICS

Mathematics textbooks and programs for elementary school abound. So how do educators decide which program has the best approach in light of what we know about how the human brain learns mathematics. Although the research is still in its early stages, it seems clear that the young mind is more likely to be successful in displaying mathematical talent if educators are aware of three characteristics:

Multi-Step Learning

Too often, elementary mathematics is presented in textbooks (and therefore taught) as a collection of separate one-step skill operations or routines. Genuine mathematical problems are typically multistep, however, requiring the learner to identify intermediate steps in order to move from what is known to what is sought. These steps should be discovered by students as the teacher guides them along. Some drill and practice are necessary, but too much of these will encourage the memorization of single-step routines, carried out procedurally with little understanding. Thus, a mathematical topic for gifted students should give rise to a rich source of problems that require the integration of several basic steps for analysis and for solving problems.

Making Connections

Gifted students should experience mathematics as a collection of relationships among distinct themes, and not as a body of unrelated methods and rules. The teacher's role here is to help students look for connections among seemingly unrelated ideas. Recognizing that new methods and problems are often more familiar than they seem at first is a basic insight that gifted students need to experience regularly.

ELEMENTARY SCHOOL MATHEMATICS—Continued

Logic and Proof

One important component of understanding the connections between different parts of elementary mathematics is the notion that these connections have a logical basis, and thus must be established by exact calculation. These calculations, or proofs, establish whether some mathematical relationship really is true. Teachers should cultivate in gifted students an understanding of the need for proof and help them recognize that, in mathematics, it is exact calculation (or proof) that determines correctness. By gaining this understanding, students realize that the solutions to mathematical problems can be determined objectively and are not subject to the arbitrary whim of any person.

APPLICATIONS

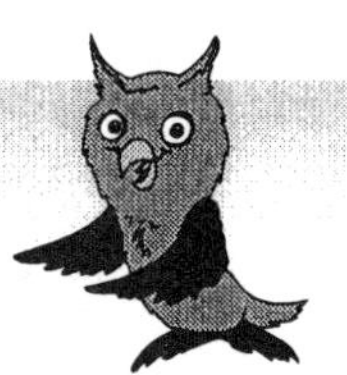

SELECTING TEACHING STRATEGIES FOR MATHEMATICS

Teaching strategies in mathematics for gifted students should aim to

- Develop deeper understanding
- Lay stronger foundations
- Foster a willingness to seek out the connections between different aspects of mathematics
- Involve higher-level thinking skills
- Cultivate a desire to understand why particular mathematical methods are correct.

The following points also need to be considered:

- Strategies should develop higher-level thinking by challenging students to observe, compare, hypothesize, criticize, classify, interpret, and summarize.
- Teachers should use open-ended problems and make clear what areas the students should pursue, what processes should be involved, and what outcomes are achievable and expected.
- Teachers should not expect gifted students to work in undirected and unsupported ways for extended periods of time.
- Strategies should have clear objectives and be designed to increase the students' ability to analyze and solve problems, to stimulate creativity, and to encourage initiative and self-direction.
- Care should be taken in selecting supplemental strategies so that students see their work as challenging and not as drudgery.
- Be sure to offer opportunities for extended research in areas of student interest.

APPLICATIONS

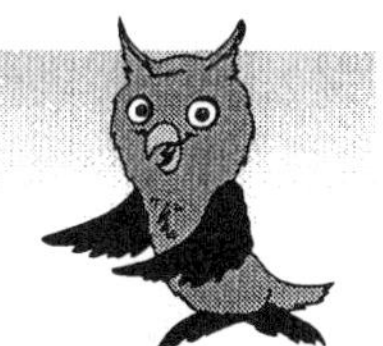

TALENT SEARCHES AVAILABLE FOR THE MATHEMATICALLY GIFTED

Talent searches are valuable opportunities for meeting the needs of mathematically gifted elementary and secondary students. Rotigel and Lupkowski-Shoplik (1999) describe the process and benefits of these searches. Over 200,000 students nationwide take advantage of the programs offered annually by nearly a dozen sponsoring universities (see list in **Resources**). Through its selection process, the talent search can not only help teachers identify mathematically gifted students, but can also give guidance for designing educational experiences appropriate to the students' ability levels.

School personnel should realize that talent searches are not restricted to just the most highly gifted, nor just to mathematics. Students who score in the top 5 percent of their age group in just one area (e.g., mathematics) are eligible. Sometimes, these students have not been identified for the school's gifted program because their talent lies in just one area, or because they do not receive high scores in language arts.

The Testing Process

Students who score at or above the 95th percentile on the Composite or Math Total, Vocabulary, Reading, Language Total, or Science subtest on a nationally normed achievement test (e.g., Iowa Test of Basic Skills) are recommended for additional testing. An above-level test is administered next, usually two to five grade-levels above the grade placement of the student. This allows the student to demonstrate mastery of more advanced concepts and results in a greater spread of scores, which can be used by teachers for educational planning. Examples of above-level tests are the Scholastic Assessment Test (SAT), the American College Testing program (ACT), or the EXPLORE test.

Using the Test Results

The above-level test helps to identify the level of a student's mathematical ability. A student who scores in the 95th percentile on the grade-level test may have demonstrated all he or she knows. Consequently, this student's performance on the above-level test will be low. For another student, the

TALENT SEARCHES FOR THE MATHEMATICALLY GIFTED—Continued

above-level test may show high scores in some or all areas, indicating exceptional achievement and ability.

For example, let's say that two 3rd-graders, Student A and Student B, both scored in the 99th percentile on their grade-level test. However, on the above-level 8th-grade test, Student A scores at the 26th percentile and Student B, at the 96th percentile, compared to other 8th graders. Although the two students' abilities seemed similar on the grade-level test, the above-level results show a very different picture. Both students are in their school's gifted program (as they should be) and both need more challenging activities. Student A needs more enrichment in mathematics, participation in contests, group work with students of similar aptitude in mathematics, and curriculum compacting (perhaps, 2 years of mathematics in one). Student B needs all the same options as Student A, plus individually-paced instruction as well as course- and grade-skipping. Student B may also be an excellent candidate for a university-sponsored Elementary Student Talent Search.

Benefits of Talent Search Participation

Accuracy of Diagnosis. Because above-level tests have a higher ceiling than grade-level tests, they more accurately measure students' abilities, thereby allowing for the development of specific educational plans for each identified student.

Development of Specific Educational Plans. The scores that the students receive on the above-level assessment lead to the development of specific recommendations that best match the students' demonstrated achievement and abilities. Suggestions can range from enrichment to honors classes to acceleration (see Table 5.3).

Opportunities to Participate in University-Sponsored Talent Searches. Students who enter talent search programs have a broad range of options including summer, weekend, and online programs as well as correspondence courses. These opportunities offer students a chance to study topics that may not be available at their home schools. The summer programs offer the chance for like-minded students to live together for several weeks and to study subjects intensively at a pace consistent with their interests and capabilities.

Learning About Themselves. Students in talent searches gain more insight into their abilities and achievement, putting them in a better position to

TALENT SEARCHES FOR THE MATHEMATICALLY GIFTED—Continued

make important choices, such as which college to attend or which career to pursue.

Recognition of Their Abilities. Some talent search programs recognize students' outstanding abilities through scholarships, awards, and honors. Several colleges and universities that sponsor talent searches, for example, also offer scholarships for students to participate in college courses while still attending high school.

Continuing Information. Talent search programs continue to provide participants with newsletters and other printed information about research findings, scholarships, and other educational opportunities. Studies show that, when compared to gifted nonparticipants, talent search participants pursue more rigorous courses of study, accelerate their education to a greater extent, and participate in more extracurricular activities (Olszewski-Kubilius, 1998).

On the following page, Table 5.3 shows some guidelines for developing the educational plan for students who achieve different scores on the above-level tests (Rotigel and Lupkowski-Shoplik, 1999).

TALENT SEARCHES FOR THE MATHEMATICALLY GIFTED—Continued

Table 5.3 Educational Planning Guidelines for Students Who Have Taken Above-Level Tests

Tests and Scores	EXPLORE-Mathematics Scale score 1-13 (taken in 4th grade) OR SAT-Mathematics Score of 200-500 (taken in 7th grade)	EXPLORE-Mathematics Scale score 14-20 (taken in 4th grade) OR SAT-Mathematics Score of 510-630 (taken in 7th grade)	EXPLORE-Mathematics Scale score 21-25 (taken in 4th grade) OR SAT-Mathematics Score of 640-800 (taken in 7th grade)
Components of the Plan	Academic counseling and development of an educational plan In-school enrichment; participation in competitions and contests Supplemental course work; Summer programs for enrichment Algebra I in 7th grade; AP calculus in 11th grade; College-level mathematics courses in 12th grade	Academic counseling and development of an educational plan Curriculum compacting (taking 2 years of mathematics in one year) Summer program of fast-paced classes in mathematics Algebra I in 6th grade; AP calculus in 10th grade; College-level mathematics courses in 11th and 12th grades	All of the options in the previous column, plus: An individualized program of study based on diagnostic testing in mathematics Consider grade skipping, early admission to high school, and taking college classes early Mentorships for advanced study in mathematics

6

Musical Talent

Most people view musical talent as a gift. But there is mounting scientific evidence that all of us have some musical capability, and that our recognition of music begins shortly after birth (if not before). A study in Japan used 2-day-old infants of congenitally deaf and homebound parents to ensure that the infants had not been exposed to music before birth (Masataka, 1999). The infants heard two types of songs: those that were recorded when sung to infants and those sung for adults. By measuring response times, the researchers found that the infants had a distinct preference for the songs directed toward infants. Because these infants had no pre-natal or post-natal exposure to music, these findings may indicate that infants are born with an innate preference for music—the type they are likely to hear from their parents.

Another study conducted experiments with 72 adults who had no musical training or education (nonmusicians) and used electroencephalography (EEG) to measure their responses to various musical chords (Koelsch, Gunter, and Friederici, 2000). The subjects listened to chord sequences that infrequently contained chords that did not fit their sound expectations. Brain activity increased when they heard the improper chord and decreased when the expected chord was played. When asked, the subjects could not explain their responses. Apparently, these subjects with no musical training still had an innate and subconscious expectation of which chords did or did not fit a musical sequence.

Every normal brain is a musical brain.

The study also showed that as the musical keys changed, the subjects could still identify which chord fit which key, and their brain activity increased when a chord did not fit the key. This occurred even though the subjects knew nothing about musical keys or the fit of chords to those keys. The researchers concluded that the subjects' brains were interpreting complex musical relationships, setting up musical expectations, and detecting violations of those expectations with no conscious realization or effort on the part of their owners. The results strengthen the notion that the human brain has innate musical ability. Music may become even more important to us as we age. Researchers have found that the debilitating effects of cognitive dementia and Alzheimer's disease often diminish when one learns to play a musical instrument.

Frankly, we really did not need science to tell us that the normal brain is a musical brain. Just think of how easily our brain takes a sequence of mixed tones presented at different tempos, groups the sounds, and perceives coherent music. We can detect a wrong note in a musical string, pick out melody and harmony, and respond to tempo and timbre. We can anticipate which note should complete a musical phrase. We can unwittingly memorize tunes and lyrics with no conscious effort and have that tune play incessantly in our head. Moreover, we do all this without conscious thought.

WHY ARE HUMANS MUSICAL?

Music *is* everywhere and everyone is musical. Anthropologists have never discovered a culture that did not have music. Although the styles of singing and the type of musical instruments very widely, some form of music exists in all cultures, from Eskimo villages to the tropical rainforests. Of course, the notion that music is innate to all humans raises an interesting question: Why? Some psychologists think music is a useless frill that developed when our neural circuits became more sophisticated. But others feel that the importance of music goes much deeper, given the role it has played in the development of our diverse cultures over thousand of years. The oldest musical instrument found to date is a crude bone flute, discovered in southern Germany with human remains that are about 36,000 years old.

Charles Darwin speculated in 1871 that music evolved as part of courtship. Just as birds sing to attract mates, Darwin suggested that early humans used music to attract and retain sexual partners. Subsequent psychologists support Darwin's ideas but propose that the power of music began at the cradle. Because young humans take so long to develop, anything that bonded mother and infant, such as music, would have immediate survival benefit and genetic staying power. In nearly all cultures today, adults carry on sing-song conversations with babies, often with both ending up in duets and rhythmic movements. Music is also used to bond groups of families into tribes. Listening to the same music, or singing and dancing together, can unite teams, villages, and cultures into a productive cluster or a dangerous mob. Music can also be a catharsis, allowing rage or grief to be channeled to public release, as in the case of those singing the national anthem in the days following the collapse of the World Trade Center towers (Milius, 2001).

Although no one knows for sure why humans are musical animals, several theories abound. But, based on historical and evolutionary records as well as the increasingly convincing evidence from neuroscience, the best explanation seems to be that, just as in other primates, singing helped primitive humans find mates, communicate and care for their young, and bond with others in the tribe. All the other benefits of music are secondary but no less enjoyable.

Music helped primitive humans find mates, communicate, and care for their young as well as bond with others in the tribe.

The idea that all human beings are musical has tremendous implications for the teaching of music. Music education should be available to all members of the school community and not just for students with obvious musical talent or whose parents deem it important.

WHAT IS MUSICAL TALENT? ■

Listening to music is one thing, but being able to *create* music is something else. Most people can process musical input and detect complex rhythm and phrases, as well as produce passable vocal music. But far fewer people seem to possess the capacity to master a musical instrument. Why is that? If music is innate, shouldn't most of us be able to learn how to play musical instruments almost as quickly as running or singing? Is it possible that the skills necessary to play a musical instrument require different brain structures? In other words, is the brain's ability to create music a distinct talent whose development is directed by genetic predispositions not found in most people? The question of how much influence genes have on talent of any kind is currently being questioned by scientists.

An extensive study by Richard Howe at the University of Exeter in England has stirred debate over how much of talent is the result of genetic predisposition and how much is a matter of sustained and rigorous practice (Howe, Davidson, and Sloboda, 1998). According to Howe and his colleagues, popular belief in Western cultures holds that talent has four components:

- People are born with the capacity to attain high levels of achievement in various activities, such as mathematics, music, literatures, and sports.
- These talents will be exhibited to some extent early in life.
- Only a small minority of people are born with these talents.
- Talent comes in different amounts, so that the "talented" are only those who achieve the highest levels of expertise or success.

Nature or Nurture?

This "either you are born with it or not" approach to explaining talent is often supported by circular reasoning: "He plays so well because he is talented. How do we know he is talented? Because he plays so well." Music is especially rich in folklore that supposedly substantiates the genetic source of musical achievement. The examples of child prodigies, such as Mozart and Artur Rubenstein, are often used to support the idea that talents appear early in life. Adding to the notion that these children are born with special capabilities, these people cite that perfect pitch (more accurately, absolute pitch) also is innate in these high achievers. Still others refer to the discovery that some parts of the brain in great achievers are larger than normal, suggesting that the talent resulted from prenatal changes in brain development.

Table 6.1 Is Musical Talent Genetic?

Pros	Alternative Possibilities
Child prodigies are evidence that innate talent appears early.	Child prodigies are rare; many professional musicians were not prodigies.
Perfect pitch is innate and a sign of special capability.	Perfect pitch may be acquired early through extensive musical training.
Larger brain areas cause musical talent.	Musical experience and practice cause larger brain areas.

Howe suggests that these arguments are weak evidence to support talent as purely genetic and that there may be alternative explanations (Table 6.1). First, he notes that much of what is written about child prodigies is anecdotal, and there are very few musical prodigies compared to the larger number of highly successful professional musicians who did not display early signs of talent. Mozart's father, Leopold, was a musician. Would the young Wolfgang have become such a musical wonder had he not been exposed to music from birth? Second, there is evidence that perfect pitch appears in young children who have been given extensive musical training. Consequently, it is just as likely that perfect pitch may be acquired early in life rather than be innate. Third, because brain growth can be affected by experience, increased brain size could be the *result* of musical experiences and practice, rather than being the cause of musical achievement.

Accordingly, is seems that activities, such as practice, accomplished *after* birth may have a significant effect on musical achievement. To examine the power of practice, John Sloboda and his colleagues interviewed 257 young musicians between the ages of eight and 18 about their performance history from the start of playing a musical instrument (Sloboda, Davidson, Howe, and Moore, 1996). Ninety-four of these students kept a diary for a period of 42 weeks to record the

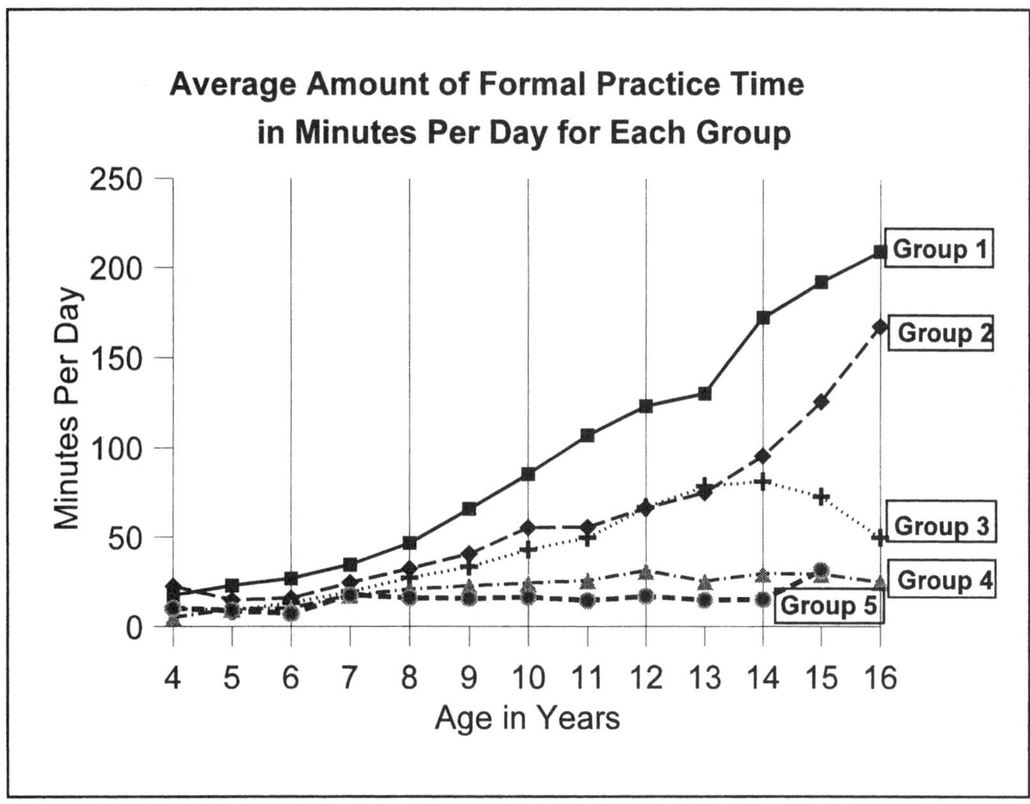

Figure 6.1 The graph shows the average practice time in minutes per day for the five groups (Sloboda, et al., 1996).

amount of time devoted to practice and other activities. The sample included participants with a broad range of musical achievement, from students who were attending a highly selective music school to individuals who had abandoned their playing after a year or less of formal instruction. Music achievement was measured by their degree of skill in playing their musical instruments through an externally validated performance examination.

Participants were divided into five groups on the basis of their level of musical competence. Group 1 was the target group, comprising students enrolled in a highly selective music school. Group 2 were students who had applied for but had not been accepted to the music school. Students in Group 3 had expressed interest in attending a music school but had not followed through with a formal application. Group 4 consisted of students who were learning a musical instrument at a nonspecialist school. Students who had been unsuccessful at instrumental music were in Group 5, having not played for at least one year prior to the study.

Not surprisingly, the researchers found a strong relationship between musical achievement and the amount of formal practice undertaken (Figure 6.1). High achievers practiced the most (Groups 1 and 2), moderate achievers practiced a moderate amount of time (Group 3), and low achievers barely practiced at all (Groups 4 and 5). Furthermore, the researchers found that high achievers who practiced less were *no more successful than low achievers*. Another important finding was that differences in practice patterns began very early in age and from the time of starting to learn an instrument. Those who practiced a lot when they were young also practiced a lot when they were older, and vice versa. These results support the premise that formal, intense practice is a major determinant of musical achievement.

What Has Science Discovered?

As the nature versus nurture debate over musical achievement continues, scientists have been making some interesting observations about music and the human brain. Table 6.2 shows some of their findings. At first glance, getting involved with music, especially at an early age, seems to have significant impact on the growing brain. That may be true. But it is important to point out that probably anything we do at an early age affects brain organization and development. For example, a comparison of the brains of mathematicians to nonmathematicians, of professional dancers to non-dancers, would likely also show structural, and perhaps functional, differences.

Formal, intense practice is a major determinant of musical achievement.

Table 6.2 Some Findings from Science on Musical Ability

Study	Findings
Elbert, et al., 1995; using PET	Compared to nonplayers, string players had greater cerebral activity and a larger area of the right motor cortex that controls the fingers of the left hand. The effects were greater for those who began playing at an early age.
Pascual-Leone, et al., 1995; using MEG	The area of the motor cortex controlling the fingers increased in size in response to piano exercises.
Schlaug, Jancke, Huang, and Steinmetz, 1995; using PET	(1) Musicians had greater activity in left temporal lobes than nonmusicians. (2) Musicians with perfect (absolute) pitch had greater activity in left temporal lobe than musicians without perfect pitch.
Pantev, et al., 1998; using PET	The auditory cortex was 25 percent larger in experienced musicians than in nonmusicians, and the effect was greater for those who started studying music at an early age.

Table 6.2 (Continued) Some Findings from Science on Musical Ability

Study	Findings
Gregersen, 1998	In-depth reviews of genetic data showed evidence of a genetic predisposition to perfect (absolute) pitch, which could be expressed as a result of childhood exposure to music. Some children with perfect pitch also demonstrated exceptional mathematical ability.
Glassman, 1999	Harmonic relationships in music may account for the dynamics and limitations of working memory.
Ohnishi, et al., 2001; using fMRI	(1) Musicians processed music in brain areas that were different from the brain areas of nonmusicians. Musicians showed more activation in the left temporal lobe but nonmusicians had more brain activity in the right temporal lobe. (2) The degree of activation for musicians was correlated with the age at which the individual started musical training; the younger the starting age, the greater the activation. (3) Trained musicians with perfect pitch had greater activation than those without this ability. These findings suggest that early music training influences the brain to organize networks in the left hemisphere to process the analytical data needed to create music.
Itoh, Fujii, Suzuki, and Nakada, 2001; using fMRI	These colleagues reaffirmed the role of the left hemisphere when playing an instrument. The left parietal lobe was more highly activated than the right when musically trained subjects played the piano, regardless of whether they used their left or right hand separately, or used both hands.
Schlaug and Christian, 2001; using MRI	Musicians trained at an early age showed larger gray matter volumes in the left and right sensory and motor cortex regions and the left parietal lobe.

So, Where Are We?

Researchers have to speculate on possible explanations for their findings. At this time, these explanations do not resolve the nature versus nurture debate and may not for the foreseeable future. Even musically talented students have mixed views on the heritability of their own musical achievement. Tremblay and Gagné (2001) asked 80 musically talented students to use a 100-point Likert-type scale to rate the extent to which they believed seven components of musical ability could be inherited. The heritability scale ranged from *Not at all* to *Completely*. The seven components were as follows: auditory (ability to recognize and discriminate sounds), creativity (ability to improvise or compose melody), interpretation (ability

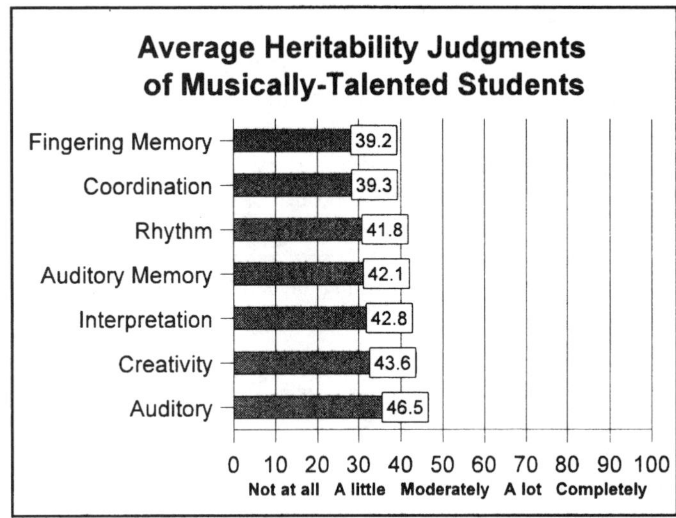

Figure 6.2 The average scores of musically-talented students on their beliefs that these musical abilities are inherited (Tremblay and Gagné, 2001).

to play a musical piece with feeling), auditory memory (ability to memorize a melody quickly), rhythm (ability to reproduce beats, duration of sounds, pauses, and tempo of a melody), coordination (ability to move hands on the instrument and to synchronize both hands), and fingering memory (ability to memorize fingering). Most students' scores fell in the moderate portion of the scale, ranging from 39.2 to 46.5 (Figure 6.2). Apparently, the music students believed that musical ability is inherited to a moderate degree and that practice and experience did not account totally for their musical achievement.

Ironically, the judgments of these talented musicians may be closer than the scientific studies to explaining what really accounts for musical achievement. On the one hand, the belief that talent is entirely innate has been overworked and, unfortunately, has led people to avoid the challenge of playing a musical instrument altogether. Too often, students invoke the absence of innate talent as the excuse for their failure and readiness to abandon their efforts. "It's not my fault. No one in my family is any good at (fill in the blank, here)," is not an uncommon excuse heard in today's classrooms. However, many accomplished musicians who displayed no early musical talent have become successful through their efforts at regular and determined practice. Granted, they may not be concert virtuosos, but their music can still provide enjoyment for themselves and others.

On the other hand, science cannot discount the possibility of a genetic predisposition to music. This genetic influence, for example, could be in the form of a larger auditory cortex capable of greater sensitivity to, and discrimination of, patterns of sounds. Another possibility is the development of a strong voice box and enhanced breathing musculature to produce powerful and melodic vocal music. Whatever the genetic contribution, such individuals, especially in a strong musical environment, will likely reach exceptionally high levels of musical achievement.

Although our understanding of how music affects the human brain is still far from complete, some of the following points can still be made:

- In most people, the brain has an innate ability to process music from birth.
- When listening to music, the processing may affect and enhance other cerebral functions, such as mathematical operations, kinesthetic performance, and memory recall.
- In most people, musical achievement may result more from efforts at regular and sustained practice than from genetic influences.
- A few people may be born with genetic predispositions which, in the right environment, will allow them to become extraordinary musical performers.
- The musical brain is highly resilient and persists even in people with profound mental and emotional disabilities.

READING AND MEMORIZING MUSIC

Reading Music

Highly successful musicians need to read musical notes and lyrics rapidly in order to produce fluent vocal and instrumental sound. Yet, some of these musically talented individuals have only average abilities in the reading of text.

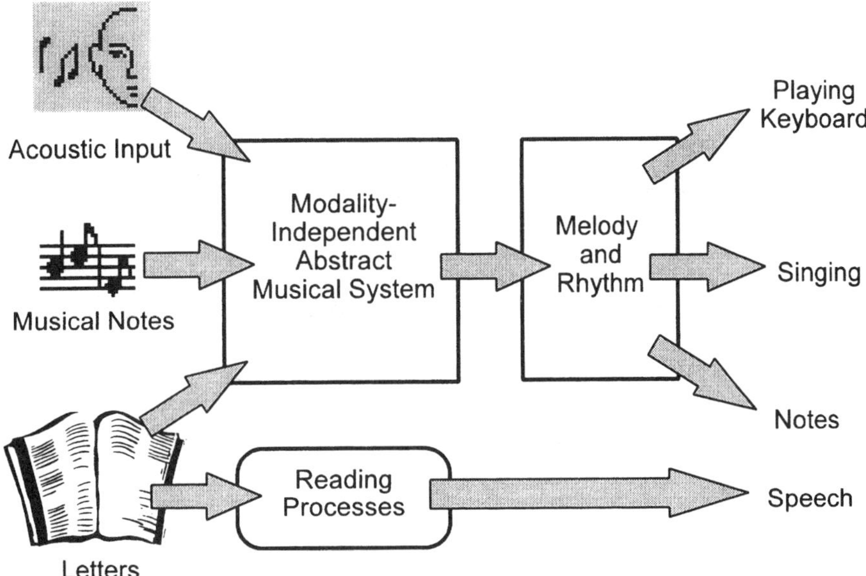

Figure 6.3 This diagram shows that the processing of musical notes and letters (lyrics) is functionally distinct from reading text and requires different cognitive operations (Stewart and Walsh, 2001).

How can this be? Should not the ability to read music with incredible speed also apply to reading text or vice versa? Apparently, this is not the case. A series of brain imaging studies on how the brain processes music in normal and brain-damaged musicians revealed that the ability to read or write music is a functionally distinct process from reading or writing text (Cappelletti, Waley-Cohen, Butterworth, and Kopelman, 2000; Stewart and Walsh, 2001). When the musicians read music, the notes and letters were integrated in the brain along with the acoustic input of what had just been played or sung. A network of brain regions, which Cappelletti and his colleagues called the *abstract musical system*, converted the input into melody and rhythm to produce the playing, singing, or writing of the next musical notes (Figure 6.3). During this process, the PET studies showed that the lower occipital and the rear part of the parietal lobes were the most activated areas (Figure 6.4). Damage to these regions resulted in the loss of the ability to read music, but not text. Apparently, different cerebral areas process text that is not related to music, but used instead for the production of speech. These findings may also suggest that there are different memory systems for storing music and nonmusical text. If so, it would explain why some patients with Alzheimer's disease, who have lost their ability to speak, are still able to sing songs and their lyrics with few or no errors.

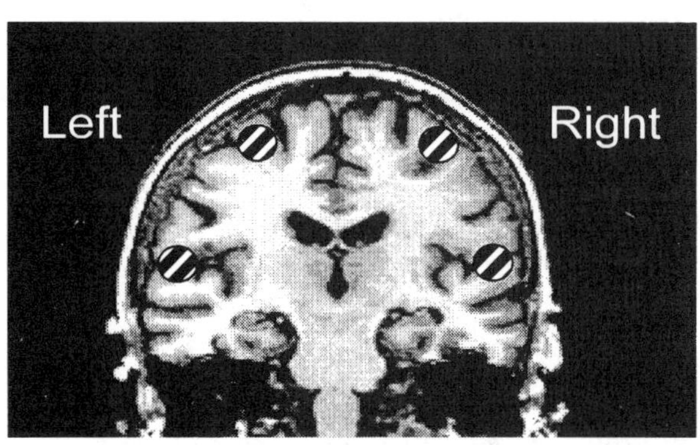

Figure 6.4 The circles in this representation of a PET scan show the areas of the occipital and parietal lobes that were most activated while a musician was reading music (Cappelletti, et al., 2000).

The results of the latest studies seem to be leading away from the earlier theory that music was essentially a right hemisphere function. It seems that music processing is spread throughout the brain and that selectively changing the focus of attention dramatically alters the patterns and intensity of cerebral activation.

Memorizing Music

Professional vocal and instrumental musicians often need to memorize large amounts of music if they want to perform publically. Although musical performance involves recall mainly from long-term memory, working memory is employed whenever the performers begin to improvise on the stored music. Yet, working memory is thought to have a functional limit of about seven chunks in most adults (Sousa, 2001a)—a capacity that would seem far too small to explain the rapid and varied modifications that some musicians display during a performance. To do this, they must have some means of binding more items within the chunks, thereby increasing the total item count in working memory. (Although working memory has a functional capacity of only so many chunks it can process at one time, there appears to be no functional limit to the number of items that can be combined into a chunk.)

Musicians brains may be much better at chunking information than the brains of nonmusicians.

Some researchers now speculate that harmonic frequencies of brain waves may be the binding medium. This hypothesis holds that (1) items bond into a chunk because some specific property synchronizes and unifies them, and (2) harmonic frequencies within an octave band of brain waves are the synchronizing mechanisms (Glassman, 1999). This theory also suggests that because trained musicians are more attuned and responsive to harmonics, their brains are much better at increasing chunk size than the brains of nonmusicians, thereby raising the item count in working memory and significantly improving the efficiency of the transfer of chunks between working and long-term memories.

Music As Another Way of Knowing

Neuroscience research into music supports the notion that music is disassociated from linguistic and other types of cognitive processing. Thus, processing music offers a unique way of acquiring nonverbal information. By studying how the brain processes music, scientists can learn things about the brain that they cannot get from other cognitive processes. Moreover, music allows us to know, discover, express, and share aspects of the human condition that we cannot experience through any other means. For that reason alone, we should be grateful for the music that talented performers create to help us all get a deeper understanding of what it means to be human.

Music allows us to know, discover, express, and share aspects of the human condition that we cannot experience through any other means.

DEVELOPING MUSICALLY TALENTED STUDENTS

The Identification Process

Identifying musically talented students requires a set of effective criteria and procedures deemed valid by professionals who work with these types of students. Haroutounian (2000) surveyed over 140 teachers, musicians, and arts specialists who work with musically talented students. The following are the most common criteria for identifying musical talent:

Musical Awareness and Discrimination

- Perceptual awareness of sound: internally senses sound and listens discriminately
- Rhythmic sense: fluidly responds to rhythm and maintains a steady pulse
- Sense of pitch: discriminates pitches; remembers and repeats melodies

Creative Interpretation

- Experiments with and manipulates sound
- Performs and reacts to music with personal expression and involvement
- Is aware of the aesthetic qualities of sound

Commitment

- Perseveres in musical activities
- Works with focused concentration and internal motivation
- Refines ideas, constructively critiques musical work of others and self

The identification process should also reach beyond the school to include recommendations from peers, private teachers, music directors, and other community members familiar with the student's musical abilities. An audition would also be appropriate.

The Nature of Practice

The extensive practice required of most musically talented students requires continuing encouragement by parents and teachers. Parents are there at the beginning and establish the routine and habits of practice from the onset. These routines set the work ethic, which can make the difference between the student reaching high or only moderate levels of mastery.

The teacher's role is critical to progressive musical development. As a tutor, the teacher provides a one-on-one environment where there are no limits to the student's progress. Being part of a performance group, such as a band, orchestra, or chorus, can greatly motivate student musicians to try more challenging musical pieces. To do so necessitates a form of practice that requires the student to work at optimal intensity. This is called *deliberate practice*, and teachers often provide the direction and encouragement that will help students recognize its value. As we discussed earlier in this chapter, the amount of practice time per week needed to produce high levels of mastery depends on the intensity of practice done in the student's early years. Musically talented teenagers who have learned the strategies of deliberate practice can achieve maximum results in less time.

Music teaching in the elementary grades is designed to reach all students. However, in the secondary schools, music classes are elective courses attracting students who have some degree of interest in vocal and instrumental music. They may represent a wide range of musical abilities, from passing interest to extraordinary talent. Given this mix, the music teacher may opt for a performance-based approach, hoping that it will appeal to a majority of the students. Furthermore, public performance helps to highlight the music curriculum and perhaps to garner community support during times when budgets are tight. This single-minded approach, however, is usually not sufficient to meet the needs of students who have already discovered their musical ability, nor will it entice those who have yet to realize their potential in music.

Looking for New Approaches to Teaching Music

Some music educators are examining the research findings in cognitive science and suggesting newer approaches to teaching music in secondary schools. Specifically, attention is focused on three factors that are influencing classroom instruction (Haroutounian, 2000;Webster, 2000):

(1) *Shifting from a teacher-centered, didactic format to a student-centered, constructivist approach.* The performance-oriented approach requires that the teacher constantly play the role of director, preparing for the next competition, festival, or concert. As a result, performance takes precedence over sharing the process of making musical decisions with students. Constructivism is an instructional format that emphasizes the importance of keeping the learner as an active participant rather than a passive receiver. Guided by the teacher, the students are engaged in creative activities that allow them to show mastery of music through their actions.

(2) *Expanding the use of technology and the Internet.* Computer software and the Internet provide many new resources for students to deal with music creatively rather than just practicing a musical piece to the teacher's specifications. With project-centered learning, teachers can encourage students to use computers and synthesizers to experiment creatively with sound.

(3) *Using creative thinking skills and metaperception.* One of the major goals of music education is to engage students' imaginations. This is more likely to occur in classrooms where teachers regularly involve students in divergent experiences that require creative thinking. Teachers will help students see music as an art form when they encourage them to create music thoughtfully through composition, performance, improvisation, and active listening. As students absorb abstract musical concepts, they learn to make creative decisions to solve musical problems. In essence, they are combining fine-tuned discrimination of the senses with high cognitive functioning to solve artistic problems. This process, sometimes called *metaperception*, is the artistic equivalent of metacognition. It includes sensing sound internally, remembering this sound, and manipulating the sound to communicate an emotional interpretation to others.

Academic Achievement Versus Musical Study

As musically talented students in secondary schools reach higher levels of performance, they begin to think about the possibility of a career in music. They crave practice time, expand their playing ability to additional instruments, and get involved in more musical performances. Parents, meanwhile, who had been so supportive when the student was younger, may not now welcome the notion of music as their child's career choice. Ironically, the student is then torn between coping with the demands of additional practice and performance time, while simultaneously trying to satisfy parental desires for more intense academic studies to keep career options open. Although it is true that many musically talented students are also gifted academically, this combined pressure can sometimes be too much. As a result, some musically talented students end their music lessons to relieve the pressure.

Working with parents, music teachers may be able to help their talented students deal with this difficult situation by looking at flexible scheduling that allows the student to pursue music lessons at other times. Programs such as MusicLink help schools develop individualized curriculums for talented students.

Implications for Teaching Music in Secondary Schools

Musically talented secondary school students have reached the intermediate to advanced level of talent development. Curriculum programs should be independently developed to meet the needs of these students (Haroutounian, 2000).

Intermediate Level: Lessons should develop the technical skills needed for advancing repertoire and exploring musical structure and style. Students seek opportunities to perform outside the school and wish to do so with technical skill and accuracy. Intermediate level students	
♬	Acquire more refined practice techniques
♬	Enjoy opportunities for performing both in and outside of school
♬	Develop technical proficiency
♬	Desire accuracy and precision in performance
♬	Experience a cognitive shift in musical thinking from active to interpretive understanding
♬	Expand performing opportunities to include occasional judged competitions
♬	Prefer instruction on musical understanding and technical development
♬	Delicately balance input from teachers, parents, and other students on competition, practice, and performance

Advanced Level: Lessons should be designed to hone already-developed technical skills and to enhance personal interpretations appropriate to the style, dynamic qualities, and aesthetic nature of the music. These students are usually already engaged in competition-level performances. Advanced level students	
♬	Analyze musical history, theory, and structure
♬	Understand stylistic differences along with various interpretations that reflect these styles
♬	Develop creative interpretation and artistic reasoning
♬	Fine-tune practice techniques and make maximum use of time for musical problem solving
♬	Use technical skills to create subtle qualities of tonal color
♬	Develop confidence through performances in professional-type settings
♬	Demonstrate subtlety and sensitivity in the critique of music performed by themselves and others

Differentiated Curriculum

Different levels of musical talent development in secondary schools can be addressed though differentiated curriculum. For a variety of reasons, the musical talents of some students do not emerge until they reach high school. Many vocal musicians, for example, do not begin taking singing lessons until adolescence, usually at the urging of a school choral director. Potential composers emerge when they start using computers to manipulate music in creative ways. Wind or brass instrument players often do not get serious about their musical studies until high school. And then there are the self-taught musicians, who are more likely to be discovered displaying their skills outside the school setting. Because these students are at varying levels of development, the music curriculum must be sufficiently flexible to meet their different needs. Haroutounian (2000) separates these students into five categories and suggests different curriculum options for each.

Advanced students who are conservatory-bound. Maximum practice time should be allotted to exceptionally talented students who are serious about pursuing a musical career. If they plan to attend a conservatory, the entrance audition is likely to be the major determinant for admissions. Consequently, the demands of intense practice may result in less time devoted to other academic studies. Guidance counselors can be helpful in developing curricular options for these exceptional talents. Although some of these students attend Saturday classes and lessons at conservatories, those who remain in a normal high school setting need independent study options to allow sufficient flexibility for practice.

Advanced students not yet committed to a career. Advanced musically talented students who have not yet committed to a performance career should have curricular options that extend beyond performance. These options could include creative work in composition, improvisation, and even collaborative projects with other art forms. The goal is to move these students out of a performance-based focus from time to time, getting them involved in creative ventures rarely offered in the traditional high school music curriculum.

Self-taught students. The talents of self-trained students lie outside the traditional secondary school music program. They have learned to develop their skills in a haphazard way, rather than through formal training. Offering instruction in the traditional studio setting may not be successful. The differentiated curriculum for self-taught students should investigate topics such as creative composition exploration, which can also include instruction in basic musical notation.

The critical listener. Critical listeners translate musical ideas into words. Their written or verbal critiques demonstrate astute musical awareness and creative verbal talents. Differentiated curriculum for critical listeners should offer comparative listening and critique of professional recordings, mentoring with a professional music critic, and opportunities for writing music reviews for the school paper.

The musical history student. Outstanding history students with musical training may be fascinated with the musical significance of historical eras, musical styles emerging from cultural influences, or other musicological connections. The curricular framework for these students should aim to link music and history in independent study or projects located within the regular gifted education program.

Conclusion

All students can develop their knowledge, understanding, and skills in music. Some may need more help than others, but that is true in any subject. Students who are generally gifted will need challenging musical contexts that will enable them to extend and apply their more general abilities. Music provides a context in which generally gifted students can deal with a range of complex factors and bring them together when making and responding to music. Generally gifted students already have the ability to think quickly and assimilate information, so these talents will also be evident when engaging in music. Furthermore, because music is abstract, it provides a means of identifying and developing skills that are not dependent on language skills. Thus, music can help teachers recognize giftedness in students who are not yet strong in language, especially those students whose first language is not English. Students who display strong musical interest and are vocally or instrumentally accomplished will need special attention so that the school environment continues to develop their talents.

Music can help teachers recognize giftedness in students who are not yet strong in language, especially those students whose first language is not English.

Musically talented students should have every opportunity to complete their talent development through high school, regardless of their future career decisions. They should be allowed to engage in challenging curricular experiences in their specialized field of interest. Schools can offer differentiated curriculum through student-developed interdisciplinary and independent study options, accelerated learning in performance classes, and courses in musical theory, composition, and music history. Teachers working with these students can serve as liaisons between the school and community to ensure student access to community resources related to music.

APPLICATIONS

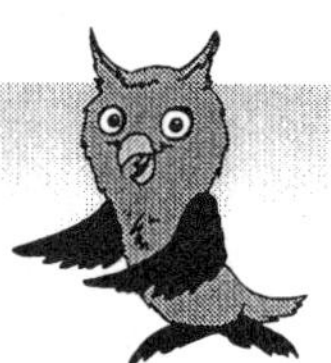

IDENTIFYING YOUNG STUDENTS WITH MUSICAL TALENT

Identifying musical capabilities in young students is not easy because most children enjoy making music, especially when listening to it. But there are some general characteristics that are likely to identify those individuals who have a greater than average interest in music. When trying to determine if a specific student has musical talent, rate the individual on the degree to which they possess the characteristics listed below. This instrument works best with elementary school children. The list is by no means exhaustive. But if the child rates high on most of the items, talk with the parents and other professional for their input.

The student...	A little Some A lot
1. Is captivated by sound and engages fully with music.	1 — 2 — 3 — 4 — 5
2. Selects an instrument with care and is unwilling to relinquish it.	1 — 2 — 3 — 4 — 5
3. Memorizes music quickly without any apparent effort.	1 — 2 — 3 — 4 — 5
4. Can repeat, usually after just one hearing, complex melodic phrases given by the teacher.	1 — 2 — 3 — 4 — 5
5. Can sing and/or play music with a natural awareness of musical phrasing.	1 — 2 — 3 — 4 — 5
6. Often responds physically to music.	1 — 2 — 3 — 4 — 5
7. Demonstrates the ability to communicate through music.	1 — 2 — 3 — 4 — 5
8. Shows a sustained inner drive to make music.	1 — 2 — 3 — 4 — 5

APPLICATIONS

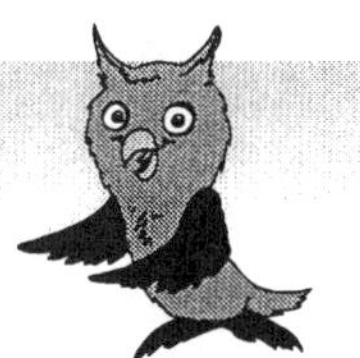

SUGGESTIONS FOR ENCOURAGING MUSICALLY TALENTED STUDENTS

Research studies indicate that the earlier individuals begin to use their musical talents, the more likely they are to continue their practice through their adolescence and young adulthood. Although musical talent generally appears in the younger years, there may be secondary school students whose talents have not yet been recognized. One of the goals of working with students who have already developed skills playing an instrument is to develop broader musical skills, as well as inspiring a deeper knowledge and understanding of music. This can occur in nearly all elementary classrooms whenever teachers feel comfortable addressing the skills of musically talented children.

The teacher helps build these skills and talent by

- Setting up challenging musical tasks and expecting a high-quality response. Students tend to meet the expectations that are set for them.
- Allowing students to take the lead in a class activity, such as starting a song or conducting the class.
- Including quick recall activities whereby students echo increasingly complex patterns given by the teacher. This choral response approach should be used sparingly, but it does encourage participation by those young students who may be shy.
- Encouraging special instruction in voice or on an instrument.
- Providing open-ended tasks or new contexts in which students can apply previously learned skills. Musically talented students usually seek out ways to apply their musical interests to classroom projects.
- Allowing opportunities in the classroom for students to use skills, such as instrumental skills, that they have learned outside the classroom.

MUSICALLY TALENTED STUDENTS—Continued

- Enabling students to use improvisation in their work, within certain limits identified by the teacher. Improvisation is an important component of creativity in music.

- Asking students, when appropriate, to analyze and evaluate music in relation to how it is constructed and produced. Further discussions can include identifying how music can be affected by different influences and the various ways that music can affect us.

- Encouraging students to participate in school choirs, bands, and orchestras.

- Providing opportunities for students to perform outside of school at public events throughout the community.

- Ensuring that students experience live professional musical presentations at regular intervals, followed by an analysis and constructive critique of the performances.

The Importance of In-School and Out-of-School Musical Activities

Teachers can often be a positive force in convincing students to get involved with musical groups. Participation by musically talented students in both in-school and out-of-school activities involving music contributes significantly to their musical achievement, especially in the elementary and early secondary grades. In 1997, the National Assessment of Educational Progress (NAEP) conducted a major study of the arts in the schools, using the 8th grade as the benchmark (Persky, Sandene, and Askew, 1999). The study assessed the students' ability to perform three processes: creating, performing, and responding. Responding refers to observing, describing, analyzing, and evaluating works of art.

MUSICALLY TALENTED STUDENTS—Continued

Figures 6.5 and 6.6 show the percentage of 8th grade students who scored at the three levels of a scale of music achievement relating their in-school and out-of-school activities in music. Clearly, participating in musical activities seems closely aligned with student achievement in music. However, the study did not specifically identify highly gifted musical students as a separate population.

In-School Music Activities (Figure 6.5). Students who participated in music activities within the school community were much more likely to score in the upper level of the responding scale in music achievement. The greatest gains were by students who owned a musical instrument, sang in school vocal groups, or played in a school band.

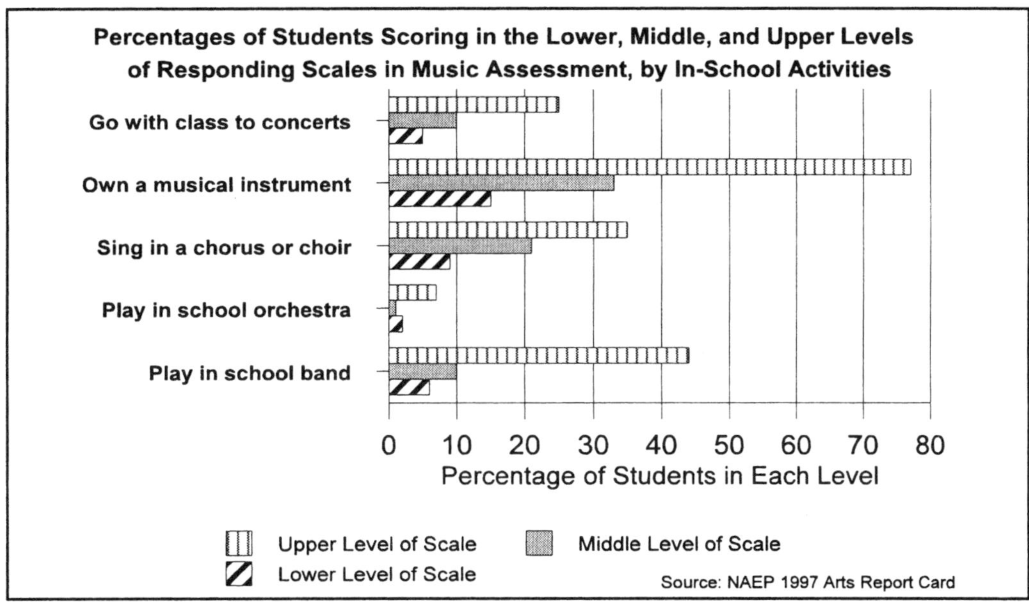

Figure 6.5 This graph shows the percentage of 8th grade students who scored in the lower, middle, and upper levels of the responding scale in music assessment, listed by their in-school activities in music.

Out-of-School Music Activities (Figure 6.6). Students who participated in out-of-school music activities were also more likely to score in the upper level of the responding scale in music achievement. The greatest gains were by students who played a musical instrument and took private music lessons.

MUSICALLY TALENTED STUDENTS—Continued

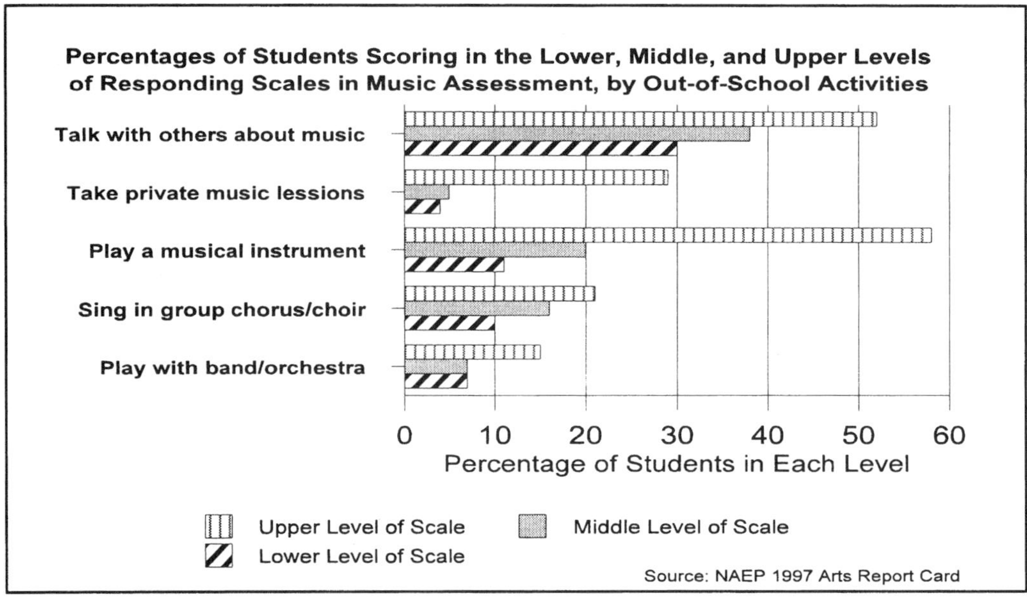

Figure 6.6 This graph shows the percentage of 8th grade students who scored in the lower, middle, and upper levels of the responding scale in music assessment, listed by their out-of-school activities in music.

APPLICATIONS

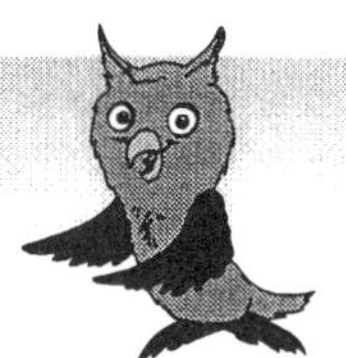

TEACHING MUSICALLY TALENTED STUDENTS IN SECONDARY SCHOOLS

Music educators are suggesting that discoveries in cognitive science should have an impact on the teaching of music in today's schools. Webster (2000) suggests that the following three factors need to be considered by music teachers in designing their lessons for musically talented students in secondary schools.

- **Constructivism.** This instructional approach focuses lesson design on activities that engage students in creative experiences so that they can construct their own understanding of the learning with the teacher's guidance. For example, instead of teaching music reading, listening, and movement through a teacher-centered approach with fact- and skill-oriented content, use small, interactive groups where students can discuss and create ways of including composition and improvisation. Other strategies might include asking students to write reports about the music they are playing, discussing the music content ("Why did the composer use this key?"), or even using student conductors on the podium.

- **Technology and the Internet.** Computers, software, synthesizers, and the Internet are just some of the new ways that students can manipulate musical sounds. Music sequencing notation and digital audio software allow students to compose music in ways that were not possible just a few years ago. For example, a software program available on the Internet, known as *Making More Music* (http://voyager.learntech.com), permits student groups to use a painting metaphor to draw layers with musical gestures. The program translates the drawings into musical notation and allows students to experiment with tempo, dynamics, and choice of timbre. As the students become more familiar with revision and

TEACHING STUDENTS IN SECONDARY SCHOOLS—Continued

other musical ideas, the program allows them to manipulate motives and phrases. Another source of real-world examples of technological applications to music can be found at the Music Teachers and Technology web page sponsored by George Reese, School of Education, the University of Illinois at Urbana-Champaign (*http://www-camil.music.uiuc.edu/mtt/default.htm*).

♫ **Creative Thinking Skills.** When teachers resort to problem-centered learning, students are able to pursue tasks that have more than one correct answer. Working alone or in groups, students are allowed to create their own examples of musical structures rather than be limited just to the teacher's example. This balance of convergent and divergent activities can be especially effective in performance venues by encouraging students to give their opinions about interpretations, by asking probing questions about the musical works they are performing, and by requiring them to practice music that creates solutions to various problems of performance. Internet resources, such as *HyperStudio*, can extend these activities further. With this approach, students of all ability levels get a deeper understanding of the learning because they are directly involved in solving problems. Moreover, these types of projects allow students to make judgments about musical content and context, use their creative thinking skills, constructively criticize others' works, and develop with other students a collective understanding of the music being studied. Although all students benefit, divergent activities such as these are particularly meaningful for the more musically talented students.

7

Underachieving Gifted Students

The phrase "underachieving gifted students" may sound like an oxymoron. But they do exist, and some educators and critics of education see underachievement as a major crisis in our nation's schools, not just for the gifted, but for all children. Underachievement can result when a gifted student acquires—for whatever reasons—some complex behaviors that erode academic performance. Whether it occurs quickly or slowly, underachievement prevents gifted students from reaching their potential. Consequently, it is an issue that must be addressed and remedied as much as any other obstacle to learning.

WHAT IS UNDERACHIEVEMENT? ■

Defining underachievement is not easy, especially among gifted students. Part of the problem lies in the definition of giftedness. Each school district has its own definition, although most rely on the use of an intelligence or achievement test score and teacher recommendations. These measures are not always reliable because few mentally gifted students truly excel in all subjects and on all academic tasks. Another problem is the definition of *underachievement*. Most commonly, it is a discrepancy between performance and an ability index, usually an IQ score. Ford (1996) reviewed over 100 studies and noted that many different instruments and criteria were used to measure underachievement, further thwarting attempts to establish a common definition.

Gifted underachievers generally display any of three behavioral responses to the school setting: noncommunicative and withdrawn, passively compliant, and aggressive/disruptive. Behaviors in all three groups reflect a belief in their inability to influence outcomes in school, a low or unrealistic self-concept, and negative attitudes toward school in general. They also tend to be easily distracted, supersensitive, and socially isolated (Achor and Tarr, 1996).

Underachievement is a pattern as complicated as the children to whom this label is applied. Consequently, some researchers believe that a more accurate way to define underachievement is to consider its various components (Delisle and Berger, 1990):

- *Underachievement Is a Behavior.* Underachievement is a behavior, not an attitude or set of work habits. Behaviors change over time and can be more directly modified than attitudes or habits. By referring to underachieving behaviors, we help these students recognize those aspects of their lives that they can change.

- *Underachievement Is Content and Situation Specific.* Gifted students can succeed in some situations and not in others. Those who may not be successful in school, for example, are often successful in outside activities, such as sports, music, or after-school jobs. Labeling a student as an underachiever ignores the positive outcomes of those areas in which the student *does* succeed. It makes more sense to label the area of underachievement, not the student (e.g., the student is underachieving in mathematics or social studies).

- *Underachievement Is Defined Differently by Different People.* As long as a student is passing, some students, parents, or teachers will not see underachievement. To others, getting a lower grade than expected is considered underachievement. Understanding the erratic nature of what constitutes success and failure is necessary to recognizing why some students underachieve.

- *Underachievement Is Tied to Self-Concept.* Self-concept can become a self-fulfilling prophesy. If students see themselves as failures, they eventually place self-imposed limits on what is possible. Good grades are dismissed as accidents or luck, but poor grades serve to reinforce a negative self-concept. Students with this attitude often give up trying because they assume that failure is inevitable. The results are low self-concept and limited incentive to change.

SOME CAUSES OF UNDERACHIEVEMENT ■

A combination of factors, both in the home and at school, can cause underachievement. Of all the possible causes, the following seem most prevalent.

- *Lack of Nurturing of Intellectual Potential.* Families with low socioeconomic status often fail to provide the environment that develops and stimulates high-level thinking. Enriching experiences, such as educational activities, travel, and shared problem solving, are few. Low-income students may come from specific ethnic or cultural groups that do not encourage intellectual development, from economically disadvantaged urban sites, or from isolated rural areas.

- ***Over-Empowerment and Over-Expectation.*** Giving children too much power too soon can lead to underachievement. Children from single-parent households, and first and only children, are the most likely candidates. Parents may also have overly exaggerated or misplaced expectations of their child's abilities, causing the child to become withdrawn in school participation. By labeling their children as the athlete, the social one, or the creative one, parents can add to competitive pressures.

- *Conflict in Values.* Students may withdraw from participating in school if they sense a conflict between the values of the school and the gifted program and those of the culture from which they come. For example, female students may underachieve because their culture may not value or expect females to pursue a college education or career. Other gifted students may underachieve because they do not want to be perceived as bookworms or nerds by their peers.

- *Lack of Motivation.* Prevailing instructional methods may not be compatible with the learning style of highly gifted students. The level of instruction may be below these students' capabilities, and classroom rules and restrictions may discourage their full participation. Classrooms that are over-competitive or under-competitive may also lead to achievement problems.

- *Learning Disabilities.* It is possible that underachieving gifted students may have psychological or physical problems that can interfere with learning. Developmental delays (physical, social, and emotional), neurological impairments (brain injury), and deficits in specific academic skills can all lead to poor academic performance. (See Chapter 8 on the twice-exceptional student.)

Adjusting to Giftedness

Some gifted students, especially adolescents between the ages of 11 and 15, may underachieve because they have serious problems adjusting to their giftedness. Perfectionism, urealistic appraisal of their gifts, rejection from peers, competitiveness, and confusion over mixed messages about their talents can all erode their achievement in school. Buescher (1990) identifies seven obstacles that can interfere with an adolescent's adjustment to giftedness.

- *Ownership of Talents.* It is not unusual for some talented adolescents to deny their talent, often because of peer pressure to conform and the adolescent's sense of being predictable. These individuals lack self-esteem and have doubts about the objectivity of their parents or teachers in identifying their gifts.

- *Giving of Themselves.* Because they have received gifts in abundance, talented adolescents sometimes feel that they must give of themselves in abundance and that their abilities belong to their teachers, parents and society.

- *Dissonance.* Gifted adolescents have learned to set high standards, to expect to do more, and to be more than their abilities might allow. In this drive toward perfection, these students experience real dissonance between how well they expect to accomplish something and how well it is actually done. This dissonance can be far greater than teachers or parents may realize.

- *Taking Risks.* Gifted adolescents are less likely to take the risks they took at an earlier age because they are more aware of the repercussions of their activities. Thus, they tend to be more cautious in weighing the advantages and disadvantages of possible choices, and in examining alternatives. They may even reject all risk taking, such as enrolling in advanced courses, competitions, or public presentations.

- *Competing Expectations.* The expectations of others (parents, teachers, peers, siblings, and friends) may compete with the gifted adolescent's own plans and goals. In effect, the adolescent's own expectations must face the onrush of the demands and desires of others. The greater the talent, the greater the expectations of others and outside interference. Trying to meet these expectations can drain energy and dampen the desire to succeed.

- *Impatience.* Gifted students can be just as impatient as other adolescents when looking for quick solutions to difficult questions or trying to develop social relationships. The impulsiveness makes them intolerant of ambiguity and unresolved situations. They can get angry if their hasty solutions fail, especially if other less capable students gloat over these failures. A string of such failures may prompt these students to withdraw.

- *Premature Identity.* For gifted adolescents, the weight of competing expectations, a low tolerance for ambiguity, and the pressure of multiple options all contribute to very early attempts to achieve an adult-like identity, even while in their early to middle teens. In an attempt to complete this identity, they may reach out for career choices that are inappropriate for their true age and that may interfere with the normal processes of identity resolution and acceptance.

IDENTIFYING GIFTED UNDERACHIEVERS

The problem of unidentified gifted underachievers has become more evident in recent years. Typical changes in school systems include the following:

- Use of more sophisticated and varied measures of intelligence and achievement
- A jump in the number of teacher referrals for special education services because of behavioral and learning problems
- Increase in efforts to recognize and develop the potential abilities of culturally different and minority children

- More reports by parents of out-of-school behaviors that demonstrate advanced interests and skills.

General Characteristics

Some of the most common characteristics and patterns of underachievement in gifted—as well as other—students are shown in the box to the left. Because gifted underachievers continue to fail in some areas, they tend to exhibit two general behavior patterns: *aggressive* or *withdrawn*. Aggressive behavior is characterized by stubbornly refusing to comply with requests, disrupting others, rejecting drill activities, alienating peers, and lack of self-direction in decision making. In contrast, withdrawn behavior patterns include lack of communication, working alone, little attempt to justify behavior, and little participation in classroom activities.

Characteristics of Gifted Underachievers
(Not all characteristics may be present in the same person.)

- high IQ score
- lack of effort
- a skill deficit in at least one subject area
- frequently unfinished work
- inattentiveness to current task
- low self-esteem
- poor work and study habits
- intense interest in one area
- seeming inability to concentrate
- failure to respond to usual motivating techniques

Studies classify underachieving gifted students into five types. The first type has low grades in general but high test scores (often on both criterion- and norm-referenced tests). In contrast, the second type displays low test scores but high course grades. The third type performs consistently below the level of capability in all subjects, and the fourth type underachieves only in certain subjects. Students whose underachievement goes unnoticed while in school comprise the fifth type. The existence of this type is most disconcerting because it means that these students will go through school seldom experiencing the educational opportunities that could have challenged them to reach their true potential.

Five Types of Gifted Underachievers

1. Low grades, high test scores
2. Low test scores, high grades
3. Low performance in all subjects
4. Low performance in certain subjects
5. Unnoticed

Dependence and Dominance

Underachieving gifted students often protect themselves by developing defense mechanisms. These temporary adaptations use dependency and domination patterns. Sylvia Rimm (1996) is a pediatric psychologist who suggests that underachievers can adopt patterns of behavior that fall on one spectrum that describes their dependence or dominance and another spectrum that represents their degree of conformity. The interaction of these elements results in a chart of quadrants (see Figure 7.1).

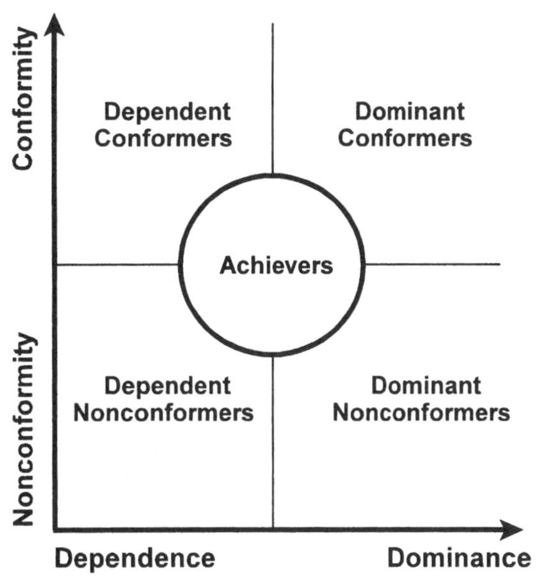

Figure 7.1 The quadrants represent different types of underachievers. (Adapted from Rimm, 1996).

According to Rimm, dependent children (left side of figure) have learned how to manipulate adults and get so much help from adults that they lose self-confidence. Because they do less, parents and teachers expect less. As a result, they can become overly sensitive, anxious, and even depressed. These children often go unnoticed.

In contrast, the dominant children (right side of figure) select only those activities they feel they can master. They manipulate adults by trapping them into arguments which can be about almost anything. Rimm maintains that if these children lose arguments, they develop enmity toward adults and use that as an excuse not to do their work or take on responsibilities. When the adults respond negatively to the manipulation, these dominant children complain that the adults do not like or understand them.

The upper and lower portions of the figure (conformity to nonconformity) represent the degree of severity of these children's problems. Those in the upper quadrants have minor problems and are likely to outgrow them. If they do not, however, then they may slip into the lower quadrants and their problems become more severe. Most dependent children will change to dominant by adolescence, although some retain a dependent-dominant mix, varying their response according to the situation.

Rimm believes that teachers and parents are often frustrated by these underachievers and inadvertently reinforce the undesirable patterns. Although children should be encouraged to be independent and creative, they should not be over-empowered so that adult guidance becomes impossible. Underachievement can be reversed, and in Rimm's model, that means adopting strategies that move the underachievers into the central circle of achievers—those children who are not dependent on defense mechanisms but who have confidence, an internal locus of control and who are resilient.

Spatially Gifted Students

Because language skills remain the most frequently used measure of academic giftedness, students who are strong in visual-spatial skills are often perceived as underachievers. Consequently, if they are poor in language skills, their teachers are more likely to focus on remediation and overlook any hint of giftedness. One major study at the University of Illinois in Urbana-Champaign found that, compared with other gifted students, students gifted in spatial ability were performing below their capabilities. Furthermore, this group had interests that were less compatible with traditional course work and received less college guidance from school counselors. The students were also less motivated by their educational experience and generally aspired to, and achieved, lower levels of academic and occupational success (Gohm, Humphreys, and Yao, 1998).

Underachievement: A Case Study
(Reis, Hébert, Díaz, Maxfield, and Ratley, 1995)

A 3-year study of 35 high-ability and underachieving students in an urban high school found the following:

- No relationship between underachievement and poverty, parental divorce, or family size.
- Underachievement began in elementary school due to lack of challenge.
- Underachievers were often not resilient enough to overcome urban problems, such as gangs and drugs.
- Abilities of underachievers were often not recognized by their parents, teachers, and guidance counselors during their elementary years.

Despite the increased awareness of underachievement in gifted students, educators need to work harder to insure that these students are identified as early as possible for several reasons. The most obvious one is the potential loss of their contributions to society. The second—and less obvious reason—is the underachiever's vulnerability to significant social and mental health problems. It is not uncommon for the gifted underachiever to become a major behavioral problem at school and at home. This behavior results from the conflict between the individual's personal psychological needs and the lack of appropriate learning opportunities in the school. Additionally, having a better chance at reversing the patterns of underachievement is another reason for early identification of these students.

UNDERACHIEVEMENT AMONG GIFTED MINORITY STUDENTS ■

Many studies have found an under-representation of minority students in gifted programs. As efforts continue to identify more minority gifted students, attention must also be focused on underachievement among the minority student population, especially African American as well as culturally and linguistically different students. Estimates of the number of gifted African American students who underachieve vary. One study of 149 middle and high school African American students found that almost 40 percent of gifted and potentially gifted students were underachievers (Ford, 1995). The study also revealed that the most effective variables for discriminating between the achievers and underachievers were: (1) attitudes of the students toward science, reading, and mathematics; (2) the perceptions that students had of their parents' desire for school success; and (3) the students' feelings about their own achievement.

Bernal (2002) maintains that no national data are available on the number of culturally and linguistically different students who underachieve or fail to get into gifted programs. But, on the basis of a sampling during the 1999-2000 school year of Texas school districts along the Mexican border, Bernal suggests that about 60 percent of these potentially gifted students were excluded from gifted programs and could be considered underachievers.

Several factors must be explored to understand why minority students underachieve. Ford and Thomas (1997) suggest that these factors fall into three categories: sociopsychological, family-related, and school-related.

- *Sociopsychological Factors.* Low academic self-concept and poor self-esteem are major contributors to underachievement. Racial identity must also be explored as a possible contributor. For example, How do students feel about their racial and ethnic heritage? Do they have a strong positive racial identity? If not, they may be especially vulnerable to negative comments by peers, such as "acting white" or "selling out," which contributes to low effort and low achievement. Specifically, many of these students must choose between their need for achievement and the need for peer affiliation. Too often, the need for affiliation wins.

  Minority students need to choose between their need for achievement and the need for peer affiliation. Too often, the need for affiliation wins.

  Minority students can attribute their outcomes to external factors, such as discrimination, and may thus put forth less effort than students who attribute outcomes to internal factors, such as ability and effort. Those minority students who substitute their belief in the power of work with their beliefs in glass ceilings and social injustices are not likely to reach their potential in school.

- *Family-Related Factors.* Numerous studies of gifted programs have found that family variables can influence the success of gifted students in school. The few studies that have examined the family influence on underachieving Black students found that the parents
  - expressed feelings of helplessness and hopelessness
  - were less involved and assertive in their children's education
  - set unclear and unrealistic expectations for their children
  - were less confident of their parenting skills.

- *School-Related Factors.* Factors in schools can influence the achievement of gifted minority students. Underachieving Black students often report
  - less positive student-teacher relations
  - too little time to understand the material
  - less supportive classroom climate
  - being disinterested and unmotivated in school.

Teacher expectations pay a big role in student achievement. Teachers who lack objectivity or training in gifted education and multicultural education may have different views of giftedness and underachievement, and thus are less likely to refer minority students for gifted education programs. Some teachers may have lower expectations for minority and low-income students than for other students. Consequently, minority students may not be identified as either gifted or underachieving. Eventually, these students underachieve due to frustration, disinterest, and lack of challenge.

Some research studies have identified key attributes of minority students' learning styles. For example, Black students tend to be field-dependent, concrete, and visual learners, but schools often emphasize abstract and verbal approaches. This mismatch between learning and teaching styles can result in confusion, frustration, and underachievement.

REVERSING PATTERNS OF UNDERACHIEVEMENT

Approaches to reversing patterns of underachievement are successful if they are based on the view that the poor performance has been shaped by forces within the school that can be changed. These forces include the social messages communicated by the teacher and peers that invite or discourage the student to participate, and the degree to which the curriculum and instructional strategies are compatible with the learning style of the underachiever. Thus, successful interventions will create positive forces that shape achievement behavior. These interventions must address three critical questions.

(1) What does it mean to be gifted and what are the associated problems?

(2) What are constructive ways of coping with the inevitable conflict that arises by the significant gap between performance level and cognitive ability?

(3) How can a student develop a healthier, more realistic self-concept?

Despite the frustration of working with students who are performing below their potential, strategies do exist that are effective in reversing underachievement. Three types of strategies are worth considering (Delisle and Berger, 1990).

- *Supportive Strategies.* These strategies focus on allowing students to feel that they are part of a group where problems and concerns can be discussed, and where curriculum activities can be chosen based on student needs and interests. Students may also be allowed to omit assignments for which they have already shown competency.

- *Intrinsic Strategies.* By accepting the notion that students' desires to achieve academically are closely linked to their self-concepts as learners, teachers use this type of strategy to encourage attempts, not just successes. Teachers also invite students to provide input on classroom rules and responsibilities. Students may also be allowed to evaluate their own work before submitting it to the teacher.

- *Remedial Strategies.* Underachievement is more likely to be reversed when teachers recognize that students make mistakes, and students can have individual strengths and weaknesses in addition to their intellectual, social, and emotional needs. Remedial strategies, therefore, are designed to allow students to excel in their areas of strength and interest. At the same time, teachers provide opportunities in the specific areas of each student's learning deficiencies. The classroom climate is one in which mistakes are considered part of the learning process for teacher and student alike.

Reversing Underachievement in Minority Students

Ford and Thomas (1997) suggest than additional efforts need to be made to reverse or prevent underachievement in gifted minority students. These interventions should

- Use valid and reliable measures for determining underachievement in minority populations
- Improve students' skills in organization, studying, time management, and taking tests
- Build self-esteem, social and academic self-concept, and racial identity
- Involve family members as partners in the educational process
- Provide appropriate school staff with training in gifted and multicultural education, which includes strategies for improving classroom climate and teacher expectations.

Bernal (2002) maintains that an effective way to improve achievement in gifted culturally and linguistically different (CLD) students is to change the nature of traditional gifted programs so that more of these students will qualify. He proposes the following remedies to address this problem of underrepresentation:

- *Evaluation:* Districts that have already had success in admitting and retaining CLD students need to evaluate their programs and share their data. The evaluation should focus on questions, such as
  - Who are the students that the program currently admits?
  - What are the students like who succeeded, and who failed?
  - What modifications have been made to the gifted program to accommodate these students and what have been the outcomes?

- *Multicultural Curriculum:* For CLD students to be successful in a gifted program, the curriculum must be multicultural. Districts need to train teachers in multicultural methodologies. This training should show teachers how to
  - Use examples from different cultures to make learning more

interesting to a wider group of students

- Demonstrate how new knowledge is influenced by ethnicity, history, and individual perspectives
- Use cooperative learning groups to promote positive interaction among students of diverse backgrounds, and
- Establish a classroom climate that makes CLD students feel wanted.

- *Recruitment:* Schools need to recruit authentic representatives of their respective minority groups into the gifted program's teaching staff. These individuals model some of the intellectual content and values of their cultural traditions for the benefit of all gifted students.

Other researchers have suggested using a variety of assessment approaches to enhance the identification of gifted minority students. Adams (1990) and Rhodes (1992) advocated the case study approach to the identification of gifted minority students. This approach uses a variety of information sources including rating scales, checklists, referrals, and peer nominations. Both Adams and Rhodes maintained that peer nomination forms are valuable because children can often identify their bright peers, and that they may be less biased toward cultural differences than their teachers.

Peer nomination instruments are often criticized for their lack of reliability and validity. However, a study involving 670 students in grades four through six did show that a peer nomination form designed to identify gifted Hispanic students had sufficient reliability and validity to warrant its use (Cunningham, Callahan, Plucker, Roberson, and Rapkin, 1998). The researchers recommended that the instrument be used with other minority groups, e.g., African Americans, Native Americans, and Asian Americans. A copy of the form used in this study can be found in **Applications** at the end of this chapter.

There is no simple answer to the problem of underachievement among gifted students. Some gifted students are high achievers in a highly-structured environment, but are underachievers if they have low self-esteem and cannot focus on a selected number of activities, establish priorities, and set long-term goals. Teachers and parents must remember that achievement and resilience can be taught. By doing so, they build the competencies and confidence that students will need as they grow and mature.

APPLICATIONS

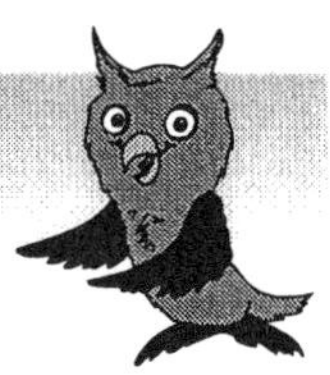

PROGRAMMING COMPONENTS FOR REVERSING UNDERACHIEVEMENT IN GIFTED STUDENTS

Programs designed specifically to reverse underachievement in gifted students can occur in the regular classroom, in resource rooms, or through the development of a plan that involves a mentor in the school or community. Achor and Tarr (1996) suggest that the program should contain at least the following five elements.

Teacher The teacher's perception of the student's problem is critical to the program's success. Consequently, the teachers must accept the fact that the student is gifted, does not want to underachieve or fail, needs to develop constructive coping skills, and has low self-esteem. To be successful, the teacher should be skilled in guidance techniques, have an accurate understanding of the nature of giftedness, and possess a positive attitude toward the challenge of working with this type of student.

Curriculum Program success is more likely if the curriculum is challenging, relevant, and rewarding to the student. The curriculum should have a balance between basic skill development and more advanced exploration of the arts and sciences. Critical elements also include the development of personal interests and career possibilities. There should be plenty of opportunities for challenge and success.

PROGRAMMING COMPONENTS—Continued

Instruction	Instructional techniques should include minimal memorization and drill/practice activities and maximal opportunities for inquiry, creative production, and scientific inquiry. Nurturing the student's self-discipline is important, as well as encouraging self-directed learning activities. The instructional climate should foster anticipation, excitement, low pressure, and personal satisfaction.
Peer Group	The peer group should include at least a few other gifted students, possibly underachievers, who can become good friends. The group must be accepting of individual differences and diversity. Their interactions can help develop needed social skills.
Special Services	Appropriate special services should be provided for gifted underachievers who are also handicapped, for those requiring remedial instruction, and for group counseling. These students sometimes require family counseling as well as supplemental medical and psychological services.

APPLICATIONS

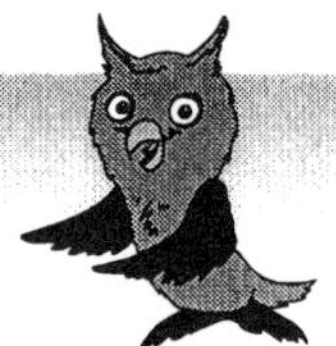

STRATEGIES FOR UNDERACHIEVING GIFTED STUDENTS

The following types of strategies are effective in preventing and reversing underachievement behavior in gifted students. They can be used by both teachers and parents (Delisle and Berger, 1990).

- **Supportive Strategies**
  - Do not assume that advanced intellectual ability also means advanced social and emotional skills.
  - Provide an atmosphere that is non-authoritarian, flexible, mutually respectful and questioning.
  - Establish reasonable rules and guidelines for behavior.
  - Give consistently positive feedback.
  - Provide strong support and encouragement.
  - Help them to accept their limitations as well as those of others, and to help others as a means of developing tolerance, understanding, empathy, and acceptance of human limitations.
  - Be a sounding board and listen to their questions without comment.
  - When it is time for solving problems, suggest possible solutions and encourage students to come up with their own solutions and strategies for choosing the best one.
  - Show enthusiasm for students' interests, observations, goals, and activities.
  - Avoid solving problems that the student is capable of managing.
  - Avoid establishing unrealistic expectations.
  - Provide a wide variety of opportunities for the students to experience success and to gain confidence in themselves.
  - Reserve time to have fun and to share daily activities.

UNDERACHIEVING GIFTED STUDENTS—Continued

- **Intrinsic Strategies**
  - Recognize that intellectual growth and development is a requirement for these children, and not merely an interest or a temporary phase that they are going through.
  - Avoid giving assignments that are too easy or too difficult.
  - Because learning style can affect achievement, ensure that these students are placed in programs that are sufficiently flexible and that have teachers who can address various learning style strengths and weaknesses. For example, gifted children are often strong in visual-spatial ability and weak in sequencing skills. They may also not do well in spelling, foreign languages, and mathematics, especially if they are taught in the traditional way.
  - Look for opportunities that allow students to explore topics in-depth, to participate in hands-on learning, and to develop adult expert-mentor relationships.
  - Encourage students to pursue their interests, recognizing, however, that some students will spend hours on a project and fail to submit required work. They need to be reminded that others may not be sympathetic to tardy or incomplete work.
  - Early career guidance can help these students set short- and long-term goals, complete required assignments, and plan for college.
  - Be aware of the fine line between encouragement and pressure. Encouragement emphasizes the process, steps, and effort used to achieve a goal; appraisal and evaluation are left to the student (intrinsic rewards). In contrast, pressure to perform focuses on outcomes and grades for which the student receives praise (extrinsic reward). Underachieving gifted students often reject praise as artificial and not authentic.

UNDERACHIEVING GIFTED STUDENTS—Continued

- **Remedial Strategies**
  - Be cautious about statements that may discourage the student, such as "Why did you get a C? You know you are gifted." Statements like these are rarely effective.
  - Avoid putting these students in situations where they are either winner or losers, and avoid comparing them to others. Rather, show them how to function in competition and how to deal with losing.
  - Special tutoring may help concerned students who are experiencing short-term academic difficulties. The tutor should be carefully selected to match the interests and learning style of the student.
  - Long-term underachievers rarely benefit from special tutoring or from study skills and time management courses. Other interventions that more directly address the *causes* of the underachievement need to be explored.

APPLICATIONS

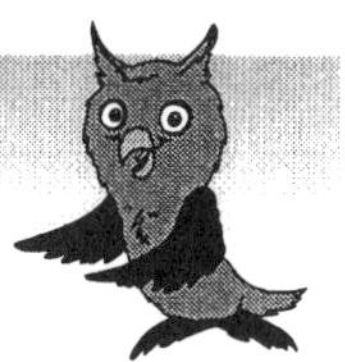

ADDITIONAL STRATEGIES FOR UNDERACHIEVING MINORITY STUDENTS

In addition to the strategies suggested in the previous pages, Ford (1996) offers some other considerations for enhancing achievement in minority students.

Supportive: Provide opportunities for these students to discuss their concerns with teachers and counselors who are trained in gifted and multicultural education. Classroom activities should focus more on cooperation than competition, and these students should get genuine positive reinforcement and praise when appropriate. Use activities that include multicultural components, mentors, and role models (such as teachers) from different ethnic and racial groups. Find substantive ways to involve family members and suggest ways that they can encourage the student at home.

Intrinsic: Allow students to have choices in selecting projects and in areas of interest. Vary teaching style to accommodate different learning styles. Use biographies of minority role models when appropriate. Include curriculum components that are multicultural, relevant, and personally meaningful to students.

Remedial: Implement academic counseling as soon as needed. Include tutoring and the teaching of study, time-management, organizational, and test-taking skills. Individual learning contracts and learning journals are also helpful.

APPLICATIONS

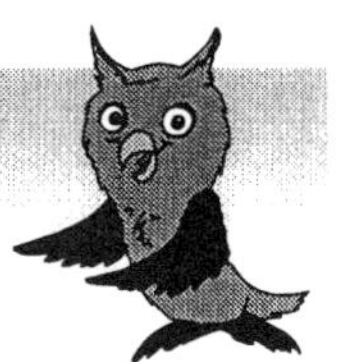

USING PEER NOMINATION FORMS TO IDENTIFY GIFTED MINORITY STUDENTS

Cunningham, et al. (1998) used the following peer nomination form in a major study to help identify gifted Hispanic students in grades four through six. Because of the instrument's high reliability and validity in their study, the researchers recommend that the instrument also be used with other minority groups, e.g., African Americans, Native Americans, and Asian Americans.

The 10 questions address intellectual abilities (questions 1, 2, 3, 9, and 10) and creative and artistic abilities (questions 4, 5, 6, 7, and 8). The directions on the form ask students to consider all of the peers in their classes, and the instructions ensure the confidentiality of their responses. The form gathers different information from that provided by standardized tests and should be just one part of a multiple assessment process.

The researchers suggest that the items on the form be used independently or in appropriate clusters to nominate students. Therefore, rather than using an overall cut-off score, students should be considered for selection on the basis of the proportion of nominations (i.e., the number of nominations divided by the class size) in the area of giftedness—intellectual abilities or creative and artistic abilities.

USING PEER NOMINATION FORMS—Continued

Peer Referral Form Cunningham, Callahan, Plucker, Roberson, and Rapkin, 1998 (Reprinted With Permission)
Teacher's Name______________________________
I am going to ask you to think of your classmates in a different way than you usually do. Read the questions below and try to think of which child in your class best fits each question. Think of the boys and girls, quiet kids and noisy kids, best friends and those with whom you don't usually play. You may only put down one name for each question. You may leave a space blank. You can use the same name for more than one question. You may not use your teacher's name or names of other adults. Please use first and last names. You do not have to put your name down on this form, so you can be completely honest.
1. What boy OR girl learns quickly, but doesn't speak up in class very often?
2. What girl OR boy will get interested in a project and spend extra time and take pride in his or her work?
3. What boy OR girl is smart in school, but doesn't show off about it?
4. What girl OR boy is really good at making up dances?
5. What boy OR girl is really good at making up games?
6. What girl OR boy is really good at making up music?
7. What boy OR girl is really good at making up stories?
8. What girl OR boy is really good at making up pictures?
9. What boy OR girl would you ask first if you needed any kind of help at school?
10. What girl OR boy would you ask to come to your house to help you work on a project? (Pretend that there would be someone to drive that person to your house.)
Note: Adapted from *Peer Referral as a Process for Locating Hispanic Students Who May Be Gifted* (unpublished doctoral dissertation, University of Arizona), by A. J. Udall, 1987.

8

The Twice-Exceptional Brain

The notion that a gifted child can have learning disabilities seems bizarre. As a result, many children who are gifted in some ways and deficient in others go undetected and unserved by our schools. Only in recent years have educators begun to recognize that high abilities and learning problems can coexist in the same person. But even with this recognition, many school districts still do not have procedures in place to screen, identify, and serve the needs of children with dual exceptionalities. What makes dual exceptionalities even possible is that the individual's strengths and weaknesses lie in different areas. Early observations of these students led to the term *paradoxical learners*, due to the many discrepancies in their school performance. Today, they are more commonly referred to as the twice-exceptional student.

■ IDENTIFYING TWICE-EXCEPTIONAL STUDENTS

Toll (1993) and Baum (1994) have suggested that gifted children who display learning problems fall into three distinct groups:

1. *Identified gifted, but also learning disabled.* The first group includes students identified as gifted but who exhibit learning difficulties in school. They often have poor spelling and handwriting and may appear disorganized or sloppy in their work. Through low motivation, laziness, or low self-esteem, they perform poorly and are often labeled as underachievers. Teachers expect them to achieve because they are labeled as gifted. As a result, their learning disabilities remain unrecognized until they lag behind their peers.

2. *No identification.* The second—and perhaps largest—group represents those children whose abilities and disabilities mask each other. They often function at grade level, are considered average students, and do not seem to have problems or any special needs. A majority of these students are unassertive, doing what is expected of them but not volunteering information about their abilities or interests. Although they may be seem to be performing well, they are in fact functioning well below their potential. In later high school years, as course work becomes more difficult, learning difficulties may become apparent, but their true potential will not be realized. Because neither exceptionality is identified, students in this group will not receive the educational programs necessary to meet their needs.

3. *Identified learning disabled, but also gifted.* The third group includes students who have already been diagnosed with learning disabilities but whose high abilities have never been recognized. This may be a larger group than one might believe at first. They are often placed in a learning-disabilities classroom where their difficulties suppress their intellectual performance. Little attention is given to their interests and strengths. Over time, they may become disruptive and find ways to use their creative abilities to avoid tasks. If their high ability remains unrecognized, then it never becomes part of their educational program, and these children never benefit from services to gifted children.

Children in all three groups are at risk for social and emotional problems when either their potential or learning disabilities go unrecognized. The problem is further compounded by the identification process because the activities used to select students for either learning disability or gifted services tend to be mutually exclusive. Consequently, these students often fail to meet the criteria for either type of service.

The Difficulties of Identification

Conservative estimates are that about 2 to 10 percent of students enrolled in gifted programs have learning disabilities (Dix and Schafer, 1996). The number of possible combinations of intellectual giftedness and learning disabilities is so great that any attempt to devise a single set of reliable measures is probably futile.

For example, gifted children with language or speech impairments cannot respond to tests requiring verbal answers. Children with hearing problems may neither be able to respond to oral directions nor possess the vocabulary necessary to express complex thoughts. Vision problems could prevent some children from understanding written vocabulary words. Learning disabilities could prevent some children from expressing themselves through speech or in writing. Moreover, dual exceptionality children often use their gifts to hide their disabilities, further complicating the identification process.

Nonetheless, researchers agree that a battery of measurements should be developed to assess these students. Assessment should include an achievement battery, an intelligence test, indicators of cognitive processing, and behavioral observations. Teachers should be given lists of characteristics (e.g., the "Characteristics of Gifted Children with Learning Disabilities" at the end of this chapter) to increase their awareness of behaviors displayed by students who are gifted and learning disabled. Parent interviews, self-concept scales, and talent checklists are just some of the tools that can be used to assess whether a child is gifted. The goal is early identification and intervention for gifted students with learning disabilities so that their needs and talents are recognized and appropriately addressed by the school staff.

Cline and Hegeman (2001) propose that the identification of gifted students with disabilities is particularly difficult for the following reasons:

Focus on Assessing the Disability. Assessment of the disability should include looking for particular strengths, such as superior mental or artistic ability, and creativity. Besides medical information, test administrators should look at participation in extracurricular activities and performance in music, visual arts, drama, or dance.

Stereotypic Expectations. The long-held perception that gifted children are motivated and mature while learning disabled children are unmotivated and sluggish needs to be overcome if we are to successfully identify this population.

Developmental Delays. Delays in a student's cognitive development may result in disabilities that mask talents. Students with visual impairments, for example, will have difficulty with any abstract thinking that requires visual representation, but may have high capabilities in other areas of language expression.

Experiential Deficits. Children in families with limited resources may not have had many opportunities for a variety of learning experiences (e.g., travel), thus inhibiting the expression of their unique abilities.

Narrow Views of Giftedness. Too many educators still hold a narrow view of giftedness as intellectual potential in mathematics and language. However, the works of Howard Gardner, Robert Sternberg (see Chapter 2), and others have provided broader conceptions of intelligence that may help in the identification of gifted students with learning disabilities.

Disability-Specific Concerns. Because a specific disability may affect a student's performance in certain parts of the testing process, test administrators may need to make adaptations or accommodations to the testing procedures. These alterations should be appropriate to the specific disability and could include omitting certain questions or extending the time for taking the test.

The Potential for Misdiagnosis

As psychologists and educators become more aware of the behaviors that suggest learning disabilities, concerns are now being raised that gifted students may be misdiagnosed as having psychological disorders as a result of the very behaviors that make them gifted. For example, many gifted children are intense in their work, engage in power struggles with adults, and are extremely sensitive to emotional situations. They are often impatient with themselves and others, displaying an intense idealism and concern for moral and social issues, which can create depression and anxiety. Further, gifted children are often bored in the regular classroom and their peer relations can be difficult. These problems, which can be associated with the characteristic strengths of gifted students, can be mislabeled and ultimately lead to misdiagnosis.

Gifted students may be misdiagnosed as having psychological disorders as a result of the very behaviors that make them gifted.

Psychologist James Webb has long been interested in the misdiagnosis of gifted students. Table 8.1 lists a few of the possible problems that he suggests may be linked to the typical strengths of gifted children (Webb, 2000). Webb contends that inexperienced health professionals are misreading the problems and mistakenly diagnosing some gifted children with attention-deficit hyperactivity disorder (ADHD), oppositional defiant disorder, bipolar disorder, and obsessive-compulsive disorder. No doubt, giftedness can coexist in students who have psychological disorders, but Webb believes that number is far smaller than currently diagnosed.

Table 8.1 Possible Problems Linked to the Typical Strengths of Gifted Children	
Strengths	**Possible Problems**
Quickly acquires and retains information.	Looks bored; gets impatient with slowness of others.
Enjoys intellectual activities and can conceptualize and synthesize abstract concepts.	May question teachers' procedures; resists practice and drill; omits details.
Seeks to organize things and people.	May be seen as rude or domineering.
Is self-critical and evaluates other critically.	Intolerant toward others; may become depressed.
Enjoys inventing new ways of doing things.	May reject what is already known; seen by others as different.
Strong desire to be accepted by others; has empathy for others.	Expects others to have similar values; sensitive to peer criticism; may feel alienated.
Has diverse interests and abilities.	Frustrated over lack of time; may appear disorganized.
Strong sense of humor.	Often sees the absurdities of situation; humor may not be understood by others; becomes class clown to get attention.
Displays intense efforts, high energy, eagerness, and alertness.	Eagerness may disrupt others; frustrated with inactivity; may be seen as hyperactive.

Similarly, some gifted students are being misdiagnosed with learning disabilities. According to Webb (2000) and Winner (2000), this can happen when health professionals misinterpret any of the following as a sign of learning dysfunction:

- large differences between the verbal IQ and performance IQ on the Wechsler intelligence tests
- large differences between the individual subscales on the intelligence and achievement sections of the Wechsler Intelligence Scale for Children
- poor handwriting
- poor sleep habits
- parental reports that the child is strong-willed, impertinent, weird, argumentative, and intense

Misdiagnosing Giftedness as Attention-Deficit Hyperactivity Disorder (ADHD)

In looking at Table 8.1, it is apparent that many of the possible problem behaviors linked to gifted students can readily be associated with the characteristics of attention-deficit hyperactivity disorder (ADHD). Specifically, the gifted characteristics of high motor activity, sensitivity, intensity, and impatience can easily be mistaken for ADHD. Surely, some gifted children suffer from ADHD, but many do not. So how do health and education professionals determine whether a child's behavior is merely the expression of giftedness or the sign of a gifted child with ADHD? Answering this question requires considering the settings and situations in which the child displays the problem behavior, as well as other potential explanations.

- *Consider the Setting and the Situation.* Gifted children do not exhibit the problem behaviors in all settings. For example, they may appear ADHD-like in one class, but not in another; or they may have problems on the ball field, but not at their music lessons. By contrast, children with ADHD exhibit their problem behaviors in all settings, although the intensity of their display may vary from one situation to another.

  Gifted children may be perceived as being off-task when their behavior might be related to boredom, mismatched learning style, lack of challenge in the curriculum, or other environmental factors. Providing more challenge will usually get them back to work. ADHD children have a difficult time focusing on their work no matter how interesting it may be.

  Hyperactivity is a common characteristic of gifted and ADHD children. However, for the gifted, their activity is highly focused and usually results in productive work or achievement of a specific goal. For ADHD children, their hyperactivity is found across all different types of situations and is often unfocused and unproductive.

- *Consider Other Sources.* Clinical studies report that a small percentage of gifted students suffer from borderline hypoglycemia (low blood sugar) and from various kinds of allergies (Webb, 2000; Silverman, 1993). Physical reactions in these conditions, coupled with the sensitivity and intensity characteristics of gifted children, can result in behavior that mimics ADHD. Once again, the intensity of their display will vary with diet, time of day, and other environmental factors.

One recent study found that highly gifted boys exhibit levels of behavior problems similar to boys who are learning disabled (Shaywitz, Holahan, Fletcher, Freudenheim, Makuch, Shaywitz, 2001). Surely, some gifted children have true learning disabilities, and their dual exceptionality should be addressed. However, health care professionals need to become more familiar with aspects of giftedness so that they are less likely to conclude that certain inherent characteristics of gifted children are signs of pathology.

Some highly gifted boys exhibit levels of behavior problems similar to boys who are learning disabled.

Guidance and Counseling Interventions

School counselors can provide guidance and counseling services that benefit gifted students with learning disabilities. These services can often help students develop positive social relationships, raise their self-esteem, and improve their overall behavior. Furthermore, counselors can advocate on behalf of these students by raising awareness of their unique needs. By assisting in the identification process, using individual and group counseling, consulting with parents, and sharing academic strategies, counselors become important collaborators and facilitators in ensuring the academic success of gifted students with learning disabilities (McEachern and Bornot, 2001).

Because of the difficulties of accurately identifying and diagnosing gifted children with learning disabilities, no reliable data are currently available on the number of gifted children who are also diagnosed with specific learning deficits. Nevertheless, the following sections examine some of the more common combinations of giftedness and associated learning disabilities.

■ GIFTEDNESS AND ATTENTION-DEFICIT HYPERACTIVITY DISORDER (ADHD)

Some gifted children do have ADHD. Unfortunately, this dual exceptionality often means that such children are not recognized as having either exceptionality. Therefore, their needs for an appropriate education often go unmet.

What Is ADHD?

Attention-deficit hyperactivity disorder (ADHD) is a syndrome that interferes with an individual's ability to focus (inattention), regulate activity level (hyperactivity), and inhibit behavior (impulsivity). It is one of the most common learning disorders in children and adolescents. About 2 to 3 times more boys than girls are affected. ADHD usually becomes evident in preschool or early elementary years, frequently persisting into adolescence and occasionally into adulthood.

Although most children have some symptoms of hyperactivity, impulsivity, and inattention, there are those in whom these behaviors persist and become the rule rather than the exception. These individuals need to be assessed by health care professionals with input from parents and teachers. No specific test exists for ADHD. The diagnosis results from a thorough review of a physical examination, a variety of psychological tests, and the observable behaviors in the child's everyday settings. A diagnosis of ADHD requires that six or more of the symptoms for inattention or for hyperactivity-impulsivity be present for at least 6 months, appear before the age of 7, and be evident across at least two of the child's environments (e.g., at home, in school, on the playground, etc.). Recently, ADHD has been classified into three subtypes: predominantly inattentive, predominantly hyperactive-impulsive, and the combined type (Sousa, 2001b).

About 2 to 3 times more boys than girls are affected by ADHD.

What Causes ADHD?

The exact causes of ADHD are unknown. Scientific evidence indicates that this is a neurologically based medical problem for which there may be several causes. Some research studies suggest that the disorder results from an imbalance in certain neurotransmitters (most likely dopamine and serotonin) that help the brain regulate focus and behavior. ADHD has been associated with symptoms in children after difficult pregnancies and problem deliveries. Maternal smoking as well as exposure to environmental toxins, such as dioxins, during pregnancy also increase the risk of an ADHD child. Other studies indicate that the ADHD brain consumes less glucose—its main fuel source—than the non-ADHD brain, especially in the frontal lobe regions. Brain imaging studies have revealed structural differences in adults with ADHD, suggesting that the disorder may have a genetic component (Sousa, 2001b).

The Attention Loop

Because one of the main characteristics of ADHD (as well as attention deficit disorder, ADD) is the inability to control attention, recent research has focused on how the brain attends to incoming and internal stimuli. Attention seems to be the result of a loop-like process that involves the brain stem, the posterior (rear) cortex, and the prefrontal cortex (Figure 8.1). The brain stem collects the incoming data and sends it to the posterior cortex which integrates the data. Interpreting the data is the job of the prefrontal cortex, and its interpretation can modify what the brain stem transmits, thus completing the loop. Any breakdown in this loop will interfere with attention, and the degree of breakdown will affect the nature of the attention deficit, some with and others without hyperactivity (Goldberg, 2001).

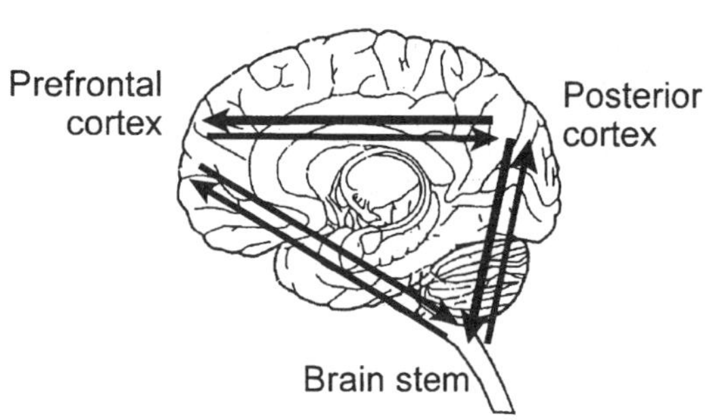

Figure 8.1 The attention loop involves the brain stem, the prefrontal cortex, and the posterior cortex.

Because gifted children have a higher functioning prefrontal cortex than their average peers, breakdowns in the attention loop are more likely to occur in the posterior cortex (sensory integration and emotional input) and in the brain stem. This may explain why gifted children with ADHD are more prone to have social and emotional problems rather than cognitive ones.

Characteristics of Gifted Children With ADHD

Assuming proper diagnosis, gifted children with ADHD do differ from *average* children with ADHD in the following ways (Lovecky, 1999).

- *Testing*. Gifted children with ADHD show great variability on tests of achievement and intelligence. Their performance is scattered and they miss many easy items while answering the difficult items correctly. Because of their excellent memory, they tend to score high on the subtests involving mathematics. They also tend to score high in abstract reasoning ability.

- *Study Skills*. These children often learn more rapidly and exhibit more mature metacognitive strategies (e.g., using of mnemonics;

grouping by category, patterns, or spatial characteristics; and recalling by association) than their age peers. However, they sometimes forget to use the strategies or may not use them efficiently. They tend to have more problems with study skills, such as note taking, organizing ideas, and outlining.

- *Developmental Issues*. Gifted children with ADHD show greater differences in their degree of social and emotional development than their average peers. They may behave less maturely than their peers in some situations and more maturely in others. They form friendships with those who will share their complex interests with the same intensity. However, they often misread social cues and show poor understanding of group dynamics and goals. They tend to be more emotional and show greater sensitivity than their age peers.

- *Interests*. Compared to their age peers, these children usually have more specialized interests and seek out activities that have greater complexity. Their interests are generally intense and last for years.

Gifted children with ADHD differ from other *gifted* children in that they

- Show greater degrees of differences in development across cognitive, social, and emotional areas and in their ability to act maturely.
- Have less ability to think sequentially and to use working memory adequately.
- Experience greater difficulty solving problems that use part-to-whole relationships because they have trouble selecting the main points among data.
- Tend to complete less work, hurry through it, take too long to complete simple things, and often change topics on projects.
- Find it difficult to work in groups, even with groups of gifted children.
- Do not feel a high degree of satisfaction or intrinsic reward for completing a project.

GIFTEDNESS AND AUTISM

To understand this twice-exceptional population, let us first examine the nature of autism and then look at some unique characteristics of individuals who are both gifted and autistic.

What Is Autism?

In autistic disorder (or autism), neurological problems develop that make it difficult for a person to communicate and form relationships with others. It is a spectrum disorder that runs the gamut from mild to severe. About 10 percent of people with autism are relatively high functioning (called high-functioning autism, or autistic savants), while others are mentally retarded or have serious language delays.

Approximately 10 percent of people with autism are high functioning and display savant skills.

Autism affects about one person in 500, and 4 out of 5 of those affected are males. Although it may appear that the incidence of autism is increasing in American children, the medical community believes it is more likely that the prevalence of autism has been underestimated in the past.

The symptoms of autism usually appear before the age of 3. Children with autism do not interact well with others and may avoid eye contact. They may resist attention and affection, and they rarely seem upset when a parent leaves or show pleasure when the parent returns. Understanding the cues of others—such as a smile, wink, or grimace—is difficult for them as well. Some children with autism also tend to be physically aggressive at times, particularly when they are in a strange or overwhelming environment. At times they will break things, attack others, or harm themselves. There is no general agreement on the causes of autism, and given that this is a spectrum disorder, it is likely that there are multiple causes. Researchers have found that autism may be associated with genetic defects (autistic characteristics tend to run in families), with structural abnormalities in the frontal lobes and brain stem, or with low concentrations of serotonin (Sousa, 2001b).

Types of Autism

Although autism is officially classified in the Fourth Edition of the Diagnostic and Statistical Manual of Mental Disorders (commonly referred to as the DSM-IV, 2000) as only one type of pervasive developmental disorder, there is no clear consensus on this view. Other researchers believe that autism may be more closely related to social, sensory, or cognitive deficits. Despite the controversy, four types or autism have been identified on the basis of differences in behaviors:

- *Kanner-Type:* Sometimes called classic autism or early infantile autism, this type is characterized by the early onset of symptoms, lack of eye contact, late speech, repetitive behaviors, and possible mental retardation.

- *Asperger's Syndrome:* A pervasive developmental disorder on the autism spectrum characterized by social deficits, relatively normal cognitive and language development, and the presence of intense, idiosyncratic interests.

- *Pervasive Developmental Disorder–Not Otherwise Specified.* This classification is used when a child does not meet the defining criteria before the age of 3 years. Sometimes this classification is used when the condition appears less severe or inconsistent with the general criteria. It is usually more closely aligned with Kanner- Type autism than with Asperger's Syndrome.

- *Regressive/Epileptic Type.* This type is characterized by the inability to understand others, mixing of sensory inputs, abnormal EEG readings, mental retardation, and high anxiety levels.

For the purposes of this book, we will focus on Kanner-type autism and Asperger's syndrome because these are the two types that are most likely to coexist with giftedness.

Impact of Giftedness on Individuals With Classic (Kanner-Type) Autism

Giftedness also runs on a spectrum from mildly gifted to genius. It is sometimes difficult to separate high functioning individuals with mild autism from those who are gifted because they can share many similar traits. For example, both the gifted and autistic tend to focus intently on objects, behaviors, and activities. They display similar negative behaviors, such as stubbornness, indifference to socialization and dress, discourteousness, and resistance to teacher authority. Both groups are powerful visual thinkers and have keen senses. Individuals who are *both* gifted and autistic are difficult to identify because their strengths and weaknesses can mask each other. Nonetheless, they have to manage and adjust to their environment. Having these dual exceptionalities brings with it positive and negative impacts (Cash, 1999).

- *Positive Impacts.* The key to the success of gifted/autistic individuals often starts in school where they can learn compensatory strategies to manipulate their autistic weaknesses and tendencies. Through behavior modification programs and by using metacognitive strategies, they can gain acceptance and credibility, and be more easily accepted by society.

- *Negative Impacts.* Gifted/autistic individuals frequently move from one environment that praises their strengths to another that misunderstands and fears their unusual and perplexing characteristics. In school, gifted/autistic students may be placed in classes where their seemingly contradictory behaviors and non-traditional social interactions often confuse uninformed teachers and peers. As a result, the gifted/autistic students may be criticized and suffer social rejection. Although some of these dual-exceptional students are insensitive to the lack of connectedness (a typical autistic characteristic), others are frustrated by the ostracism.

Too often, gifted/autistic individuals do not receive intellectual opportunities and are frequently placed in classes with mentally-challenged students. The school focuses on addressing only their weaknesses and remediation becomes the sole educational goal. Consequently, these students can suffer from depression, low self-esteem, and lack of motivation. On the other hand, more educators are becoming aware that some autistic children may also be gifted, and are exploring interventions, such as early identification and screening, the use of diagnostic instruments, coordinated teacher and parent training, parent support networks, behavior modification programs, and learning theory reform. If prompt identification and appropriate interventions begin in school, there is a greater likelihood that gifted/autistic individuals can develop into important and contributing adults (Cash, 1999).

Too often, gifted/autistic individuals do not receive intellectual opportunities and are frequently placed in classes with mentally-challenged students.

Asperger's Syndrome

Identified in 1944 by Austrian physician Hans Asperger, this syndrome is a developmental disorder with many of the same symptoms of autism. Asperger's syndrome (AS) may occur in as many as 26 out of 10,000 children (Note: Classic autism occurs in about 4 out of every 10,000 children.). The number of occurrences is changing as AS becomes better known and as the number of professionals diagnosing it increases. AS is usually referred to as *high-functioning autism* because people with the disorder generally display higher mental performance than those with typical autism.

In classic autism, the male to female ratio is 4:1. In high-functioning Asperger's syndrome, that ratio is 9:1.

Like autism, AS is a lifelong condition. The condition usually appears after the age of 18 months and is characterized by poor motor coordination and late mobility. As the child develops, other symptoms appear, such as routinized obsessive-compulsive behaviors, poor motor coordination with clumsy gait, strong attachments to places, poor eye contact, difficulty in relating to people, lack of empathy for others, and depression. Speech is often repetitive and pedantic, with monotone intonation and the absence of first person pronouns.

Savant skills are not present in all AS individuals. But they are common and usually involve extraordinary memory and preoccupation with the mastery of one or two subjects, such as history trivia, sports statistics, weather, and train schedules, often at the exclusion of learning in all other areas. Although their general language abilities are limited, they can carry on extensive discourse in their areas of special expertise but may have little grasp of the meaning of the words they are using. Some AS individuals have a history of *hyperlexia*, which is rote reading at a precocious age.

That AS individuals have problems with social interaction can be a particularly burdensome characteristic because it carries into adulthood, causing social isolation and frustration. AS children are often unable to understand the social customs associated with dating or to pick up on nonverbal social cues, such as eye contact, voice intonation, or gesturing. As a result, AS individuals often devise a set of rules to cope with social interactions. The rules are generally inflexible and serve only to further isolate these individuals rather than help them succeed in social situations. Several programs have been devised to help AS students enhance their social skills.

Genetic Components

There is growing evidence that both autism and AS have genetic components. First, in classic autism, the male to female ratio is 4:1; in high functioning AS, that ratio is 9:1. These gender differences are far too great to be explained entirely by differences in socialization. They more likely reflect developmental differences between the two sexes regulated by genetic information. Second, there is an increased incidence of AS profiles among relatives of children with AS. Third, there is an increased incidence of other developmental disorders among the siblings of AS children. One study investigated the genetic connection through a series of cognitive performance tasks to test whether the parents of children diagnosed with AS displayed similar cognitive traits (Baron-Cohen and Hammer, 1997). Mothers and fathers of AS children performed better than the control subjects on those tasks associated with AS strengths, but worse on the tasks associated as weakness in AS profiles. This finding lent support to the notion that parents of AS children carry mild forms of the disorder. Another finding was that male parents performed lower on all tasks than female parents, suggesting that the genetic factors that contribute to AS are more closely linked to males. However, it is likely that AS results from many contributing factors, including genetic ones.

Brain Imaging

Only a handful of studies have used brain imaging techniques to examine differences in cerebral functions of AS children compared to non-AS children. Using fMRI, one study found some differences in frontal lobe activity of AS and non-AS children during a task involving social judgment (Oktem, Diren, Karaagaoglu, and Anlar, 2001). However, more studies are needed to understand the sources and implications of these differences in activity levels.

General Characteristics of AS

More studies on AS have been undertaken in recent years as researchers try to further understand this exceptionality. A survey of these studies found that children and adolescents with AS tended to have the following characteristics (Barnhill, 2001; Henderson, 2001):

- An IQ range similar to the general public
- High oral language skills; low written language skills
- Fluent verbalization but poor problem-solving skills
- Knowledge of simple vocabulary but difficulty with inferences and abstract language

- Pronounced emotional difficulties recognized by others but not by themselves
- An approach to new learning that resembles a learned helplessness
- Low sensory thresholds causing a sensory overload that may be overwhelming
- Low ability to plan use of time or estimate time passage
- Difficulty with social/emotional cues
- Difficulty acknowledging that a perspective different from their own can exist

Direct and specific skill strategies can be used to help AS individuals cope with the challenges posed by these characteristics, especially in school and social situations.

Identification of Gifted Students with AS

Until recently, AS was generally diagnosed later than classic autism, most likely because AS individuals had relatively normal early development. As practitioners become more familiar with AS, earlier diagnosis means earlier intervention and appropriate services. Early diagnosis becomes even more important for gifted AS individuals so that programs can be devised to address their gifts as well as their disabilities. Finding the measure to accurately identify gifted AS students has not been easy. However, Henderson (2001) reports that the behavioral patterns, motor skills, gifted and talented characteristics, and leadership can be measured reliably by various instruments.

To parents and teachers, AS appears a serious disability, especially because it inhibits social interaction. Yet, individuals with AS develop deep interests in narrow topics and can often succeed in areas where attention to detail is critical and social discourse minimal. When given educational support and appropriate opportunities, many AS students are academically successful and attend college. Many AS persons are drawn to science, inventions, mathematics, and computers and can have successful careers in these areas. The December 2001 issue of *Wired* magazine, for instance, reported on the high number of AS people who are gainfully employed in computer or related industries in the Silicon Valley area of California. Areas of focused research also provide AS individuals with opportunities for career success.

When given educational support and appropriate opportunities, many students with Asperger's syndrome are academically successful and attend college.

Misdiagnosis of AS

Someone not familiar with the asynchronous development of gifted children could mistake these characteristics as signs of Asperger's syndrome.

Just as the characteristics of giftedness can be misread as signs of psychological disorders and learning disabilities, so can they lead to a misdiagnosis of Asperger's syndrome (Amend, 2000). Intense fascination with a specific subject, an uneven profile of abilities, original problem-solving methods, and exceptional concentration are not only components of AS, but of giftedness as well. Someone not familiar with the asynchronous development of gifted children could mistake these characteristics as signs of AS.

Programs for the Troubled Gifted

Because of the complexities and possible combinations of dual exceptionalities, planning a program of instruction for these students can be complicated. But all of these students require programs that will nurture their gifts, address their disability, and provide the emotional support necessary to deal with any inconsistent abilities (Baum, 1994).

One common programming approach is for students to receive primary instruction in the regular classroom and also to attend a resource pullout program, a gifted pullout class, or a combination of both. In a study conducted by Nielsen and Morton-Albert (1989), the self-concepts of gifted students with learning disabilities varied with the type of educational services they were receiving. Not surprisingly, students had a lower self-concept when they primarily received learning disability services. In contrast, when these students also received gifted services that focused on their strengths, their self-concept scores closely matched the scores of gifted students without handicaps.

The researchers did find an exception to these findings: The self-concept scores of gifted students with learning disabilities and who were in self-contained learning disabled/gifted classes more closely matched those of students with learning disabilities than those of gifted students. Apparently, the self-concept of these students is influenced by their perceptions of how they are compared to other students by their parents and their peers.

SAVANT SYNDROME ■

In the 1880s, J. Langdon Down (known for naming Down's syndrome) described individuals he called "idiot savants," who were mentally retarded yet displayed extraordinary talents far beyond their handicaps. Now called Savant syndrome, it is a rare condition in which persons with various developmental disabilities have abilities that are remarkable considering their handicap (called *talented savants*) to those rarer individuals whose brilliance would be spectacular even in a normal person (called *prodigious savants*). About 10 percent of persons with autism have some savant abilities. This group represents about one-half of the savant population; the other half have some other form of developmental disability, such as mental retardation.

Treffert (2000a) describes their skills as falling within a narrow range including music (they have perfect pitch and usually play the piano), spatial skills, high-speed calculating and mathematical ability, calendar calculating, art (sculpture and drawing), and mechanical abilities. Other rare abilities occasionally emerge, such as unusual language skills, map memorization, and enhanced sense of touch and smell. The skills tend to be associated with right cerebral hemisphere activities (nonsymbolic, directly perceived) rather than the left hemisphere (sequential, logical, and language specialization (see Chapter 2). Regardless of the nature of the special skills, they are always linked to a phenomenal memory system that is very narrow but deep. This system, according to Treffert, is at the automatic level of procedural memory rather than at the higher level of cognitive memory common in normal individuals.

What Causes Savant Syndrome?

Because many savants display skills associated with right hemisphere lateralization, researchers speculated that the syndrome could be the result of injury to the left brain, either before, during, or shortly after birth. Recent CT and MRI imaging studies do reveal left hemisphere damage in savants, especially in areas near the frontal lobe (Treffert, 2000b). These findings suggest that savant syndrome is caused by damage to the left frontal hemisphere, which stimulates right hemisphere compensation. The damage also causes memory circuits to compensate by shifting from high-level, frontal lobe cognitive memory to low-level procedural memory (Figure 8.2). In prodigious savants, genetic factors may also be involved because practice alone cannot account for the extraordinary mastery of their savant skills.

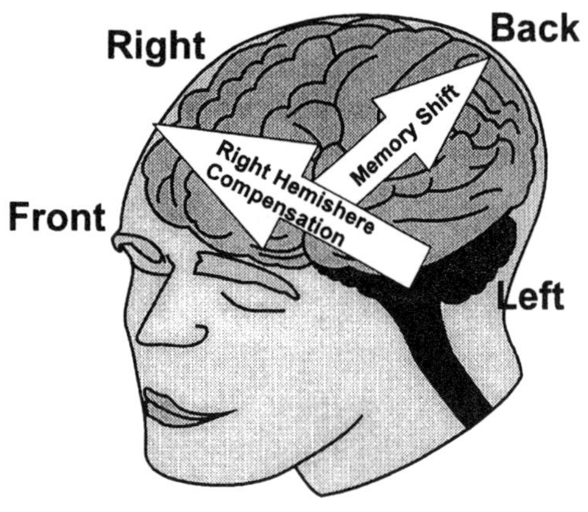

Figure 8.2 Damage to the left frontal hemisphere results in right hemisphere compensation and the shifting of memory circuits to low-level procedural memory.

One of the explanations offered for pre-natal brain injury lies in the potentially toxic effects of circulating testosterone in the fetus. Because the left hemisphere of the brain is slower in development than the right hemisphere, it is more vulnerable to testosterone's toxicity, which may explain the high male-to-female ratio in savant syndrome, autism, and other learning disabilities. As for injuries occurring after birth, Carter (1999) reported on one 9-year-old boy who was transformed from an average student to a mechanical genius after part of this left brain was destroyed by a bullet.

Dealing With Autistic Savants

As with most people who have dual exceptionalities, the question becomes: Do we train the talent or eliminate the deficit? But appropriate therapies do not have to take an either/or approach. Training the talent can lessen the effects of the deficits. With properly trained educators leading the way, a greater number of autistic savants are succeeding in the classroom and in the workplace.

■ HYPERLEXIA

Hyperlexia is a term applied to children who exhibit precocious reading skills but have significant problems with learning and language as well as impaired social skills. Hyperlexic children may also be diagnosed with autism, pervasive development disorder, attention deficit disorder, or Asperger's syndrome. Others receive no diagnosis and are considered just precocious. Controversy currently exists as to whether hyperlexia is a form of autism or a separate and distinct language disorder.

Controversy currently exists as to whether hyperlexia is a form of autism or a separate and distinct language disorder.

Identification of Hyperlexia

Children are suspected of having hyperlexia if they exhibit the following three characteristics (Kupperman, Bligh, Barouski, 2002):

- *Precocious Reading Ability.* By the age of 18 to 24 months, parents are amazed by the child's ability to name letters and numbers. This skill was not taught to the child by parents. By 3 years of age, these children see printed words and read them, sometimes before they have really learned to talk. They are fascinated by the printed word.

- *Peculiar Language Learning Disorders.* Of those children who talk (there are also nonverbal hyperlexics), nearly all display echolalic speech (repeating what others have said) and good auditory memory for songs learned by rote, the alphabet, and numbers. They also show impairment in the ability to initiate or sustain a conversation, despite adequate speech.

- *Problems in Social Development.* The behaviors that may be observed include the following: noncompliance, extreme need for sameness, difficulty with transitions, difficulty in socializing with peers, and impaired ability to make peer friendships.

Types of Hyperlexia

Because behavioral symptoms subside in many children as their language comprehension and expression improve, identification of true hyperlexia is difficult. The studies on hyperlexia seem to indicate that there are three types (Treffert, 2000a; Kupperman, et al., 2002):

- *Just Precocious.* These are children who have very precocious reading skills and who are normal in all other aspects of development. They do not display any long-lasting autistic behaviors. Rather, these are normal children who just enjoy reading and whose brains are considerably more active when reading (Figure 8.3).

- *Precocious Reading/Autistic-Like Behaviors*. These children display exceptional reading skills coupled with autistic-like behaviors, such as echolalia, and impaired social skills. But these children are *not* autistic and may represent the group where a specific diagnosis of hyperlexia is most appropriate. The long-term outlook for this group is good.

- *Savant Behavior*. These children have such extraordinary reading skills that they display savant skills, associated with autism or some other developmental disorder. In this case, the hyperlexia is but one symptom of a more serious spectrum disorder.

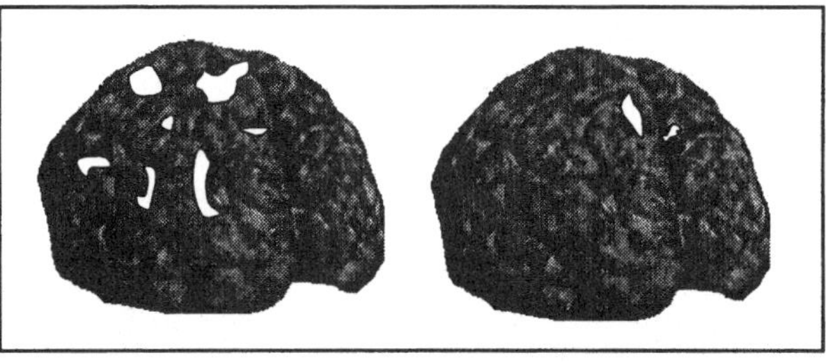

Figure 8.3 This representation of PET scans shows how the brain of a young hyperlexic reader (left) is much more active (white areas) than that of an age-matched control (Restak, 2001).

Dealing With Hyperlexia

Because of the various types of hyperlexia, a comprehensive assessment by a knowledgeable team is essential for proper diagnosis. For instance, it is important to differentiate these children from those whose language disorders may be related to a hearing loss, autism mental retardation, or emotional disturbance. Although hyperlexic children are like other children with language learning disorders, they are more fortunate in that they have the reading skill to use as a supportive resource. Nonetheless, hyperlexia is puzzling because it raises questions about the relationship between reading and language. A child may display exceptional reading ability while also presenting a collection of linguistic, behavioral, and social deficits.

Kupperman and her colleagues (2002) report that most of the children with hyperlexia show remarkable improvement from the time they are first diagnosed at the age of 2 or 3 until they enter 2nd grade. At first, their behavior looks autistic (i.e., they are echolalic and not able to understand much language). However, as their language comprehension and expressive language improve, these children emerge out of their autism. By the time they reach 1st or 2nd grade, they lose most of their autistic characteristics but may still

Most children with hyperlexia lose their autistic-like characteristics by 2nd or 3rd grade.

remain aloof from other children. At this point, they can be taught social skills. Emphasis should be placed on intensive speech and language therapy because the success of these children depends on the development of their comprehension and use of language.

APPLICATIONS

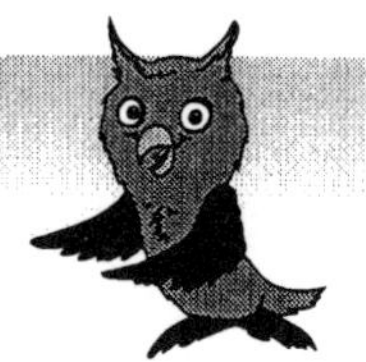

CHARACTERISTICS OF GIFTED CHILDREN WITH DISABILITIES

Although recognizing giftedness in children with disabilities is no easy task, some characteristics do emerge that can help educators (and parents) in this process. Tables 8.1 and 8.2 on the following pages are adapted from the work of Colleen Willard-Holt (1999) who surveyed the research literature and collected characteristics of children with dual exceptionalities.

Table 8.1 shows the characteristics of gifted students who also have physical, hearing, and vision impairments. Table 8.2 describes the characteristics of gifted students who also have learning disabilities and attention problems. It is important to note that some students are misdiagnosed with attention-deficit hyperactivity disorder (ADHD) when in fact they are gifted and are reacting to an inappropriate learning environment (Sousa, 2001b, p. 51).

One way to distinguish between the two is to examine the persistence and pervasiveness of the problem behavior. Gifted children are more likely to act out in specific situations where they are not challenged. Students who display problem behavior in all situations may have ADHD. It is also possible for a child to be both gifted and have ADHD.

GIFTED CHILDREN WITH DISABILITIES—Continued

Table 8.1 Characteristics of Gifted Students with Physical, Hearing, and Vision Impairments
(Adapted from C. Willard-Holt, 1999, *Dual Exceptionalities,* ERIC Clearinghouse on Disabilities and Gifted Education, Arlington, VA)

Gifted with Physical Disabilities	Gifted with Hearing Impairments	Gifted with Vision Impairments
❑ Development of compensatory skills ❑ Creative in finding alternative ways of communicating and accomplishing tasks ❑ Impressive store of knowledge ❑ Good sense of humor ❑ Superior memory ❑ Insightful ❑ Ability to set and strive for long-term goals ❑ Advanced academic skills ❑ Good problem-solving skills ❑ Persistence and patience ❑ Greater maturity than age mates ❑ High motivation to achieve ❑ Self-criticism and perfectionism ❑ Possible difficulty with abstractions ❑ Possible limited achievement due to pace of work	❑ Development of speech and reading skills without instruction ❑ Early reading ability ❑ Function in regular school setting ❑ High reasoning ability ❑ Rapid grasp of ideas ❑ Excellent memory ❑ Nontraditional ways of getting information ❑ Self-starter ❑ Intuitive ❑ Ingenuity in problem solving ❑ Delays in concept attainment ❑ Symbolic language abilities ❑ Wide range of interests ❑ Good sense of humor ❑ Enjoys manipulating the environment	❑ Fast rate of learning ❑ Excellent memory ❑ Superior verbal communication skills and vocabulary ❑ Advanced problem-solving skills ❑ Motivation to know ❑ Excellent ability to concentrate ❑ Creative production of thought that progresses more slowly than sighted students ❑ Slower rate of cognitive development than sighted students

GIFTED CHILDREN WITH DISABILITIES—Continued

Table 8.2 Characteristics of Gifted Students with Learning Disabilities and Attention Problems

(Adapted from C. Willard-Holt, 1999, *Dual Exceptionalities,* ERIC Clearinghouse on Disabilities and Gifted Education, Arlington, VA)

Gifted With Learning Disabilities	Gifted Who Are Bored	Gifted With ADHD
❑ High abstract reasoning ❑ Advanced vocabulary ❑ Good mathematical skills ❑ Sophisticated sense of humor ❑ Keen visual memory and spatial skills ❑ Insightful ❑ Creative ❑ Imaginative ❑ Good problem-solving skills ❑ High performance in science, music, arts ❑ Difficulty with memorization, computation, phonics, spelling ❑ Grasp of metaphors and satire ❑ Understanding of complex systems and models ❑ Often fails to complete assignments ❑ Difficulties with sequential tasks	❑ Poor attention and daydreaming ❑ Low tolerance with tasks that seem irrelevant ❑ Question school customs, rules and traditions ❑ High activity level ❑ May need less sleep ❑ Begin many projects but take few to completion ❑ Lose or forget homework ❑ Disorganized ❑ Judgment lags behind intellectual growth ❑ Intensity may lead to power struggle with authorities ❑ May appear careless ❑ Difficulty restraining desire to talk ❑ High sensitivity to criticism ❑ Do not exhibit problem behavior in all settings	❑ Poor sustained attention ❑ Shift from one uncompleted activity to another ❑ Diminished persistence on tasks not having immediate consequences ❑ Impulsive ❑ Poor delay of gratification ❑ More active and more restless than other children ❑ Often talk excessively ❑ Poor adherence to requests to regulate behavior in social settings ❑ Inattentive to details ❑ Often interrupt or intrude on others ❑ Highly sensitive to criticism ❑ Often lose things required for tasks at school or at home ❑ Problem behaviors exist in *all* settings, but are more severe in some ❑ High variability in task performance and in time used to accomplish tasks

APPLICATIONS

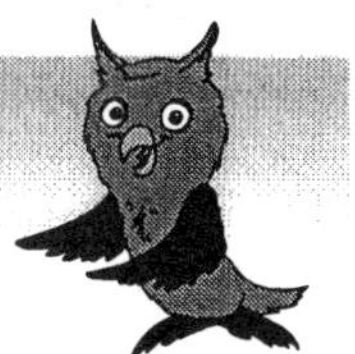

SOME TEACHING STRATEGIES FOR GIFTED/LEARNING DISABLED STUDENTS

Several successful teaching strategies and practices have been suggested in the literature. These should be considered in addition to providing supplemental gifted services for students who are both gifted and learning disabled (Dix and Schafer,1996; Rivera, Murdock, and Sexton,1995; Silverman, 1989a).

Instruction:

- *Staff Development.* Ongoing staff development is necessary to ensure that educators have the information they need to screen, identify, and successfully teach gifted/learning disabled students.

- *Basic Skills.* Teachers should continue with their instruction in basic skills because these students often have learning problems in these areas.

- *Technology.* Incorporate technology into lessons whenever possible. Equipment such as cameras, calculators, computers, and audio and video recorders can help students reach their potential and produce quality work.

- *Student Strengths and Weaknesses.* Students already know their weaknesses; help them find, appreciate, and use their strengths. Offer options that allow students to use their strengths and preferred ways of learning.

- *Classroom Materials.* When possible, students need to select from a variety of classroom materials to show mastery of the learning in a manner that matches their strengths. A variety of assessment tools, such as performance measures and portfolios, should also be available.

SOME TEACHING STRATEGIES FOR GIFTED/LEARNING DISABLED STUDENTS—Continued

- *Compensation Strategies.* Teachers should neither focus on students' weaknesses nor ignore them. Students need to be taught compensation strategies to address their weaknesses. For example, they can learn calculator skills to do math computation or learn to use a computer and a spell checker to compensate for poor spelling.

- *Instructional Approaches.* Emphasize higher-order abstract thinking, creativity, and a problem-solving approach. Promote active inquiry, discussion, and experimentation.

- *Teaching Strategy and Learning Disability.* Whenever possible, match the teaching strategy to address the learning disability. For example, if a student has auditory processing difficulties, avoid a quick-response format as these students will need more time to respond to verbal inquiries.

- *Number of Instructions.* Remember the capacity limits of working memory and limit the number of instructions given at any one time.

- *Chalkboard.* Many of these students need visual tools to help them remember directions or steps in a procedure.

- *Modeling.* Allow students to observe others who are successfully performing a task before they try it themselves. Develop models that demonstrate different ways of thinking and communicating.

- *Visual and Hands-On Procedures.* Classroom strategies that include visual and hands-on activities take advantage of these students' learning strengths.

- *Self-Concept.* Find opportunities to assist in strengthening the students' self-concept.

- *Time.* Provide for individual pacing in areas of the students' strengths and disabilities.

SOME TEACHING STRATEGIES FOR GIFTED/LEARNING DISABLED STUDENTS—Continued

Classroom Dynamics:

- *Proximity and Quiet.* Place students with attention problems near the teacher, and provide for them a quiet space with a minimum of distractions.

- *Eye Contact.* These students often have short attention spans and are easily distracted. Before giving individual instructions, make eye contact with the student to ensure that attention is focused on you.

- *Expectations.* Expect students to participate in all activities and strive for normal peer interactions whenever possible. Facilitate acceptance and demand respect for all members of the class. Treat a student with a disability the same way you would treat a student without that disability.

- *Differences.* Model ways to celebrate individual differences. Discuss the implications of talents and disabilities with the class.

APPLICATIONS

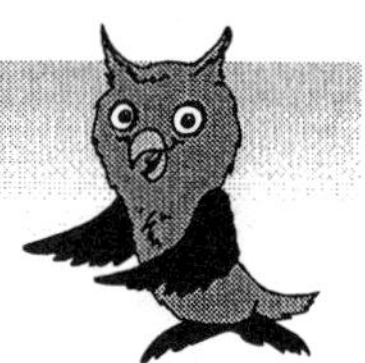

SOME COUNSELING STRATEGIES FOR GIFTED/LEARNING-DISABLED STUDENTS

School counselors can play an important role in helping gifted/learning-disabled students adjust and succeed in school. McEachern and Bornot (2001) suggest that counselors can contribute in the following ways.

- *Consulting With Parents.* Parents seek answers as to why their child can exhibit intellectual abilities while having difficulty in school performance. Counselors can do the following:
— Provide parents with information on the diagnosis and suggest strategies that support the education of their child when at home.
— Reduce tension between parents, teachers, and students and suggest appropriate emotional responses.
— Set up support groups among parents so they can share similar concerns, discuss strategies for change, and gain confidence in parenting.

- *Sharing Academic Strategies With Teachers.* Counselors can work with teachers to design curriculum and instruction activities that are more likely to keep gifted/learning-disabled students engaged and successful. Here are some ways that counselors can help:
— Urge that the curriculum focus on exploratory, discovery, and investigative learning, including provisions for the various learning styles of these students. Activities that involve art, photography, drama, and other self-directed and unconventional methods should be encouraged.
— Include technology in the curriculum, such as using computers for word processing, to improve language and writing skills, and for individualized instruction and introducing calculators and tape recorders (audio and video) as instructional tools.
— Advise teachers to develop student strengths as well as to remedy student weaknesses. Overemphasis on student weaknesses will lower their self-esteem and confidence. Advise teachers, too, on the importance of providing emotional encouragement and assurance

SOME COUNSELING STRATEGIES FOR GIFTED/LEARNING-DISABLED STUDENTS—Continued

that tell students they can be successful.

— Use film, videos, books, and guest speakers to expose these students to local and nationally known role models of gifted individuals with learning disabilities who have been successful.

— Collaborate with teachers of the gifted to discuss ways of supporting the social and psychological needs of these students. These teachers may also agree to conduct small-group counseling sessions and behavior modification interventions in the classroom, so that students do not have to be taken out of class for such activities.

— Increase teachers' understanding of gifted/learning-disabled students by facilitating and coordinating workshops that offer guest speakers who can give expert information and resources. Counselors can prepare special materials that will help teachers identify these students for referral as well as select and incorporate learning strategies that are likely to be successful.

- *Individual and Group Counseling With Students.* Gifted/learning-disabled students often have difficulty facing the fact that they have some areas of high performance and others in which they are less capable than their peers. Teachers sometimes tell these students that they are bright but lazy and that they are not living up to their potential. The pressure to excel and meet others' expectations often puts these students at greater risk for stress, self-blame, depression, and suicide. Counselor interventions—individual or group, as appropriate—can include the following:

  — Helping these students understand that inadequacy in one area or skill does not mean inadequacy in all areas. Offer ideas on ways to use their strengths to build up their weaknesses.

  — Discouraging negative thinking by helping students rephrase the negativism into positive expressions. Suggest both stress-reduction strategies and healthy coping behaviors.

  — Using art therapy as a creative and symbolic way for relieving the pressure these students feel and for discussing problems and setting goals.

  — Conducting sessions on the use of problem-solving strategies to identify and address areas of strengths and weakness. Also helpful

SOME COUNSELING STRATEGIES FOR GIFTED/LEARNING-DISABLED STUDENTS—Continued

are sessions to teach about constructive peer interactions, goal-setting, and positive study habits, such as note taking, summarizing, and preparing for tests.

- *Advocacy*. Counselors can become effective advocates for gifted/learning-disabled students by
  — Discussing with other school personnel the problems and general needs of these students.
  — Monitoring the progress of these students through their school experiences, assuring that their courses are consistent with their career goals, and encouraging that they are participating in appropriate extracurricular activities.
  — Using peers as tutors in the academic areas for which the gifted/learning-disabled students need assistance.
  — Assuring, as members of the child study team, that these students receive appropriate services, including referrals to outside agencies, if necessary.

School counselors are in a unique position to serve as facilitators, teachers, and advocates for the under-served population of gifted students with learning disabilities.

APPLICATIONS

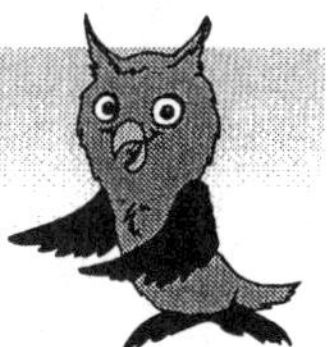

WORKING WITH GIFTED CHILDREN WITH ADHD

Interventions for gifted children with ADHD have to be somewhat different from those recommended for average children with ADHD. Here are some items to consider when developing the Individualized Education Plan (IEP) for these children (Lovecky, 1999):

- *Acceleration.* These children may need acceleration while being taught the metacognitive skills to support the higher level of thinking required for more challenging work. This suggests a differentiated program rather than just being placed in an advanced class.

- *Enhance Strengths, Build on Weaknesses.* Gifted children with ADHD need academic programs that will allow them to enhance their strengths while building on their weaker areas. For example, they may need to be taught organizational and study skills in the context of their high-level work—learnings that their gifted peers without ADHD usually acquire without difficulty. Their program should also provide mentors in their areas of strength to maintain the stimulation and complexity needed to enhance their cognitive development.

- *Team Approach.* Without a comprehensive educational plan that includes addressing their cognitive, social, and emotional needs, these children will not enhance their ability to focus and sustain attention. Further, they may develop ineffective work habits and achieve less. If they lose their interest in learning, emotional and behavioral problems may emerge that can further affect their achievement. A team of specialists with expertise in both giftedness and ADHD is an effective approach for meeting the unique needs of these children.

APPLICATIONS

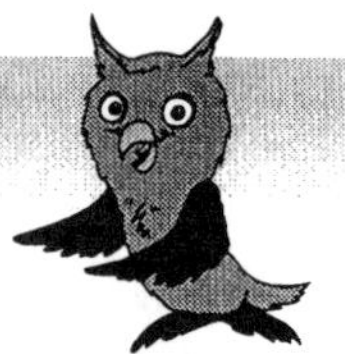

MANAGING STUDENTS WITH ASPERGER'S SYNDROME

Although students with Asperger's syndrome (AS) can be managed in the regular classroom, they often need educational support services. Occasionally, the resource room or tutoring can be helpful by providing individualized instruction and review. However, some students with high-functioning AS are able to adapt and function in school with educators who are understanding, knowledgeable, and flexible. Here are some suggestions for managing AS students in an instructional setting (Bauer, 1996).

- Keep classroom routines as consistent, predictable, and structured as possible because AS students do not like surprises.
- Prepare students in advance for any changes or transitions, such as vacation days and holiday breaks.
- Apply rules carefully. Rules should be clearly expressed and written down. However, they should be applied with some flexibility. That is, instructions do not need to be exactly the same for AS students as for the rest of the class. This approach also models tolerance for student peers.
- Use visuals (e.g., charts, schedules, lists, and pictures) and emphasize the visual cues that can be used for retention. Although many AS students have strong visual preferences as part of their learning-style profile, they also have poor visual memory.
- Take full advantage of the student's special area of interest when teaching. Allowing the student access to special interest areas can also be used as a reward for completing other tasks or for displaying appropriate behavior.
- Protect the student from bullying. One approach is to educate peers about learning differences so that the class becomes a supportive social as well as educational environment.
- Look for ways to take advantage of the special interest areas of AS students, such as using them occasionally to help other students. This technique can help the AS student gain acceptance from peers, who begin to recognize the value of the AS students' capabilities.

MANAGING STUDENTS WITH ASPERGER'S SYNDROME—Continued

- Help the student gain proficiency in frontal lobe executive functions by teaching strategies to improve their organizational skills and study habits.
- Avoid escalating power struggles. Displays of authority may cause these students to become rigid and stubborn, and their behavior can rapidly get out of control. If that occurs, it is often better to back away and let the situation cool down. Of course, preventative measures, such as negotiating and offering choices at the outset may avoid the confrontation entirely.
- Keep the teaching on a concrete level because AS students have difficulty understanding abstract language forms, such as metaphors, idioms, figurative speech, and sarcasm. When possible, try to recast abstract concepts into simpler and more concrete components.
- Ensure that other members of the school staff who come in contact with AS students are properly trained in management approaches and are aware of their needs.
- Work closely with the student's parents because they are usually familiar with the management and instructional strategies that have worked in the past. Frequent communication regarding challenges and areas of progress is more likely to result in parents and educators working toward similar and productive solutions.

APPLICATIONS

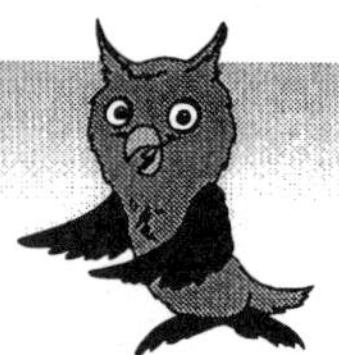

ENHANCING THE SOCIAL INTERACTION SKILLS OF ASPERGER'S SYNDROME STUDENTS

Students with Asperger's syndrome (AS) usually have difficulty engaging in the social interactions expected for their age. This often leads to social isolation and frustration. Marjorie Bock (2001) has developed a social behavioral learning strategy for AS students to guide their social interactions. The strategy is composed of four components and is called SODA, an acronym for Stop, Observe, Deliberate, and Act. Each component contains three to five questions or statements that can be individualized to meet the specific needs and age level of students.

STOP

This component helps the student understand the social setting, determine the sequence of events that will occur, and select a low-traffic area to complete the rest of the tasks. The typical questions are

What is the room arrangement?
What is the activity schedule or routine?
Where should I go to observe?

OBSERVE

The second component helps students note social cues by observing what the people are doing. If they can hear what people are saying, they should listen for similarities across conversations, note the length of a typical conversation, as well as what the people do when the conversation ends. The typical questions are

What are the people doing?
What are the people saying?
What is the length of a typical conversation?
What do the people do after they have visited?

ENHANCING THE SOCIAL INTERACTION SKILLS OF ASPERGER'S SYNDROME STUDENTS—Continued

DELIBERATE

The third component helps the students decide what they would like to do and say as well as look for cues to let them know if the people would like to visit longer or end the visit. The typical questions are

What would I like to do?
What would I like to say?
How will I know when others would like to visit longer or would like to end this conversation?

ACT

The last component helps students interact with others. They select the person with whom they would like to converse and present a greeting. They then listen to the speaker and decide what they would like to learn more about. They share some of their own related experiences and then look for cues to decide if the person wants to continue talking or end the visit. The typical statements are

Approach person(s) with whom I like to visit.
Say, "Hello, how are you?"
Listen to person(s) and ask related questions.
Look for cues that this person would like to end or continue the visit.

This is the basic SODA format. Other questions can be added to each component as needed. Bock suggests that teaching SODA should involve at least one session to present and explain the model, and at least three sessions to demonstrate each component. Students then practice the strategy in class for three sessions, followed by at least three out-of-class situations. The goal here is to get AS students to replace their inflexible and ineffective social interaction rules with SODA so that they can recognize and attend to social cues, selecting the appropriate response to various social situations.

APPLICATIONS

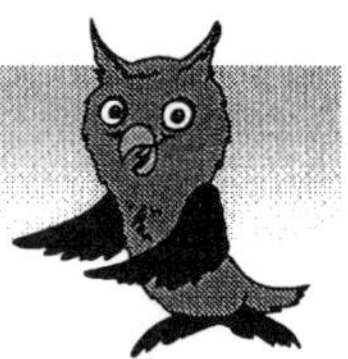

HELPING STUDENTS WITH HYPERLEXIA

Educators are just beginning to recognize that children who enter school diagnosed with hyperlexia need some special attention. Early intervention seems to be the best remedy for improving their comprehension and use of language as well as their social skills. The American Hyperlexia Association recommends the following considerations in designing school programs for hyperlexic children (Kupperman, et al., 2002).

Placement	Although hyperlexic children can spell, decode, and write at much higher levels than their peers, their language comprehension and socialization may preclude them from regular school programs. However, their verbal language skills are the reverse of normal development, and special education teachers need to be adequately trained for this unusual developmental situation.
Educational Goals	Instruction should aim to • Facilitate accommodation to school structure and group learning • Develop language comprehension and expression • Improve social interaction with peers • Develop alternative learning strategies • Address behavioral issues
Classroom Conditions	Classrooms (regular or special) that include hyperlexic students should • Be small so that these students are not overwhelmed with too much peer input • Contain a strong language development component that includes expressive, receptive, and written and oral language activities • Have a structured but not rigid class routine. These children do best when they can anticipate what is happening next and when they get help for schedule changes. • Use a variety of behavioral interventions. Too rigid a behavioral modification system may be frustrating, and these children may not accept behavioral rewards. • Use visual and manipulative materials • Provide opportunities for social interactions with an appropriate peer group • Include opportunities for mainstreaming in areas such as arts, music, athletics, recess, and lunch • Offer the services of speech/language pathologists

HELPING STUDENTS WITH HYPERLEXIA—Continued

Types of Classrooms

KINDERGARTEN

Regular kindergarten: Some hyperlexic children adjust easily to regular kindergarten with supportive services, such as an aide. Adjustment is easier if these students are given both written and verbal instructions, and given individual as well as group directions. Large class size is often a problem.

Developmental kindergarten: Although the smaller class size and more individualized program can be helpful, other children in the class may have difficulties in areas that are strengths for the hyperlexic child (e.g., working on letter recognition or shapes). There also may be too much emphasis on the development of pre-reading skills.

PRIMARY GRADES

Regular Education: This format can work for hyperlexic children who have had early intervention on language and behavioral skills. The regular education teacher and the class need to be prepared for the hyperlexic child. Support services and parent involvement may be necessary.

Communication Disorders Classroom: Because of their strong emphasis on language intervention and academic orientation, these classes are usually appropriate for hyperlexic children. Mainstreaming into regular education is possible, and generally there is enough variety in the peer group to include hyperlexic children with age-appropriate social skills.

Learning Disabilities Classes: Some hyperlexic children succeed in these classes where the academic work is highly individualized. However, because hyperlexic children are quite different from the typical learning-disabled child who has trouble reading, the focus should be on language and socialization issues.

Behavior Disorders and Emotionally Handicapped Classes: These classes are generally inappropriate for hyperlexic children because their behavioral issues are related to their language disorder. As language skills improve, so does the behavior.

9

Putting It All Together

In the preceding chapters, we have discussed the nature of the gifted brain and suggested strategies that can help gifted students succeed in school. We have looked at general giftedness as well as at some of the specific types of giftedness in the areas of language, mathematics, and music. The problem of underachieving and twice-exceptional students was also examined, including specific strategies to meet their atypical needs.

As educators reflect on how to best meet the needs of gifted students, they must do so at a time when changes are occurring in the structure and organization of schools and classrooms. Inclusion policies are returning more students with special needs to the regular education program, and budget cuts are trimming pull-out programs targeted for identified gifted and talented students. Consequently, teachers are now faced with trying to address curriculum standards while dealing with a range of student abilities that is broader than ever. Although resources are available both in and outside the school for gifted students, the regular classroom teacher is most likely to be their primary educator. With that reality in mind, this chapter suggests how teachers can identify gifted students, establish an effective learning environment to meet their needs, and incorporate relevant teaching strategies within the context of the inclusive classroom.

> **In today's schools, the regular classroom teacher is likely to be the primary educator of gifted students.**

IDENTIFYING GIFTED STUDENTS

Because some students do not begin to show their gifts until after entering school, teachers may be the first to recognize potential areas of giftedness. As teachers observe their students, they begin to assess intellectual potential along with other factors, such as emotional and social needs.

Preliminary Assessment for Giftedness

The first indications that a student may be gifted will most likely come from observations of high performance in one or more of the following areas:

- *General intellectual ability:* Students who have high intelligence test scores, usually two standard deviations above the mean, on individual and group measures.
- *Specific academic aptitude:* Students who show outstanding performance in a specific area (e.g., language arts, science, or mathematics) and who score above the 95th percentile in achievement tests.
- *Leadership ability:* Students who can direct individuals or groups to a common decision or action. They can negotiate and adapt in difficult situations.
- *Creative and productive thinking:* Students who can produce new ideas by bringing together dissimilar or independent elements, and who have the aptitude for developing new meanings that have social value.
- *Psychomotor ability:* Students who have outstanding motor abilities such as practical, mechanical, spatial, and physical skills.
- *Visual and performing arts:* Students who demonstrate talent in visual art, dance, music, drama, or related studies.

Follow-Up Assessments

If there is evidence of high intellectual or performance ability, the teacher must determine whether the student is truly gifted. Before submitting the student to a barrage of tests, the teacher should assess the student's capabilities on a number of characteristics that the research literature associates with giftedness.

The Characteristics of Giftedness Scale in the **Applications** section at the end of this chapter identifies 25 characteristics that are common among gifted students. Using this scale may help the teacher make a more valid preliminary judgment about a specific student's abilities (Silverman, Chitwood, and Waters, 1986).

Students who are gifted in the performing arts usually display many of the characteristics of giftedness in addition to their advanced skills in the main area of competence. Thus, the scale can be used to identify students who are talented in different domains. Although these characteristics can distinguish between gifted and average students, they have not been shown to distinguish different levels of giftedness.

Some students who score high on the characteristics scale do not get high scores on tests of achievement. These students may have other problems, such as hearing and vision deficits that impair their classroom participation and depress scores on standardized tests. In this event, it helps to look at the subtest scores to determine areas of strength and weakness. Gifted children often score high on subtests that measure abstract reasoning.

Identifying Minority Students

Minority students continue to be underrepresented in gifted programs. One reason for this situation is not that they are less talented than the other classmates, but that their different experiences, values, and beliefs have prevented them from demonstrating their abilities through the assessment instruments that are commonly used for selection into gifted education programs. These students often do better on nontraditional assessments.

Because the goal of gifted education is inclusivity, not exclusivity, Schwartz (1997) suggests that the following methods be used to identify giftedness so that all students receive fair consideration for gifted education opportunities.

Standardized Tests. More recent standardized tests are designed to reduce cultural bias. They include Mercer's System of Multicultural Pluralistic Assessment, Renzulli and Hartman's Scale for Rating Behavioral Characteristics of Superior Students, and Bruch's Abbreviated Binet for the Disadvantaged.

Observation. Information from parents, educators, and classmates can draw attention to the talents of others. Parents can notice their child's degree of interest in intellectual tasks. Teacher observations allow for the evaluation of a child's development over time. How students use their time, how they solve problems, and what interests them can all be indicators of giftedness. Also, just asking students who is the most helpful among them can turn a teacher's attention to an otherwise unnoticed child.

Self-Identification. Students can sometimes reveal through interest inventories the talents they display in nonschool settings, such as participation in community theater or music groups. They may also describe the type of role they play in the family at home.

Portfolios. Materials in student portfolios often show the learning, progress, and applications of knowledge that these students have made. Also, unlike standardized tests, portfolios permit the assessment of students' creativity. An assessment rubric that has been mutually developed by student and teacher can help to make the evaluation of portfolios easier and more objective.

Educators should ensure that procedures are in place to identify the special talents of students from diverse backgrounds. Moreover, the gifted education programs should reflect and respect their culture and learning styles. Doing so will help these students obtain the enriching educational experiences and materials they need to fully reach their potential.

DEVELOPING THE LEARNING ENVIRONMENT ■

Some teachers deal with a widely heterogeneous class by establishing greater control, reducing flexibility of assignments, and presenting more teacher-centered lessons. Although this approach may work for some students, gifted students need to develop their knowledge and practice their skills in a flexible and secure learning environment that

- Encourages students to use a variety of resources, ideas, tasks, and methods as they pursue learning goals. By having these options, the gifted students can continue to pursue learning objectives on their own while the teacher attends to other students who may need more help in the inclusive classroom.

- Is student-centered and that values and accepts the variety of student interests and learning styles. The more heterogeneous the class, the greater the variety of learning styles among students.

- Encourages students to be open to ideas and initiatives offered by others.

- Allows students to work in a variety of interactive settings, such as individually, in pairs, in small groups, or with students in other classes, as appropriate. Also, using gifted students as mentors for other students can enhance the spirit of learning as a cooperative venture.

- Supports student independence and autonomy within reasonable limits that are mutually set by the students and teacher, where appropriate.

- Is not constrained by subject boundaries or other conventional curricular limitations. Gifted students often have strong interests in specific areas. Look for ways to connect the curriculum to their interests.

- Encourages students to reflect on the processes they use to learn and on the factors that help them to make progress.

STRATEGIES FOR THE GIFTED IN THE INCLUSIVE CLASSROOM

Although much research is available on meeting the needs of gifted students in the inclusive classroom, few studies examine the effects of instructional strategies on both gifted and non-gifted students. However, Johnsen and Ryser (1996) describe five areas of differentiation and six strategies that do emerge from those studies that affect the performance of gifted students in regular classrooms. They suggest that teachers need to differentiate by

- Modifying curriculum content
- Allowing for student preferences
- Altering the pace of instruction
- Creating a flexible classroom environment
- Using specific instructional strategies

The following six strategies have shown to increase critical thinking, creativity, and problem solving abilities:

- Posing open-ended questions that require higher-level thinking
- Modeling thinking strategies, such as decision making and evaluation
- Accepting ideas and suggestions from students and expanding on them
- Facilitating independent and original problems and solutions
- Helping student identify rules, principles, and relationships
- Taking time to explain the nature of errors

Westberg and Archambault (1998) conducted an extensive study on teaching elementary gifted students in inclusive settings and identified the themes and common approaches used by these teachers. The following strategies occurred most frequently:

- Establishing high standards for all students in the classroom
- Making curriculum modifications to increase the level of challenge
- Finding mentors for students in their areas of intense interest
- Encouraging independent investigations and projects as often as possible
- Creating flexible instructional groups to maintain interest and to keep students engaged

More strategies on specific curriculum topics will be found in the **Application** sections of previous chapters.

WHERE DO WE GO FROM HERE?

Researchers and practitioners in gifted education are concerned that gifted students are not being adequately identified or challenged in our schools (Winner, 1996). Parents complain that their children are usually bored and unengaged in school. These students are often underachievers and tend to be highly critical of their teachers, who they feel know less than they do. In many instances, teachers fail to recognize a student as gifted and may think the student is unmotivated or learning disabled. If the student is recognized as gifted, the teacher may have few opportunities to offer curriculum at the appropriate level, and the student may have to learn independently. Surely, we can do better than this.

Why Are We Not Doing More for Gifted Students?

Why are schools not doing more for our most gifted students? In my opinion, several major factors are contributing to the lack of progress.

Budget Constraints

Although some school districts are making valiant efforts to maintain high quality programs for gifted and talented students, the reality is that budget constraints are forcing cutbacks on programs already in place or preventing new programs from getting off the ground. As the number of students with learning disabilities grows, more funds must be shifted to that area, often reducing the amount available for other programs. This "rob Peter to pay Paul" approach is lamentable, but it is still the way most school districts allocate budgetary resources when expenses are rising faster than revenues.

The Egalitarian Compromise

Shifting funds from gifted programs to special education needs is sometimes justified by our need to maintain an egalitarian society. However, we too often see little reason for helping the gifted—presuming that they already have an advantage—and turn our attention primarily to students at the other end of the ability spectrum.

The obstacles to doing more for our gifted students are

- **Budget constraints**
- **Egalitarianism**
- **Anti-intellectualism**

But the truth is that many potentially gifted students come from families who do not have the financial means to provide all the resources necessary to fulfill their child's potential. These parents must rely on the public schools to perform that important task. The notion that "those bright kids don't need more money" is not only wrong, but it undermines the mission of public schools: to help all children fully develop into learned citizens.

Anti-intellectualism

Students with different gifts and talents get a different slice of the educational dollar. Talented athletes and musicians usually have their sports and music activities fully funded and often have plenty of additional opportunities outside of school. Students who are intellectually gifted, on the other hand, usually get placed in a pull-out enrichment program that meets once or twice a week. This is a weak program compared to the opportunities available to the athletically or musically gifted.

Some Considerations for Helping Gifted Students

Intellectual giftedness, of course, runs on a spectrum from mildly to moderately to profoundly gifted. The mildly gifted stay in regular classes because they often fail to meet the minimum scores necessary for selection into the gifted programs. The moderately gifted (usually IQ scores of around 130) can become candidates for gifted programs if other conditions (e.g., teacher recommendations) are met. This group represents the vast majority of the gifted students who participate in gifted education programs. Students who are profoundly gifted (generally with IQ scores of 160 and higher) are not challenged by current public education gifted programs and probably will not find appropriate educational experiences until they reach college.

Are Pull-Out Programs Worth It?

If the reality is that there will be limited funding for gifted education programs in the foreseeable future, then we need to look carefully at how we are spending the money that is available. Although pull-out programs are popular at the elementary level, they allow only a few hours a week of instruction for moderately gifted students. Typically, these classes offer little continuity, rarely allow students to study something in depth, and usually offer just one kind of curriculum to all gifted children, no matter where their gifts lie. Research on these programs has shown them to be of modest benefit. In actuality, these classes are not much different from good classes for ordinary children. Students of any ability level would probably benefit from the kinds of open-ended, project-based learning that goes on in the best enrichment classes. So, is this the best way to be spending the limited funds for gifted education?

The educational benefits of part-time pull-out programs for gifted students are modest at best.

Are Full-Time Gifted Classes Better?

A few school districts have established full-time gifted classes that include moderate grade skipping. Because the entrance requirement for these classes is typically a score of 130 or higher on an IQ test, these programs serve moderately gifted students. Research studies show that students in these classes do achieve more than equally gifted children who remain in a mixed-ability classroom; the benefits are modest, but better than the part-time pull-out programs. As for grade skipping, studies of moderate skipping show that this kind of acceleration has beneficial effects for students and is not harmful socially or emotionally.

Raising Standards for All

The needs of moderately gifted children can be met not only by the various special programs I have mentioned in this book but also by raising the standards for all children. Numerous research studies have shown that when standards are raised in classrooms, achievement rises for all levels of students, including the brightest. Thus, the ongoing nationwide movement to raise standards for all students may be the single most effective beginning step for improving the educational experience for those who are moderately gifted, provided they also have access to other educationally challenging opportunities.

Winner (1996) believes that another strong piece of evidence that raising standards results in higher achievement levels for all students comes from international comparisons of student achievement. It is well known that American children fare poorly on achievement tests compared with children in most other developed countries in Western Europe and Asia. The only plausible explanation for the higher performance of average students in other countries is that these students are held to higher expectations.

What Do We Do for the Profoundly Gifted?

Programs for gifted students, as currently formatted, do not address the needs of the profoundly gifted. First, these students need to be evaluated in terms of their specific talents rather than by a composite IQ score, which often reveals nothing about a student's unique abilities. Second, school districts should develop fast-paced and intensive courses for these students, either during the school year or in the summer. Many of the talent search programs sponsored by universities suggest model programs to address the needs of these extremely gifted students (see the section on **Resources**). Allocating resources and devising courses for the profoundly gifted need not mean sacrificing the needs of the moderately gifted. For, if we elevate our standards, the moderately gifted also would be appropriately challenged.

Schools need to do more to address the needs of profoundly gifted students.

Teacher Training

Teacher training institutions must recognize that gifted education is the responsibility of all teachers, not just the few who specialize in that particular area. At least some training in gifted education should be provided to undergraduates and graduate students who plan to become professional educators. School administrators, too, must endeavor to ensure that policies on meeting the needs of gifted students are developed and translated into practice within each classroom. Only through our concerted efforts will we be certain that our schools are doing their best to meet the needs of our brightest students.

CONCLUSION ■

Neuroscientists are continually probing the human brain to discover the mechanisms and networks that allow it to carry out its many functions. They are exploring concepts as diverse as intuition, psychic phenomena, mind-body connections, and how the brain manages the information that creates consciousness. Surely the revelations that are to come will offer a deeper understanding of how the brain learns so that we can be more successful in helping all our children reach their fullest potential.

APPLICATIONS

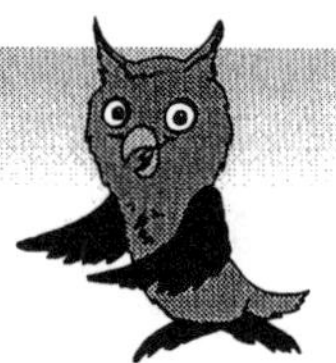

THE CHARACTERISTICS OF GIFTEDNESS SCALE

The following scale may help the teacher make a more valid preliminary judgment about a specific student's abilities. Research studies conducted in the 1980s identified 25 characteristics of gifted individuals (Silverman, Chitwood, and Waters, 1986). More recent experimental and clinical studies continue to support these characteristics.

Guidelines:

- On this scale, the teacher should rate each characteristic by circling a number from 1 to 5 that best describes how often that characteristic is evident. The scale is just a guide and is by no means a definitive measure of giftedness. However, if the teacher scores the student at the 4 or 5 end of the scale on more than half of the characteristics, further assessment is warranted.

- Students gifted in the performing arts usually display many of the characteristics of giftedness on this scale in addition to their advanced skills in the main area of competence. Thus, the scale can be used to identify students who are talented in different domains.

- Although these characteristics can distinguish between gifted and average students, they have not been shown to distinguish different levels of giftedness.

- Students who score high on the characteristics scale but who do not get high scores on tests of achievement may have other problems, such as hearing and vision deficits that impair their classroom participation and depress scores on standardized tests. In this case, look at the subtest scores to determine areas of strength and weakness.

THE CHARACTERISTICS OF GIFTEDNESS SCALE—Continued

CHARACTERISTICS OF GIFTEDNESS (Adapted from Silverman, Chitwood, and Waters, 1986)	
Compared to other students in the class, this student...	Seldom Occasionally Often
1. Has a longer attention span.	1 ----- 2 ----- 3 ----- 4 ----- 5
2. Displays an excellent memory.	1 ----- 2 ----- 3 ----- 4 ----- 5
3. Has keen powers of observation.	1 ----- 2 ----- 3 ----- 4 ----- 5
4. Displays ability with numbers.	1 ----- 2 ----- 3 ----- 4 ----- 5
5. Perseveres, when interested.	1 ----- 2- ---- 3 ----- 4 ----- 5
6. Is concerned with justice and fairness.	1 ----- 2 ----- 3 ----- 4 ----- 5
7. Shows high intensity in studies.	1 ----- 2 ----- 3 ----- 4 ----- 5
8. Has a wide range of interests.	1 ----- 2 ----- 3 ----- 4 ----- 5
9. Uses an extensive vocabulary.	1 ----- 2 ----- 3 ----- 4 ----- 5
10. Displays personal sensitivity.	1 ----- 2 ----- 3 ----- 4 ----- 5
11. Shows a high degree of creativity.	1 ----- 2 ----- 3 ----- 4 ----- 5
12. Tends to be a perfectionist.	1 ----- 2 ----- 3 ----- 4 ----- 5
13. Has a preference for older companions.	1 ----- 2 ----- 3 ----- 4 ----- 5
14. Is good at jigsaw puzzles.	1 ----- 2 ----- 3 ----- 4 ----- 5
15. Has good problem solving and reasoning abilities.	1 ----- 2 ----- 3 ----- 4 ----- 5
16. Displays a vivid imagination.	1 ----- 2 ----- 3 ----- 4 ----- 5
17. Shows compassion for others.	1 ----- 2 ----- 3 ----- 4 ----- 5
18. Makes judgments mature for age.	1 ----- 2 ----- 3 ----- 4 ----- 5
19. Has an excellent sense of humor.	1 ----- 2 ----- 3 ----- 4 ----- 5
20. Demonstrates unusual curiosity.	1 ----- 2 ----- 3 ----- 4 ----- 5
21. Has high degree of energy.	1 ----- 2 ----- 3 ----- 4 ----- 5
22. Shows early or avid reading ability.	1 ----- 2 ----- 3 ----- 4 ----- 5
23. Tends to question authority.	1 ----- 2 ----- 3 ----- 4 ----- 5
24. Demonstrates moral sensitivity.	1 ----- 2 ----- 3 ----- 4 ----- 5
25. Appears to learn rapidly.	1 ----- 2 ----- 3 ----- 4 ----- 5

Glossary

Acceleration. Presenting information at a fast pace that corresponds more closely to the pace at which gifted students learn.

Adaptive decision making. The process of solving a problem that has multiple solutions depending on the context and priorities of the moment, as in, "What gift should I buy for my nephew's birthday?"

Alphabetic principle. The notion that written words are composed of letters of the alphabet that intentionally and systematically represent segments of spoken words.

Amygdala. The almond-shaped structure in the brain's limbic system that encodes emotional messages to long-term storage.

Angular gyrus. A brain structure that decodes visual information about words so they can be matched to their meanings.

Asperger's syndrome. A developmental disorder also known as high functioning autism because people with the disorder generally display higher mental performance.

Attention-deficit hyperactivity disorder (ADHD). A syndrome that interferes with an individual's capacity to regulate activity level, inhibit behavior, and attend to tasks in developmentally appropriate ways.

Autism. A spectrum disorder that affects an individual's ability to communicate, form relationships with others, and relate appropriately to the environment.

Axon. The neuron's long and unbranched fiber that carries impulses away from the cell to the next neuron.

Bloom's Taxonomy of the Cognitive Domain. A model developed by Benjamin Bloom in the 1950s for classifying the complexity of human thought into six levels.

Brain stem. One of the major parts of the brain, it receives sensory input and monitors vital functions such as heartbeat, body temperature, and digestion.

Broca's area. A region in the left frontal lobe of the brain believed responsible for generating the vocabulary and syntax of an individual's native language.

Cerebellum. One of the major parts of the brain, it coordinates muscle movement.

Cerebrum. The largest of the major parts of the brain, it controls sensory interpretation, thinking, and memory.

Chunking. The ability of the brain to perceive a coherent group of items as a single item or chunk.

Compacting. Eliminating drill and repetitious material from the curriculum so that gifted students can move on to more challenging material.

Computerized tomography (CT, formerly CAT) scanner. An instrument that uses X-rays and computer processing to produce a detailed cross-section of brain structure.

Constructivism. This theory of learning states that active learners use past experiences and chunking to construct sense and meaning from new learning, thereby building larger conceptual schemes.

Corpus callosum. The bridge of nerve fibers that connects the left and right cerebral hemispheres and allows communication between them.

Cortex. The thin but tough layer of cells covering the cerebrum that contains all the neurons used for cognitive and motor processing.

Dendrite. The branched extension from the cell body of a neuron that receives impulses from nearby neurons through synaptic contacts.

Electroencephalograph (EEG). An instrument that charts fluctuations in the brain's electrical activity via electrodes attached to the scalp.

Frontal lobe. The front part of the brain that monitors higher-order thinking, directs problem solving, and regulates the excesses of the emotional (limbic) system.

Functional magnetic resonance imaging (fMRI). An instrument that measures blood flow to the brain to record areas of high and low neuronal activity.

Glial cells. Special "glue" cells in the brain that surround each neuron providing support, protection, and nourishment.

Gray matter. The thin but tough covering of the brain's cerebrum also known as the cerebral cortex.

Hemisphericity. The notion that the two cerebral hemispheres are specialized and process information differently.

Hippocampus. A brain structure that compares new learning to past learning and encodes information from working memory to long-term storage.

Hyperlexia. A term describing children who have precocious reading skills but who also have significant problems with learning and language.

Imagery. The mental visualization of objects, events, and arrays.

Immediate memory. A temporary memory where information is processed briefly (in seconds) and subconsciously, then either blocked or passed on to working memory.

Inclusion. Grouping students into a regular classroom without regard to ability.

Limbic system. The structures at the base of the cerebrum that control emotions.

Long-term storage. The areas of the cerebrum where memories are stored permanently.

Magnetic resonance imaging (MRI). An instrument that uses radio waves to disturb the alignment of the body's atoms in a magnetic field to produce computer-processed, high-contrast images of internal structures.

Motor cortex. The narrow band across the top of the brain from ear to ear that controls movement.

Myelin. A fatty substance that surrounds and insulates a neuron's axon.

Neuron. The basic cell making up the brain and nervous system, consisting of a globular cell body, a long fiber called an axon which transmits impulses, and many shorter fibers called dendrites which receive them.

Neurotransmitter. One of nearly 100 chemicals stored in axon sacs that transmit impulses from neuron to neuron across the synaptic gap.

Phonemes. The smallest units of sound in a language that combine to make syllables.

Positron emission tomography (PET) scanner. An instrument that traces the metabolism of radioactively tagged sugar in brain tissue producing a color image of cell activity.

Prefrontal cortex. The foremost part of the brain's frontal lobes, responsible for coordinating all cognitive and executive functions.

Prodigy. A child of high intelligence who is able to perform a specific skill at an adult level of competence, and is aware of thinking strategies.

Rehearsal. The reprocessing of information in working memory.

Retention. The preservation of a learning in long-term storage in such a way that it can be identified and recalled quickly and accurately.

Reticular activating system (RAS). The dense formation of neurons in the brain stem that controls major body functions and maintains the brain's alertness.

Savant. An individual with an exception ability to perform a specific skill, usually artistic, musical, or mathematical, but who often displays flat emotions and is unaware of thinking strategies.

Self-concept. Our perception of who we are and how we fit into the world.

Synapse. The microscopic gap between the axon of one neuron and the dendrite of another.

Thalamus. A part of the limbic system that receives all incoming sensory information, except smell, and shunts it to other areas of the cortex for additional processing.

Twice-Exceptional. A term used to describe gifted individuals who also have a learning disability.

Underachievement. A significant difference between an individual's ability and performance.

Veridical decision making. The process of solving a problem that has only one correct answer, as in, "What is my dentist's telephone number?"

Wernicke's area. A section in the left temporal lobe of the brain believed responsible for generating sense and meaning in an individual's native language.

White matter. The support tissue that lies beneath the cerebrum's gray matter (cortex).

Working memory. The temporary memory wherein information is processed consciously.

References

Achor, T., and Tarr, A. (1996, Spring). *Underachieving gifted students*. Arlington, VA: ERIC Clearinghouse on Disabilities and Gifted Children.

Adams, K. (1990). *Examining black underrepresentation in gifted programs*. Arlington, VA: ERIC Clearinghouse on Disabilities and Gifted Children.

Alexander, J., Carr, M., and Schwanenflugel, P. (1995). Development of metacognition in gifted children. *Developmental Review, 15*, 1-37.

Alexander, J. E., O'Boyle, M. W., and Benbow, C. P. (1996, August-September). Developmentally advanced EEG alpha power in gifted male and female adolescents. *International Journal of Psychophysiology, 23*, 25-31.

Amend, E. R. (2000). *Misdiagnosis of Asperger's disorder in gifted youth*. In Webb, J. T. (2000, August 7) *Mis-diagnosis and dual diagnosis of gifted children: Gifted and LD, ADHD, OCD, Oppositional Defiant Disorder*. Paper presented at the annual convention of the American Psychological Association, Washington, DC, August 7, 2000.

American Psychiatric Association (APA). (2000). *Diagnostic and Statistical Manual of Mental Disorders*, Fourth Edition, Text Revision (DSM-IV). Washington, DC: American Psychiatric Publishing Group.

Barnhill, C. (2001, May). What's new in AS research: A synthesis of research conducted by the Asperger syndrome project. *Intervention in School and Clinic, 36*, 300-305.

Baron-Cohen, S., and Hammer, J. (1997). Parents of children with Asperger's syndrome: What is the cognitive phenotype? *Journal of Cognitive Neuroscience, 9*, 548-554.

Baum, S. (1994). Meeting the needs of gifted/learning disabled students. *The Journal of Secondary Gifted Education, 5*, 6-16.

Bauer, S. (1996). Asperger syndrome. *Online Asperger Syndrome Information and Support* [Online]. Available at http://www.udel.edu/bkirby/asperger.

Beatty, J. (2001). *The human brain: Essentials of behavioral neuroscience*. Thousand Oaks, CA: Sage Publications.

Benbow, C. P., and Stanley, J. C. (1983). Sex differences in mathematical reasoning ability: More facts. *Science, 222*, 1029-31.

Bernal, E. M. (2002). Three ways to achieve a more equitable representation of culturally and linguistically different students in GT programs. *Roeper Review, 24*, 82-88.

Berns, G. S., Cohen, J. D., and Mintun, M. A. (1997). Brain regions responsive to novelty in the absence of awareness. *Science, 276*, 1272-1275.

Bischoff-Grethe, A., Proper, S. M., Mao, H., Daniels, K. A., and Berns, G. S. (2000). Conscious and unconscious processing of nonverbal predictability in Wernicke's area. *Journal of Neuroscience, 20*, 1975-81.

Blanton, R. E., Levitt, J. G., Thompson, P. M., Narr, K. L., Capetillo-Cunliffe, L., Nobel, A., Singerman, J. D., McCracken, J. T., and Toga, A. W. (2001, July). Mapping cortical asymmetry and complexity patterns in normal children. *Psychiatry Research, 107*, 29-43.

Bloom, B. S. (1956). *Taxonomy of educational objectives (cognitive domain)*. New York: Longman.

Bock, M. (2001, May). SODA strategy: Enhancing the social interaction skills of youngsters with Asperger's syndrome. *Intervention in School and Clinic, 36*, 272-278.

Buckner, R. L., Kelley, W. M., and Petersen, S. E. (1999, April). Frontal cortex contributions to human memory formation. *Nature Neuroscience, 2*, 311-314.

Buescher, T. M., and Higham, S. (1990). *Helping adolescents adjust to giftedness*. Arlington, VA: ERIC Clearinghouse on Disabilities and Gifted Education.

Burruss, J. D. (1999). Problem-based learning. *Science Scope, 22*, 46-49.

Cappelletti, M., Waley-Cohen, H., Butterworth, B., and Kopelman, M. (2000). A selective loss of the ability to read and write music. *Neurocase, 6*, 332-341.

Carr, M., Alexander, J., Schwanenflugel, P. (1996). Where gifted children do and do not excel on metacognitive tasks. *Roeper Review, 18*, 212-217.

Carter, R. (1999, September 10). Tune in turn off. *New Scientist, 164*, 30-35.

Cash, A. B. (1999, September). A profile of gifted individuals with autism: The twice-exceptional learner. *Roeper Review, 22*, 22-27.

Ceci, S. (2001, July/August). Intelligence: The surprising truth. *Psychology Today*, 46-53.

Chiang, W. C., and Wynn, K. (2000) Infants' tracking of objects and collections. *Cognition, 77*, 169-195.

Chochon, F., Cohen, L., van der Moortele, P. F., and Dehaene, S. (1999). Differential contributions of the left and right inferior parietal lobules to number processing. *Journal of Cognitive Neuroscience, 11*, 617-630.

Clark, G., and Zimmerman, E. (1998). Nurturing the arts in programs for gifted and talented students. *Phi Delta Kappan, 79*, 747-751.

Cline, S., and Hegeman, K. (2001, Summer). Gifted children with disabilities. *Gifted Child Today, 24*, 16-24.

Cobine, G. (1995). *Effective use of student journal writing*. Bloomington, IN: Indiana University, ERIC Clearing House on Reading, English, and Communication.

Cunningham, C. M., Callahan, C. M., Plucker, J. A., Roberson, S. C., and Rapkin, A. (1998). Identifying Hispanic students of outstanding talent: Psychometric integrity of a peer nomination form. *Exceptional Children, 64*, 197-209.

Dapretto, M., and Bookheimer, S. Y. (1999). Form and content: Dissociating syntax and semantics in sentence comprehension. *Neuron, 2*, 427.

Dehaene, S., Spelke, E., Pinel, P., Stanescu, R., and Tsivkin, S. (1999, May 7). Sources of mathematical thinking: Behavioral and brain-imaging evidence. *Science, 284*, 970-974.

Dehaene-Lambertz, G. (2000). Cerebral specialization for speech and non-speech stimuli in infants. *Journal of Cognitive Neuroscience, 12*, 449-460.

Delisle, I. (1996). Multiple intelligences: Convenient, simple, wrong. *Gifted Child Today Magazine, 19*, 12-13.

Delisle, J. R., and Berger, S. L. (1990). *Underachieving gifted students*. Arlington, VA: ERIC Clearinghouse on Disabilities and Gifted Education.

Dix, J., and Schafer, S. (1996). From paradox to performance: Practical strategies for identifying and teaching GT/LD students. *Gifted Child Today, 19*, 22-25, 28-31.

Elbert, T., Pantev, C., Weinbruch, C., Rockstrub, B., and Taub, E. (1995). Increased cortical representation of the fingers of the left hand in string players. *Science, 270*, 305-307.

Engle, R. W., Laughlin, J. E., Tuholski, S. W., and Conway, R. A. (1999, September). Working memory, short-term memory, and general fluid intelligence: a latent-variable approach. *Journal of Experimental Psychology, 128*, 309-331.

Field, T., Harding, J., Yando, R., Gonzales, K., Lasko, D., Bendell, D., and Marks, C. (1998, Summer). Feelings and attitudes of gifted students. *Adolescence, 33*, 331-342.

Ford, D. Y. (1995). *A study of achievement and underachievement among gifted, potentially gifted, and average African-American students* (Research Monograph 95128). Storrs, CT: University of Connecticut, The National Research Center on the Gifted and Talented.

Ford, D. Y. (1996). *Reversing underachievement among gifted black students: Promising practices and programs*. New York: Teachers College Press.

Ford, D. Y., and Thomas, A. (1997, June). *Underachievement among gifted minority students: Problems and promises*. Arlington, VA: ERIC Clearinghouse on Disabilities and Gifted Children.

Francis, R., and Underhill, R. G. (1996). A procedure for integrating math and science. *School Science and Mathematics, 96*, 114-119.

Frasier, M. and Passow, A. H. (1994) *Toward a new paradigm for identifying talent potential*. Storrs, CT: University of Connecticut, National Research Center on the Gifted and Talented.

Frederikse, M. E., Lu, A., Aylward, E., Barta, P., and Pearlson, G. (1999, December). Sex differences in the inferior parietal lobule. *Cerebral Cortex, 9*, 896-901.

Gagne, F. (1985). Giftedness and talent: Reexamining a reexamination of the definitions. *Gifted Child Quarterly, 29*, 103-112.

Galuske, R. A. W., Schlote, W., Bratzke, H., and Singer, W. (2000). Interhemispheric asymmetries of the modular structure in human temporal cortex. *Science, 289*, 1946-1949.

Gamoran, A., Nystrand, M., Berends, M., and LePore, P. C. (1995, Winter). An organizational analysis of the effects of ability grouping. *American Educational Research Journal,* 32, 687-715.

Gardner, H. (1983). *Frames of mind: The theory of multiple intelligences.* New York: Basic Books.

Gentry, M, and Kettle, K. (1998, Winter). Distinguishing myths from realities: NRC/GT research. *National Research Center on the Gifted and Talented Newsletter.*

Gilger, J. W., Ho, H., Whipple, A. D., and Spitz, R. (2001). Genotype-environment correlations for language-related abilities. *Journal of Learning Disabilities, 34*, 492-502.

Glass, G. V., McGaw, B., and Smith, M.L. (1981). *Meta-analysis in social research.* Beverly Hills, CA: Sage.

Glassman, R. B. (1999). Hypothesized neural dynamics of working memory: Several chunks might be marked simultaneously by harmonic frequencies within an octave band of brain waves. *Brain Research Bulletin, 50*, 77-93.

Gohm, C. L., Humphreys, L. G., and Yao, G. (1998, Fall). Underachievement among spatially gifted students. *American Educational Research Journal, 35*, 515-531.

Goldberg, E. (2001). *The executive brain: Frontal lobes and the civilized mind.* New York: Oxford University Press.

Goleman, D. (1995). *Emotional intelligence: Why it can matter more than I.Q.* New York: Bantam Books.

Gollub, J. P., Bertenthal, M. W., Labov, J. B., and Curtis, P. C. (Eds.). (2002). *Learning and understanding: Improving advanced study of mathematics and science in U.S. high schools.* Washington, DC: National Academy Press.

González, M. A., Campos, A., and Pérez, M. J. (1997). Mental imagery and creative thinking. *Journal of Psychology, 13*, 357-364.

Gregersen, P. K., (1998). Instant recognition: The genetics of pitch perception. *American Journal of Human Genetics, 62*, 221-223.

Grigorenko, E. L. and Sternberg, R. J. (1997, Spring). Styles of thinking, abilities, and academic performance. *Exceptional Children, 63*, 295-312.

Gur, R. C., Turetsky, B. I., Matsui, M., Yan, M., Bilker, W., Hughett, P., and Gur, R. E. (1999, May 15). Sex differences in brain gray matter and white matter in healthy young adults: Correlations with cognitive performance. *Journal of Neuroscience, 19*, 4065-4072.

Halsted, J. W. (1990). *Guiding the gifted reader.* Arlington, VA: ERIC Clearinghouse on Disabilities and Gifted Education.

Haroutounian, J. (2000). The delights and dilemmas of the musically talented teenager. *Journal of Secondary Gifted Education, 12*, 3-14.

Henderson, L. M. (2001, Summer). Asperger's syndrome in gifted individuals. *Gifted Child Today, 24*, 28-35.

Henson, R., Shallice, T., and Dolan, R. (2000). Neuroimaging evidence for dissociable forms of repetition priming. *Science, 287*, 1269-1272.

Hittmair-Delazer, M., Semenza, C., and Denes, G. (1994). Concepts and facts in calculation. *Brain, 117*, 715-728.

Hoeflinger, M. (1998, May-June). Mathematics and science in gifted education: Developing mathematically promising students. *Roeper Review, 20*, 224-227.

Howe, R., Davidson, J., and Sloboda, J. (1998). Innate talents: Reality or myth? *The Behavioral and Brain Sciences, 21*, 399-407.

Itoh, K., Fujii, Y., Suzuki, K., and Nakada, T. (2001). Asymmetry of parietal lobe activation during piano performance: A high field functional magnetic resonance imaging study. *Neuroscience Letters, 309*, 41-44.

Jausovec, N. (2000, September). Differences in cognitive processes between gifted, intelligent, creative, and average individuals while solving complex problems: An EEG study. *Intelligence, 28*, 213-240.

Johnsen, S. K., and Ryser, G. R. (1996). An overview of effective practices with gifted students in general-education settings. *Journal of Education for the Gifted, 19*, 379-404.

Johnson, D. T. (2000, April). *Teaching mathematics to gifted students in a mixed-ability classroom.* Arlington, VA: ERIC Clearinghouse on Disabilities and Gifted Education.

Kalchman, M., and Case, R. (1999). Diversifying the curriculum in a mathematics classroom streamed for high-ability learners: A necessity unassumed. *School Science and Mathematics, 99*, 320-329.

Kenny, D. A., Archambault, F. X., and Hallmark, B. W. (1994). *The effects of group composition on gifted and non-gifted elementary students in cooperative learning groups*. Storrs, CT: University of Connecticut, the National Research Center on the Gifted and Talented.

Koelsch, S., Gunter, T., and Friederici, A. D. (2000). Brain indices of music processing: "Nonmusicians" are musical. *Journal of Cognitive Neuroscience, 12*, 520-541.

Kupperman, P., Bligh, S., Barouski, K. (2002). Hyperlexia. *Center for Speech and Language Disorders* [Online]. Available at http://www.csld.org.

Lando, B. Z., and Schneider, B. H. (1997). Intellectual contributions and mutual support among developmentally advanced children in homogeneous and heterogeneous work discussion groups. *Gifted Child Quarterly, 41*, 44-57.

Leahey, E., and Guo, G. (2001). Gender differences in mathematical trajectories. *Social Forces, 80*, 713-732.

LeDoux, J. E. (2002). Emotions, memory and the brain. *Scientific American, 12*, 62-71.

Lovecky, D. V. (1999, October). *Gifted children with AD/HD*. Arlington, VA: ERIC Clearinghouse on Disabilities and Gifted Children.

Martin, A., Wiggs, C. L., and Weisberg, J. (1997). Modulation of human medial temporal lobe activity by form, meaning, and experience. *Hippocampus*, *7*, 587-593.

Masataka, N. (1999). Preference for infant-directed singing in 2-year-old hearing infants of deaf parents. *Developmental Psychology, 35*, 1001-1005.

Mayseless, O. (1993). Gifted adolescents and intimacy in close same-sex relationships. *Journal of Youth and Adolescence, 22*, 135-46.

McEachern, A. G., and Bornot, J. (2001, October). Gifted students with learning disabilities: Implications and strategies for school counselors. *Professional School Counseling, 3*, 34-41.

M.I.N.D. Institute. (2002, January). Major strides toward math literacy. *M.I.N.D. Newsletter, 1*, 1-11.

Milius, S. (2001). Face the music: Why are we such a musical species—and does it matter? *Natural History, 110*, 48-58.

Mingus, T. T. Y., and Grassi, R. M. (1999). What constitutes a nurturing environment for the growth of mathematically gifted students? *School Science and Mathematics, 99*, 286-293.

Miyake, A., Friedman, N. P., Rettinger, D. A., Shah, P., and Hegarty, M. (2001, December). How are visuospatial working memory, executive functioning, and spatial abilities related? A latent-variable analysis. *Journal of Experimental Psychology, 130*, 621-640.

Mueller, C. M., and Dweck, C. S. (1998). Praise for intelligence can undermine children's motivation and performance. *Journal of Personality and Social Psychology, 75*.

National Association for Gifted Children (NAGC). (1998). *Pre-K-Grade 12 gifted program standards*. Washington, DC: Author.

National Center for Education Statistics (NCES). (1999). *Highlights from the Third International Mathematics and Science Study (TIMSS): Overview and key findings across grade levels*. Washington, DC: Author.

National Center for Education Statistics (NCES). (2001). *Highlights from the Third International Mathematics and Science Study-Repeat (TIMSS-R)*. Washington, DC: Author.

Nielsen, M. E., and Morton-Albert, S. (1989). The effects of special education on the self-concept and school attitude of learning-disabled/gifted students. *Roeper Review, 12*,29-36.

Ohnishi, T., Matsuda, H., Asada, T., Aruga, M., Hirakata, M., Nishikawa, M., Katoh, A., and Imabayashi, E. (2001). Functional anatomy of musical perception in musicians. *Cerebral Cortex, 11*, 754-760.

Oktem, F., Diren, B., Karaagaoglu, E., and Anlar, B. (2001, April). Functional magnetic resonance imaging in children with Asperger's syndrome. *Journal of Child Neurology, 16*, 253-256.

Olszewski-Kubilius, P. (1998). Talent search: Purposes, rational, and role in gifted education. *Journal of Secondary Gifted Education, 9*, 106-113.

Pallas, A. M., Entwisle, D. R., Alexander, K. L., and Stluka, M. F. (1994, January). Ability-group effects: Instructional, social, or institutional? *Sociology of Education, 67*, 27-46.

Pantev, C., Oostenveld, R., Engelien, A., Ross, B., Roberts, L. E., and Hoke, M. (1998, April 23). Increased auditory cortical representation. *Nature, 392*, 811-813.

Pascual-Leone, A., Dang, N., Cohen, L., Brasil-Neto, J., Cammarota, A., and Hallett, M. (1995). Modulation of muscle responses evoked by transcranial magnetic stimulation during the acquisition of new fine motor skills. *Journal of Neurophysiology, 74*, 1037-1045.

Persky, H. R., Sandene, B. A., and Askew, J. M. (1999). *The NAEP 1997 Arts Report Card*. Washington, DC: National Center for Education Statistics.

Powell, T., and Siegle, D. (2000, Spring). Teacher bias in identifying gifted and talented students. *National Research Center on the Gifted and Talented Newsletter*, 13-15.

Purves, D. (Ed.). (2001). *Neuroscience,* (2nd ed.). Sunderland, MA: Sinauer.

Reis, S. M., Burns, D. E., and Renzulli, J. S. (1992a). *Curriculum compacting: The complete guide to modifying the regular curriculum for high ability students*. Mansfield Center, CT: Creative Learning Press.

Reis, S. M., Burns, D. E., and Renzulli, J. S. (1992b). *A facilitator's guide to help teachers compact curriculum*. Storrs, CT: University of Connecticut, The National Research Center on the Gifted and Talented.

Reis, S. M., Hébert, T. P., Díaz, E. I., Maxfield, L. R., and Ratley, M. E. (1995). *Case studies of talented students who achieve and underachieve in an urban high school* (Research Monograph 95120). Storrs, CT: University of Connecticut, The National Research Center on the Gifted and Talented.

Reis, S. M., Westberg, K. L., Kulikowich, J. M., and Purcell, J. H. (1998, Spring). Curriculum compacting and achievement test scores: What does the research say? *Gifted Child Quarterly, 42*, 123-129.

Renzulli, J. (1978). What makes giftedness? Reexamining a definition. *Phi Beta Kappan, 60*, 180-184, 261.

Renzulli, J. (1986). The three-ring conception of giftedness: A developmental model for creative productivity. In Sternberg, R. J., and Davidson, E. (Eds.), *Conceptions of giftedness* (53-92). New York: Cambridge University Press.

Restak, R. M. (2001). *The secret life of the brain*. Washington, DC: John Henry Press.

Rhodes, L. (1992). Focusing attention on the individual in identification of gifted black students. *Roeper Review, 14*, 108-110.

Rimm, S. B. (1996). *Dr. Sylvia Rimm's smart parenting: How to raise a happy achieving child*. New York: Crown Publishers.

Rittle-Johnson, B., and Alibali, M. W. (1999). Conceptual and procedural knowledge of mathematics: Does one lead to the other? *Journal of Educational Psychology, 91*, 175.

Rivera, D. B., Murdock, J., and Sexton, D. (1995). Serving the gifted/learning disabled. *Gifted Child Today, 18*, 34-37.

Robinson, A. and Clinkenbeard, P. R. (1998, August). Giftedness: An exceptionality examines. *Annual Review of Psychology, 49*, 117-139.

Rodgers, J. L., Cleveland, H. H., van den Oord, E., and Rowe, D. C. (2000, June). Resolving the debate over birth order, family size, and intelligence. *American Psychologist, 55*, 599-612.

Rogers, K. B. (1998). Using current research to make "good" decisions about grouping. *NASSP Bulletin, 82*, 38-46. Research data is also available online at http://www.educ.state.mn.us/gifted.

Rotigel, J. V., and Lupkowski-Shoplik, A. (1999). Using talent searches to identify and meet the educational needs of mathematically gifted youngsters. *School Science and Mathematics, 99*, 330-337.

Scarr, S., and McCartney, K. (1983). How people make their own environments. *Child Development, 54*, 424-435.

Schacter, D. L. (2001). *The seven sins of memory: How the mind forgets and remembers*. New York: Houghton Mifflin.

Schlaug, G., Jancke, L., Huang, Y., and Steinmetz, H. (1995). In vivo evidence of structural brain asymmetry in musicians. *Science, 267*, 699-701.

Schlaug, G., and Christian, G. (2001, May 8). *Musical training during childhood may influence regional brain growth*. Paper presented at the 53rd Annual Meeting of the American Academy of Neurology, Philadelphia.

Schwartz, W. (1997, May). Strategies for identifying the talents of diverse students. *ERIC Clearinghouse on Urban Education Digest, 122*, 1-6.

Shadmehr, R. and Holcomb, H. H. (1997). Neural correlates of motor memory consolidation. *Science, 277*, 821-825.

Shaywitz, B. A., Shaywitz, S. E., and Gore, J. (1995). Sex differences in the functional organization of the brain for language. *Nature, 373*, 607-609.

Shaywitz, S. E., Holahan, J. M., Fletcher, J. M., Freudenheim, D. A., Makuch, R. W., and Shaywitz, B. A. (2001, Winter). Heterogeneity within the gifted: Higher IQ boys exhibit behaviors resembling boys with learning disabilities. *Gifted Child Quarterly, 45*, 16-23.

Shore, B. M., and Delcourt, M. A. B. (1996). Effective curricular and program practices in gifted education and the interface with general education. *Journal of Education for the Gifted, 20*, 138-154.

Silverman, L. K. (1989a). Invisible gifts, invisible handicaps. *Roeper Review, 12*, 37-42.

Silverman, L. K. (1989b). The visual-spatial learner. *Preventing School Failure, 34,* 15-20.

Silverman, L. K. (1993). *Counseling the gifted and talented*. Denver: Love Publishing.

Silverman, L. K., Chitwood, D. G., and Waters, J. L. (1986). Young gifted children: Can parents identify giftedness? *Topics in Early Childhood Education, 6*, 23-38.

Sloboda, J. A., Davidson, J. W., Howe, M. J. A., and Moore, D. G. (1996). The role of practice in the development of performing musicians. *British Journal of Psychology, 87*, 287-309.

Smutny, J. F. (2000, May). *Teaching young gifted children in the regular classroom.* Arlington, VA: ERIC Clearinghouse on Disabilities and Gifted Children.

Smutny, J. F. (2001, June). *Creative strategies for teaching language arts to gifted students (K-8).* Arlington, VA: ERIC Clearinghouse on Disabilities and Gifted Children.

Sousa, D. A. (2001a). *How the brain learns*, (2nd ed.). Thousand Oaks, CA: Corwin Press.

Sousa, D. A. (2001b). *How the special needs brain learns.* Thousand Oaks, CA: Corwin Press.

Southern,W. T., Jones, E. D., and Stanley, J. C. (1993). Acceleration and enrichment: The context and development of program options. In Heller, K. A., Monks, F. J., and Passow, A. H. (Eds.), *International handbook of research and development of giftedness and talent* (387-409). Oxford: Pergamon.

Sowell, E. R., Thompson, P. M., Holmes, C. J., Jernigan, T. L., and Toga, A. W. (1999). In-vivo evidence for post-adolescent brain maturation in frontal and striatal regions. *Nature: Neuroscience, 2*, 859–861.

Squire, L. R. and Kandel, E. R. (1999). *Memory: From mind to molecules.* New York: W. H. Freeman.

Sternberg, R. J. (1985). *Beyond IQ: A triarchic theory of human intelligence.* New York: Cambridge University Press.

Sternberg, R. J. (2000, December). Identifying and developing creative giftedness. *Roeper Review, 23*, 60-64.

Sternberg, R. J. and Zhang, L. (1995, September). What do we mean by giftedness? A pentagonal implicit theory. *Gifted Child Quarterly, 39*, 88-94

Sternberg, R. J., Ferrari, M., Clinkenbeard, P. R., and Grigorenko, E. L. (1996). Identification, instruction, and assessment of gifted children: A construct validation of a triarchic model. *Gifted Child Quarterly, 40*, 129-137.

Sternberg, R. J., Grigorenko, E. L., Jarvin, L., Clinkenbeard, P., Ferrari, M., and Torfi, B. (2000, Spring). The effectiveness of triarchic teaching and assessment. *National Research Center on the Gifted and Talented Newsletter,* 3-8.

Stewart, L., and Walsh, V. (2001). Music of the hemispheres. *Current Biology, 11,* R125- R127.

Swiatek, M. A. (1995). An empirical investigation of the social coping strategies used by gifted adolescents. *Gifted Child Quarterly, 39,* 154-160.

Sytsma, R. E. (2001, November). *Gifted education in America's high schools: National survey results.* Paper presented at the meeting of the National Association for Gifted Children, Cincinnati, OH.

Thompson, M. (1999). Developing verbal talent. *Center for Talent Development* [Online]. See http://www.ctd.northwestern.edu/.

Thompson, P. M., Cannon, T.D., Narr, K. L., van Erp, T., Poutanen, V., Huttanen, M., Lönnqvist, J., Standertskjöld-Nordenstam, C., Kaprio, J., Khaledy, M., Dail, R., Zoumalen, C., and Toga, A. (2001, December 1). Genetic influences on brain structure. *Nature Neuroscience, 4,* 1253-1258.

Tomlinson, C. A. (1995). *How to differentiate instruction in mixed-ability classrooms.* Alexandria, VA: Association for Supervision and Curriculum Development.

Tomlinson, C. A. (1999). *The differentiated classroom: Responding to the needs of all learners.* Alexandria, VA: Association for Supervision and Curriculum Development.

Toll, M. F. (1993). Gifted learning disabled: A kaleidoscope of needs. *Gifted Child Today, 16,* 34-35.

Treffert, D. A. (2000a). *Extraordinary people: Understanding savant syndrome.* Lincoln, NE: iUniverse Press.

Treffert, D. A. (2000b). The savant syndrome in autism. In Accardo, P., Magnusen, C., and Capute, A. (Eds.). *Autism: Clinical and research issues.* Baltimore: York Press.

Tremblay, T., and Gagné, F. (2001). Beliefs of students talented in academics, music, and dance concerning the heritability of human abilities in these fields. *Roeper Review,23,* 173-177.

Tuholski, S. W., Engle, R. W., and Baylis, G. C. (2001, April). Individual differences in working memory capacity and enumeration. *Memory and Cognition, 29,* 484-492.

Tyler-Wood, T. L., Mortenson, M., Putney, D., and Cass, M. A. (2000). An effective mathematics and science curriculum option for secondary gifted education. *Roeper Review, 22*, 266-269.

Udall, A. J. (1987). *Peer referral as a process for locating Hispanic students who may be gifted.* Unpublished doctoral dissertation, University of Arizona.

Udall, A. J. and Passe, M. (1993). Gardner-based performance-based assessment notebook. Charlotte, NC: Charlotte-Mechlenburg Schools.

Van Rooy, C., Stough, C., Pipingas, A., Hocking, C., and Silberstein, R. B. (2001, October). Spatial working memory and intelligence biological correlates. *Intelligence, 29*, 275-292.

VanTassel-Baska, J., Johnson, D. T., Hughes, C. E., and Boyce, L. N. (1996). A study of language arts curriculum effectiveness with gifted learners. *Journal of Education for the Gifted, 19*, 461-480.

Wagner, A. D., Schacter, D. L., Rotte, M., Koutstaal, W., Maril, A., Dale, A. M., Rosen, B. R., and Buckner, R. L. (1998, August 21). Building memories: Remembering and forgetting of verbal experiences as predicted by brain activity. *Science, 281*, 1188–1191.

Wakeley, A., Rivera, S., and Langer, J. (2000). Can young infants add or subtract? *Child Development, 71*, 1525-1534.

Webb, J. T. (2000, August 7). *Mis-diagnosis and dual diagnosis of gifted children: Gifted and LD, ADHD, OCD, Oppositional Defiant Disorder*. Paper presented at the annual convention of the American Psychological Association, Washington, DC.

Webster, P. (2000). Reforming secondary music teaching in the new century. *Journal of Secondary Gifted Education, 12*, 17-24.

Westberg, K. L., and Archambault, F. X., Jr. (1997). A multi-site case study of successful classroom practices for high ability students. *Gifted Child Quarterly, 41*, 42-51.

Whalen, J., McCloskey, M., Lesser, R. P., and Gordon, B. (1997). Localizing arithmetic processes in the brain: Evidence from a transient deficit during cortical stimulation. *Journal of Cognitive Neuroscience, 9*, 409-417.

White, D. A. and Breen, M. (1998). Edutainment: Gifted education and the perils of misusing multiple intelligences. *Gifted Child Today, 21*, 12-14, 16-17.

Willard-Holt, C. (1999, May). *Dual exceptionalities*. Arlington, VA: ERIC Clearinghouse on Disabilities and Gifted Education.

Winebrenner, S. (2000, September). Gifted students need an education, too. *Educational Leadership, 58*, 52-55.

Winebrenner, S., and Devlin, B. (2001, March). *Cluster grouping of gifted students: How to provide full-time services on a part-time budget: Update 2001*. Arlington, VA: ERIC Clearinghouse on Disabilities and Gifted Children.

Winner, E. (1996). *Gifted children: Myths and realities*. New York: Basic Books.

Winner, E. (2000). The origins and ends of giftedness. *American Psychologist, 55*, 159-169.

Witelson, S. F., Kigar, D. L., and Harvey, T. (1999, June 19). The exceptional brain of Albert Einstein. *The Lancet, 353*, 2149-2153.

Wynn, K. (1992). Addition and subtraction in human infants. *Nature, 358*, 749-750.

Wynn, K. (1998). Psychological foundations of number: Numerical competence in human infants. *Trends in Cognitive Sciences, 2*, 296-303.

Resources

TEXTS

Assouline, S., Colangelo, N., Lupkowski-Shoplik, A., and Lipscomb, J. (1999). *Iowa acceleration scale manual: A guide for whole-grade acceleration (K-8)*. Scottsdale, AZ: Great Potential Press.

Bireley, M. (1995). *Crossover children: A sourcebook for helping children who are gifted and learning disabled.* Reston, VA: Council for Exceptional Children.

Cline, S., and Schwartz, D. (1999). *Diverse populations of gifted children: Meeting their needs in the regular classroom and beyond.* Upper Saddle River, NJ: Prentice Hall.

Colangelo, N., and Davis, G. A. (Eds.) (1997). *Handbook of gifted education*. Boston: Allyn and Bacon.

Kay, K. (Ed.) (2000). Uniquely gifted: Identifying and meeting the needs of the twice exceptional student. Gilsum, NH: Avocus Publishing.

Rogers, K. B. (2002). Re-forming gifted education: Matching the program to the child. Scottsdale, AZ: Great Potential Press.

Smutny, J. F., Walker, S. Y., and Meckstroth, E. A. (1997). *Teaching young gifted children in the regular classroom: Identifying, nurturing, and challenging ages 4-9.* Minneapolis, MN: Free Spirit Publishing.

Sousa, D. A. (2001a). How the brain learns, (2nd ed.). Thousand Oaks, CA: Corwin Press.

Sternberg, R. J. (1997). *Successful intelligence*. New York: Plume.

Strip, C. A., and Hirsch, G. (2000). Helping gifted children soar: A practical guide for parents and teachers. Scottsdale, AZ: Great Potential Press.

Tomlinson, C. A. (1999). The differentiated classroom: Responding to the needs of all learners. Alexandria, VA: Association for Supervision and Curriculum Development.

Tomlinson, C. A., Kaplan, S. N., Renzulli, J. S., Purcell, J., Leppien, J., and Burns, D. (2002). *The parallel curriculum.* Thousand Oaks, CA: Corwin Press.

Winner, E. (1996). Gifted children: Myths and realities. New York: Basic Books.

ORGANIZATIONS

American Hyperlexia Association
195 West Spangler, Suite B
Elmhurst, Illinois 60126
Tel. (630) 415-2212
Web: www.hyperlexia.org

The Association for the Gifted
Indiana Academy for Science, Mathematics, and Humanities
Ball State University
Muncie, IN 47306-0580
Tel. (765) 285-7455
Web: www.cectag.org

Center for Excellence in Education (Applications of Technology)
Indiana University
201 North Rose Avenue
Bloomington, IN 47405-1006
Tel. (812) 856-8210
Web: http://cee.indiana.edu

Council for Exceptional Children
1110 North Glebe Road, Suite 300
Arlington, VA 22201-5407
Tel. (888) CEC-SPED (888-232-7733)
Web: www.cec.sped.org

Davidson Institute for Talent Development (Resources for Profoundly Gifted Youth)
9665 Gateway Drive, Suite B
Reno, Nevada 89521
Tel. (775) 852-3483
Web: www.davidson-institute.org

ERIC Clearinghouse on Disabilities and Gifted Education
1110 North Glebe Road
Arlington, VA 22201-5704
Tel. 1-800-328-0272
Web: www.ericec.org

The Gifted Child Society
190 Rock Road
Glen Rock, NJ 07452-1736
Tel. (201) 444-6530
Web: www.gifted.org

Gifted Development Center
1452 Marion Street
Denver, CO 80218
Tel. (303) 837-8378
Web: www.gifteddevelopment.com

National Association for Gifted Children
1707 L Street NW, Suite 550
Washington, DC 20036
Tel. (202) 785-4268
Web: www.nagc.org

National Research Center on the Gifted and Talented
University of Connecticut
2131 Hillside Road, Unit 3007
Storrs, CT 06269-3007
Tel. (860) 486-4826
Web: www.gifted.uconn.edu/nrcgt.html

Supporting Emotional Needs of the Gifted
P.O. Box 6550
Scottsdale, AZ 85261
Tel. (206) 498-6744
Web: www.sengifted.org

World Council for Gifted and Talented Children, Inc.
18401 Hiawatha Street
Northridge, CA 91326
Tel. (818) 368-7501
Web: www.worldgifted.org

TALENT SEARCH PROGRAMS

Program	Address and Web Site	Type of Talent Search
Academic Talent Search	California State University 6000 J Street Sacramento, CA 95819-6098 http://edweb.csus.edu/projects/ats	Elementary and middle school students in northern California
Rocky Mountain Talent Search	University of Denver Office of Academic Youth Programs 1981 South University Boulevard Denver, CO 80208 www.du.edu/education/ces/rmts.html	For 6th through 9th graders in Colorado, Nevada, Idaho, Montana, New Mexico, Utah, and Wyoming
Center for Talent Development	Northwestern University 617 Dartmouth Place Evanston, IL 60208-4175 http://ctdnet.acns.nwu.edu	For 3rd to 8th graders in surrounding states
Iowa Talent Search	Iowa State University (OPPTAG) 310 Pearson Hall Ames, IA 50011 www.public.iastate.edu/~opptag_info	For 7th graders in and around Iowa
The Belin-Blank Center for Gifted Education and Talent Development	University of Iowa 210 Lindquist Center Iowa City, IA 52242 www.uiowa.edu/~belinctr	For 4th through 9th graders nationwide

Program	Address and Web Site	Type of Talent Search
Center for Talented Youth	Johns Hopkins University 3400 North Charles Street Baltimore, MD 21218 www.cty.jhu.edu	For 2nd through 8th graders nationwide
Talent Identification Program	Duke University (TIP) Box 90747 Durham, NC 27708 www.tip.duke.edu	Elementary and middle school students nationwide
Carnegie Mellon Institute for Talented Elementary Students	Carnegie Mellon University (C-MITES) 4902 Forbes Avenue, #6261 Pittsburgh, PA 15213-3890 http://www.cmu.edu/cmites	For 3rd through 6th graders in Pennsylvania
Halbert and Nancy Robinson Center for Young Scholars	University of Washington Box 351630 Seattle, WA 98195 http://depts.washington.edu/cscy	For 5th through 8th graders in Washington
Canada: Center for Gifted Education	University of Calgary 170 Education Block 2500 University Drive NW Calgary, Alberta, T2N 1N4, Canada http://www.acs.ucalgary.ca/~gifteduc/talent.html	For 4th, 5th, and 6th graders in Calgary and Edmonton

WEBSITES

This list of websites is just a sampling of the various resources that are available for obtaining information about gifted programs. Some sites offer puzzles, problems, and games for challenging gifted children. The list is by no means complete, but it will serve as a useful starting point for exploring the vast number of resources that are available on the Internet. Nearly all of the websites have hyperlinks to other sites. The website addresses were accurate as of time of publication.

Center for the Improvement of Early Reading Achievement (CIERA)
www.ciera.org

Creative Learning Press
www.creativelearningpress.com

Edward deBono's Official Website
Provides information about his teaching materials and games as well as other resources to enhance creativity and lateral thinking ability. If you are familiar with de Bono's work, you'll find all those resources described here. There are also pre-seminar materials at the deBono Institute. Finding your way around the site is an interesting lateral thinking puzzle in itself.
Web: www.edwdebono.com/

Future Problem Solving Program
www.fpsp.org

HighIQWorld,
Articles and links related to gifted education.
www.s-2000.com/hi-iq/intelligence/gifted_kids.html

Hoagie's Gifted Education Page,
Includes the latest research on parenting and education (including academic acceleration or enrichment, home schooling, traditional programs, the highly gifted, etc.)
Web: www.hoagiesgifted.org

Hollingworth Center for Highly Gifted Children
Web: www.hollingworth.org

International Baccalaureate Organization
Web: www.ibo.org

Mensa Foundation for Gifted Children (MFGC)
Resources for Very Able and Gifted Children
Includes links to:
Support Groups for Very Able and Gifted Children
Advice for Parents and Teachers
Educational Resource Links
Distance Learning and Educational Materials
Web: www.mfgc.org.uk/mfgc/links.html

Mindspring.Com
Includes the latest research on academic acceleration or enrichment, home schooling, traditional programs, the highly gifted.
Web: www.mindspring.com/~mensa/pages

National Conference of Governors' Schools
Web: www.ncogs.org

Odyssey of the Mind
Web: www.odyssey.org

Online Asperger Syndrome Information and Support (O.A.S.I.S.)
Web: www.udel.edu/bkirby/asperger

Portfolio usage suggestions from ERIC
The portfolio and its use: Developmentally appropriate assessment of young children.
Web: www.ed.gov/databases/ERIC_Digests/ed351150.html

Smarter Kids.com
An array of educational books, software and games; fill out the free Learning Style Survey to find out how your child learns best; explore the Parent Resource Center, which includes activities, tips and a collection of SmarterSites, providing materials for Advanced Students.
Web: www.smarterkids.com

Index

Page numbers in **boldface** are **Applications**.

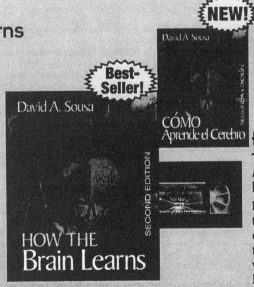

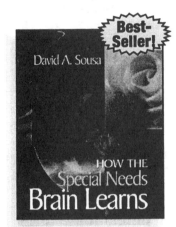

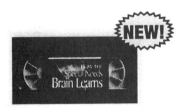

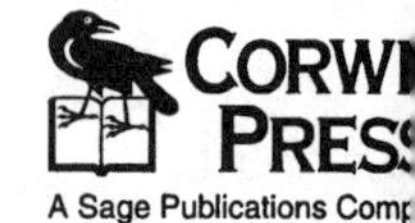

CORWI
PRESS
A Sage Publications Comp

HOW THE Brain Learns

THIRD EDITION

HOW THE Brain Learns

THIRD EDITION

David A. Sousa

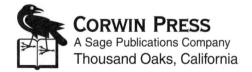

For information:

Corwin Press
A Sage Publications Company
2455 Teller Road
Thousand Oaks, California 91320
www.corwinpress.com

Sage Publications Ltd
1 Oliver's Yard
55 City Road
London EC1Y 1SP
United Kingdom

Sage Publications India Pvt. Ltd.
B-42, Panchsheel Enclave
Post Box 4109
New Delhi 110 017 India

Printed in the United States of America on acid-free paper

Library of Congress Cataloging-in-Publication Data

Sousa, David A.
How the brain learns / David A. Sousa.— 3rd ed.
p. cm.
Includes bibliographical references and index.
ISBN 1-4129-3660-8 (cloth) — ISBN 1-4129-3661-6 (pbk.)
1. Learning, Psychology of. 2. Learning—Physiological aspects. 3. Brain. I. Title.
LB1057.S65 2006
370.15'23—dc22

2005029776

05 06 07 08 10 9 8 7 6 5 4 3 2 1

Acquisitions editor: Robert D. Clouse
Editorial assistant: Jingle Vea
Production editor: Sanford Robinson
Typesetter: C&M Digitals (P) Ltd.
Cover designer: Tracy Miller
Production artist: Lisa Miller

Contents

List of Practitioner's Corners

About the Author

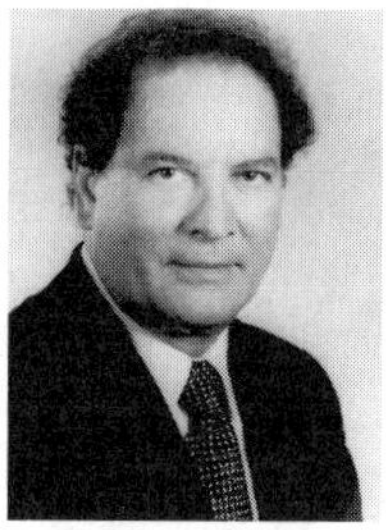

David A. Sousa, Ed.D., is an international educational consultant. He has made presentations at national conventions of educational organizations and has conducted workshops on brain research and science education in hundreds of school districts and at several colleges and universities across the United States, Canada, Europe, and Asia.

Dr. Sousa has a bachelor of science degree in chemistry from Massachusetts State College at Bridgewater, a master of arts in teaching degree in science from Harvard University, and a doctorate from Rutgers University. His teaching experience covers all levels. He has taught junior and senior high school science, served as a K–12 director of science, and was Supervisor of Instruction for the West Orange, New Jersey, schools. He then became superintendent of the New Providence, New Jersey, public schools. He has been an adjunct professor of education at Seton Hall University, and a visiting lecturer at Rutgers University. He was president of the National Staff Development Council in 1992.

Dr. Sousa has edited science books and published numerous books and articles in leading educational journals on staff development, science education, and brain research. He has received awards from professional associations and school districts for his commitment and contributions to research, staff development, and science education. He received the Distinguished Alumni Award and an honorary doctorate in education from Bridgewater (Mass.) State College.

He has appeared on the NBC Today show and on National Public Radio to discuss his work with schools using brain research. He makes his home in south Florida.

Who dares to teach
must never cease to learn.

—John Cotton Dana

Preface to the Third Edition

Since the publication of the second edition of this book, neuroscientists have continued to make remarkable discoveries about how the human brain grows, develops, and learns. Scanning technologies are more sophisticated and are able to track brain activity faster and more accurately than ever before. Perhaps the greatest discovery of neuroscientists that has benefitted many children has been the improved understanding of how the brain acquires language and learns to read. These research insights have allowed scientists to design educational interventions that are amazingly successful in actually rewiring the brains of young struggling readers so that their reading skills improve dramatically. Can you imagine that? We can now rewire young brains!

For this third edition, I have made some changes in the text as a result of new knowledge about the brain. Specifically, I have

- Updated the Information Processing Model to reflect newer terminology and understandings about memory systems
- Updated the exciting research about language acquisition and how the brain learns to read
- Expanded the chapter on thinking skills and included the recently revised version of Bloom's Taxonomy
- Added more examples of how emotions influence learning and memory
- Added two Practitioner's Corners
- Added a section on resources that includes additional books and Internet sites
- Included more primary sources for those who wish to review the actual research studies

When the first edition of this book was published over a decade ago, not too many educators were familiar with the growing knowledge base in cognitive neuroscience. Today, most educators are very familiar with the explosion of current research on the brain. There is little doubt that some of the findings of this exciting research have implications for what we do in schools and classrooms. But there is also a lot of hype about the brain these days and not all of it is accurate. Educators must avoid the hype and use caution when deciding whether new knowledge can improve our practice.

I firmly believe that science will continue to reveal deeper understandings about how the brain learns. As educators become more familiar with these revelations, I also believe they will ensure that brain-compatible schools provide opportunities for all learners to succeed.

—David A. Sousa

Acknowledgments

Corwin Press gratefully acknowledges the contribution of the following people:

Elizabeth F. Day
Teacher of the Year
Mechanicville Middle School
Mechanicville, NY

Janice Ferguson
Professor, Exceptional Education
Department of Special Instruction Programs
Western Kentucky University
Bowling Green, KY

Janet Steck
Part-Time Faculty
Department of Early Childhood,
Physical and Special Education
The University of Toledo
Toledo, OH

Nicola Salvatico
Teacher of the Year
General Wayne Elementary School
Malvern, PA

Randy J. Wormald
Teacher of the Year
Belmont High School
Belmont, NH

Carrie Jane Carpenter
Teacher of the Year
Hugh Hartman Middle School
Redmond, OR

Jensi Kellogg-Andrus
Teacher of the Year
Watertown High School
Watertown, SD

Marguerite Lawler-Rohner
Teacher of the Year
Westcott Junior High School
Portland, ME

Introduction

You start out as a single cell derived from the coupling of a sperm and egg; this divides into two, then four, then eight, and so on, and at a certain stage there emerges a single cell which will have as all its progeny the human brain. The mere existence of that cell should be one of the great astonishments of the earth.

—Lewis Thomas,
The Medusa and the Snail

The human brain is an amazing structure—a universe of infinite possibilities and mystery. It constantly shapes and reshapes itself as a result of experience, yet it can take off on its own without input from the outside world. How does it form a human mind, capture experience, or stop time in memory? Although it does not generate enough energy to light a simple bulb, its capabilities make it the most powerful force on Earth.

For thousands of years, humans have been delving into this mysterious universe and trying to determine how it accomplishes its amazing feats. How fast does it grow? What impact does the environment have on its growth? What is intelligence? How does it learn language? How does it learn to read?

Just how the brain learns has been of particular interest to teachers for centuries. Now, in the 21st century, there is new hope that our understanding of this remarkable process called teaching and learning will improve dramatically. A major source of that understanding is coming from the sophisticated medical instruments that allow scientists to peer inside the living—and learning—brain.

LOOKING INSIDE THE BRAIN

New technologies for looking inside and seeing the workings of the living brain have advanced faster than scientists predicted just 10 years ago. The more we learn about the brain, the more remarkable it seems. Hardly a week goes by when some major news story about the brain appears in the press or on television. Consequently, most of us have heard about the imaging technologies, and some readers may have even experienced a brain scan. Because we will be mentioning brain scans throughout this book, here is a brief review of the more common scanning instruments that have contributed to our understanding of brain structure and function.

Types of Brain Imaging

The imaging technologies fall into two major categories: those that look at brain *structure* and those that look at brain *function*. When aimed at the brain, computerized axial tomography (CAT) and magnetic resonance imaging (MRI) are very useful diagnostic tools that produce computer images of the brain's internal structure. For example, they can detect tumors, malformations, and the damage caused by cerebral hemorrhages.

Different technologies, however, are required to look at how the brain works. An alphabet soup describes the five most common procedures that can be used to isolate and identify the areas of the brain where distinct levels of activity are occurring. The scanning technologies for looking at brain function are the following:

- Electroencephalography (EEG)
- Magnetoencephalography (MEG)
- Positron Emission Tomography (PET)
- Functional Magnetic Resonance Imaging (fMRI)
- Functional Magnetic Resonance Spectroscopy (fMRS)

Here is a brief explanation of how each one works. A summary chart follows.

- **Electroencephalography (EEG) and Magnetoencephalography (MEG).** These two techniques are helpful in determining how quickly something occurs in the brain. To do that, they measure electrical and magnetic activity occurring in the brain during mental processing. In an EEG, anywhere from 19 to 128 electrodes are attached to various positions on the scalp with a conductive gel so electrical signals can be recorded in a computer. In a MEG, about 100 magnetic detectors are placed around the head to record magnetic activity. EEGs and MEGs can record changes in brain activity that occur as rapidly as one millisecond (one-thousandth of a second), typical times when the brain is processing language. When a group of neurons responds to a specific event (like a word), they activate and their electrical and magnetic activity can be detected above the noise of the nonactivated neurons. This response is called an *Event-Related Potential* or ERP. ERP evidence has provided information about the time needed for the brain to do mathematical calculations or process reading. EEG and MEG do not expose the subject to radiation and are not considered hazardous.
- **Positron Emission Tomography (PET).** The first technology to observe brain functions, it involves injecting the subject with a radioactive solution that circulates to the brain. Brain regions of higher activity accumulate more of the radiation, which is picked up by a ring of detectors around the subject's head. A computer displays the concentration of radiation as a picture of blood flow in a cross-sectional slice of the brain regions that are aligned with the

detectors. The picture is in color, with the more active areas in reds and yellows, the quieter areas in blues and greens. Two major drawbacks to PET scans are the invasive nature of the injection and the use of radioactive materials. Consequently, this technique is not used with normal children because the radioactive risk is too high.

- **Functional Magnetic Resonance Imaging (fMRI).** This newer technology is rapidly replacing PET scans because it is painless, noninvasive, and does not use radiation. The technology helps to pinpoint the brain areas of greater and lesser activity. Its operation is based on the fact that when any part of the brain becomes more active, the need for oxygen and nutrients increases. Oxygen is carried to the brain cells by hemoglobin. Hemoglobin contains iron, which is magnetic. The fMRI uses a large magnet to compare the amount of oxygenated hemoglobin entering brain cells with the amount of deoxygenated hemoglobin leaving the cells. The computer colors in the brain regions receiving more oxygenated blood and can locate the activated brain region to within one centimeter (less than a half-inch).
- **Functional Magnetic Resonance Spectroscopy (fMRS).** This technology involves the same equipment as fMRI but uses different computer software to record levels of various chemicals in the brain while the subject is thinking. Like the fMRI, fMRS can precisely pinpoint the area of activity, but it can also identify whether certain key chemicals are also present at the activation site. fMRS has been used to study language function in the brain by mapping the change in specific chemicals, such as lactate, that respond to brain activation during tasks involving language.

Researchers are also learning much more about several dozen brain chemicals called *neurotransmitters.* These substances bathe the brain cells and either permit signals to pass between them or inhibit them. Wide fluctuations in the concentration of neurotransmitters in certain brain areas can change our mood, affect our movement, diminish or enhance our alertness, and interfere with our ability to learn.

To determine which parts of the brain control various functions, neurosurgeons use tiny electrodes to stimulate individual nerve cells and record their reactions. Besides the information collected by these techniques, the growing body of case studies of individuals recovering from various types of brain damage is giving us new evidence about and insights into how the brain develops, changes, learns, remembers, and recovers from injury.

IMPLICATIONS FOR TEACHING

As we examine the clues that this research is yielding about learning, we recognize its importance to the teaching profession. Every day teachers enter their classrooms with lesson plans, experience, and the hope that what they are about to present will be understood, remembered, and useful to their students. The extent that this hope is realized depends largely on the knowledge base that these teachers use in designing those plans and, perhaps more important, on the instructional techniques they select during the lessons. Teachers try to change the human brain every day. The more they know about how it learns, the more successful they can be.

Techniques for Mapping Brain Functions		
Technique	**What It Measures**	**How It Works**
Electroencephalography (EEG) Magnetoencephalography (MEG)	The electrical and magnetic activity occurring in the brain during mental processing. The spikes of activity are called Event-Related Potentials (ERP).	In EEG, multiple electrodes are attached to the scalp to record electrical signals in a computer. In MEG, magnetic detectors are placed around the head to record magnetic activity. EEGs and MEGs record changes in brain activity that occur as rapidly as one millisecond. When a group of neurons responds to a specific event, they activate and their electrical and magnetic activity can be detected. This response is called an Event-Related Potential or ERP.
Positron Emission Tomography (PET)	Amount of radiation present in brain regions	The subject is injected with a radioactive solution that circulates to the brain. Brain regions of higher activity accumulate more radiation, which is picked up by a ring of detectors. A computer displays the concentration of radiation in a cross-sectional slice of the brain regions aligned with the detectors. The picture shows the more active areas in reds and yellows, the quieter areas in blues and greens.
Functional Magnetic Resonance Imaging (fMRI)	Levels of deoxygenated hemoglobin in brain cells	Any part of the brain that is thinking requires more oxygen, which is carried to the brain cells by hemoglobin. The fMRI uses a large magnet to compare the amount of oxygenated hemoglobin entering brain cells with the amount of deoxygenated hemoglobin leaving the cells. The computer colors in the brain regions receiving more oxygenated blood and locates the activated brain region to within one centimeter (half-inch).
Functional Magnetic Resonance Spectroscopy (fMRS)	Levels of specific chemicals present during brain activity	This technology involves the same equipment as fMRI but uses different computer software to record levels of various chemicals in the brain while the subject is thinking. fMRS can precisely pinpoint the area of activity, but it can also identify whether certain key chemicals are also present at the activation site.

Educators in recent years have become much more aware that neuroscience is finding out a lot about how the brain works, and that some of the discoveries have implications for what happens in schools and classrooms. There is a growing interest among educators in the biology of learning and how much an individual's environment can affect the growth and development of the brain. Teacher training institutions are beginning to incorporate brain research into their courses. Staff development programs are devoting more time to this area, more books about the brain are available, brain-compatible teaching units are sprouting up, and the journals of most major educational organizations have devoted special issues to the topic. These are all good signs. I believe this focus on recent brain research can improve the quality of our profession's performance and its success in helping others learn.

> ***Teachers try to change the human brain every day. The more they know about how it learns, the more successful they can be.***

Some Important Findings

As research continues to provide a deeper understanding of the workings of the human brain, educators need to be cautious about how they apply these findings to practice. There are critics who believe that brain research should not be used at this time in schools and classrooms. Some critics say it will be years before this has any application to educational practice. Others fear that unsubstantiated claims are being made, and that educators are not sufficiently trained to tell scientific fact from hype. The concerns are understandable but should not prevent educators from learning what they need to know to decide whether a research study has applications to their practice. For those who wonder how recent discoveries about the brain can affect teaching and learning, we can tell them that this research has:

- Reaffirmed that the human brain continually reorganizes itself on the basis of input. This process, called *neuroplasticity*, continues throughout our life but is exceptionally rapid in the early years. Thus, the experiences the young brain has in the home and at school help shape the neural circuits that will determine how and what that brain learns in school and later.
- Revealed more about how the brain acquires spoken language.
- Developed scientifically based computer programs that dramatically help young children with reading problems.
- Shown how emotions affect learning, memory, and recall.
- Suggested that movement and exercise improve mood, increase brain mass, and enhance cognitive processing.
- Tracked the growth and development of the teenage brain to better understand the unpredictability of adolescent behavior.
- Developed a deeper understanding of circadian cycles to explain why teaching and learning can be more difficult at certain times of day.
- Studied the effects of sleep deprivation and stress on learning and memory.
- Recognized that intelligence and creativity are separate abilities, and that both can be modified by the environment and schooling.

Other researchers strongly disagree with the critics and support the increased attention that educators are giving to neuroscience. Several universities here and abroad have established dedicated research centers to examine how discoveries in neuroscience can affect educational practice. As a result, educational theory and practice will become much more research-based, similar to the medical model.

There is, of course, no panacea that will make teaching and learning a perfect process—and that includes brain research. It is a long leap from making a research finding in a laboratory to the changing of schools and practice because of that finding. These are exciting times for educators, but we must ensure that we don't let the excitement cloud our common sense.

WHY THIS BOOK CAN HELP IMPROVE TEACHING AND LEARNING

What I have tried to do here is report on research (from neuroscience as well as the behavioral and cognitive sciences) that is sufficiently reliable that it can inform educational practice. This is hardly a novel idea. Madeline Hunter in the late 1960s introduced the notion of teachers using what science was learning about learning and modifying traditional classroom procedures and instructional techniques accordingly. Her program at the UCLA School of Education came to be called "Instructional Theory Into Practice," or ITIP. Readers familiar with that model will recognize some of Dr. Hunter's work here, especially in the areas of transfer and practice. I had the privilege of working periodically with her for nine years, and I firmly believe that she was the major force that awakened educators to the importance of continually updating their knowledge base and focusing on research-based strategies and the developing science of learning.

This book will help answer questions such as:

- When do students remember best in a learning episode?
- How can I help students understand and remember more of what I teach?
- Why is focus so important, and why is it so difficult to get?
- How can I teach motor skills effectively?
- How can humor and music help the teaching-learning process?
- How can I get students to find meaning in what they are learning?
- Why is transfer such a powerful principle of learning, and how can it destroy a lesson without my realizing it?
- What classroom strategies are more likely to appeal to the brain of today's student?
- What important questions should I be asking myself as I plan daily and unit lessons?

Chapter Contents

Chapter 1. Basic Brain Facts and Brain Development. Because we are going to talk a lot about the brain, we should be familiar with some of its anatomy. This chapter discusses some of the majors structures of the human brain and their functions. It explores how the young brain grows and develops, focusing on those important windows of opportunity for learning in the early years. There is an explanation of how students' brains today are very different from those of just a few years ago, especially in what they expect from their school experiences.

Chapter 2. How the Brain Processes Information. Trying to develop a simple model to describe the complex process of learning is not easy. The model at the heart of this chapter outlines what cognitive researchers believe are the critical steps involved in the brain's acquisition and processing of information. The components of the model are discussed in detail and updated from previous editions. Also included is an instrument to help you determine your sensory preferences.

Chapter 3. Memory, Retention, and Learning. Teachers want their students to remember forever what they are taught, but that does not happen too often. The third chapter focuses on the different types of memory systems and how they work. Those factors that affect retention of learning are discussed here along with ideas of how to plan lessons that result in greater remembering.

Chapter 4. The Power of Transfer. Transfer is one of the most powerful and least understood principles of learning. Yet a major goal of education is to enable students to transfer what they learn in school to solve future problems. The nature and power of transfer are examined in this chapter, including how to use past knowledge to enhance present and future learning.

Chapter 5. Brain Specialization and Learning. This chapter explores how areas of the brain are specialized to perform certain tasks. It examines hemispheric specialization and debunks some myths that have obscured the value of this work. You will be able to determine whether you have a hemispheric preference and what that means about how you think, learn, and teach. The chapter also examines the latest research on how we learn to speak and read, and the implications of this research for classroom instruction and for the curriculum and structure of schools.

Chapter 6. The Brain and the Arts. Despite strong evidence that the arts enhance cognitive development, they run the risk of being abandoned so more time can be devoted to preparing for mandated high stakes testing. Public support for keeping the arts is growing. This chapter presents the latest evidence of how the arts in themselves contribute to the growth of neural networks as well as enhance the skills needed for mastering other academic subjects.

Chapter 7. Thinking Skills and Learning. Are we challenging our students enough to do higher-level thinking? This chapter discusses some of the characteristics and dimensions of human thinking. It focuses on the recent revision of Bloom's Taxonomy, notes its continuing compatibility with current research on higher-order thinking, and explains the taxonomy's critically important relationship to difficulty, complexity, and intelligence.

Chapter 8. Putting It All Together. So how do we use these important findings in daily practice? This chapter emphasizes how to use the research presented in this book to plan lessons. It discusses different types of teaching methods, and suggests guidelines and a format for lesson design. Because neuroscience continues to reveal new information about learning, the chapter describes support systems to help educators maintain expertise in brain-compatible techniques and move toward continuous professional growth.

At the end of each chapter are the **Practitioner's Corners.** Some include activities that check for understanding of the major concepts and research presented in the chapter. Others offer my interpretation of how this research might translate into effective classroom strategies that improve the teaching-learning process. Readers are invited to critically review my suggestions and rationale to determine if they have any value for their work.

Main thoughts are highlighted in boxes throughout the book. At the very end of each chapter, you will find a page called **Key Points to Ponder**, an organizing tool to help you remember important ideas, strategies, and resources you may wish to consider later.

Where appropriate, I have explained some of the chemical and biological processes occurring within the brain. However, I have intentionally omitted complex chemical formulas and reactions, and have avoided side issues that would distract from the main purpose of this book. My intent is to present just enough science to help the average reader understand the research and the rationale for any suggestions I offer.

Who Should Use This Book?

This book will be useful to **classroom teachers** because it presents a research-based rationale for why and when certain instructional strategies should be considered. It focuses on the brain as the organ of thinking and learning, and takes the approach that the more teachers know about how the brain learns, the more instructional options become available. Increasing the options that teachers have during the dynamic process of instruction also increases the likelihood that successful learning will occur.

The book should also help **staff developers** who continually need to update their own knowledge base and include research and research-based strategies and support systems as part of their repertoire. Chapter 8 offers some suggestions to help staff developers implement and maintain the knowledge and strategies suggested here.

Principals and Head Teachers should find here a substantial source of topics for discussion at faculty meetings, which should include, after all, instructional as well as informational items. In doing so, they support the attitude that professional growth is an ongoing school responsibility and not an occasional event. More important, being familiar with these topics enhances the principal's credibility as the school's instructional leader and promotes the notion that the school is a learning organization for *all* its occupants.

This book can help teachers, staff developers, principals, college instructors, and parents.

College and university instructors should also find merit in the research and applications presented here, as both suggestions to improve their own teaching as well as information to be passed on to prospective teachers.

Some of the information in this book will be useful to **parents**, who are, after all, the child's first teachers.

Indeed, the ideas in this book provide the research support for a variety of initiatives, such as cooperative learning groups, differentiated instruction, integrated thematic units, and the interdisciplinary approach to curriculum. Those who are familiar with constructivism will recognize many similarities in the ideas presented here. The research is yielding more evidence that knowledge is not only transmitted from the teacher to the learners but is transformed in the learner's mind as a result of cultural and social mediation. Much of this occurs through elaborative rehearsal and transfer and is discussed in several chapters.

Try It Yourself—Do Action Research

Benefits of Action Research

One of the best ways to assess the value of the strategies suggested in this book is to try them out in your own classroom or in any other location where you are teaching. Conducting this action research allows you to gather data to determine the effectiveness of new strategies and affirm those you already use, to acclaim and enhance the use of research in our profession, and to further your own professional development.

Other benefits of action research are that it provides teachers with consistent feedback for self-evaluation, it introduces alternative forms of student assessment, and its results may lead to important changes in curriculum. Action research can be the work of just one teacher, but its value grows immensely when it is the consistent effort of a teacher team, department, school staff, or even an entire district. Incorporating action research as a regular part of the K–12 academic scene not only provides useful data but also enhances the integrity of the profession and gains much-needed respect from the broad community that schools serve.

Using action research provides valuable data, affirms best practices, and enhances the integrity of the profession.

Teachers are often hesitant to engage in action research, concerned that it may take too much time or that it represents another accountability measure in an already test-saturated environment. Yet, with all the programs and strategies emerging today in the name of reform, we need data to help determine their validity. The valuable results of cognitive neuroscience will continue to be ignored in schools unless there is reliable evidence to support their use. Action research is a cost-effective means of assessing the effectiveness of brain-compatible strategies that are likely to result in greater student learning.

The Outcomes of Action Research

The classroom is a laboratory in which the teaching and learning processes meet and interact. Action research can provide continual feedback on the success of that interaction. Using a solution-oriented approach, action research includes identifying the problem, systematically collecting data, analyzing the data, taking action based on the data, evaluating and reflecting on the results of those actions, and, if needed, redefining the problem (Figure I.1). The teacher is always in control of the type of data collected, the pace of assessment, and the analysis of the results. This process encourages teachers to reflect on their practices, to refine their skills as a practitioner, and to direct their

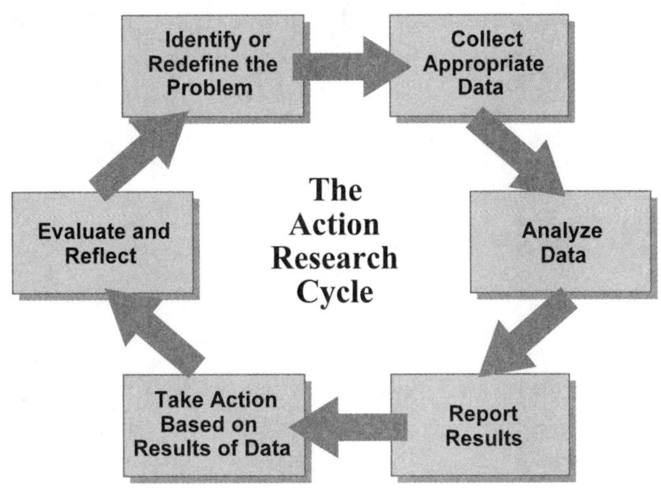

Figure I.1 The diagram illustrates the six steps in the action research cycle.

own professional development. This is a new view of the profession, with the teacher as the main agent of change.

Building administrators have a special obligation to encourage action research among their teachers. With so much responsibility and accountability being placed on schools and teachers, action research can quickly assess the effectiveness of instructional strategies. By supporting such a program, principals demonstrate by action that they are truly instructional leaders and not just building managers. See the **Practitioner's Corner** at the end of this chapter on page 13 for specific suggestions on using action research in the classroom.

Finally, this third edition of the book reflects what more I have gathered about the brain and learning at the time of publication. Because this is now an area of intense research and scrutiny, educators need to constantly read about new discoveries and adjust their understandings accordingly. As we discover more about how the brain learns, we can devise strategies that can make the teaching-learning process more efficient, effective, and enjoyable.

What's Coming Up?

As neuroscience advances, educators are realizing that some basic information about the brain must now become part of their knowledge base. Educators are not neuroscientists, but they are members of the *only* profession whose job is to change the human brain every day. Therefore, the more they know about how it works, the more likely they are to be successful at changing it. To that end, the next chapter will take the reader through a painless and easy-to-read explanation of some major brain structures and their functions as well as a peek at the brain of today's students.

> ***Educators are in the only profession whose job is to change the human brain every day.***

PRACTITIONER'S CORNER

What Do You Already Know?

The value of this book can be measured in part by how it enhances your understanding of the brain and the way it learns. Take the following true-false test to assess your current knowledge of the brain. Decide whether the statements are generally true or false and circle T or F. Explanations for the answers are identified throughout the book in special boxes.

1. T F The structures responsible for deciding what gets stored in long-term memory are located in the brain's rational system.

2. T F Learners who can perform a new learning task well are likely to retain it.

3. T F Reviewing material just before a test is a good practice to determine how much has been retained.

4. T F Increased time on task increases retention of new learning.

5. T F Two very similar concepts or motor skills should be taught at the same time.

6. T F The rate at which a learner retrieves information from memory is closely related to intelligence.

7. T F The amount of information a learner can deal with at one time is genetically linked.

8. T F It is usually not possible to increase the amount of information that the working (temporary) memory can deal with at one time.

9. T F Most of the time, the transfer of information from long-term storage is under the conscious control of the learner.

10. T F Bloom's Taxonomy has not changed over the years.

PRACTITIONER'S CORNER

How Brain Compatible Is My Teaching/School/District?

Directions: On a scale of 1 (lowest) to 5 (highest), circle the number that indicates the degree to which your teaching/school/district does the following. Connect the circles to see a profile.

1.	I/We adapt the curriculum to recognize the windows of opportunity students have during their cognitive growth.	1——2——3——4——5
2.	I/We are trained to provoke strong, positive emotions in students during the learning process.	1——2——3——4——5
3.	I/We are trained to help students adjust their self-concept to be more successful in different learning situations.	1——2——3——4——5
4.	I/We provide an enriched and varied learning environment.	1——2——3——4——5
5.	I/We search constantly for opportunities to integrate curriculum concepts between and among subject areas.	1——2——3——4——5
6.	Students have frequent opportunities during class to talk about what they are learning, while they are learning.	1——2——3——4——5
7.	I/We do not use lecture as the main mode of instruction.	1——2——3——4——5
8.	One of the main criteria I/we use to decide on classroom activities and curriculum is relevancy to students.	1——2——3——4——5
9.	I/We understand the power of chunking and use it in the design of curriculum and in daily instruction.	1——2——3——4——5
10.	I/We understand the primacy-recency effect and use it regularly in the classroom to enhance retention of learning.	1——2——3——4——5

PRACTITIONER'S CORNER

Using Action Research

Basic Guidelines

Action research helps teachers assess systematically the effectiveness of their own educational practices using the techniques of research. Because data collection is essential to this process, teachers need to identify the elements of the research question that can be measured.

- **Select the Research Question.** Because you need to collect data, choose a research question that involves elements which can be easily measured quantitatively or qualitatively. Some examples:

    1. How does the chunking of material affect the learner's retention? This can be measured by a short oral or written quiz.
    2. How does teaching material at the beginning or middle of a lesson affect learner retention? This can be measured by quizzes.
    3. How does changing the length of wait time affect student participation? This can be measured by comparing the length of the wait time to the number of subsequent student responses.
    4. Does using humor or music increase student focus? Can either be measured by number of students who are on/off task with or without humor or music.
    5. Does teaching two very similar concepts at different times improve student understanding and retention of them? This can be measured by oral questioning or quizzes after teaching each concept.

- **Collect the Data.** Remember that you need baseline data before you try the research strategy to provide a comparison. Plan carefully the methods you will use to measure and collect the data. Try not to use paper-and-pencil tests exclusively. You will collect pretrial and posttrial data.

    Pretrial. Select a control group, which is usually the same group of students that will be used with the research strategy. Collect test data without using the research strategy.

    Posttrial. Use the strategy (e.g., chunking, prime-time-1, wait time, humor) and then collect the appropriate data.

- **Analyze the Data.** Use simple analytical techniques, such as comparing the average group test scores before and after using the research strategy. What changes did you notice in the two sets of data? Did the research strategy produce the desired result? If not, why not? Was there an unexpected consequence (positive or negative) of using the strategy?

- **Share the Data.** Sharing the data with colleagues is an important component of the action research process. Too often, teachers work in isolation, with few or no opportunities to interact continuously with colleagues to design and discuss their lessons.

- **Implement the Change.** If the research strategy produced the desired results, decide how you will make it part of your teaching repertoire. If you did not get the desired results, decide whether you need to change some aspect of the strategy or perhaps use a different measure.

- **Try New Practices.** Repeat the above steps with other strategies so that action research becomes part of your ongoing professional development.

Chapter 1

Basic Brain Facts

With our new knowledge of the brain, we are just dimly beginning to realize that we can now understand humans, including ourselves, as never before, and that this is the greatest advance of the century, and quite possibly the most significant in all human history.

—Leslie A. Hart,
Human Brain and Human Learning

Chapter Highlights: This chapter introduces some of the basic structures of the human brain and their functions. It explores the growth of the young brain and some of the environmental factors that influence its development into adolescence. Whether the brain of today's student is compatible with today's schools is also discussed.

The adult human brain is a wet, fragile mass that weighs a little over three pounds. It is about the size of a small grapefruit, is shaped like a walnut, and can fit in the palm of your hand. Cradled in the skull and surrounded by protective membranes, it is poised at the top of the spinal column. The brain works ceaselessly, even when we are asleep. Although it represents only about 2 percent of our body weight, it consumes nearly 20 percent of our calories! The more we think, the more calories we burn. Perhaps this can be a new diet fad, and we could modify Descartes' famous quotation from "I think, therefore I am" to "I think, therefore I'm thin"!

Through the centuries, surveyors of the brain have examined every cerebral feature, sprinkling the landscape with Latin and Greek names to describe what they saw. They analyzed structures and

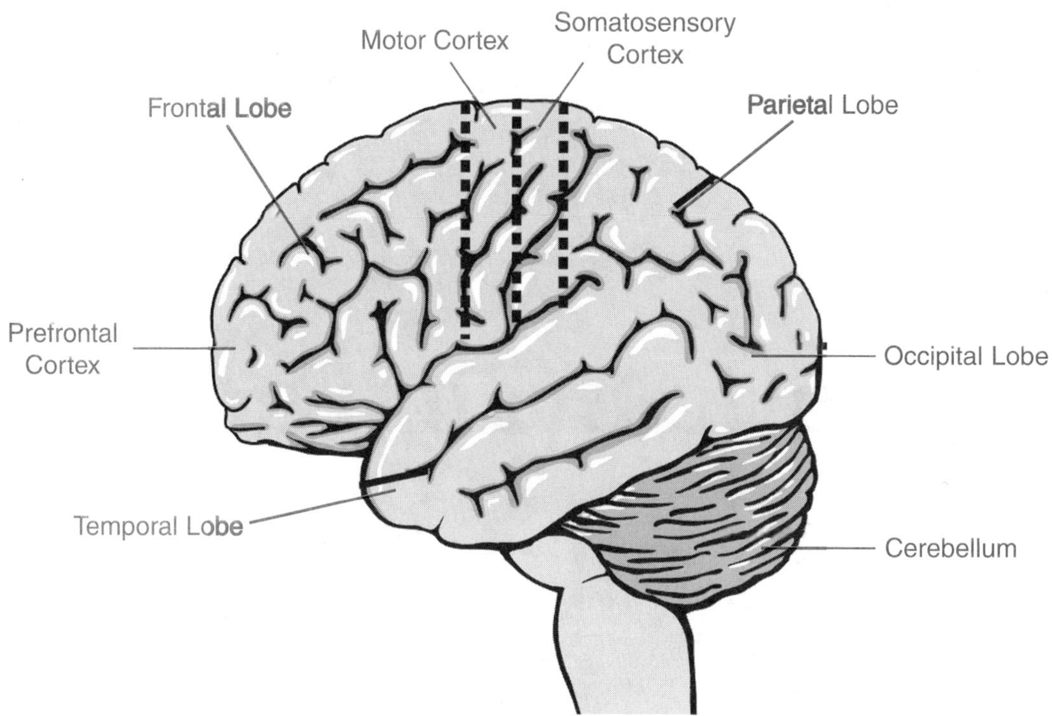

Figure 1.1 The major exterior regions of the brain.

functions and sought concepts to explain their observations. One early concept divided the brain by location—forebrain, midbrain, and hindbrain. Another, proposed by Paul MacLean in the 1960s, described the triune brain according to three stages of evolution: reptilian (brain stem), paleo-mammalian (limbic area), and mammalian (frontal lobes).

For our purposes, we will take a look at major parts of the outside of the brain (Figure 1.1). We will then look at the inside of the brain and divide it into three parts on the basis of their general functions: the brainstem, limbic system, and cerebrum (Figure 1.2). We will also examine the structure of the brain's nerve cells, called *neurons*.

SOME EXTERIOR PARTS OF THE BRAIN

Lobes of the Brain

Although the minor wrinkles are unique in each brain, several major wrinkles and folds are common to all brains. These folds form a set of four lobes in each hemisphere. Each lobe tends to specialize for certain functions.

Frontal Lobes. At the front of the brain are the *frontal lobes*, and the part lying just behind the forehead is called the *prefrontal cortex.* These lobes deal with planning and thinking. They comprise the rational and executive control center of the brain, monitoring higher-order thinking, directing problem solving, and regulating the excesses of the emotional system. The frontal lobe

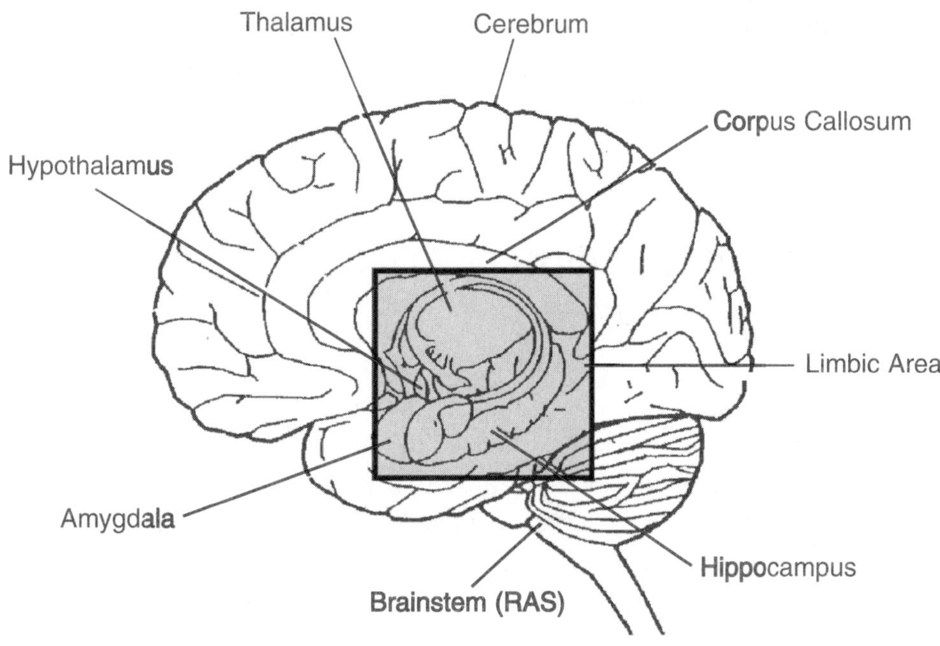

Figure 1.2 A cross section of the human brain.

also contains our self-will area—what some might call our personality. Trauma to the frontal lobe can cause dramatic—and sometimes permanent—behavior and personality changes. Because most of the working memory is located here, it is the area where focus occurs (Smith & Jonides, 1999). The frontal lobe matures slowly. MRI studies of post-adolescents reveal that the frontal lobe continues to mature into early adulthood. Thus, the capability of the frontal lobe to control the excesses of the emotional system is not fully operational during adolescence (Sowell, Thompson, Holmes, Jernigan, & Toga, 1999; Goldberg, 2001). This is one important reason why adolescents are more likely than adults to submit to their emotions and resort to high-risk behavior.

> ***Because the rational system matures slowly in adolescents, they are more likely to submit to their emotions.***

Temporal Lobes. Above the ears rest the *temporal lobes*, which deal with sound, music, face and object recognition, and some parts of long-term memory. They also house the speech centers, although this is usually on the left side only.

Occipital Lobes. At the back are the paired *occipital lobes*, which are used almost exclusively for visual processing.

Parietal Lobes. Near the top are the *parietal lobes*, which deal mainly with spatial orientation, calculation, and certain types of recognition.

Motor Cortex and Somatosensory Cortex

Between the parietal and frontal lobes are two bands across the top of the brain from ear to ear. The band closer to the front is the *motor cortex*. This strip controls body movement and, as we will learn later, works with the cerebellum to coordinate the learning of motor skills. Just behind the motor cortex, at the beginning of the parietal lobe, is the *somatosensory cortex,* which processes touch signals received from various parts of the body.

SOME INTERIOR PARTS OF THE BRAIN

Brainstem

The brainstem is the oldest and deepest area of the brain. It is often referred to as the reptilian brain because it resembles the entire brain of a reptile. Of the 12 body nerves that go to the brain, 11 end in the brainstem (the olfactory nerve—for smell—goes directly to the limbic system, an evolutionary artifact). Here is where vital body functions, such as heartbeat, respiration, body temperature, and digestion, are monitored and controlled. The brainstem also houses the reticular activating system (RAS), responsible for the brain's alertness and about which more will be explained in the next chapter.

The Limbic System

Nestled above the brainstem and below the cerebrum lies a collection of structures commonly referred to as the limbic system and sometimes called the old mammalian brain. Many researchers now caution that viewing the limbic system as a separate functional entity is outdated because all of its components interact with many other areas of the brain.

Most of the structures in the limbic system are duplicated in each hemisphere of the brain. These structures carry out a number of different functions including the generation of emotions and processing emotional memories. Its placement between the cerebrum and the brainstem permits the interplay of emotion and reason.

Four parts of the limbic system are important to learning and memory. They are:

The Thalamus. All incoming sensory information (except smell) goes first to the thalamus (Greek for "inner chamber"). From here it is directed to other parts of the brain for additional processing. The cerebrum and cerebellum also send signals to the thalamus, thus involving it in many cognitive activities.

The Hypothalamus. Nestled just below the thalamus is the hypothalamus. While the thalamus monitors information coming in from the outside, the hypothalamus monitors the internal systems to maintain the normal state of the body (called *homeostasis*). By controlling the release of a variety of hormones, it moderates numerous body functions, including sleep, food intake, and liquid intake. If body systems slip out of balance, it is difficult for the individual to concentrate on cognitive processing of curriculum material.

The Hippocampus. Located near the base of the limbic area is the hippocampus (the Greek word for "seahorse," because of its shape). It plays a major role in consolidating learning and in converting information from working memory via electrical signals to the long-term storage regions, a process that may take days to months. It constantly checks information relayed to working memory and compares it to stored experiences. This process is essential for the creation of meaning.

Its role was first revealed by patients whose hippocampus was damaged or removed because of disease. These patients could remember everything that happened before the operation, but not afterward. If they were introduced to you today, you would be a stranger to them tomorrow. Because they can remember information for only a few minutes, they can read the same article repeatedly and believe on each occasion that it is the first time they have read it. Brain scans have confirmed the role of the hippocampus in permanent memory storage. Alzheimer's disease progressively destroys neurons in the hippocampus, resulting in memory loss.

Recent studies of brain-damaged patients have revealed that although the hippocampus plays an important role in the recall of facts, objects, and places, it does not seem to play much of a role in the recall of long-term personal memories (Lieberman, 2005).

The Amygdala. Attached to the end of the hippocampus is the amygdala (Greek for "almond"). This structure plays an important role in emotions, especially fear. It regulates the individual's interactions with the environment than can affect survival, such as whether to attack, escape, mate, or eat.

Because of its proximity to the hippocampus and its activity on PET scans, researchers believe that the amygdala encodes an emotional message, if one is present, whenever a memory is tagged for long-term storage. It is not known at this time whether the emotional memories themselves are actually stored in the amygdala. One possibility is that the emotional component of a memory is stored in the amygdala while other cognitive components (names, dates, etc.) are stored elsewhere (Squire & Kandel, 1999). The emotional component is recalled whenever the memory is recalled. This explains why people recalling a strong emotional memory will often experience those emotions again. The interactions between the amygdala and the hippocampus ensure that we remember for a long time those events that are important and emotional.

Teachers, of course, hope that their students will permanently remember what was taught. Therefore, it is intriguing to realize that the two structures in the brain mainly responsible for long-term remembering are located in the *emotional* area of the brain. Understanding the connection between emotions and cognitive learning and memory will be discussed in later chapters.

Test Question No. 1: The structures responsible for deciding what gets stored in long-term memory are located in the brain's rational system.

Answer: False. These structures are located in the emotional (limbic) system.

Cerebrum

A soft jellylike mass, the cerebrum is the largest area, representing nearly 80 percent of the brain by weight. Its surface is pale gray, wrinkled, and marked by furrows called fissures. One large fissure runs from front to back and divides the cerebrum into two halves, called the *cerebral hemispheres*. For some still unexplained reason, the nerves from the left side of the body cross over to the right hemisphere, and those from the right side of the body cross to the left hemisphere. The two hemispheres are connected by a thick cable of over 250 million nerve fibers called the *corpus callosum* (Latin for "large body"). The hemispheres use this bridge to communicate with each other and coordinate activities.

The hemispheres are covered by a thin but tough laminated *cortex* (meaning "tree bark"), rich in cells, that is about 1/10th of an inch thick and, because of its folds, has a surface area of about two square feet. That is about the size of a large dinner napkin. The cortex is composed of six layers of cells meshed in about 10,000 miles of connecting fibers per cubic inch! Here is where most of the action takes place. Thinking, memory, speech, and muscular movement are controlled by areas in the cerebrum. The cortex is often referred to as the brain's gray matter.

The neurons in the thin cortex form columns whose branches extend down through the cortical layer into a dense web below known as the white matter. Here, neurons connect with each other to form vast arrays of neural networks that carry out specific functions.

Cerebellum

The cerebellum (Latin for "little brain") is a two-hemisphere structure located just below the rear part of the cerebrum, right behind the brainstem. Representing about 11 percent of the brain's weight, it is a deeply folded and highly organized structure containing more neurons than all of the rest of the brain put together. The surface area of the entire cerebellum is about the same as that of one of the cerebral hemispheres.

This area coordinates movement. Because the cerebellum monitors impulses from nerve endings in the muscles, it is important in the performance and timing of complex motor tasks. It modifies and coordinates commands to swing a golf club, smooth a dancer's footsteps, and allow a hand to bring a cup to the lips without spilling its contents. The cerebellum may also store the memory of automated movements, such as touch-typing and tying a shoelace. Through such automation, performance can be improved as the sequences of movements can be made with greater speed, greater accuracy, and less effort. The cerebellum also is known to be involved in the mental rehearsal of motor tasks, which also can improve performance and make it more skilled. A person whose cerebellum is damaged slows down and simplifies movement, and would have difficulty with finely-tuned motion, such as catching a ball, or completing a handshake.

Recent studies indicate that the role of the cerebellum has been underestimated. Researchers now believe that it also acts as a support structure in cognitive processing by coordinating and fine-tuning our thoughts, emotions, senses (especially touch), and memories. Because the cerebellum is connected also to regions of the brain that perform mental and sensory tasks, it can perform these skills automatically, without conscious attention to detail. This allows the conscious part of the

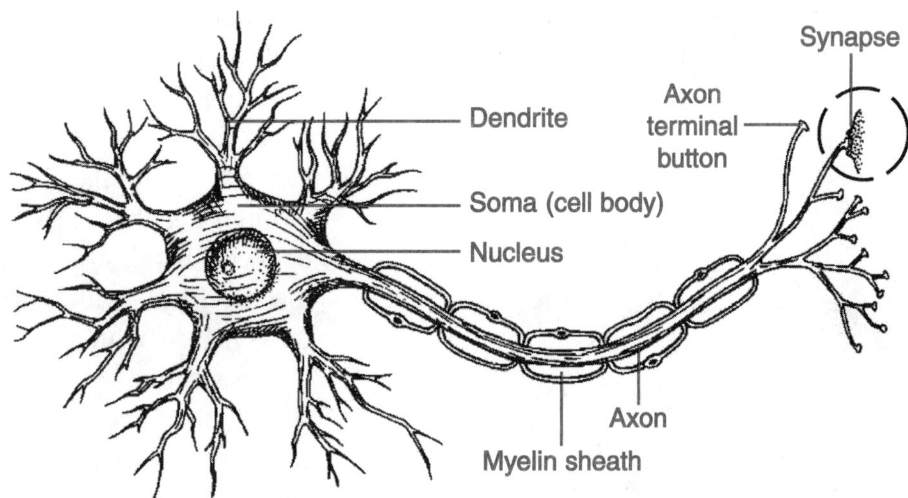

Figure 1.3 Neurons transmit signals along an axon and across the synapse (in dashed circle) to the dendrites of a neighboring cell. The myelin sheath protects the axon and increases the speed of transmission.

brain the freedom to attend to other mental activities, thus enlarging its cognitive scope. Such enlargement of human capabilities is attributable in no small part to the cerebellum and its contribution to the automation of numerous mental activities.

Brain Cells

The brain is composed of a trillion cells of at least two known types, nerve cells and glial cells. The nerve cells are called *neurons* and represent about one-tenth of the total—roughly 100 billion. Most of the cells are *glial* (Greek for "glue") cells that hold the neurons together and act as filters to keep harmful substances out of the neurons. Very recent studies indicate that some glial cells, called *astrocytes*, have a role in regulating the rate of neuron signaling. By attaching themselves to blood vessels, astrocytes also serve to form the blood-brain barrier, which plays an important role in protecting brain cells from blood-borne substances that could disrupt cellular activity.

The neurons are the functioning core for the brain and the entire nervous system. Neurons come in different sizes, but the body of each brain neuron is about 1/100th the size of the period at the end of this sentence. Unlike other cells, the neuron (see Figure 1.3) has tens of thousands of branches emerging from its core, called *dendrites* (from the Greek word for "tree"). The dendrites receive electrical impulses from other neurons and transmit them along a long fiber, called the *axon* (Greek for "axis"). There is normally only one axon per neuron. A layer called the *myelin sheath* surrounds each axon. The sheath insulates the axon from the other cells and increases the speed of impulse transmission. This impulse travels along the neurons through an electrochemical process and can move through the entire length of a 6-foot adult in 2/10ths of a second. A neuron can transmit between 250 and 2,500 impulses per second.

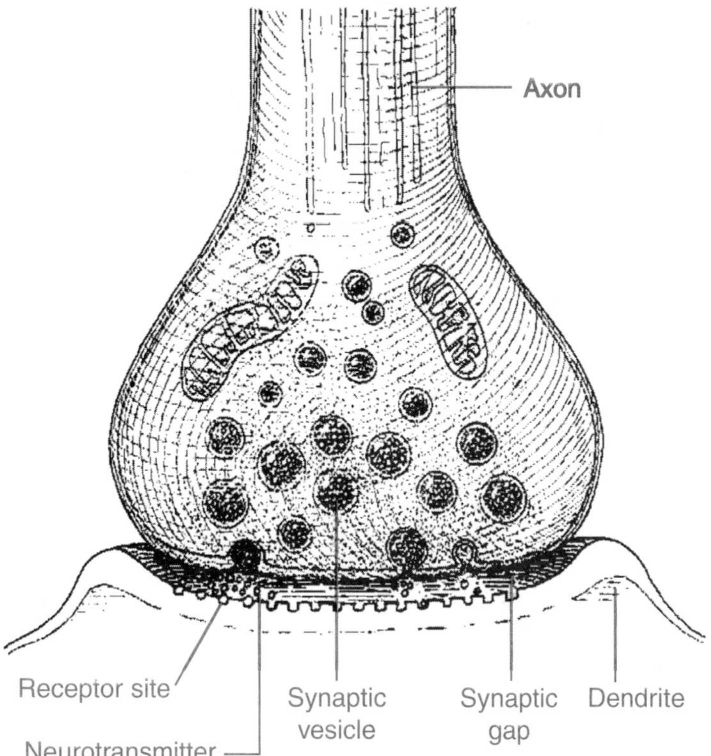

Figure 1.4 The neural impulse is carried across the synapse by chemicals called neurotransmitters that lie within the synaptic vesicles.

Neurons have no direct contact with each other. Between each dendrite and axon is a small gap of about a millionth of an inch called a *synapse* (from the Greek, meaning "to join together"). A typical neuron collects signals from others through the dendrites, which are covered at the synapse with thousands of tiny bumps, called *spines*. The neuron sends out spikes of electrical activity (impulses) through the axon to the synapse where the activity releases chemicals stored in sacs (called *synaptic vesicles*) at the end of the axon (Figure 1.4). These chemicals, called *neurotransmitters*, either excite or inhibit the neighboring neuron. More than 50 different neurotransmitters have been discovered so far. Some of the common neurotransmitters are acetylcholine, epinephrine, serotonin, and dopamine. Learning occurs by changing the synapses so that the influence of one neuron on another also changes.

A direct connection seems to exist between the physical world of the brain and the work of the brain's owner. Recent studies of neurons in people of different occupations (e.g., professional musicians) show that the more complex the skills demanded of the occupation, the more dendrites were found on the neurons. This increase in dendrites allows for more connections between neurons resulting in more sites in which to store learnings.

There are about 100 billion neurons in the adult human brain—about 16 times as many neurons as people on this planet and about the number of stars in the Milky Way. Each neuron can have up to 10 thousand dendrite branches. This means that it is possible to have up to one quadrillion (that's a one followed by 15 zeros) synaptic connections in one brain. This inconceivably large number allows the brain to process the data coming continuously from the senses; to store decades of memories, faces, and places; to learn languages; and to combine information in a way that no other individual on this planet has ever thought of before. This is a remarkable achievement for just three pounds of soft tissue!

> ***Believe it or not, the number of potential synaptic connections in just one human brain is about 1,000,000,000,000,000.***

Conventional wisdom has been that neurons were the only body cells that never regenerate. However, researchers have discovered that the adult human brain does generate neurons in at least one site—the hippocampus. This discovery raises the question of whether neurons regenerate in other parts of the brain and, if so, if it might be possible to stimulate them to repair and heal damaged brains, especially for the growing number of people with Alzheimer's disease. Research into Alzheimer's disease is exploring ways to stop the deadly mechanisms that trigger the destruction of neurons.

Mirror Neurons

Scientists using fMRI technology recently discovered clusters of neurons in the premotor cortex (the area in front of the motor cortex that plans movements) firing just before a person carries out a planned movement. Curiously, these neurons also fired when a person saw someone else perform the movement. For example, the firing pattern of these neurons that preceded the subject grasping a cup of coffee, was identical to the pattern when the subject saw someone else do that. Thus, similar brain areas process both the production and perception of movement. Neuroscientists believe these *mirror neurons* may help an individual to decode the intentions and predict the behavior of others. They allow us to re-create the experience of others within ourselves, and to understand others' emotions and empathize. Seeing the look of disgust or joy on other people's faces cause mirror neurons to trigger similar emotions in us. We start to feel their actions and sensations as though we were doing them.

Mirror neurons probably explain the mimicry we see in young children when they imitate our smile and many of our other movements. We have all experienced this phenomenon when we attempted to stifle a yawn after seeing someone else yawning. Neuroscientists believe that mirror neurons may explain a lot about mental behaviors that have remained a mystery. For instance, there is experimental evidence that children with autism may have a deficit in their mirror-neuron system. That would explain why they have difficulty inferring the intentions and mental state of others (Oberman et al., 2005). Researchers also suspect that mirror neurons may play a role in our ability to develop articulate speech.

Brain Fuel

Brain cells consume oxygen and glucose (a form of sugar) for fuel. The more challenging the brain's task, the more fuel it consumes. Therefore, it is important to have adequate amounts of these substances in the brain for optimum functioning. Low amounts of oxygen and glucose in the blood can produce lethargy and sleepiness. Eating a moderate portion of food containing glucose (fruits are an excellent source) can boost the performance and accuracy of working memory, attention, and motor function (Korol & Gold, 1998; Scholey, Moss, Neave, & Wesnes, 1999).

> ***Many students (and their teachers) do not eat a breakfast with sufficient glucose, nor drink enough water during the day for healthy brain function.***

Water, also essential for healthy brain activity, is required to move neuron signals through the brain. Low concentrations of water diminish the rate and efficiency of these signals. Moreover, water keeps the lungs sufficiently moist to allow for the efficient transfer of oxygen into the bloodstream.

Many students (and their teachers, too) do not eat a breakfast that contains sufficient glucose, nor do they drink enough water during the day to maintain healthy brain function. Schools should have breakfast programs and educate students on the need to have sufficient blood levels of glucose during the day. Schools should also provide frequent opportunities for students and staff to drink plenty of water. The current recommended amount is one eight-ounce glass of water a day for each 25 pounds of body weight.

NEURON DEVELOPMENT IN CHILDREN

Neuron development starts in the embryo shortly after conception and proceeds at an astonishing rate. In the first four months of gestation, about 200 billion neurons are formed, but about half will die off during the fifth month because they fail to connect with any areas of the growing embryo. This purposeful destruction of neurons (called *apoptosis*) is genetically programmed to ensure that only those neurons that have made connections are preserved, and to prevent the brain from being overcrowded with unconnected cells. Any drugs or alcohol that the mother takes during this time can interfere with the growing brain cells, increasing the risk of fetal addiction and mental defects.

The neurons of a newborn are immature; many of their axons lack the protective myelin layer and there are few connections between them. Thus, most regions of the cerebral cortex are quiet. Understandably, the most active areas are the brainstem (body functions) and the cerebellum (movement).

The neurons in a child's brain make many more connections than those in adults. A newborn's brain makes connections at an incredible pace as the child absorbs its environment. Information is entering the brain through "windows" that emerge and taper off at various times. The richer the environment, the greater the number of interconnections that are made. Consequently, learning can take place faster and with greater meaning.

As the child approaches puberty, the pace slackens and two other processes begin: Connections the brain finds useful become permanent; those not useful are eliminated (apoptosis) as the brain selectively strengthens and prunes connections based on experience. This process continues throughout our lives, but it appears to be most intense between the ages of three and 12. Thus, at an early age, experiences are already shaping the brain and designing the unique neural architecture that will influence how it handles future experiences in school, work, and other places.

Windows of Opportunity

Windows of opportunity represent important periods in which the young brain responds to certain types of input to create or consolidate neural networks. Some windows are critical, and are called *critical periods* by pediatric researchers. For example, if even a perfect brain doesn't receive visual stimuli by the age of two, the child will be forever blind, and if it doesn't hear words by the age of 12, the person will most likely never learn a language. When these critical windows close, the brain cells assigned to those tasks may be pruned or recruited for other tasks (Diamond & Hopson, 1998).

Other windows are more plastic, but still significant. It is important to remember that learning can occur in each of the areas for the rest of our lives, even after a window tapers off. However, the

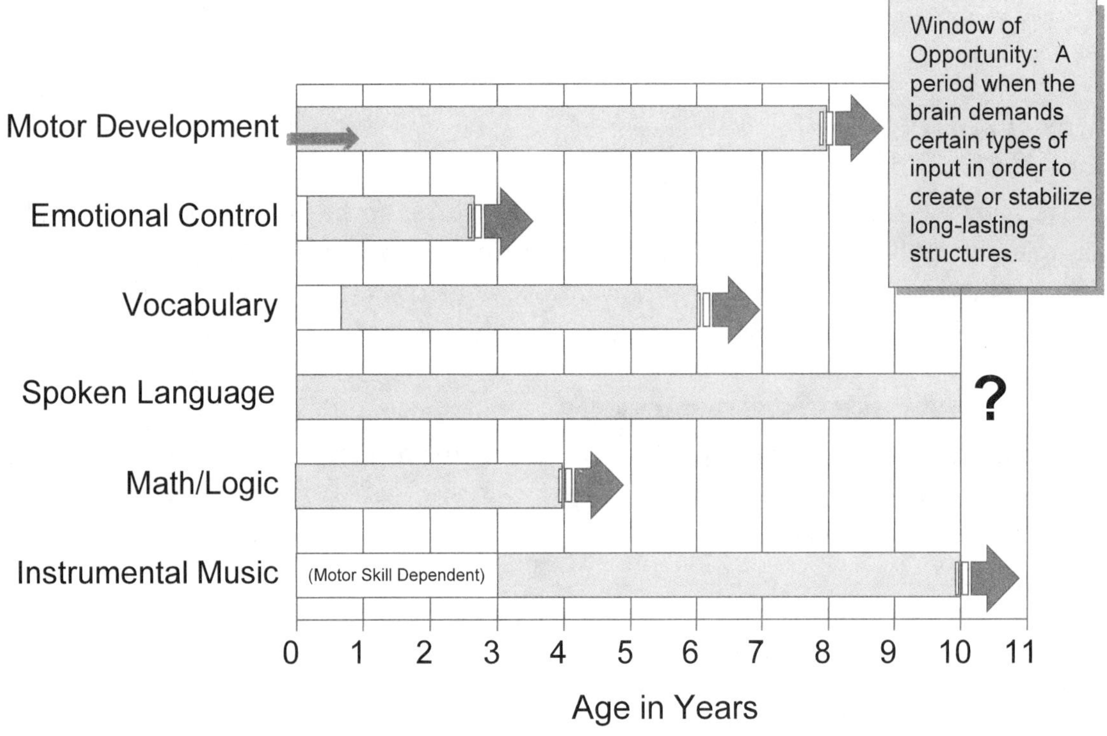

Figure 1.5 The chart shows some of the sensitive periods for learning during childhood, according to current research. Future studies may modify the ranges shown in the chart. It is important to remember that learning occurs throughout our entire life.

skill level probably will not be as high. This ability of the brain to continually change during our lifetime in subtle ways as a result of experience is referred to as *plasticity*.

An intriguing question is why the windows taper off so early in life, especially since the average life span is now over 75 years of age. One possible explanation is that these developmental spurts are genetically determined and were set in place many thousands of years ago when our life span was closer to 20 years. Figure 1.5 shows just a few of the windows which we will examine to understand their importance.

Motor Development

This window opens during fetal development. Those who have borne children remember all too well the movement of the fetus during the third trimester as motor connections and systems are consolidating. The child's ability to learn motor skills appears to be most pronounced in the first eight years. Such seemingly simple tasks as crawling and walking require complicated associations of neural networks, including integrating information from the balance sensors in the inner ear and output signals to the leg and arm muscles. Of course, a person can learn motor skills after

> ***What is learned while a window of opportunity is opened will most likely be learned masterfully.***

the window tapers off. However, what is learned while it is open will most likely be learned masterfully. For example, most concert virtuosos, Olympic medalists, and professional players of individual sports (e.g., tennis and golf) began practicing their skills by the age of eight.

Emotional Control

The window for developing emotional control seems to be from two to 30 months. During that time, the limbic (emotional) system and the frontal lobe's rational system are evaluating each other's ability to get its owner what it wants. It is hardly a fair match. Studies of human brain growth suggest that the emotional (and older) system develops faster than the frontal lobes (Figure 1.6) (Beatty, 2001; Goldberg, 2001; Gazzaniga, Ivry, & Mangun, 2002; Luciana, Conklin, Hooper, & Yarger, 2005; Paus, 2005; Restak, 2001; Steinberg, 2005). Consequently, the emotional system is more likely to win the tug-of-war for control. If tantrums almost always get the child satisfaction when the window is open, then that is likely the method the child will use when the window tapers off. This constant emotional-rational battle is one of the major contributors to the "terrible twos." Certainly, one can learn to control emotions after that age. But what the child learned during that open window period will be difficult to change, and it will strongly influence what is learned after the window tapers off.

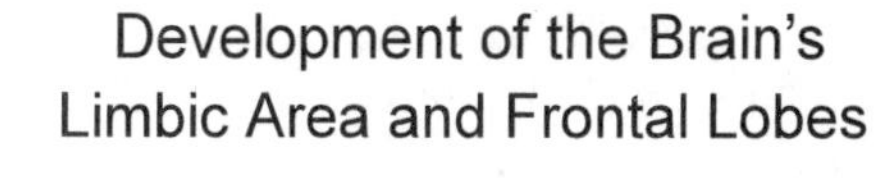

The struggle between the emotional and rational systems is a major contributor to the "terrible twos."

In an astonishing example of how nurturing can influence nature, there is considerable evidence confirming that how parents respond to their children emotionally during this time frame can encourage or stifle genetic tendencies. Biology is not destiny, so gene expression is not necessarily inevitable. To produce their effects, genes must be turned on. The cells on the tip of your nose contain the same genetic code as those in your stomach lining. But the gene that codes for producing stomach acid is activated in your stomach, yet idled on your nose. For example, shyness is a trait that seems to be partially hereditary. If parents are overprotective of their bashful young daughter, the toddler is likely to remain shy. On the other hand, if they encourage her to interact with other toddlers, she may overcome it. Thus, genetic tendencies toward intelligence, sociability, or schizophrenia and aggression can be ignited or moderated by parental response and other environmental influences (Reiss, Neiderheiser, Hetherington, & Plomin, 2000).

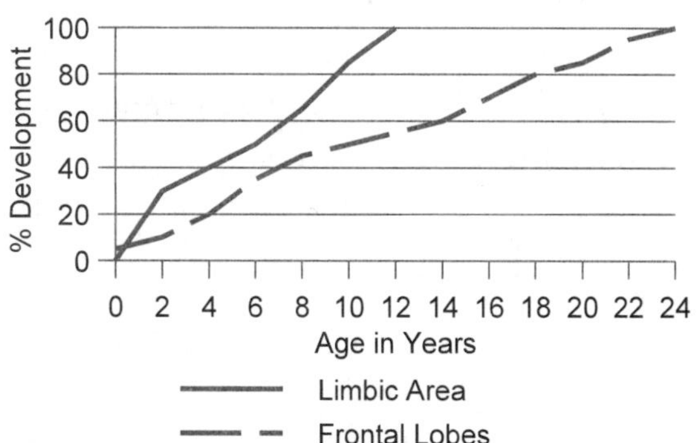

Figure 1.6 Based on research studies, this chart suggests the possible degree of development of the brain's limbic area and frontal lobes. The 10- to 12-year lag in the full development of the frontal lobes (the brain's rational system) explains why so many adolescents and young adults get involved in risky situations.

Vocabulary

Because the human brain is genetically predisposed for language, babies start uttering sounds and babble nonsense phrases as early as the age of two months. By the age of eight months, infants begin to try out simple words like "mama" and "dada." The language areas of the brain become really active at 18 to 20 months. A toddler can learn 10 or more words per day, yielding a vocabulary of about 900 words at age three, increasing to 2,500 to 3,000 words by the age of five.

Here's testimony to the power of talk: Researchers have shown that babies whose mothers talked to them more had significantly larger vocabularies. Knowing a word is not the same as understanding its meaning. So it is crucial for parents to encourage their children to use new words in a context that demonstrates they know what the words mean. Children who know the meaning of most of the words in their large vocabulary will start school with a greater likelihood that learning to read will be easier and quicker.

Language Acquisition

The newborn's brain is not the *tabula rasa* (blank slate) we once thought. Certain areas are specialized for specific stimuli, including spoken language. The window for acquiring spoken language opens soon after birth and tapers off around the ages of 10 to 12 years. Beyond that age, learning any language becomes more difficult. The genetic impulse to learn language is so strong that children found in feral environments often make up their own language. There is also evidence that the human ability to acquire grammar may have a specific window of opportunity in the early years (Diamond & Hopson, 1998). Knowing this, it seems illogical that many schools still wait to *start* new language instruction in middle school or high school rather than in the primary grades. Chapter 5 deals in greater detail with how the brain acquires spoken language.

Mathematics and Logic

How and when the young brain understands numbers is uncertain, but there is mounting evidence that infants have a rudimentary number sense which is wired into certain brain sites at birth (Butterworth, 1999). The purpose of these sites is to categorize the world in terms of the "number of things" in a collection, that is, they can tell the difference between two of something and three of something. We drive along a road and see horses in a field. While we are noticing that they are brown and black, we cannot help but see that there are four of them. Researchers have also found that toddlers as young as two recognize the relationships between numbers as large as 4 and 5, even though they are not able to verbally label them. This research shows that fully functioning language ability is not needed to support numerical thinking (Brannon & van der Walle, 2001).

Instrumental Music

All cultures create music, so we can assume that it is an important part of being human. Babies respond to music as early as two to three months of age. A window for creating music may be open at birth, but obviously neither the baby's vocal chords nor motor skills are adequate to sing or to play an instrument. Around the age of three years, most toddlers have sufficient manual dexterity to play a piano (Mozart was playing the harpsichord and composing at agc four). Several studies have shown that children ages three to four years who received piano lessons scored significantly higher in spatial-temporal tasks than a group who did not get the instrumental music training. Further, the increase was long-term. Brain imaging reveals that creating instrumental music excites the same regions of the left frontal lobe responsible for mathematics and logic. See Chapter 6 for more on the effects of music on the brain and learning.

School districts should communicate with the parents of newborns and offer their services and resources to help parents succeed as the first teachers of their children.

Research on how the young brain develops suggests that an enriched home and preschool environment during the early years can help children build neural connections and make full use of their mental abilities. Because of the importance of early years, I believe school districts should communicate with the parents of newborns and offer their services and resources to help parents succeed as the first teachers of their children. Such programs are already in place on a statewide basis in Michigan, Missouri, and Kentucky, and similar programs sponsored by local school districts are springing up elsewhere. But we need to work faster toward achieving this important goal.

THE BRAIN AS A NOVELTY SEEKER

Part of our success as a species can be attributed to the brain's persistent interest in novelty, that is, changes occurring in the environment. The brain is constantly scanning its environment for stimuli. When an unexpected stimulus arises—such as a loud noise from an empty room—a rush of adrenalin closes down all unnecessary activity and focuses the brain's attention so it can spring into action. Conversely, an environment that contains mainly predictable or repeated stimuli (like some classrooms?) lowers the brain's interest in the outside world and tempts it to turn within for novel sensations.

Environmental Factors That Enhance Novelty

We often hear teachers remark that students are more different today in the way they learn than ever before. They seem to have shorter attention spans and bore easily. Why is that? Is there something happening in the environment of learners that alters the way they approach the learning process?

The Environment of the Past

The home environment for many children several decades ago was quite different from that of today. For example,

- The home was quieter—some might say boring compared to today.
- Parents and children did a lot of talking and reading.
- The family unit was more stable and ate tegether, and the dinner hour was an opportunity for parents to discuss their children's activities as well as reaffirm their love and support.
- If the home had a television, it was in a common area and controlled by adults. What children watched could be carefully monitored.
- School was an interesting place because it had television, films, field trips, and guest speakers. Because there were few other distractions, school was an important influence in a child's life and the primary source of information.
- The neighborhood was also an important part of growing up. Children played together, developing their motor skills as well as learning the social skills needed to interact successfully with other children in the neighborhood.

The Environment of Today

In recent years, children have been growing up in a very different environment.

- Family units are not as stable as they once were. Single-parent families are more common, and children have fewer opportunities to talk with the adults who care for them. Their dietary habits are changing as home cooking is becoming a lost art.
- They are surrounded by media: cell phones, multiple televisions, movies, computers, video games, e-mail, and the Internet. Teens spend nearly 17 hours a week on the Internet and nearly 14 hours a week watching television (Guterl, 2003).
- Many 10- to 18-year olds can now watch television and play with other technology in their own bedrooms, leading to sleep deprivation. Furthermore, with no adult present, what kind of moral compass is evolving in the impressionable pre-adolescent mind as a result of watching programs containing violence and sex on television and the Internet?
- They get information from many different sources beside school.
- The multi-media environment divides their attention. Even newscasts are different. In the past, only the reporter's face was on the screen. Now, the TV screen I am looking at is loaded with information. Three people are reporting in from different corners of the world. Additional non-related news is scrolling across the bottom, and the stock market averages are changing in the lower right-hand corner just below the local time and temperature. For me, these tidbits are distracting and are forcing me to split my attention into several components. I find myself missing a reporter's comment because a scrolling item caught my attention. Yet, children have become accustomed to these information-rich and rapidly changing messages.

They can pay attention to several things at once, but they do not go into any one thing in depth.

- They spend much more time indoors with their technology, thereby missing outdoor opportunities to develop gross motor skills and socialization skills necessary to communicate and act personally with others. One unintended consequence of spending so much time indoors is the rapid rise in the number of overweight children and adolescents, now more than 15 percent of 6- to 19-year olds.
- Young brains have responded to the technology by changing their functioning and organization to accommodate the large amount of stimulation occurring in the environment. By acclimating itself to these changes, brains respond more than ever to the unique and different—what is called *novelty*. There is a dark side to this increased novelty-seeking behavior. Some adolescents who perceive little novelty in their environment may turn to mind-altering drugs, such as ecstasy and amphetamines, for stimulation. This drug dependence can further enhance the brain's demand for novelty to the point that it becomes unbalanced and resorts to extremely risky behavior.
- Their diet contains increasing amounts of substances that can affect brain and body functions. Caffeine is a strong brain stimulant, considered safe for most adults in small quantities. But caffeine is found in many of the foods and drinks that teens consume daily. Too much caffeine causes insomnia, anxiety, and nausea. Some teens can also develop allergies to aspartame (an artificial sugar found in children's vitamins and many "lite" foods) and other food additives. Possible symptoms of these allergic reactions include hyperactivity, difficulty concentrating, and headaches (Bateman, et al., 2004; Millichap & Yee, 2003).

When we add to this mix the changes in family lifestyles and the temptations of alcohol and drugs, we can realize how very different the environment of today's child is from that of just 15 years ago.

Have Schools Changed With the Environment?

Many educators are recognizing the characteristics of the new brain, but they do not always agree on what to do about it. Granted, teaching methodologies are changing, new technologies are being used, and teachers are even introducing pop music and culture to supplement traditional classroom materials. But schools and teaching are not changing fast enough. In high schools, lecturing continues to be the main method of instruction, primarily because of the vast amount of required curriculum material and the pressure of increased accountability and testing. Students remark that school is a dull, nonengaging environment that is much less interesting than what is available outside school.

> ***As we continue to develop a more scientifically based understanding about today's novel brain, we must decide how this new knowledge should change what we do in schools and classrooms.***

Despite the recent efforts of educators to deal with this new brain, many high school students still do not feel challenged. In a 2004 survey of 90,000 high school students in 26 states, 55 percent of students said they devoted three hours a week or less to classroom preparation, but 65 percent reported getting grades of A or B. Survey administrators reported that many students said they did not feel challenged to do their best work and thus were more likely to spend time doing personal reading online than doing assigned reading for their classes (HSSSE, 2005).

In another survey of 10,500 high school students, conducted by the National Governors Association, more than one-third of the students said their school had not done a good job challenging them to think critically and analyze problems. About 11 percent said they were thinking of dropping out of school. Over one-third of this group said they were leaving because they were "not learning anything" (NGA, 2005).

The Gallup Poll asked nearly 800 students ages 13 to 17 in an online survey to select three adjectives that best described how they felt about school. Half the students chose "bored" and 42 percent chose "tired" (Gallup, 2004a).

Clearly, we educators have to rethink now, more than ever, how we must adjust schools to accommodate and maintain the interest of this new brain. As we continue to develop a more scientifically based understanding about today's novel brain and how it learns, we must decide how this new knowledge should change what we do in schools and classrooms.

What's Coming Up?

Now that we have reviewed some basic parts of the brain, and discussed how the brain of today's student has become acclimated to novelty, the next step is to look at a model of how the brain processes new information. Why do students remember so little and forget so much? How does the brain decide what to retain and what to discard? The answers to these and other important questions about brain processing will be found in the next chapter.

PRACTITIONER'S CORNER

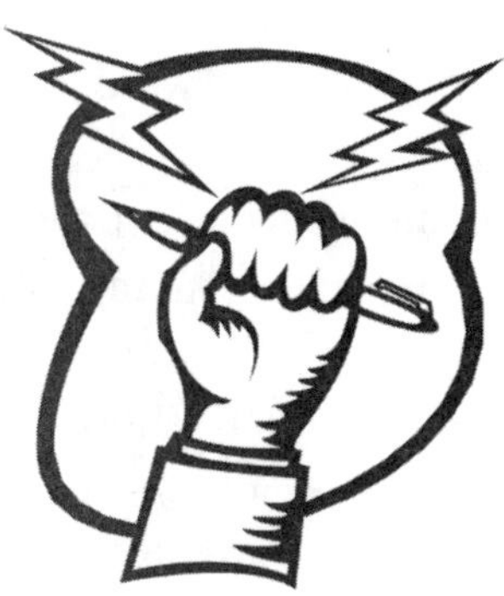

Fist for a Brain

This activity shows how you can use your fists to represent the human brain. Metaphors are excellent learning and remembering tools. When you are comfortable with the activity, share it with your students. They are often very interested in knowing how their brain is constructed and how it works. This is a good example of novelty.

1. Extend both arms with palms open and facing down and lock your thumbs.

2. Curl your fingers to make two fists.

3. Turn your fists inward until the knuckles touch.

4. While the fists are touching, pull both toward your chest until you are looking down on your knuckles. This is the approximate size of your brain! Not as big as you thought? Remember, it's not the size of the brain that matters; it's the number of connections between the neurons. Those connections form when stimuli result in learning. The thumbs are the front and are crossed to remind us that the left side of the brain controls the right side of the body, and the right side of the brain controls the left side of the body. The knuckles and outside part of the hands represent the **cerebrum** or thinking part of the brain.

5. Spread your palms apart while keeping the knuckles touching. Look at the tips of your fingers, which represent the **limbic** or emotional area. Note how this area is buried deep within the brain, and how the fingers are mirror-imaged. This reminds us that most of the structures of the limbic system are duplicated in each hemisphere.

6. The wrists are the **brainstem** where vital body functions (such as body temperature, heart beat, blood pressure) are controlled. Rotating your hands shows how the brain can move on top of the spinal column, which is represented by your forearms.

PRACTITIONER'S CORNER

Review of Brain Area Functions

Here is an opportunity to assess your understanding of the major brain areas. Write in the table below your own key words and phrases to describe the functions of each of the eight brain areas. Then draw an arrow to each brain area on the diagram below and label it.

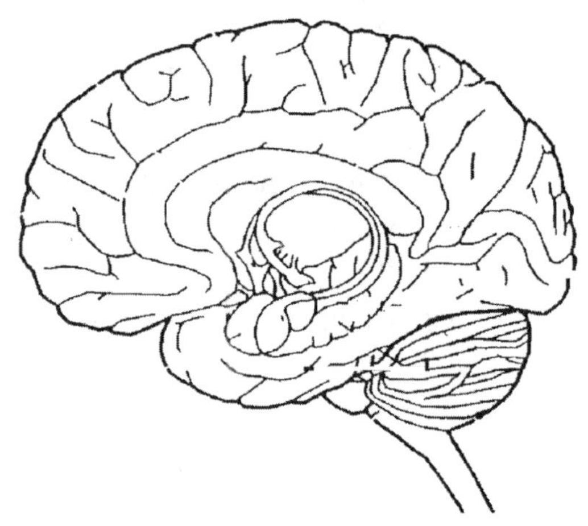

Cerebrum:
Frontal Lobe:
Thalamus:
Hypothalamus:
Hippocampus:
Amygdala:
Cerebellum:
Brainstem:

PRACTITIONER'S CORNER

Using Novelty in Lessons

Using novelty does *not* mean that the teacher needs to be a stand-up comic or the classroom a three-ring circus. It simply means using a varied teaching approach that involves more student activity. Here are a few suggestions for incorporating novelty in your lessons.

- **Humor.** There are many positive benefits that come from using humor in the classroom at *all* grade levels. See the **Practitioner's Corner** in Chapter 2 (p. 63) which suggests guidelines and beneficial reasons for using humor.

- **Movement.** When we sit for more than twenty minutes, our blood pools in our seat and in our feet. By getting up and moving, we recirculate that blood. Within a minute, there is about 15 percent more blood in our brain. We do think better on our feet than on our seat! Students sit too much in classrooms, especially in secondary schools. Look for ways to get students up and moving, especially when they are verbally rehearsing what they have learned.

- **Multi-Sensory Instruction.** Today's students are acclimated to a multi-sensory environment. They are more likely to give attention if there are interesting, colorful visuals and if they can walk around and talk about their learning.

- **Quiz Games.** Have students develop a quiz game or other similar activity to test each other on their knowledge of the concepts taught. This is a common strategy in elementary classrooms, but underutilized in secondary schools. Besides being fun, it has the added value of making students rehearse and understand the concepts in order to create the quiz questions and answers.

- **Music.** Although the research is inconclusive, there are some benefits of playing music in the classroom at certain times during the learning episode. See the **Practitioner's Corner** in Chapter 6 (p. 235) on the use of music.

PRACTITIONER'S CORNER

Preparing the Brain for Taking a Test

Taking a test can be a stressful event. Chances are your students will perform better on a test of cognitive or physical performance if you prepare the brain by doing the following:

- **Exercise.** Get the students up to do some exercise for just two minutes. Jumping jacks are good because the students stay in place. Students who may not want to jump up and down can do five brisk round trip walks along the longest wall of the classroom. The purpose here is to get the blood oxygenated and moving faster.

- **Fruit.** Besides oxygen, brain cells also need glucose for fuel. Fruit is an excellent source of glucose. Students should eat about 2 ounces (over 50 grams) of fruit. Dried fruit, such as raisins, is convenient. Avoid fruit drinks as they often contain just fructose, a fruit sugar that does not provide immediate energy to cells. The chart below shows how just 50 grams of glucose increased long-term memory recall in a group of young adults by 35 percent and recall from working memory by over 20 percent (Korol & Gold, 1998).

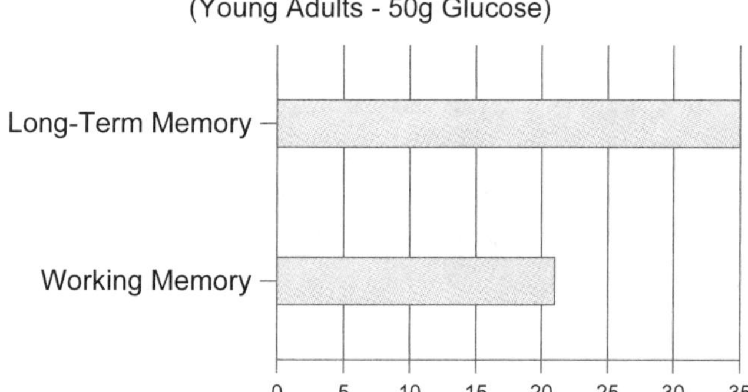

- **Water.** Wash down the fruit with an 8-ounce glass of water. The water gets the sugar into the bloodstream faster and hydrates the brain.

Wait about five minutes after these steps before giving the test. That should be enough time for the added glucose to fire up the brain cells. The effect lasts for only about 30 minutes, so the steps need to be repeated periodically for longer tests.

Chapter 1—Basic Brain Facts

Key Points to Ponder

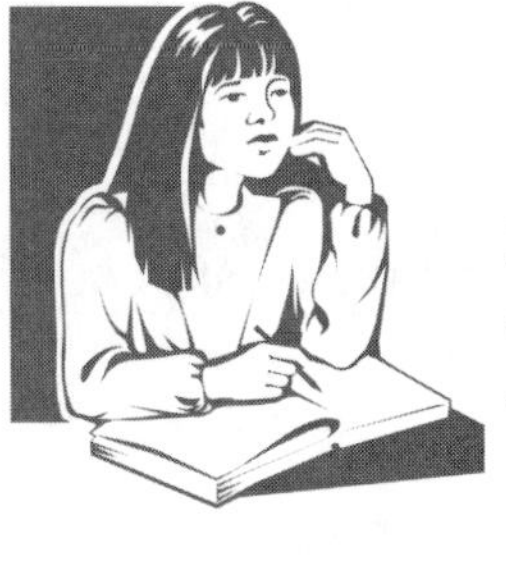

Jot down on this page key points, ideas, strategies, and resources you want to consider later. This sheet is your personal journal summary and will help to jog your memory.

Chapter 2

How the Brain Processes Information

There are probably more differences in human brains than in any other animal partly because the human brain does most of its developing in the outside world.

—Robert Ornstein and Richard Thompson, *The Amazing Brain*

Chapter Highlights: This chapter presents a modern dynamic model of how the brain deals with information from the senses. It covers the behavior of the two temporary memories, the criteria for long-term storage, and the impact of the self-concept on learning.

Although the brain remains largely a mystery beyond its own understanding, we are slowly uncovering more about its baffling processes. Using scanning technologies, researchers can display in vivid color the differences in brain cell metabolism that occur in response to different types of brain work. A computer constructs a color-coded map indicating what different areas are doing during such activities as learning new words, analyzing tones, doing mathematical calculations, or responding to images. One thing is clear: The brain calls selected areas into play depending on what the individual is doing at the moment. This knowledge encourages us to construct models that explain data and behavior, but models are useful only when they contain some predictability about specific operations. In choosing a model, it is necessary to select those specific operations that can be meaningfully depicted and represented in a way that is consistent with more recent research findings.

THE INFORMATION PROCESSING MODEL

Several models exist to explain brain behavior. In designing a model for this book, I needed one that would accurately represent the complex research of neuroscientists in such a way as to be understood by educational practitioners. I recognize that a model is just one person's view of reality, and I readily admit that this particular information processing model comes closest to *my* view of how the brain learns. It differs from other models in that it escapes the limits of the computer metaphor and recognizes that learning, storing, and remembering are dynamic and interactive processes. Beyond that, the model incorporates much of the recent findings of research and is sufficiently flexible to adjust to new findings as they are revealed. I have already made several changes in this model since I began working with it nearly 25 years ago. A few additional changes are the result of new information learned since the second edition of this book was published. My hope is that classroom teachers will be encouraged to reflect on their methodology and decide if there are new insights here that could affect their instruction and improve learning.

Origins of the Model

The precursor of this model was developed by Robert Stahl (1985) of Arizona State University in the early 1980s. Stahl's more complex model synthesized the research in the 1960s and 1970s on cognitive processing and learning. His goal was to convince teacher educators that they should use his model to help prospective teachers understand how and why learning occurs. He also used the model to develop an elaborate and fascinating learning taxonomy designed to promote higher-order thinking skills. Certain components of the model needed to be altered as a result of subsequent discoveries in neuroscience.

Usefulness of the Model

The model discussed here (Figure 2.1) has been updated so that it can be used by the widest range of teacher educators and practitioners. It uses common objects to represent various stages in the process. Even this revised model does not pretend to include all the ways that researchers believe the human brain deals with information, thought, and behavior. It limits its scope to the major cerebral operations that deal with the collecting, evaluating, storing, and retrieving of information—the parts most useful to educators.

The model starts with information from our environment and shows how the senses reject or accept it for further processing. It then explains the two temporary memories, how they operate, and

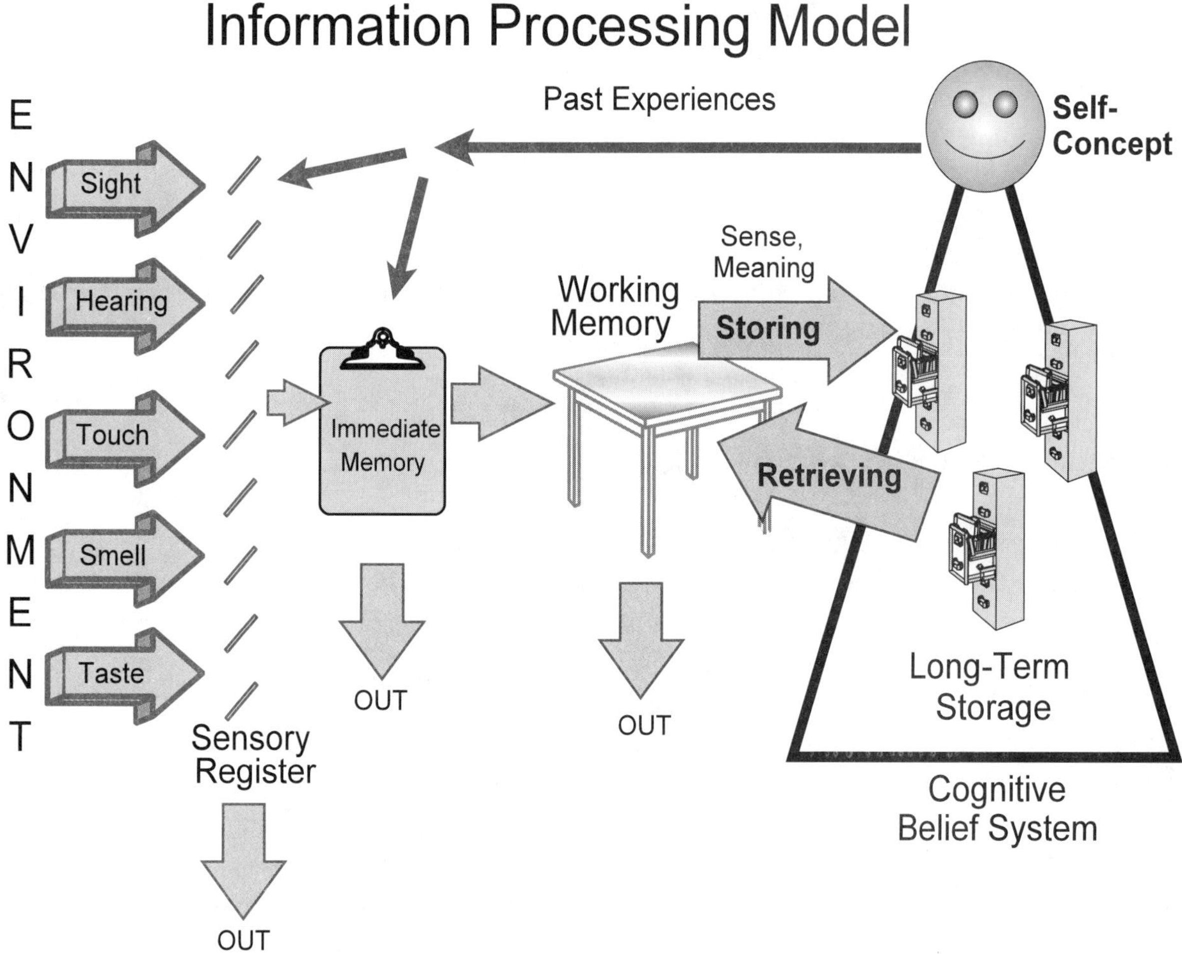

Figure 2.1 The Information Processing Model represents a simplified explanation of how the brain deals with information from the environment. Information from the senses passes through the sensory register to immediate memory and then on to working memory for conscious processing. If the learner attaches sense and meaning to the learning, it is likely to be stored. The self-concept often determines how much attention the learner will give to new information.

the factors that determine if a learning is likely to be stored. Finally, it shows the inescapable impact that experiences and self-concept have on future learning. The model is simple, but the processes are extraordinarily complex. Knowing how the human brain seems to process information and learn can help teachers plan lessons that students are more likely to understand and remember.

Limitations of the Model

Although the explanation of the model will follow items going through the processing system, it is important to note that this linear approach is used solely for simplicity and clarity. Much of the recent evidence on memory supports a model of parallel processing. That is, many items are processed quickly and simultaneously (within limits), taking different paths through and out of the

> ***The brain changes its own properties as a result of experience.***

system. Memories are dynamic and dispersed, and the brain has the capacity to change its own properties as the result of experience. Even though the model may seem to represent learning and remembering as a mechanistic process, it must be remembered that we are describing a *biological process*. Nonetheless, I have avoided a detailed discussion of the biochemical changes that occur within and between neurons. That would not contribute to the understanding necessary to convert the fruits of research and this model into successful classroom practice, which is, after all, our goal.

Inadequacy of the Computer Model

The rapid proliferation of computers has encouraged the use of the computer model to explain brain functions. This is indeed tempting, especially as computers become more complex. Using the analogy of input, processing, and output seems so natural, but there are serious problems with such a model. Certainly, the smallest hand-held calculator can out-tally the human brain in solving complex mathematical operations. Larger computers can play chess, translate one language into another, and correct massive manuscripts for most spelling and grammatical errors in just seconds. The brain performs more slowly because of the time it takes for a nerve impulse to travel along the axon, synaptic delays, and because the capacity of its working memory is limited. But computers cannot exercise judgment with the ease of the human brain. Even the most sophisticated computers are closed linear systems limited to binary code, the 0s and 1s in linear sequences that are the language of computer operations.

The human brain has no such limitations. It is an open, parallel-processing system continually interacting with the physical and social worlds outside. It analyzes, integrates, and synthesizes information and abstracts generalities from it. Each neuron is alive and altered by its experiences and its environment. As you read these words, neurons are interacting with each other, reforming and dissolving storage sites, and establishing different electrical patterns that correspond to your new learning.

> ***As you read these words, neurons in your brain are interacting with each other in patterns that correspond to your new learning.***

How the brain stores information is also very different from a computer. The brain stores sequences of patterns, and recalling just one piece of a pattern can activate the whole. We can also identify the same thing in different forms, such as recognizing our best friend from behind or by her walk or voice. Computers cannot deal well with such variations (Hawkins & Blakeslee, 2004). Moreover, emotions play an important role in human processing and creativity. And the ideas generated by the human brain often come from images, not from logical propositions. For these and many other reasons, the computer model is, in my opinion, inadequate and misleading.

At first glance, the model may seem to perpetuate the traditional approach to teaching and learning—that students repeat newly learned information in quizzes, tests, and reports. On the contrary, the new research is revealing that students are more likely to gain greater understanding of and derive greater pleasure from learning when allowed to *transform* the learning into creative thoughts and products. This model emphasizes the power of transfer during learning and the importance of moving students through higher levels of complexity of thought. This will be explained further in Chapters 4 and 5.

The Senses

Our brain takes in more information from our environment in a single day than the largest computer does in a year. That information is detected by our five senses. (Note: Apart from the five classical senses of sight, hearing, smell, touch, and taste, our body has special sensory receptors that detect internal signals. For example, we have receptors inside the ear and body muscles that detect the body's movement and position in space; sensory hairs in the ear that detect balance and gravity; stretch receptors in muscles to help the brain coordinate muscular contraction; and pain receptors throughout the body. For the purposes of the model, however, I have focused on the classical senses because they are the major receptors of *external* stimuli.)

All sensory stimuli enter the brain as a stream of electrical impulses that result from neurons firing in sequence along the specific sensory pathways. The brain sits in a black box (the skull) and does not see light waves or hear sound waves. Rather, certain specialized modules of neurons process the electrical impulses created by the light and sound waves into what the brain *perceives* as vision and sound.

The senses do not all contribute equally to our learning. Over the course of our lives, sight, hearing, and touch (including kinesthetic experiences) contribute the most. Our senses constantly collect tens of thousands of bits of information from the environment every second, even while we sleep. That number may seem very high, but think about it. The nerve endings on your skin are detecting the clothes you are wearing. Your ears pick up sounds around you, the rods and cones in your eyes are reacting to this print as they move across the page, you may still be tasting recent food or drink, and your nose may be detecting an odor. Put these data together and you see how they can add up. Of course, the stimuli must be strong enough for the senses to detect and record them.

Sensory Register

Imagine if the brain had to give its full attention to all those bits of data at once. We would blow the cerebral equivalent of a fuse! Fortunately, the brain has evolved a system for screening all these data to determine their importance to the individual. This system involves the *thalamus* (located in the limbic system) and a portion of the brain stem known as the *reticular activation system* (RAS). This system, which is also referred to as the *sensory register*, is drawn in the model as the side view of Venetian blind slats (see the slashes in Figure 2.1). Like the blinds, the sensory register filters incoming information to determine how important it is.

All incoming sensory information (except smell) is sent first to the thalamus, which briefly monitors the strength and nature of the sensory impulses for survival content and, in just milliseconds (a millisecond is 1/1,000th of a second), uses the individual's past experiences to determine the data's degree of importance. Most of the data signals are unimportant, so the sensory register allows them to drop out of the processing system. Have you ever noticed how you can be in a room studying while there is construction noise outside? Eventually, it seems that you no longer hear the noise. Your sensory register is blocking these repetitive stimuli, allowing your conscious brain to focus on more important things. This process is called *perceptual* or *sensory filtering*, and, to a large degree, we are consciously unaware of it.

The sensory register does hold sensory information for a very brief period of time (seconds). This is referred to as *sensory memory.* Let's say you are intently watching a football game during the final minutes of play. Your spouse comes in and starts talking about an important matter. After a few minutes, your spouse says, "You're not listening to me!" Without batting an eye you say, "Yes, I am," and then proceed to repeat your spouse's last sentence word for word. Fortunately, you captured this sensory memory trace just before it decayed, and nipped a potential argument in the bud.

Short-Term Memory

As researchers gain greater insight into the brain's memory processes, they have had to devise and revise terms that describe the various stages of memory. *Short-term memory* is used by cognitive neuroscientists to include all of the early steps of temporary memory that will lead to stable long-term memory. Short-term memory primarily includes *immediate memory* and *working memory* (Gazzaniga, et al., 2002; Squire & Kandel, 1999).

Immediate Memory

Sensory data that are not lost move from the thalamus to the sensory processing areas of the cortex and through the first of two temporary memories, now called *immediate memory*. The idea that we seem to have two temporary memories is a way of explaining how the brain deals with large amounts of sensory data, and how we can continue to process these stimuli subconsciously for many seconds beyond the sensory register's time limits. Indeed, some neuroscientists equate sensory memory and immediate memory, arguing that separating them is more a convenience rather than a biological necessity.

For our purposes, we will represent immediate memory in the model as a clipboard, a place where we put information briefly until we make a decision on how to dispose of it. Immediate memory operates subconsciously or consciously and holds data for up to about 30 seconds. (Note: The numbers used in this chapter are averages over time. There are always exceptions to these values as a result of human variations or pathologies.) The individual's experiences determine its importance. If the item is of little or no importance within this time frame, it drops out of the system. For example, when you look up the telephone number of the local pizza parlor, you usually can remember it just long enough to make the call. After that, the number is of no further importance and drops out of

You cannot recall information that your brain does not retain.

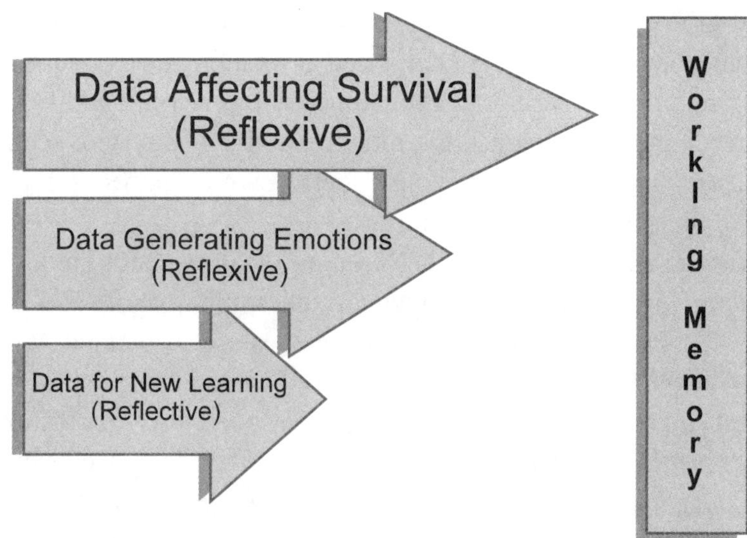

Figure 2.2 Data affecting survival and data generating emotions are processed ahead of data for new learning, which in school is called curriculum.

immediate memory. Later on, you will have little success in remembering the entire number because you cannot recall information that your brain does not retain.

Examples of Immediate Memory at Work. Here are two other examples to understand how the processing occurs up to this point. Suppose you decide to wear a new pair of shoes to work today. They are snug, so when you put them on, the receptors in your skin send pain impulses to the sensory register. For a short time you feel discomfort. After a while, however, as you get involved with work, you do not notice the discomfort signals anymore. The sensory register is now blocking the impulses from reaching your consciousness. Should you move your foot in a way that causes the shoe to pinch, however, the sensory register will pass this pain stimulus along to your consciousness and you become aware of it.

Another example: You are sitting in a classroom and a police car with its siren wailing passes by. Experience reminds you that a siren is an important sound. Signals from the sensory register pass the auditory stimuli over to immediate memory. If over the next few seconds the sound of the siren gets fainter, experience signals the immediate memory that the sound is of no further importance and the auditory data are blocked and dropped from the system. All this is happening subconsciously while your attention is focused on something else. If asked about the sound 15 minutes later, you will not remember it. You cannot recall what you have not stored.

Suppose, on the other hand, that the siren sound gets louder and suddenly stops, followed by another siren that gets louder and stops. Experience will now signal that the sounds are important because they are nearby, may affect your survival, and therefore require your attention. At this point, the now-important auditory data move rapidly into working memory for conscious processing so that you can decide what action to take.

Threats and Emotions Affect Memory Processing. This last example illustrates another characteristic of brain processing: There is a hierarchy of response to sensory input (Figure 2.2). Any input that is of higher priority diminishes the processing of data of lower priority. The brain's main job is to help its owner survive. Thus, data interpreted as posing a threat to the survival of the individual, such as a burning odor, a snarling dog, or someone threatening bodily injury, are processed immediately. Upon receiving the stimulus, the reticular activating system sends a rush of adrenaline throughout the brain. This reflexive response shuts down all unnecessary activity and directs the brain's attention to the source of the stimulus.

Emotional data also take high priority. When an individual responds emotionally to a situation, the older limbic system (stimulated by the amygdala) takes a major role and the complex cerebral processes are suspended. We have all had experiences when anger, fear of the unknown, or joy quickly overcame our rational thoughts. This reflexive override of conscious thought can be strong enough to cause temporary inability to talk ("I was dumbfounded") or move ("I froze"). This happens because the hippocampus is susceptible to stress hormones that can inhibit cognitive functioning and long-term memory.

> ***Students must feel physically safe and emotionally secure before they can focus on the curriculum.***

Under certain conditions, emotions can enhance memory by causing the release of hormones that stimulate the amygdala to signal brain regions to strengthen memory. Strong emotions can shut down conscious processing during the event while enhancing our memory of it. Emotion is a powerful and misunderstood force in learning and memory. Another way of stating the hierarchy illustrated in Figure 2.2 is that before students will turn their attention to cognitive learning (the curriculum), they must feel physically safe and emotionally secure.

Over the years, most teacher-training classes have told prospective teachers to focus on reason, cover the curriculum, and avoid emotions in their lessons. Now, we need to enlighten educators about how emotions consistently affect attention and learning. Districts must ensure that schools are free of weapons and violence. Teachers can then promote emotional security in the classroom by establishing a positive climate that encourages students to take appropriate risks. Students must sense that the teacher wants to help them be right rather than catch them being wrong.

> ***How a person "feels" about a learning situation determines the amount of attention devoted to it.***

Moreover, superintendents and board members need to examine their actions, which set the emotional climate of a district. Is it a place where people want to come to work? Does the district reward or frown on appropriate risk taking?

How a person "feels" about a learning situation determines the amount of attention devoted to it. Emotions interact with reason to support or inhibit learning. To be successful learners and productive citizens, we need to know how to use our emotions intelligently. Thus, we need to explore what and how we teach students about their emotions. For example, we could teach about controlling impulses, delaying gratification, expressing feelings, managing relationships, and reducing stress. Students should recognize that they can manage their emotions for greater productivity and can develop emotional skills for greater success in life.

Working Memory

Working memory is also a temporary memory and the place where conscious, rather than subconscious, processing occurs. The information processing model represents working memory as a work table, a place of limited capacity where we can build, take apart, or rework ideas for eventual storage somewhere else. When something is in working memory, it generally captures our focus and demands our attention. Information in working memory can come from the sensory/immediate memories or be retrieved from long-term memory. Brain imaging studies show that most of working memory's activity occurs in the frontal lobes, although other parts of the brain are often called into action.

In recent years, researchers have compiled studies suggesting that the functioning of working memory can be explained by a three-part system (Figure 2.3) containing a *central control* (executive) *mechanism* and two subordinate components involved in rehearsal (Baddeley, 1995; Gazzaniga et al., 2002). The central control mechanism manages the interactions between the two subordinate systems and long-term memory. The *phonological loop* is the mechanism that uses auditory signals to code information into working memory, such as when we are talking about what we are learning. The *visuospatial sketchpad* allows for encoding information into working memory in solely visual or as a combination of visual and spatial (visuospatial) codes. This three-part model suggests that auditory and visual rehearsal *occurring during learning* increase working memory's interactions with long-term memory, raising the probability it will be stored.

There is also experimental evidence that when working memory is processing new information, the visuospatial component can become so activated that it has difficulty filtering out non-related images (de Fockert, Rees, Frith, & Lavie, 2001). This finding could have implications for cellular phone use in cars. If the phone conversation requires sufficient thought processing, it may sufficiently stimulate working memory so that the driver becomes distracted by irrelevant sights along the road.

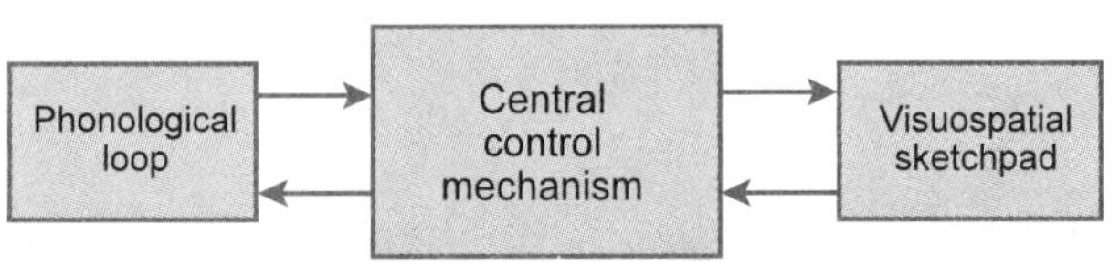

Figure 2.3 This model represents the three-part system that comprises working memory. The central control mechanism manages the phonological loop and the visuospatial sketchpad (Baddeley, 1995).

Capacity of Working Memory. Miller (1956) discovered years ago that working memory can handle only a few items at once. This functional capacity changes with age. Table 2.1 shows how the capacity of working memory increases as one passes through the major growth spurts in cognitive development. Preschool infants can deal with about two items of information at once. Preadolescents can handle three to seven items, with an average of five. Through adolescence, further cognitive expansion occurs and the capacity increases to a range of five to nine, with an average of seven. For most people, that number remains constant throughout life.

More recent research has raised questions about the exact capacity limit of working memory. Some studies suggest that it now may be as low as four items for adults. A few others say it is difficult to state an actual number because variables such as interest, mental time delays, and distractions

Table 2.1 Changes in Capacity of Working Memory With Age

Approximate Age Range in Years	Capacity of Working Memory in Number of Chunks		
	Minimum	**Maximum**	**Average**
Younger Than 5	1	3	2
Between 5 and 14	3	7	5
14 and Older	5	9	7

may undermine and invalidate experimental attempts to find a capacity limit (Cowan, 2001). Nonetheless, most of the research evidence to date supports the notion that working memory has a functional limit, and the number seven continues to be accepted as a workable guideline for adolescents and adults.

Let's test this notion. Get a pencil and a piece of paper. When ready, stare at the number below for seven seconds, then look away and write it down. Ready? Go.

9217053

Check the number you wrote down. Chances are you got it right. Let's try it again with the same rules. Stare at the number below for seven seconds, then look away and write it down. Ready? Go.

4915082637

Again, check the number you wrote down. Did you get all 10 of the digits in the correct sequence? Probably not. Because the digits were random, you had to treat each digit as a single item, and your working memory just ran out of functional capacity.

This limited capacity explains why we have to memorize a song or a poem in stages. We start with the first group of lines by repeating them frequently (a process called *rehearsal*). Then we memorize the next lines and repeat them with the first group, and so on. It is possible to increase the number of items within the functional capacity of working memory through a process called *chunking*. This process will be explained in the next chapter.

Keep the number of items in a lesson objective within the capacity limits of students and they are likely to remember more of what they learned. Less is more!

Why would such a sophisticated structure like the human brain exhibit such severe limitations in working memory capacity? No one knows for sure. One possible explanation is that it is unlikely during the development of the brain thousands of years ago that our ancestors had to process or identify more than one thing at a time. It is also unlikely that they had to make several split-second decisions at the same time. Even in fight-or-flight situations, there probably was only one enemy or predator at a time. Today, however, people are often trying to do several things at once during their workday, making the memory's capacity limits more obvious.

Implications for Teaching. Can you see the implication this functional capacity has on lesson planning? It means that the elementary teacher who expects students to remember in one lesson the eight rules for using the comma is already in trouble. So is the high school or college teacher who wants students to learn in one lesson the names and locations of the 10 most important rivers in the world. Keeping the number of items in a lesson objective within the appropriate capacity limit increases the likelihood that students will remember more of what they learned. Less is more!

Time Limits of Working Memory. Working memory is temporary and can deal with items for only a limited time. How long is that time? This intriguing question has been clinically investigated for over a century, starting with the work of Hermann Ebbinghaus (1850-1909) during the 1880s. He concluded that we can process items intently in working memory (he called it short-term memory) for up to 45 minutes before becoming fatigued. Because Ebbinghaus mainly used himself as the subject to measure retention in laboratory conditions, the results are not readily transferable to the average high school classroom.

Any discussion of time limits for processing new information has to include motivation. People who are intensely motivated about a subject can spend hours reading and processing it. They are not likely to quit until they are physically tired. That is because motivation is essentially an emotional response, and we already know that emotions play an important part in attention and learning. Students are not equally motivated in all subjects. Therefore, these time limits are more likely to apply to students who are in learning episodes that they do not find motivating.

Peter Russell (1979) shows this time span to be much shorter and age dependent. Although his work was done nearly 30 years ago, the time limits for the novelty-seeking brain of today are very similar. For preadolescents, it is 5 to 10 minutes, and for adolescents and adults, 10 to 20 minutes. These are average times, and it is important to understand what the numbers mean. An adolescent (or adult) normally can process an item in working memory *intently* for 10 to 20 minutes before mental fatigue (as opposed to physical fatigue) or boredom with that item occurs and the individual's focus drifts. For focus to continue, there must be some change in the way the individual is dealing with the item. For example, the person may switch from thinking about it to physically using it, or making different connections to other learnings. If something else is not done with the item, it is likely to fade from working memory.

This is not to say that some items cannot remain in working memory for hours, or perhaps days. Sometimes, we have an item that remains unresolved—a question whose answer we seek or a troublesome family or work decision that must be made. These items can remain in working memory, continually commanding some attention and, if of sufficient importance, interfere with our accurate processing of other information.

Implications for Teaching. These time limits suggest that packaging lessons into 15- to 20-minute components are likely to result in maintaining greater student interest than one 40-minute lesson. It seems that, with many lessons, shorter is better! We'll talk more about lesson length and memory in Chapter 3.

Criteria for Long-Term Storage

Now comes the most important decision of all: Should the items in working memory be encoded to long-term storage for future recall, or should they drop out of the system? This is an important decision because we cannot recall what we have not stored. Yet teachers teach with the hope that students will retain the learning objective for future use. So, if the learner is ever to recall this information in the future, it has to be stored.

What criteria does the working memory use to make that decision? Figure 2.2 can help us here. Information that has survival value is quickly stored. You don't want to have to learn every day that walking in front of a moving bus or touching a hot stove can injure you. Strong emotional experiences also have a high likelihood of being permanently stored. We tend to remember the best and worst things that happened to us.

> ***Information is most likely to get stored if it makes sense and has meaning.***

But in classrooms, where the survival and emotional elements are minimal or absent, other factors come into play. It seems that the working memory connects with the learner's past experiences and asks just two questions to determine whether an item is saved or rejected. They are: "Does this make *sense*?" and "Does this have *meaning*?" Imagine the many hours that go into planning and teaching lessons, and it all comes down to these two questions! Let's review them.

- **"Does this make sense?"** This question refers to whether the learner can understand the item on the basis of experience. Does it "fit" into what the learner knows about how the world works? When a student says, "I don't understand," it means the student is having a problem making sense of the learning.
- **"Does it have meaning?"** This question refers to whether the item is *relevant* to the learner. For what purpose should the learner remember it? Meaning, of course, is a very personal thing and is greatly influenced by that person's experiences. The same item can have great meaning for one student and none for another. Questions like "Why do I have to know this?" or "When will I ever use this?" indicate that the student has not, for whatever reason, accepted this learning as relevant.

Here are two examples to explain the difference between sense and meaning. Suppose I tell a 15-year-old student that the minimum age for getting a driver's license in his state is age 16, but it is 17 in a neighboring state. He can understand this information, so it satisfies the sense criterion. But the age in his own state is much more relevant to him, because this is where he will apply for his license. Chances are high that he will remember his own state's minimum age (it has both sense *and* meaning) but will forget that of the neighboring state (it has sense but lacks meaning).

Suppose you are a teacher and you read in the newspaper that the average salary for dock workers last year was $60,000, whereas the average for teachers was $42,000. Both numbers make sense to you, but the average teacher's salary has more meaning because you are in that profession.

Whenever the learner's working memory decides that an item does not make sense or have meaning, the probability of it being stored is extremely low (see Figure 2.4). If either sense or meaning is

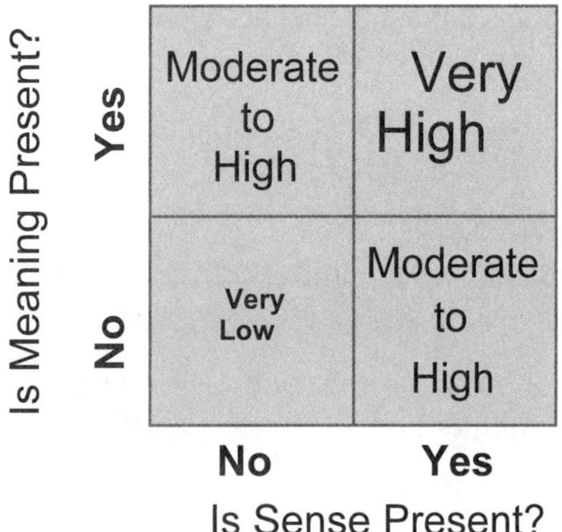

Figure 2.4 The probability of storing information varies with the degree of sense and meaning that are present.

present, the probability of storage increases significantly (assuming, of course, no survival or emotional component). If both sense *and* meaning are present, the likelihood of long-term storage is very high.

Relationship of Sense to Meaning

Sense and meaning are independent of each other. Thus, it is possible to remember an item because it makes sense but has no meaning. If you have ever played *Trivial Pursuit* or similar games, you may have been surprised at some of the answers you knew. If another player asked how you knew that answer, you may have replied, "I don't know. It was just there!" This happens to all of us. During our lifetime, we pick up bits of information that made sense at the time and, although they were trivial and had no meaning, they made their way into our long-term memory.

It is also possible to remember an item that makes no sense but has meaning. My sixth-grade teacher once asked the class to memorize Lewis Carroll's nonsense poem "Jabberwocky." It begins, *Twas brillig, and the slithy toves did gyre and gimble in the wabe.* The poem made no sense to us sixth graders, but when the teacher said that she would call on each of us the next day to recite it before the class, it suddenly had meaning. Since I didn't want to make a fool of myself in front of my peers, I memorized it and recited it correctly the next day, even though I had no idea what the sense of it was.

Brain scans have shown that when new learning is readily comprehensible (sense) and can be connected to past experiences (meaning), there is substantially more cerebral activity followed by dramatically improved retention (Maquire, Frith, & Morris, 1999).

Meaning Is More Significant. Of the two criteria, meaning has the greater impact on the probability that information will be stored. Think of all the television programs you have watched that are NOT stored, even though you spent one or two hours with the program. The show's content or story line made sense to you, but if meaning was absent, you just did not save it. It was *entertainment* and no learning resulted from it. You might have remembered a summary of the show, or whether it was enjoyable or boring, but not the details. On the other hand, if the story reminded you of a personal experience, then meaning was present and you were more likely to remember more details of the program.

Test Question No. 2: Learners who can perform a new learning task well are likely to retain it.

Answer: False. We cannot presume that because a learner performs a new learning task well, it will be permanently stored. Sense and/or meaning must be present in some degree for storage to occur.

Implications for Teaching. Now think of this process in the classroom. Every day, students listen to things that make sense but lack meaning. They may diligently follow the teacher's instructions to perform a task repeatedly, and may even get the correct answers, but if they have not found meaning after the learning episode, there is little likelihood of long-term storage. Mathematics teachers are often frustrated by this. They see students using a certain formula to solve problems correctly one day, but they cannot remember how to do it the next day. If the process was not stored, the information is treated as brand new again!

Sometimes, when students ask why they need to know something, the teacher's response is, "Because it's going to be on the test." This response adds little meaning to a learning. Students resort to writing the learning in a notebook so that it is preserved in writing, but not in memory. We wonder the next day why they forgot the lesson.

Teachers spend about 90 percent of their planning time devising lessons so that students will *understand* the learning objective (i.e., make sense of it). But to convince a learner's brain to persist with that objective, teachers need to be more mindful of helping students establish *meaning*. We should remember that what was meaningful for us as children may not be necessarily meaningful for children today.

Past experiences always influence new learning. What we already know acts as a filter, helping us attend to those things that have meaning (i.e., relevancy) and discard those that don't. If we expect students to find meaning, we need to be certain that today's curriculum contains connections to *their* past experiences, not just ours. Further, the enormous size and the strict separation of secondary curriculum areas do little to help students find the time to make relevant connections between and among subjects. Helping students to make connections between subject areas by integrating the curriculum increases meaning and retention, especially when students recognize a future use for the new learning. Meaning is so powerful that most states prohibit trial lawyers from using what is dubbed the "golden rule" argument. It asks the jury, "If you were in this person's situation, what would you have done?"

Past experiences always influence new learning.

Long-Term Storage

Storing occurs when the hippocampus encodes information and sends it to one or more long-term storage areas. The encoding process takes time and usually occurs during deep sleep. While learners may *seem* to have acquired the new information or skill in a lesson, there is no guarantee that storage will be permanent after the lesson. How do we know if retention has occurred? If the student can accurately recall the learning after a specific period of time has passed, we say that the learning has been retained. Because research on retention shows that the greatest loss of newly acquired information or a skill occurs within the first 18 to 24 hours, the 24-hour period is a reasonable guideline for determining if information was transferred into long-term storage. If a learner cannot recall new learning after 24 hours, there is a high probability that it was not permanently stored and, thus, can never be recalled. This point has implications for how we test students for retention of previously learned material. See the **Practitioner's Corner** at the end of this chapter on page 70 on how to test whether information is in long-term storage. Sometimes, we store only the gist of an experience, not the specifics. This may occur after watching a movie or television program. We store a generalization about the plot but few, if any, details.

Test Question No. 3: Reviewing material just before a test is a good practice to determine how much has been retained in long-term storage.

Answer: False. Reviewing material just before a test allows students to enter the material into working memory for immediate use. Thus, the test cannot verify that what the learner recalls actually came from long-term storage.

The long-term storage areas are represented in the model (Figure 2.1) as file cabinets— places where information is kept in some type of order. Although there are three file cabinets in the diagram for simplicity, we do not know how many long-term storage sites actually are in the brain. Memories are not stored as a whole in one place. Different parts of a memory are stored in various sites which reassemble when the memory is recalled. Long-term memory is a dynamic, interactive system that activates storage areas distributed across the brain to retrieve and reconstruct memories.

Long-Term Memory and Long-Term Storage

This is a good place to explain the difference between the terms *long-term memory* and *long-term storage,* as I use them in the model. Long-term memory refers to the process of storing and retrieving information, while long-term storage refers to the areas in the brain where the memories are kept.

The Cognitive Belief System

The total of all that is in our long-term storage areas forms the basis for our view of the world around us. This information helps us to make sense out of events, to understand the laws of nature, to recognize cause and effect, and to form decisions about goodness, truth, and beauty. This total construct of how we see the world is called the *cognitive belief system.* It is shown in the information processing model as a large triangle extending beyond the long-term storage areas (file cabinets). It is drawn this way to remind us that the thoughts and understandings that arise from the long-term storage data are greater than the sum of the individual items. In other words, one marvelous quality of the human brain is its ability to combine individual items in many different ways. As we accumulate more items, the number of possible combinations grows exponentially.

Because no two of us have the same data in our long-term storage (not even identical twins raised in the same environment have identical data sets), no two of us perceive the world in exactly the same way. People can put the same experiences together in many different ways. To be sure, there are areas of agreement: Gravity, for example (few rational people would dispute its effects), or inertia, since most people have experienced the lurch forward or backward when a moving vehicle rapidly changes speed. There can be strong disagreement, however, about what makes an object or person beautiful, or an act justified. The persistent debates over abortion and capital punishment are testimony to the wide range of perspectives that people have over any issue. These differences reflect the ways individuals use the experiences in their long-term storage areas to interpret the world around them.

The cognitive belief system is our view of the world around us and how it works.

Here is a simple example of how people's experiences can cause them to interpret the same information differently. Close your eyes and form the mental image of an "old bat." Go ahead, try it! What picture comes to mind? For some baseball fans, it might be a marred wooden club that has been in too many games. A zoologist, however, might picture an aging fruit bat as it flies haltingly among the trees. Still others might recall an old hag whose complaining made their lives unpleasant. Here are at least three very different images generated by the same two words, each one formed by individuals whose experiences are different from the others.

Self-Concept

Deep within the cognitive belief system lies the *self-concept.* While the cognitive belief system portrays the way we see the world, the self-concept describes the way we view ourselves in that world. I might conceptualize myself as a good softball player, an above average student, or a poor mathematician. These and a long list of other descriptions form part of a person's self-concept.

The self-concept is represented in the information processing model (Figure 2.1) as a face and is placed at the apex of the triangle to emphasize its importance. *Self-concept* is used here as a neutral term that can run the gamut from very positive to very negative (Figure 2.5). The face on the diagram of the model has a smile, indicating a positive self-concept. But for some people, the face might have a frown because they may not see themselves as positive beings in their world. Emotions play an important role in forming a person's self-concept.

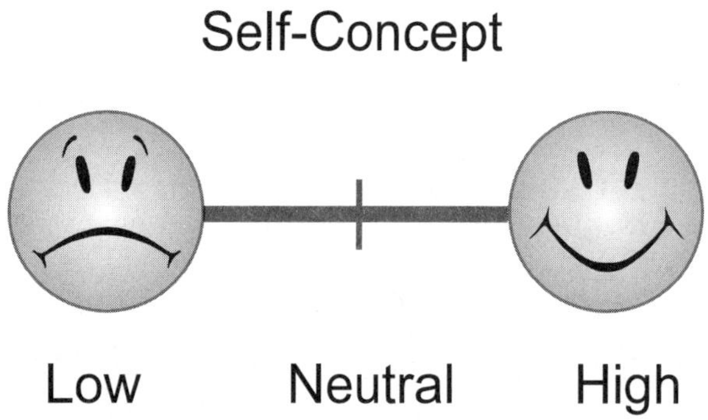

Self-Concept

Low Neutral High

Figure 2.5 Self-concept describes how we see ourselves in the world. It can range from very low to very high and vary with different learning situations.

Self-Concept and Past Experiences

Our self-concept is shaped by our past experiences. Some of our experiences, such as passing a difficult test or getting recognition for a job well done, raised our self-concept. Other experiences, such as receiving a reprimand or failing to accomplish a task, lowered our self-concept. These experiences produced strong emotional reactions that the brain's amygdala encoded and stored with the cognitive event. These emotional cues are so strong that we often reexperience the original emotion each time we recall the event. Over time, the addition of new positive and negative experiences moderate the self-concept and alter how we see ourselves in our world.

Accepting or Rejecting New Learning

Remember that the sensory register and temporary memory systems use past experiences as the guide for determining the importance of incoming stimuli to the individual. Thus, if an individual is in a new learning situation and past experience signals the sensory register that prior encounters with this information were successful, then the information is very likely to pass along to working memory. The learner now consciously recognizes that there were successes with this information and focuses on it for further processing. But if past experiences produced failure, then the sensory register is likely to block the incoming data, just as Venetian blinds are closed to block light. The learner resists being part of the unwanted learning experience and resorts to some other cerebral activity, internal or external, to avoid the situation. In effect, the learner's self-concept has closed off the receptivity to the new information. As mentioned earlier in discussing the hierarchy of data processing, when a curriculum concept struggles with an emotion, the emotion almost always wins. Of course, it is possible for the rational system (frontal lobe) to override the emotions, but that usually takes time and conscious effort.

> ***People will participate in learning activities that have yielded success for them and avoid those that have produced failure.***

Let us use an example to explain this important phenomenon. Someone who was a very successful student in mathematics remembers how that success boosted self-concept. As a result, the individual now feels confident when faced with basic mathematical problems. On the other hand, for someone who was a poor mathematics student, lack of success would lower self-concept. Consequently, such an individual will avoid dealing with mathematical problems whenever possible. People will participate in learning activities that have yielded success for them and avoid those that have produced failure.

Implications for Teaching. Students who experience self-concept shutdown in the classroom often give signs of their withdrawal—folding their arms, losing themselves in other work, or causing distraction. Too often, teachers deal with this withdrawal by reteaching the material, usually slower and louder. But they are attacking the problem from the front end of the information processing system, and this is rarely successful. It is the equivalent of putting a brighter light outside the closed Venetian blinds, hoping the light will penetrate. If the blinds are fully closed and effective, no light will get through, regardless of how bright it may be.

The better intervention is to deal with the learner's emotions and convince the learner to allow the perceptual register to open the blinds and pass the information along. But since the self-concept controls the blinds, the learner must believe that participating in the learning situation will produce new successes rather than repeat past failures. When teachers provide these successes, they encourage students to open the sensory register and, ultimately, to participate and achieve in the once-avoided learning process. In short, the self-concept controls the feedback loop and determines how the individual will respond to almost any new learning situation. Recognizing this connection gives teachers new insight on how to deal with reluctant learners.

What's Coming Up?

This completes our trip through the information processing model. Remember that the brain is a parallel processor and deals with many items simultaneously. Even though it rejects much data, it always stores some. The next chapter will examine the nature of memory and the factors that determine and help in the retention of learning.

PRACTITIONER'S CORNER

Walking Through the Brain

Directions: In this activity, students/participants will assume the roles of the different parts of the information processing model.

1. Each participant gets one of the following assignments:

   3–4 persons for the **sensory register**

   1 person for the **immediate memory**

   1 person for the **working memory**

   3–4 persons for the **long-term storage**

   rest of the group represents **incoming information**

2. In an open area of the classroom, the participants should arrange themselves in a pattern that approximates the information processing model shown earlier in Figure 2.1.

3. All participants, except those representing **incoming information**, briefly explain their role and function in the model.

4. The participants representing incoming information then move through the model one at a time, explaining what is happening at each stage.

5. **Variations**: Replay the activity demonstrating how information can be accepted or rejected by the sensory register, immediate memory, and working memory. One of the participants representing **long-term storage** can also represent the feedback loop of past experiences.

6. After demonstrating several different possibilities, discuss how this activity may have enhanced your understanding of the model. Note the positive effect that kinesthetic activities can have on learning new material.

PRACTITIONER'S CORNER

Redesigning the Information Processing Model

This activity gives the students/participants the opportunity to redesign the information processing model explained in this chapter.

Directions: In the area below redesign the information processing model using a **different** metaphor (e.g., a sports game, taking a vacation, cooking recipe). Keep the same metaphor for each of the major parts of the model. Be prepared to explain the metaphor and why you chose it.

PRACTITIONER'S CORNER

Sensory Preferences and Learning Style

Although we use all five senses to collect information from our environment, they do not contribute equally to our knowledge base. Most people do not use sight, hearing, and touch equally during learning. Just as most people develop a left- or right-handed preference, they also develop preferences for certain senses as they gather information from their environment. Some people have a preference for learning by sight, for example. They are called *visual* learners. Others who use hearing as the preferred sense are known as *auditory* learners. Still others who prefer touch or whole-body involvement in their learning are called *kinesthetic* learners. Sensory (also called *modality)* preferences are an important component of an individual's learning style. Teachers need to

- **Understand** that students with different sensory preferences will behave differently during learning.

- **Recognize** that they tend to teach the way they learn. A teacher who is a strong auditory learner will prefer this modality when teaching. Students who also are strong auditory learners will feel comfortable with this teacher's methods, but visual learners can have difficulty in maintaining focus. They will doodle or look at other materials to satisfy their visual craving.

- **Note,** similarly, that students with auditory preferences want to talk about their learning and can become frustrated with teachers who use primarily visual strategies. Strong kinesthetic learners require movement while learning or they become restless—tapping their pencils, squirming in their seats, or walking around the room.

- **Avoid** misinterpreting these variations in learning style behavior as inattention or as intentional misbehavior. The variations may, in fact, represent the natural responses of learners with different and strong preferences.

- **Understand** that a teacher's own learning style and sensory preferences can affect learning and teaching. Teachers should design lessons that include activities to address all sensory preference and learning styles.

PRACTITIONER'S CORNER

Determining Your Sensory Preferences

This checklist indicates your sensory preference(s). It is designed for adults and is one of many that are available. You should not rely on just one checklist for self-assessment. Remember that sensory preferences are usually evident only during prolonged and complex learning tasks.

Directions: For each item, circle "**A**" if you **agree** that the statement describes you most of the time. Circle "**D**" if you **disagree** that the statement describes you most of the time. Move quickly through the questions. Your first response is usually the more accurate one.

1. I prefer reading a story rather than listening to someone tell it. A D
2. I would rather watch television than listen to the radio. A D
3. I remember names better than faces. A D
4. I like classrooms with lots of posters and pictures around the room. A D
5. The appearance of my handwriting is important to me. A D
6. I think more often in pictures. A D
7. I am distracted by visual disorder or movement. A D
8. I have difficulty remembering directions that were told to me. A D
9. I would rather watch athletic events than participate in them. A D
10. I tend to organize my thoughts by writing them down. A D
11. My facial expression is a good indicator of my emotions. A D
12. I tend to remember names better than faces. A D

13. I would enjoy taking part in dramatic events like plays. A D

14. I tend to subvocalize and think in sounds. A D

15. I am easily distracted by sounds. A D

16. I easily forget what I read unless I talk about it. A D

17. I would rather listen to the radio than watch television. A D

18. My handwriting is not very good. A D

19. When faced with a problem, I tend to talk it through. A D

20. I express my emotions verbally. A D

21. I would rather be in a group discussion than read about a topic. A D

22. I prefer talking on the phone rather than writing a letter to someone. A D

23. I would rather participate in athletic events than watch them. A D

24. I prefer going to museums where I can touch the exhibits. A D

25. My handwriting deteriorates when the space becomes smaller. A D

26. My mental pictures are usually accompanied by movement. A D

27. I like being outdoors and doing things like biking, camping, swimming, hiking, etc. A D

28. I remember best what was done rather than what was seen or talked about. A D

29. When faced with a problem, I often select the solution involving the greatest activity. A D

30. I like to make models or other hand-crafted items. A D

31. I would rather do experiments than read about them. A D

32. My body language is a good indicator of my emotions. A D

33. I have difficulty remembering verbal directions if I have not done the activity before. A D

Interpreting Your Score

Total the number of "**A**" responses in items 1–11: _____
This is your visual score.

Total the number of "**A**" responses in items 12–22: _____
This is your auditory score.

Total the number of "**A**" responses in items 23–33: _____
This is your tactile/kinesthetic score.

If you scored a lot higher in any one area: This sense is *very probably* your preference during a protracted and complex learning situation.

If you scored a lot lower in any one area: This sense is *not likely* to be your preference in a learning situation.

If you have similar scores in all three areas: You can learn things in almost any way they are presented.

Reflections

A. What was your preferred sense? Were you surprised?

B. How does this preference show up in your daily life?

C. How does this preference show up in your teaching?

PRACTITIONER'S CORNER

Developing a Classroom Climate Conducive to Learning

Learning occurs more easily in environments free from threat or intimidation. Whenever a student detects a threat, thoughtful processing gives way to emotion or survival reactions. Experienced teachers have seen this in the classroom. Under pressure to give a quick response, the student begins to stumble, stabs at answers, gets frustrated or angry, and may even resort to violence.

There are ways to deal with questions and answers that reduce the fear of giving a wrong answer. The teacher could:

- Supply the question to which the wrong answer belongs:
  "You would be right if I had asked . . . "
- Give the student a prompt that leads to the correct answer.
- Ask another student to help.

Threats to students loom continuously in the classroom. The teacher's capacity to humiliate, embarrass, reject, and punish all constitute perceived threats. Many students even see grading more as a punitive than as a rewarding process. Students perceive threats in varying degrees, but the presence of a threat in *any* significant degree impedes learning. One's thinking and learning functions operate fully only when one feels secure.

Teachers can make their classrooms better learning environments by avoiding threats (even subtle intimidation) and by establishing democratic climates in which students are treated fairly and feel free to express their opinions during discussions. In these environments students:

- Develop trust in the teacher
- Exhibit more positive behaviors
- Are less likely to be disruptive
- Show greater support for school policy
- Sense that thinking is encouraged and nurtured

For Further Discussion

- What kinds of emotions in school could interfere with cognitive processing (i.e., have a negative effect on learning)?

  ____

  ____

- What strategies and structures can schools and teachers use to limit the threat and negative effects of these emotions?

  ____

  ____

- What factors in schools can foster emotions in students that promote learning (i.e., have a positive effect)?

  ____

  ____

- What strategies have you used to encourage the positive emotions that promote learning?

  ____

  ____

PRACTITIONER'S CORNER

Using Humor to Enhance Climate and Promote Retention

Humor has many benefits when used frequently and appropriately in the classroom and other school settings.

Physiological Benefits

- **Provides More Oxygen**. Brain cells need oxygen and glucose for fuel. When we laugh, we get more oxygen into the bloodstream, so the brain is better fueled.
- **Causes an Endorphin Surge**. Laughter causes the release of *endorphins* in the blood. Endorphins are the body's natural painkillers, and they also give the person a feeling of euphoria. In other words, the person enjoys the moment in body as well as in mind. Endorphins also stimulate the brain's frontal lobes, thereby increasing the degree of focus and amount of attention time.
- **Moderates Body Functions.** Scientists have found that humor decreases stress, modulates pain, decreases blood pressure, relaxes muscle tension, and boosts immune defenses. These are all desirable outcomes.

Psychological, Sociological, and Educational Benefits

- **Gets Attention**. The first thing a teacher has to do when starting a lesson is to get the students' attention or focus. Because the normal human brain loves to laugh, starting with a humorous tale (such as a joke, pun, or story) gets the learner's attention. Self-deprecating humor ("You won't believe what happened to me this weekend.") is particularly effective with teens.
- **Creates a Positive Climate**. Students are going to be together in a classroom for about 180 days. We need to find ways to help this increasingly diverse student population get along. When people laugh together, they bond and a community spirit emerges—all positive forces for an climate conducive to learning.
- **Increases Retention and Recall**. We know that emotions enhance retention, so the positive feelings that result from laughter increase the probability that students will remember what they learned and be able to recall it later.
- **Improves Everyone's Mental Health**. Schools and all their occupants are under more stress than ever. Taking time to laugh can relieve that stress and give the staff and students better

mental attitude with which to accomplish their tasks. Let's take our work seriously but ourselves lightly.

- **Provides an Effective Discipline Tool**. Good-natured humor (not teasing or sarcasm) can be an effective way of reminding students of the rules without raising tension in the classroom. Laughter also dampens hostility and aggression. Teachers who use appropriate humor are more likeable and students have a more positive feeling toward them. Discipline problems, therefore, are less likely to occur.

Using Humor as Part of Lessons. Humor should not be limited to an opening joke or story. Because of its value as an attention-getter and retention strategy, look for ways to use humor within the context of the learning objective. Droz and Ellis (1996) give many helpful suggestions on how to get students to use humor in lessons on writing, mathematics, science, and history.

Administrators and Humor. Administrators also need to remember the value of humor in their relationships with staff, students, and parents. As leaders, they set the example. In meetings and other settings, they can show that humor and laughter are acceptable in schools and classrooms.

Some Barriers to Humor in Classrooms

- **"I'm Not Funny."** Some teachers want to use humor in the classroom but don't perceive themselves as jokesters. They'll say: "I'm just not funny" or "I can't tell a joke." But the teacher doesn't have to be funny, just the material—and there's plenty of it. Books on humor are available in local stores, and don't forget that students themselves often provide humor by their responses in class and answers on tests. Be certain that you use this material appropriately, avoiding teasing or sarcasm.

- **"Students Won't Enjoy It**." Secondary teachers, particularly, believe that students won't find humor in corny jokes or that they are too sophisticated to laugh. But everyone likes to laugh (or groan) at humor. I suggest starting each class period with humor for three weeks, then stopping. I'm certain that students will say, "Hey, where's the joke?"—evidence that they *were* listening.

- **"It Takes Too Much Time**." This is a common concern. Secondary teachers often feel so pressured to cover curriculum material that they are reluctant to give time to what may seem like a frivolous activity. On the other hand, humor is an *efficient* as well as effective way to gain students' attention and improve retention of learning. It really is a useful investment of time.

Avoiding Sarcasm. All of the wonderful benefits mentioned above are the result of using wholesome humor that everyone can enjoy, and not sarcasm, which is inevitably destructive to someone. Even some well-intentioned teachers say, "Oh, I know my students very well, so they can take sarcasm." More than ever, today's students are coming to school looking for emotional support. Sarcasm is one of the factors that can undermine that support and turn students against their peers, the teacher, and the school. Besides, there are plenty of sources of good humor without sarcasm.

For a deeper look at the research on the effects of humor on the body and brain, see Cardoso (2000) and Schmidt (1995, 2002).

PRACTITIONER'S CORNER

Increasing Processing Time Through Motivation

Working memory is a temporary memory, so items have a limited time for processing. But the longer an item is processed (or rehearsed), the greater the probability that sense and meaning may be found, and therefore, that retention will occur. One way to increase processing time is through motivation, which is essentially an emotional response. Not surprisingly, recent research has validated long-standing beliefs that motivation is a key to the amount of attention devoted to a learning situation.

Motivation can come from within the individual, called *intrinsic motivation,* when an activity is related to a person's needs, values, interests, and attitudes. People spend hours on their hobbies because of intrinsic motivation. These internal attributes are so deeply rooted that they are difficult to change. But they can change over time.

Motivation that comes from the environment, such as rewards and punishment, is called *extrinsic motivation.* External motivators are used to control and reward behavior. Grades, stars, and praise are examples of external motivators used in schools. Although these incentives serve a purpose, they have little relationship to the internal process of learning. It's no secret that learning occurs best when the learner is intrinsically motivated (Wigfield & Eccles, 2002). External motivators can be of value by getting students started on a topic so that they can move toward intrinsic rewards.

Here are a few ideas about motivation for teachers to consider (Diamond & Hopson, 1998; Hunter, 2004; Moore, 2005):

- **Generate Interest.** If the learner is interested in the item, then the processing time can be extended significantly because the learner is dealing with the item in different ways and making new connections with past learnings that once were also of interest. The working memory is seeking ways to use this new learning to enhance the usefulness of the past learning. We all know students who won't give us five minutes of their undivided attention in class, but who spend hours working on a stamp collection, playing video games, or repairing a carburetor.

Teachers can identify these interests by having their students complete interest inventories at the beginning of the school year. The information gathered from these surveys can help teachers design lessons that include references to student interests as often as possible. Guidance counselors can provide information on the types and sources of interest inventories.

Today's novelty-seeking brain wants to get actively involved in the learning process. Active learning involves choices and actions that the learner finds pleasurable and effective for developing an understanding of the big picture as well as the relationship between and among the components of the learning objective. This approach stimulates intrinsic motivation and interest. Teachers, then, should:

- Make clear what the students should be able to do when the lesson objective is accomplished.
- Include provocative ideas and challenging activities.
- Involve the students in developing the criteria that will be used to assess their competency (e.g., assessment rubrics).
- Demonstrate how closely the content is connected to the real world.
- Give students choices in selecting activities and questions to pursue.

- **Establish Accountability.** When learners believe they will be held accountable for new learning, processing time increases. High school students have little difficulty staying on task in driver education classes. Not only do they have interest but they also know they will be legally accountable for their knowledge and skills long after they complete the license tests.

- **Provide Feedback.** When students get prompt, specific, and corrective feedback on the results of their thinking, they are more likely to continue processing, make corrections, and persist until successful completion. Frequent brief quizzes that are carefully corrected and returned promptly are much more valuable learning tools than the unit test, and are more likely to help students be successful. This success will improve self-concept and encourage them to try more difficult tasks. Computers are motivating because they provide immediate and objective feedback and allow students to evaluate their progress and understand their level of competence.

Another effective strategy suggested by Hunter (2004) for increasing processing time through motivation is called *level of concern.* This refers to how much the student cares about the learning. We used to think that if the students had anxiety about learning, then little or no learning occurred. But there is helpful anxiety (desire to do well) and there is harmful anxiety (feeling threatened). Having anxiety about your job performance will usually get you to put forth more effort to obtain positive results. When you are concerned about being more effective (helpful anxiety), you are likely to learn and try new strategies. This is an example of how emotions can increase learning.

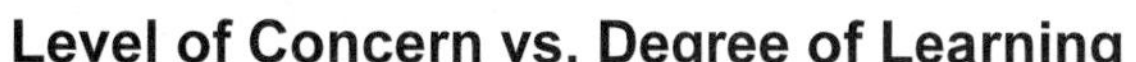

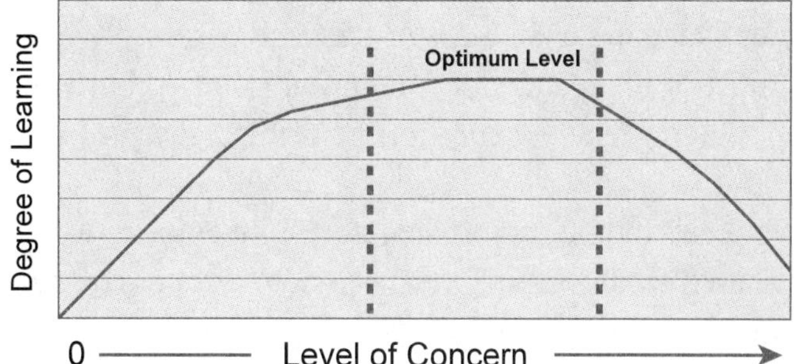

The graph shows that as the level of concern increases, so does the degree of learning. If the stress level gets too high, our focus shifts to the emotions and the consequences generated by the stress, and learning fades. Students need a certain level of concern to stimulate their efforts to learn. When there is no concern, there is little or no learning. But if there is too much concern, anxiety shuts down the learning process and adverse emotions take over. The teacher then has to seek the level of concern that produces the optimum processing time and learning. Hunter (2004) offers four ways to raise or lower the level of concern in a lesson.

- Consequences. Teachers raise the level of concern when they say "This is going to be on the test," and lower it with, "Knowing this will help you learn the next set of skills more easily."

- Visibility. Standing next to a student who is off-task will raise that student's concern; moving away from an anxious student will lower concern. Telling students their work will be displayed can also raise concern.

- Amount of Time. Giving students only a little time to complete a learning task will raise concern; extending the time will lower it.

- Amount of Help. If students have little or no help while completing a learning task, concern rises. On the other hand, if they have quick access to help, concern lowers. This can be a problem, however. If students can always get immediate help, they may become dependent and never learn to solve problems for themselves. There comes a time when the teacher needs to reduce the help and tell the students to use what they have learned to solve the problem on their own.

Reflections

A. What types of class activities increase the level of concern beyond the optimum level?

B. What strategies lower the level of concern raised by the activities in your answers to A above?

PRACTITIONER'S CORNER

Creating Meaning in New Learning

Meaning refers to the relevancy that students attach to new learning. Meaning isn't inherent in content, but rather is the result of how the students relate it to their past learnings and experiences. Questions like "Why do I need to know this?" reveal a learner who is having difficulty determining the relevancy of the new topic. Here are a few ways teachers can help students attach meaning to new learning.

- **Modeling**. Models are examples of the new learning that the learner can perceive in the classroom rather than relying on experience. Models can be concrete (an engine) or symbolic (a map). To be effective, a model should:
  - Accurately and unambiguously highlight the critical attribute(s) of new learning. A dog is a better example of a mammal than a whale.
  - Be given first by the teacher to ensure that it is correct during this period of prime time when retention is highest.
  - Avoid controversial issues that can evoke strong emotions and redirect the learner's attention.

- **Using Examples From Students' Experience.** These allow students to bring previous knowledge into working memory to accelerate making sense and attaching meaning to the new learning. Make sure that the example is clearly relevant to the new learning. This is not easy to do on the spot, so examples should be thought out in advance when planning the lesson.

- **Creating Artificial Meaning.** When it is not possible to identify exemplary elements from student experience to develop meaning, we can resort to other methods. Mnemonic devices help students associate material so they can remember it. Examples are HOMES to remember the Great Lakes and "Every good boy does fine" for the musical notes *e, g, b, d,* and *f* (See Chapter 3).

PRACTITIONER'S CORNER

Using Closure to Enhance Sense and Meaning

Closure describes the covert process whereby the learner's working memory summarizes for itself its perception of what has been learned. It is during closure that a student often completes the rehearsal process and attaches sense and meaning to the new learning, thereby increasing the probability that it will be retained in long-term storage.

- **Initiating Closure:** The teacher gives directions that focus the student on the new learning, such as "I'm going to give you about two minutes to think of the three causes of the Civil War that we learned today. Be prepared to discuss them briefly." In this statement, the teacher told the students how much quiet time they have for the cerebral summarizing to occur and identified the overt activity (discussion) that will be used for student accountability. During the discussion, the teacher can assess the quality and accuracy of what occurred during closure and make any necessary adjustments in teaching.

- **Closure Is Different From Review.** In review, the teacher does most of the work, repeating key concepts made during the lesson and rechecking student understanding. In closure, the student does most of the work by mentally rehearsing and summarizing those concepts and deciding whether they make sense and have meaning.

- **When to Use Closure.** Closure can occur at various times in a lesson.
  - It can start a lesson: "Think of the two causes of the Civil War we talked about yesterday and be prepared to discuss them."
  - It can occur during the lesson (called *procedural closure)* when the teacher moves from one sublearning to the next: "Review those two rules in your mind before we learn the third rule."
  - It should also take place at the end of the lesson (called *terminal closure)* to tie all the sublearnings together.

Closure is an investment that can pay off dramatically in increased retention of learning.

PRACTITIONER'S CORNER

Testing Whether Information Is in Long-Term Storage

Information that the learner processes during a lesson remains in working memory where it eventually will be dropped out or saved for long-term storage. Just because students act as if they have learned the new information or skill doesn't mean it will be transferred to long-term storage. Extensive research on retention indicates that 70 to 90 percent of new learning is forgotten within 18 to 24 hours after the lesson. Consequently, if the new learning survives this time period intact, it is probably destined for long-term storage and will not deteriorate further.

This time requirement confirms that the processing and transfer between working memory and long-term storage needs adequate time for the encoding and consolidation of the new information into the storage networks. Thus, tomorrow is the earliest reliable time we can confirm that what was learned today has been indeed retained.

How to Test. If teachers want to test whether information actually has been transferred to long-term storage, the test needs to

- Be given no sooner than 24 hours after the learning
- Test precisely what should have been retained
- Come as a surprise to the learner, with no warning or preparation time

Rationale. If the learners have warning about the test, they are likely to review the material just before the test. In this case, the test may determine the amount of information the learners were able to cram and hold in working memory and not what they have recalled from long-term storage. While testing without warning may seem insensitive, it is the only way teachers can be sure that long-term storage was the source of the test information that the learners provided. Unannounced quizzes, then, should help students assess what they have remembered, rather than be a classroom management device to get students back on task.

Misuse of Tests. Some teachers use unannounced tests as punishment to get students back on task. This is a misuse of a valuable tool. Another approach is for teachers to

- **Establish** sense and meaning to increase the probability that retention will occur.
- **Explain** to students that unannounced tests help them see *what* as well as *how much* they have retained and learned over a given period of time.

- **Ensure** that the test or quiz matches the rehearsal when it was first taught. If the learning required essentially rote rehearsal, give a rote type of test. If it required elaborate rehearsal, use a test that allows the students more flexibility in their responses.

Using the Test Results. It is important that teachers

- **Analyze** immediately the results of the test to determine what areas need to be retaught or practiced. If some students forgot parts, consider forming cooperative learning groups that focus on reteaching the forgotten areas.

- **Record** the grades of only a small portion of these unannounced assessments. Rather, ask students to share their results and discuss in a think-pair-share format what strategies the students used to remember their correct responses. In this way, students talk about their memory processes and have a better understanding of how they learn and remember.

- **Decide** whether memory strategies such as concept maps, mnemonics, or chunking (see following chapters) can help in retention.

The analysis might also reveal areas of the curriculum to be reworked or updated for relevance, or it might show that the lesson should be retaught in a different way. A task analysis on a failed lesson is a good way to detect false assumptions about learning that the teacher may have made, and it recasts the lesson into a new presentation that can be more successful for both students and teacher.

Using tests as tools to help students to be right, rather than to catch them being wrong, will create a supportive learning climate that results in improved student performance.

PRACTITIONER'S CORNER

Using Synergy to Enhance Learning

Synergy describes how the joint actions of people working together increase each other's effectiveness. This strategy gets students moving and talking while learning. It is effective because it is novel, is multisensory, uses active participation, is emotionally stimulating, and encourages socialization. Each participant ends up having a better understanding as a result of this interaction (synergy). It can be used from the primary grades to graduate school. Here are the guidelines:

- **Provide Adequate Time for Reflection.** After teaching a concept, ask students to quietly review their notes and be prepared to explain what they have learned to someone else. Be sure to allow sufficient time for this mental rehearsal to occur (usually 1 to 3 minutes).

- **Model the Activity.** Working with a student, show the students how you want them to behave and interact during the activity.

- **Get Students to Stand, Move, and Deliver.** Ask students to walk across the room and pair up with someone they do not usually work with or know very well. They stand face-to-face and take turns explaining what they have learned. They add to their notes anything their partners have said that they do not have. When done, all students end up with more information and ideas than they would have had if they worked alone. If they cannot agree or don't understand something, they are to ask the teacher about it when the activity is over. (Note: Make sure students stand face-to-face—rather than just looking at each other's notes—so that they must talk to their partners. Allow pairs only—one trio, if you have an uneven number of students.)

- **Keep in Motion.** Move around the room using proximity to help students stay on task. Answer questions to get them back on track, but avoid reteaching the lesson. Otherwise, students will become dependent on your reteaching rather than on each other's explanations.

- **Provide Enough Time and Adjust As Needed.** Allow adequate time for this process to be effective. Start with a few minutes, adding more time if they are still on task and reducing the time when you sense they are done.

- **Ensure Accountability.** To help keep students on task, tell them that you will call on several students at random when the activity is over to explain what they discussed.

- **Clarify Any Misunderstandings.** Ask if there were any misunderstandings or items that need further explanation, and clarify them. An inviting statement would be "Is there anything I need to clarify?" rather than "Is there anything you didn't understand?"

- **Use Variety for the Pairing.** You can pair students by birth week or month, hair or eye color, height, musical cues, similar first names, etc. Aim for random pairing as much as practicable to enhance socialization (because students tend to work more with their friends) and to avoid monotony.

Some Potential Barriers to Using Synergy

- **"The Teacher Should Be Talking."** The long-standing practice of the teachers being the "deliverers" of information is tough to overcome. For that reason, some teachers are uncomfortable with this activity because they are not "working" (read "talking"). But one of the reasons this activity can be so effective is because it shifts the work to the students' brains, increasing the likelihood that they will find sense and meaning in the new learning.

- **"It Takes Too Much Time."** The question is: What would the teacher be doing otherwise? More talking? This is a useful investment of time because the students are talking about the lesson, thereby enhancing learning and retention.

- **"The Students Will Get Off Task."** This is a common and realistic concern. However, off-task behavior can be reduced significantly if the teacher continually moves around the room, listens in and asks questions of the student pairs, and holds them accountable for the learning at the end of the activity.

PRACTITIONER'S CORNER

NeuroBingo

Directions: In this activity the entire group gets up and moves around. Each person tries to find someone who can answer one of the questions in a box. The person who answers the question initials the box. The object is to get a bingo pattern (horizontally, vertically, or diagonally). No person may initial the same sheet twice. Time limit: 15 to 20 minutes, depending on the size and age of the group.

FIND A PERSON WHO IS ABLE TO

Explain the function of the sensory register	Explain the importance of sense and meaning to learning	Define "windows of opportunity"	Explain how the brain prioritizes incoming information	Explain the functions of the frontal lobes
State the two functions of the hippocampus	Tell you the function of immediate memory	Explain the function of the amygdala	Explain what is meant by the "novel" brain	Provide an example of how self-concept affects learning
Relate the cognitive belief system to learning	Tell you the functions of the cerebellum	Tell you the functions of the cerebrum	Describe the time limits of working memory	Explain synapses
Explain the meaning of sensory preferences	Describe the capacity limits of working memory	Explain what is meant by emotional control	Explain the function of neurotransmitters	Explain the function of longterm memory
Explain the value of humor in learning	Name the five senses	Describe the sources of brain research	Explain closure	Describe a neuron

Chapter 2—How the Brain Processes Information

Key Points to Ponder

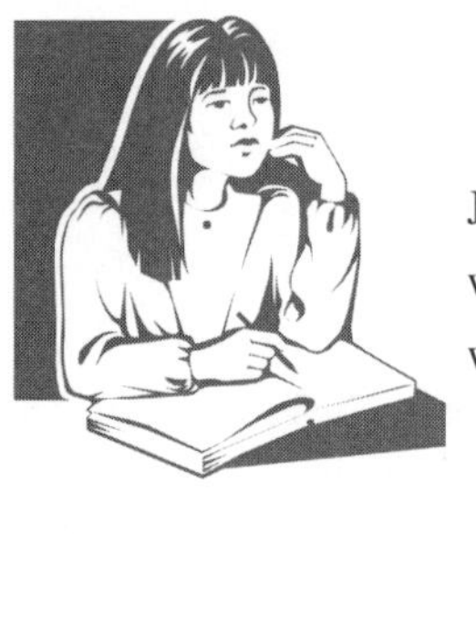

Jot down on this page key points, ideas, strategies, and resources you want to consider later. This sheet is your personal journal summary and will help to jog your memory.

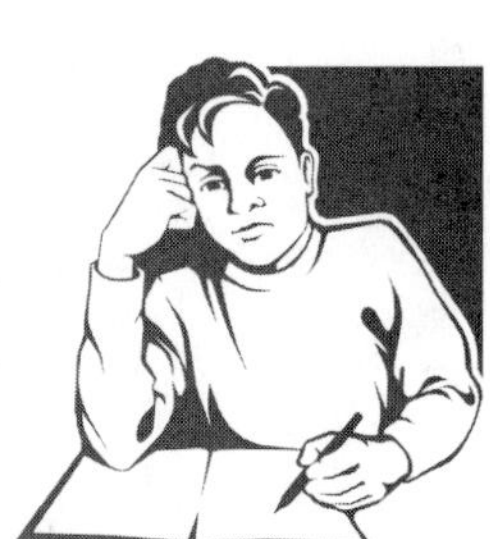

Chapter 3

Memory, Retention, and Learning

The memory should be specially taxed in youth, since it is then that it is strongest and most tenacious. But in choosing the things that should be committed to memory, the utmost care and forethought must be exercised; as lessons well learned in youth are never forgotten.

—Arthur Schopenhauer

Chapter Highlights: This chapter probes the nature of memory. It explains why our ability to retain information varies within a learning episode and with the teaching method used. It also discusses the value and pitfalls of practice, as well as techniques for increasing the capacity of working memory.

Memory gives us a past and a record of who we are and is essential to human individuality. Without memory, life would be a series of meaningless encounters that have no link to the past and no use for the future. Memory allows individuals to draw on experience and use the power of prediction to decide how they will respond to future events.

For all practical purposes, the capacity of the brain to store information is unlimited. That is, with about 100 billion neurons, each with thousands of dendrites, the number of potential neural

The brain goes through physical and chemical changes each time it learns.

pathways is incomprehensible. The brain will hardly run out of space to store all that an individual learns in a lifetime. Learning is the process by which we *acquire* new knowledge and skills; memory is the process by which we *retain* the knowledge and skills for the future. Most of what makes up our cognitive belief system, we have learned. Investigations into the neural mechanisms required for different types of learning are revealing more about the interactions between learning new information, memory, and changes in brain structure. Just as muscles improve with exercise, the brain seems to improve with use. While learning does not increase the number of brain cells, it does increase their size, their branches, and their ability to form more complex networks.

The brain goes through physical and chemical changes when it stores new information as the result of learning. Storing gives rise to new neural pathways and strengthens existing pathways. Thus, every time we learn something, our long-term storage areas undergo anatomical changes that, together with our unique genetic makeup, constitute the expression of our individuality.

HOW MEMORY FORMS

What is a memory? Is it actually located in a piece of the brain at a specific spot? Are memories permanent? How does the brain manage to store a lifetime of memories in an organ the size of a melon? Is forgetting actually losing the memory or just access to it? The definitive explanation for memory is still elusive. Nevertheless, neuroscientists have discovered numerous mechanisms that occur in the brain that, taken together, define a workable hypothesis about memory formation, storage, and recall.

The Temporary Stimulus

You will recall from Chapter 1 that a stimulus (say, the color red, a whiff of perfume, or a musical note) causes nerve impulses to travel down the axon to the gap, or synapse, where neurotransmitter chemicals are released. These chemicals cross the synapse to the dendrite of the other neuron. As the chemical messages enter the neighboring neuron, they spark a series of electrochemical reactions that cause this second neuron to generate a signal, or "fire." The reaction continues and causes more receptor sites on other neurons to fire as well. This sequence forms a pattern of neuronal connections firing together.

The firing may last only for a brief time, after which the memory decays and is lost. If the second neuron is not stimulated again, it will stay in a state of readiness for hours, or days. What is created here is a perception, and even recognition, of an outside stimulus that quickly passes. We are bombarded with thousands of such events each day. The ability for these events to decay quickly means that our brain does not get cluttered with useless memories.

Forming the Memory

On the other hand, if the pattern is repeated during this standby period (through rehearsal and practice), the tendency for the associated group to fire together is increased. The faster a neuron fires, the greater the electrical charge it generates and the more likely it is to set off its neighbors. As the neighbors fire, the surfaces of their dendrites change to make them more sensitive to stimulation. This process of synaptic awareness and sensitivity is called *long-term potentiation* or *LTP*. Eventually, repeated firing of the pattern binds the neurons together so that if one fires, they all fire, ultimately forming a new memory trace, or *engram* (Figure 3.1). These individual traces associate and form networks so that whenever one is triggered, the whole network is strengthened, thereby consolidating the memory and making it more easily retrievable (Carter, 1998; Fields, 2005; Restak, 2003; Squire & Kandel, 1999).

Memories are not stored intact. Instead, they are stored in pieces and distributed in sites throughout the cerebrum. The shape, color, and smell of an orange, for example, are categorized and stored in different sets of neurons. Activating these sites simultaneously brings together a recollection of our thoughts and experiences involving an orange. There is also evidence that the brain stores an extended experience in more than one network. Which storage sites to select could be determined by the number of associations that the brain makes between new and past learnings. The more connections that are made, the more understanding and meaning the learner can attach to the new learning, and the more likely it is that it will be stored in different networks. This process now gives the learner multiple opportunities to retrieve the new learning.

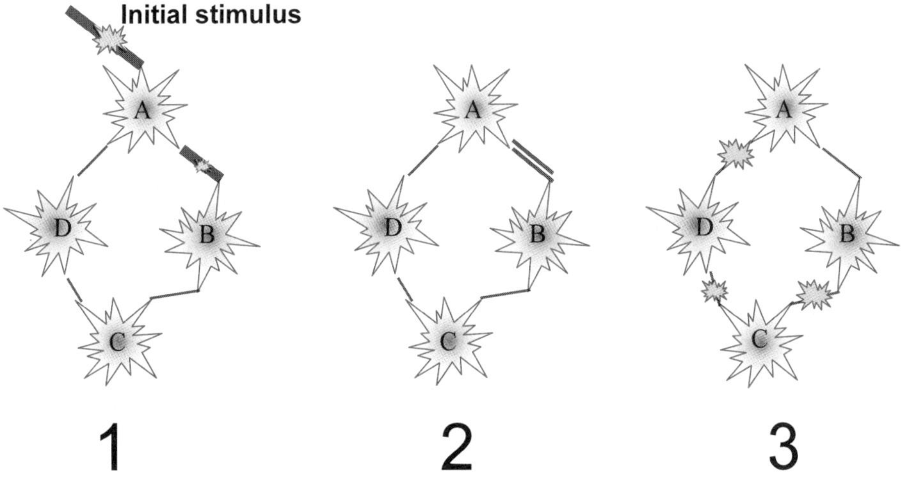

Figure 3.1 Memories are formed when a group of neurons fires together when activated. (1) Neuron A receives a stimulus, which causes it to set off neuron B. (2) If neuron A fires again soon, a link is established. Later, neuron A can just fire weakly to set off neuron B. (3) The firing of neurons A and B may set off neighboring neurons C and D. If this happens repeatedly, the four cells become a network and will fire together in the future—forming a memory.

> ***The more understanding and meaning the learner can attach to the new learning, the more likely it is that it will be stored in different networks. This process now gives the learner multiple opportunities to retrieve the new learning.***

Smart Drugs to Enhance Memory

Drugs will soon be available that enhance the ability of the neurons to form and recall engrams. Pharmaceutical companies are working on " smart drugs," several of which are already being tested on humans (Lynch, 2002). One approach is to use substances called ampakines that affect long-term potentiation to increase synaptic transmission. Another is to enhance the effectiveness of certain neurotransmitters during memory formation. Although researchers are aiming to develop drugs that will help patients with memory disorders, these same drugs will help normal people perform memory tasks, such as test taking, with greater success. This prospect will pose some interesting ethical questions for classroom teachers. How do we deal with a student who takes a legal smart drug just before we give a test?

STAGES AND TYPES OF MEMORY

Scientists have been debating for decades how best to classify forms of memory. Numerous case studies of people experiencing memory loss, the results of experiments designed to test memory, and analysis of brain scans all suggest that memories exist in different forms. The problem is getting neuroscientists to agree on a set taxonomy that defines thc stages and types of human memory. Furthermore, as new research results emerge, the taxonomy and nomenclature change accordingly. I have attempted here to present what most active researchers seem to accept as a workable model for describing memory systems at the time of publication.

Stages of Memory

The stages of memory are the following: sensory/immediate, working, and long-term. In Chapter 2, we looked at the nature of sensory/immediate and working memories, which you will recall are temporary memories. Some stimuli that are processed in these temporary memories are eventually transferred to long-term memory sites where they actually change the structure of the neurons so they can last a lifetime.

Types of Memory

Although neuroscientists are not in total agreement with psychologists as to all of the characteristics of long-term memory, there is considerable agreement on some of their types, and their description is important to understand before setting out to design learning activities accordingly. Long-term memory can be divided into two major types, *declarative memory* and *nondeclarative memory*. Figure 3.2 shows the stages of memory and the various types of long-term memory.

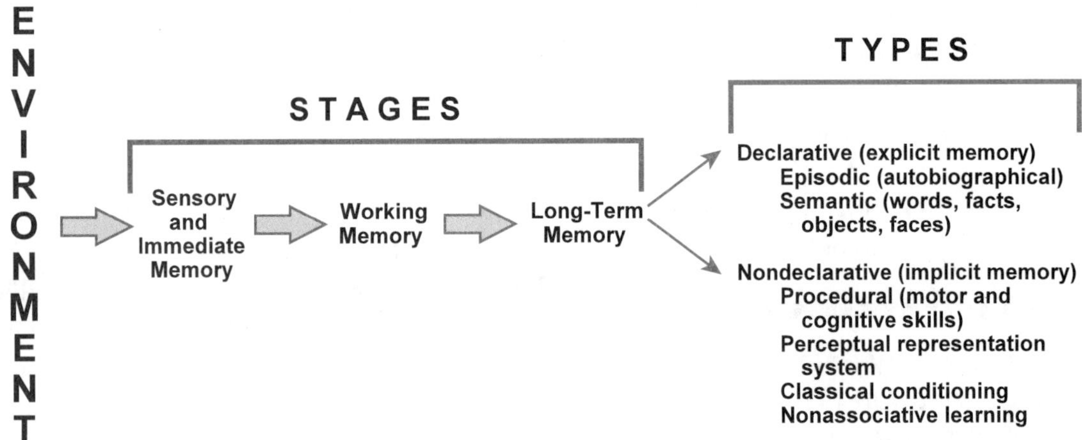

Figure 3.2 The hypothesized structure of human memory showing the relationship among different forms of memory.

Declarative Memory

Declarative memory (also called *conscious* or *explicit* memory) describes the remembering of names, facts, music, and objects (e.g., where you live and the kind of car you own), and is processed by the hippocampus and cerebrum. Think for a moment about a person who is now important in your life. Try to recall that person's image, voice, and mannerisms. Then think of an important event you both attended, one with an emotional connection, such as a concert, wedding, or funeral. Once you have the context in mind, note how easily other components of the memory come together. This is declarative memory in its most common form—a conscious and almost effortless recall. Declarative memory can be further divided into *episodic memory* and *semantic memory*.

Episodic Memory. Episodic memory refers to the conscious memory of events in our own life history, such as our sixteenth birthday party, falling off a new bicycle, or what we had for breakfast this morning. It helps us identify the time and place when an event happened and gives us a sense of self. Episodic memory is the memory of *remembering*.

Semantic Memory. Semantic memory is knowledge of facts and data that may not be related to any event. It is knowing that the Eiffel Tower is in Paris, how to tell time, how to multiply two numbers, and who the fortieth president was. Semantic memory is the memory of *knowing*. A veteran knowing that there was a Vietnam War in the 1970s is using semantic memory; remembering his experiences in that war is episodic memory.

Nondeclarative Memory

Nondeclarative memory (sometimes called *implicit* memory) describes all memories that are *not* declarative memories, that is, memories that can be used for things that cannot be declared or explained in any straightforward manner. Because nondeclarative memories do not require the intentional recall of experiences, they have been of particular interest to researchers. As a result, the descriptions and names of the categories of nondeclarative memories have changed over the last decade in light of new research. To date, the generally accepted categories of nondeclarative memory include *procedural memory, perceptual representation system, classical conditioning,* and *nonassociative learning.*

Procedural Memory. Procedural memory refers to the learning of motor and cognitive skills, and remembering *how* to do something, like riding a bicycle, driving a car, swinging a tennis racket, and tying a shoelace. As practice of the skills continues, these memories become more efficient and can be performed with little conscious thought or recall. The brain process shifts from *reflective* to *reflexive*. For example, you may remember the first time you drove an automobile by yourself. No doubt you gave a lot of conscious attention to your speed, maneuvering the vehicle, putting your foot on the correct pedal, and observing surrounding traffic (reflective thought). However, as you continued to practice this routine, the skills were stored in procedural memory and became more automatic (reflexive activity). Now, aren't you sometimes amazed at how you can drive from home to work and not even recall what happened on the road? "Did I really stop at that stop sign back there?" "What was that thump I heard a while ago?" Procedural memory was driving the car while working memory was planning your day.

Procedural memory helps us to learn things that don't require conscious attention and to habituate ourselves to the environment.

Much of what we do during the course of a day involves the performance of skills. We go through the morning grooming and breakfast rituals, read the newspaper, get to work, and shake the hand of a new acquaintance. We do all of these tasks without realizing that we have learned them and without being aware that we are using our memory. Although learning a new skill involves conscious attention, skill performance later becomes unconscious and relies essentially on nondeclarative memory.

We also learn *cognitive skills*, such as reading, discriminating colors, identifying tones in music, and figuring out a *procedure* for solving a problem. Cognitive skills are different from cognitive concept building in that cognitive skills are performed automatically and rely on procedural memory rather than declarative memory. Perceptual and cognitive skill acquisition involve some different brain processes and memory sites from cognitive concept learning. If they are learned differently, should they be taught differently?

Perceptual Representation System (PRS). The perceptual representation system (PRS) refers to the structure and form of words and objects in memory that can be prompted by prior experience, without explicit recall. The PRS used to be included as part of procedural memory. But recent studies have identified unique characteristics of this recall system that merit it a separate category. Essentially, the PRS describes our ability to complete fragments of words or tell whether objects in drawings could exist in the real world. Not surprisingly, our success at completing these tasks is much improved if we have seen the entire words and pictures on a previous occasion, even if we only glimpsed at the words and pictures and did not have time to study them intently. This is a form of implicit (nondeclarative) memory because no explicit processing of the words or pictures was involved.

Classical Conditioning. Classical conditioning (also called Pavlovian conditioning) occurs when a conditioned stimulus to an organism prompts an unconditioned response from that organism. Remember Pavlov ringing a bell as he fed his dogs? Because the response gets associated with the stimulus, this form of learning is called *associative learning.* Experienced teachers know exactly how to respond in school when the fire alarm bell sounds. They have learned to associate the sound of the alarm with the procedures needed to safely evacuate the building.

Nonassociative learning. Nonassociative learning occurs in two forms. *Habituation* helps us to learn not to respond to things that don't require conscious attention, and to accustom ourselves to the environment. Thus, we can become accustomed to the clothes we wear, the daily noisy traffic outside the school, a ticking clock in the den, or the sounds of construction. This adjustment to the environment allows the brain to screen out unimportant stimuli so it can focus on those that matter.

In *sensitization,* we increase our response to a particularly noxious or threatening stimulus. For example, Californians who have been through an earthquake respond quickly and vigorously to any weak noise or vibration thereafter, even though it may be unrelated to an earthquake.

It seems that procedural and declarative memories are stored differently. Studies of brain-damaged and Alzheimer's victims show that they may still be perfectly capable of riding a bicycle (procedural) without remembering the word, *bicycle* or when they learned to ride (declarative). Procedural and declarative memory seem to be stored in different regions of the brain, and declarative memory can be lost while procedural is spared (Rose, 2005).

Emotional Memory

Earlier taxonomies of memory systems usually listed *emotional memory* as a form of nondeclarative memory. But in refining their memory categories, scientists have identified situations requiring explicit (i.e., declarative) learning and memory. So emotional memories can be both implicit and explicit. In either case, the amygdala is heavily involved in processing emotional learning and memory. For example, sometimes, an experience is stored merely as an emotional *gist* or summary of the event, that is, we remember whether we liked it or not. A year after seeing a movie, for example, we might be able to recall only bits of the storyline (declarative memory) and perhaps its mood and our reaction (nondeclarative memory). Students often can remember whether they liked a particular topic, but cannot recall many details about it.

Emotional Memory and Learning

In Chapter 2, we learned how emotions can positively or negatively affect the acquisition of new learning. Emotions impact on learning in two distinct ways. One is the emotional climate in which the learning occurs. The other is the degree to which emotions are associated with the learning content. Figure 3.3 illustrates two ways that emotions impact directly on learning.

The Learning Climate. Emotions that students associate with a learning experience (but not the content) become part of the nondeclarative memory system. Emotional climate is directly

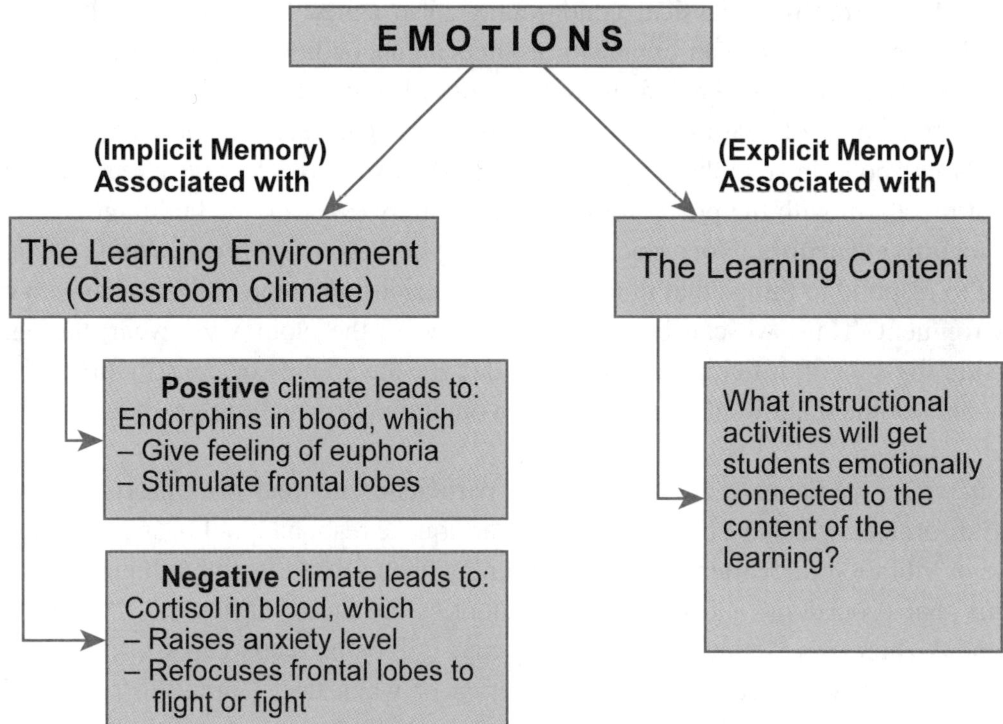

Figure 3.3 The chart shows the two ways that emotions impact on learning. One way is the emotional climate of the environment in which the learning takes place. The other deals with the emotions that the learner experiences while processing the content of the learning.

related to classroom climate, which is regulated by the teacher. Students ask: Do I have a good rapport with the teacher? Is my opinion respected? Does the teacher make me feel dumb when I ask for help? Am I the butt of sarcastic remarks? Does the teacher care whether I succeed? The answers to these questions generate emotions that determine how a student *feels* about the learning situation. These unconscious responses can turn them toward or away from their teachers and future learning experiences.

When students feel positive about their learning environment, endorphins are released in the brain. Endorphins produce a feeling of euphoria and stimulate the frontal lobes, thereby making the learning experience more pleasurable and successful. Conversely, if students are stressed and have a negative feeling about the learning environment, cortisol is released. Cortisol is a hormone that travels throughout the brain and body and activates defense behaviors, such as fight or flight. Frontal lobe activity is reduced to focusing on the cause of the stress and how to deal with it. Little attention is given to the learning task. Cortisol appears to interfere especially with the recall of emotional memories (Kuhlmann, Kirschbaum, & Wolf, 2005).

Connect Content to Emotions. Students are much more likely to remember curriculum content in which they have made an emotional investment. For this to happen, teachers often need to use strategies that get students emotionally involved with the learning content. For example, I once sat in a high school classroom where students had been asked to create some original material that showed how their study of the Civil War had affected them emotionally. Taking turns, the students sang songs, recited poems, displayed sketches and watercolors depicting battle scenes, and acted out skits of major Civil War events. I suspect that more students will remember the causes and results of that war for many years to come. Simulations, role-playing, journal writing, and real world experiences are all examples of strategies that teachers can use to help students connect emotions to content.

Flashbulb Memories

A powerful emotional experience can cause an instantaneous and long-lasting memory of an event, called a *flashbulb memory*. An example is remembering where you were and what you were doing when the *Challenger* space shuttle exploded or when the World Trade Center was attacked. Although these memories are not always accurate, they do attest to the brain's ability to record and recall emotionally significant experiences. This ability most likely results from the stimulation of the amygdala and the release throughout the body of emotion-arousing substances, such as adrenalin (Cahill & McGaugh, 1998). This process puts vivid memory tags on emotionally charged events. As a result, confidence in the recollection is high, although flashbulb memories seem to be no more accurate than the recall of memories of everyday experiences (Gazzaniga et al., 2002).

Implications for Teaching

How the learner processes new information presented in school has a great impact on the quality of what is learned and is a major factor in determining whether and how it will be retained. Memories, of course, are more than just information. They represent fluctuating patterns of associations and connections across the brain from which the individual extracts order and meaning. Teachers with a greater understanding of the types of memory and how they form can select strategies that are more likely to improve the retention and retrieval of learning.

LEARNING AND RETENTION

Learning and retention are different. Learning involves the brain, the nervous system, and the environment, and the process by which their interplay acquires information and skills. Sometimes, we need information for just a short period of time, like the telephone number for a pizza delivery, and then the information decays in just a few seconds. Thus, learning does not always involve long-term retention.

> ***Learning and retention are different. We can learn something for just a few minutes and then lose it forever.***

A good portion of the teaching done in schools centers on delivering facts and information to build concepts that explain a body of knowledge. We teach numbers, arithmetic operations, ratios, and theorems to explain mathematics. We teach about atoms, momentum, gravity, and cells to explain science. We talk about countries, famous leaders, and their trials and battles to explain history, and so on. Students may hold on to this information in working memory just long enough to take a test, after which it readily decays and is lost. (See the **Practitioner's Corner** in Chapter 2 on testing whether information is in long-term storage, p. 70.) Retention, however, requires that the learner not only give conscious attention but also build conceptual frameworks that have sense and meaning for eventual consolidation into the long-term storage networks.

FACTORS AFFECTING RETENTION OF LEARNING

Retention refers to the process whereby long-term memory preserves a learning in such a way that it can locate, identify, and retrieve it accurately in the future. As explained earlier, this is an inexact process influenced by many factors including the degree of student focus, the length and type of rehearsal that occurred, the critical attributes that may have been identified, the student's learning style, and, of course, the inescapable influence of prior learnings.

The information processing model in Chapter 2 identifies some of these factors and sets the stage for finding ways to transfer what we know into daily classroom practice. Let us look more specifically at the way the brain processes and retains information during a learning episode, how the nature of that processing affects the degree of retention, and how the degree of retention varies with the length of the episode.

Rehearsal

Rehearsal deals with the repetition and processing of information whereas practice generally refers to the repetition of motor skills.

The assignment of sense and meaning to new learning can occur only if the learner has adequate time to process and reprocess it. This continuing reprocessing of information is called *rehearsal,* and it is a critical component in the transference of information from working memory to long-term storage. Rehearsal is different from practice in that rehearsal deals with the repetition and processing of information whereas practice, for our purposes, refers to the repetition of motor skills.

The concept of rehearsal is not new. Even the Greek scholars of 400 BC knew its value. They wrote:

> *Repeat again what you hear; for by often hearing and saying the same things, what you have learned comes complete into your memory.*
>
> —from the *Dialexeis*

Two major factors should be considered in evaluating rehearsal: The amount of time devoted to it, which determines whether there is both initial and secondary rehearsal, and the type of rehearsal carried out, which can be *rote* or *elaborative.*

Time for Initial and Secondary Rehearsal

Time is a critical component of rehearsal. Initial rehearsal occurs when the information first enters working memory. If the learner cannot attach sense or meaning, and if there is no time for further processing, then the new information is likely to be lost. Providing sufficient time to go beyond the initial processing to secondary rehearsal allows the learner to review the information, to make sense of it, to elaborate on the details, and to assign value and relevance, thus increasing significantly the chance of long-term storage. When done at the end of a learning episode, this rehearsal is called closure (see Chapter 2).

Scanning studies indicate that the frontal lobe is very much involved during the rehearsal process and, ultimately, in long-term memory formation. This makes sense because working memory is also located in the frontal lobe. Several studies using fMRI scans of humans showed that during longer rehearsals the amount of activity in the frontal lobe determined whether items were stored or forgotten (Buckner, Kelley, & Petersen, 1999; Wagner et al., 1998). Students carry out initial and secondary rehearsal at different rates of speed and in different ways, depending on the type of information in the new learning and their learning styles. As the learning task changes, learners automatically shift to different patterns of rehearsal.

Rote and Elaborative Rehearsal

Rote Rehearsal. This type of rehearsal is used when the learner needs to remember and store information exactly as it is entered into working memory. This is not a complex strategy, but it is necessary to learn information or a cognitive skill in a specific form or sequence. We use rote rehearsal to remember a poem, the lyrics and melody of a song, multiplication tables, telephone numbers, and steps in a procedure.

Elaborative Rehearsal. This type of rehearsal is used when it is not necessary to store information exactly as learned, but when it is more important to associate the new learnings with prior learnings to detect relationships. This is a more complex thinking process in that the learner reprocesses the information several times to make connections to previous learnings and assign meaning. Students use rote rehearsal to memorize a poem, but elaborative rehearsal to interpret its message.

When students get very little time for, or training in, elaborative rehearsal, they resort more frequently to rote rehearsal for nearly all processing. Consequently, they fail to make the associations or discover the relationships that only elaborative rehearsal can provide. Also, they continue to believe that learning is merely the recalling of information as learned rather than its value for generating new ideas, concepts, and solutions.

Rote rehearsal is valuable for certain limited learning objectives. Nearly all of us learned the alphabet and the multiplication tables through rote rehearsal. But rote rehearsal simply allows us to acquire information in a certain sequence. It doesn't mean we understand the information or can apply it to new situations. Too often, students use rote rehearsal to memorize important terms and facts in a lesson, but are unable to use the information to solve problems. They will probably do fine on a true-false or fill-in-the-blank test. But they will find difficulty answering higher-order questions that require them to apply their knowledge to new situations.

The goal of learning is not just to acquire knowledge, but to be able to use that knowledge in a variety of different settings. To do this, students need a deeper understanding of the concepts involved in the learning. For example, we could teach students the various types of government, such as monarchy, parliamentary, republic, totalitarian state, dictatorship, and theocracy. On a test, we could ask them to write and define the types of government and even to name a country as an example of each type.

There is almost no long-term retention of cognitive concepts without rehearsal.

All this could be accomplished through rote rehearsal. But if we want students to understand why people are willing to die to change their type of government, or to make predictions about how different governments will react to a crisis, then they must have a much deeper grasp of the concepts of government and governing. That requires elaborative rehearsal. Perhaps one reason students are bored in school is that they spend too much time memorizing but not understanding.

When deciding on how to use rehearsal in a lesson, teachers need to consider the time available as well as the type of rehearsal appropriate for the specific learning objective. Keep in mind that rehearsal only contributes to, but does not guarantee that information will transfer into, long-term storage. However, there is almost no long-term retention *without* rehearsal.

Test Question No. 4: Increased time on task increases retention of new learning.

Answer: False. Simply increasing a student's time on a learning task does not guarantee retention if the student is not allowed the time and help to personally interact with the content through rehearsal.

Retention During a Learning Episode

When an individual is processing new information, the amount of information retained depends, among other things, on *when* it is presented during the learning episode. At certain time intervals during the learning, we will remember more than at other intervals. Let's try a simple activity to illustrate this point. You will need a pencil and a timer. Set the timer to go off in 12 seconds. When you start the timer, look at the list of 10 words. When the timer sounds, cover the list and write as many of the 10 words as you remember on the lines to the right of the list. Write each word on the line that represents its position on the list (i.e., the first word on line one, etc.). Thus, if you cannot remember the eighth word, but you remember the ninth, write it on line number nine.

Ready? Start the timer and stare at the word list for 12 seconds. Now cover the list and write the words you remember on the lines to the right. Don't worry if you did not remember all the words.

KEF	1.	________
LAK	2.	________
MIL	3.	________
NIR	4.	________
VEK	5.	________
LUN	6.	________
NEM	7.	________
BEB	8.	________
SAR	9.	________
FIF	10.	________

Turn to your list again and circle the words that were correct. To be correct, they must be spelled correctly and be in the proper position on the list. Look at the circled words. Chances are you remembered the first 3 to 5 words (lines 1 through 5) and the last 1 to 2 words (lines 9 and 10), but had difficulty with the middle words (lines 6-8). Read on to find out why.

Primacy-Recency Effect

Your pattern in remembering the word list is a common phenomenon that is referred to as the *primacy-recency effect* (also known as the *serial position effect*). In a learning episode, we tend to remember best that which comes first, and remember second best that which comes last. We tend to remember least that which comes just past the middle of the episode. This is not a new discovery. Ebbinghaus published the first studies on this effect in the 1880s.

> ***During a learning episode, we remember best that which comes first, second best that which comes last, and least that which comes just past the middle.***

More recent studies help to explain why this is so. The first items of new information are within the working memory's functional capacity so they command our attention, and are likely to be retained in semantic memory. The later information, however, exceeds the capacity and is lost. As the learning episode concludes, items in working memory are sorted or chunked to allow for additional processing of the arriving final items, which are likely held in working memory and will decay unless further rehearsed (Gazzanniga et al., 2002; Terry, 2005).

Figure 3.4 shows how the primacy-recency effect influences retention during a 40-minute learning episode (Buzan, 1989; Thomas, 1972). The times are approximate and averages. Note that it is a bimodal curve, each mode representing the degree of greatest retention during that time period. For future reference, I will label the first or primacy mode *prime-time-1,* and the second or recency mode *prime-time-2.* Between these two modes is the time period in which retention during the lesson is least. I will refer to that area as the *down-time.* This is not a time when no retention takes place, but a time when it is most difficult for retention to occur.

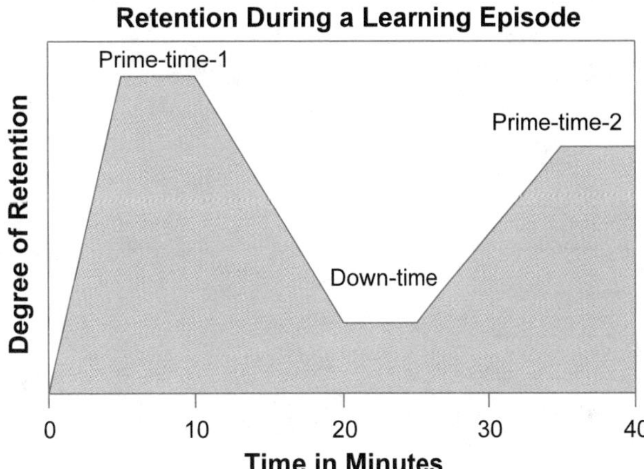

Figure 3.4 The degree of retention varies during a learning episode. We remember best that which comes first (prime-time-1) and last (prime-time-2). We remember least that which comes just past the middle.

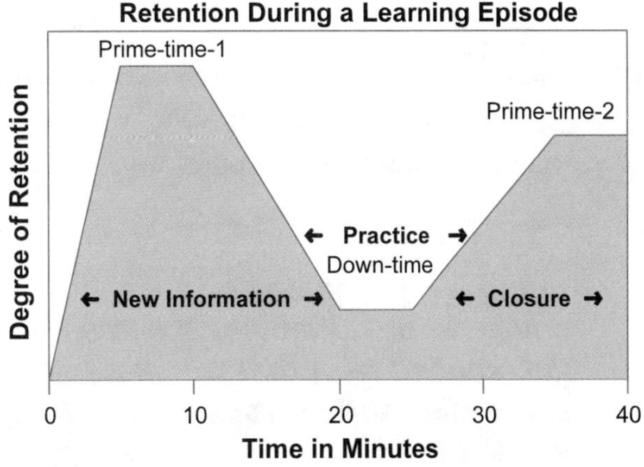

Figure 3.5 New information should be presented in prime-time-1, and closure in prime-time-2. Practice is appropriate for the down-time segment.

Implications for Teaching

Teach New Material First

There are important implications of the primacy-recency effect for teaching a lesson. The learning episode begins when the learner focuses on the teacher with intent to learn (indicated by "0" in the Figure 3.4 graph). New information or a new skill should be taught first, during prime-time-1, because it is most likely to be remembered. Keep in mind that the students will remember almost any information coming forth at this time. It is important, then, that only *correct* information be presented. This is not the time to be searching for what students may know about something. I remember watching a teacher of English start a class with, "Today, we are going to learn about a new literary form called *onomatopoeia.* Does anyone have any idea what that is?" After several wrong guesses, the teacher finally defined it. Regrettably, those same wrong guesses appeared in the follow-up test. And why not? They were mentioned during the most powerful retention position, prime-time-1.

The new material being taught should be followed by practice or review during the down-time. At this point, the information is no longer new, and the practice helps the learner organize it for further processing. Closure should take place during prime-time-2, since this is the second most powerful learning position and an important opportunity for the learner to determine sense and meaning. Adding these activities to the graph in Figure 3.5 shows how we can take advantage of research on retention to design a more effective lesson.

Misuse of Prime-Time

Even with the best of intentions, teachers with little knowledge of the primacy-recency effect can do the following: After getting focus by telling the class the day's lesson objective, the teacher takes attendance, distributes the previous day's homework, collects that day's homework, requests notes from students who were absent, and reads an announcement about a club meeting after school. By the time the teacher gets to the new learning, the students are already at the down-time. As a finale, the teacher tells the students that they were so well-behaved during the lesson that they can do anything they want during the last five minutes of class (i.e., during prime-time-2) as long as they are quiet. I have observed this scenario, and I can attest that the next day those students remembered who was absent and why, which club met after school, and what they did at the end of the period. The new learning, however, was difficult to remember because it was presented at the time of least retention. See the **Practitioner's Corner** on p. 121 on using the primacy-recency effect in the classroom.

> ***When you have the students' focus, teach the new information. Don't let prime-time get contaminated with wrong information.***

Retention Varies With Length of Teaching Episode

Another fascinating characteristic of the primacy-recency effect is that the proportion of prime-times to down-time changes with the length of the teaching episode. Look at Figure 3.6. Note that during a 40-minute lesson, the two prime-times total about 30 minutes, or 75 percent of the teaching time. The down-time is about 10 minutes, or 25 percent of the lesson time. If we double the length of the learning episode to 80 minutes, the down-time increases to 30 minutes, or 38 percent of the total time period.

As the lesson time lengthens, the percentage of down-time increases faster than for the prime-times. The information is entering working memory faster than it can be sorted or checked, and it accumulates. This cluttering interferes with the sorting and chunking processes and reduces the learner's ability to attach sense and meaning, thereby decreasing retention. Think back to some of those college classes that lasted for two hours or more. After about the first 20 minutes, didn't you find yourself concentrating more on taking notes rather than on processing and learning what was being presented?

Figure 3.6 also shows what happens when we shorten the learning time to 20 minutes. The down-time is about 2 minutes, or 10 percent of the total lesson time. As we shorten the learning episode, the down-time decreases faster than the prime-times. This finding indicates that there is a higher probability of effective learning taking place if we can keep the learning episodes short and, of course, meaningful. Thus, teaching two 20-minute lessons provides 20 percent more prime-time (approximately 36 minutes) than one 40-minute lesson (approximately 30 minutes). Note, however, that a time period shorter than 20 minutes may not give the learner sufficient time to determine the pattern and organization of the new learning, and is thus of little benefit.

Table 3.1 summarizes the approximate number of minutes in the prime-times and down-times of the learning cycle for episodes of 20, 40, and 80 minutes. Remember that the times are averages over many episodes. Nonetheless, these data confirm what we may have long suspected: More retention occurs when lessons are shorter and meaningful.

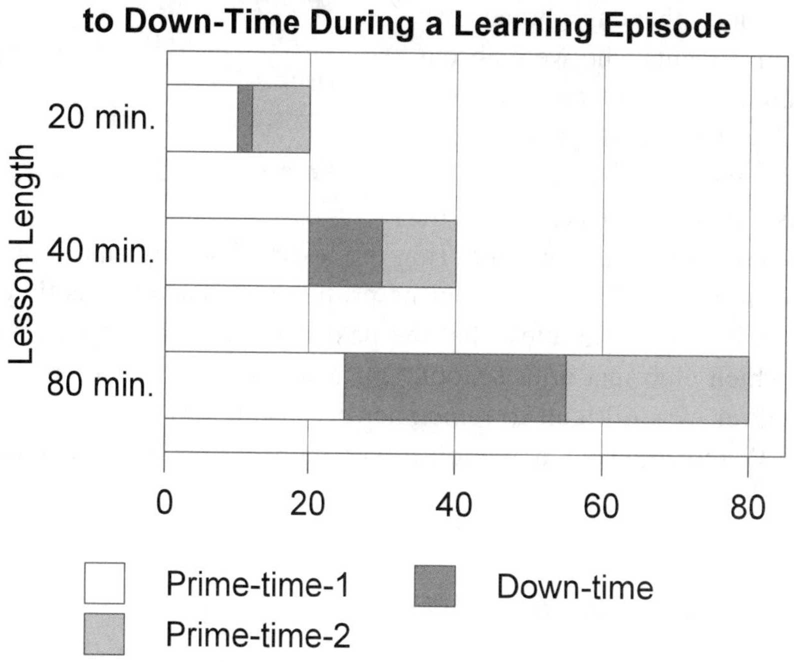

Figure 3.6 The proportion of down-time to prime-times for 20-, 40-, and 80-minute learning episodes, when taught as one lesson.

Shorter Is Better: Impact on Block Scheduling

Because today's students are accustomed to quick change and novelty in their environment, many find it difficult to concentrate on the same topic for long periods of time. They fidget, drift, send text messages to each other, and get into off-task conversations. This is particularly true if the teacher is doing most of the work, such as lecturing. The primacy-recency effect has a particularly important impact on block scheduling, in which a learning episode of 80 or more minutes can be a blessing or a disaster, depending on how the time is used. Figure 3.7 shows that a block containing four 20-minute segments will often be much more productive than one continuous lesson. Further, only one or two of the four block segments should be teacher directed. (See the **Practitioner's Corner** on p. 123 on block scheduling.)

Rest Between Block Lesson Segments

Most teachers believe that staying on-task throughout the learning period is best. During 1994-1997, while an adjunct professor at Seton Hall University, I asked secondary teachers to conduct action research projects in their block schedule classrooms to determine if going off-task between lesson segments (for example, telling a joke or story, playing music, taking a quiet rest break, or getting students up and moving around) resulted in more, less, or the same amount of attending

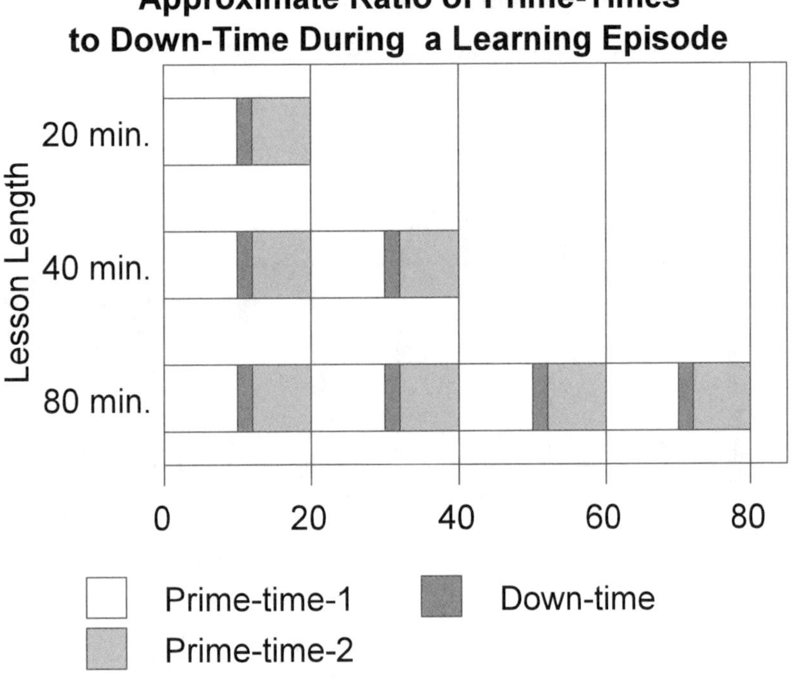

Figure 3.7 By dividing each learning episode into 20-minute segments, there is proportionately more prime-time to down time

Table 3.1 Average Prime- and Down-times in Learning Episodes

Episode Time	Prime-Times		Down-Time	
	Total Number of Minutes	Percentage of Total Time	Number of Minutes	Percentage of Total Time
20 minutes	18	90	2	10
40 minutes	30	75	10	25
80 minutes	50	62	30	38

(measured by the speed with which the students returned to task) than if they had stayed continuously on-task.

Figure 3.8 is the compilation of their results, which are similar to Tony Buzan's (1989) findings in the 1980s. The graph suggests that teachers are more likely to keep students focused *during*

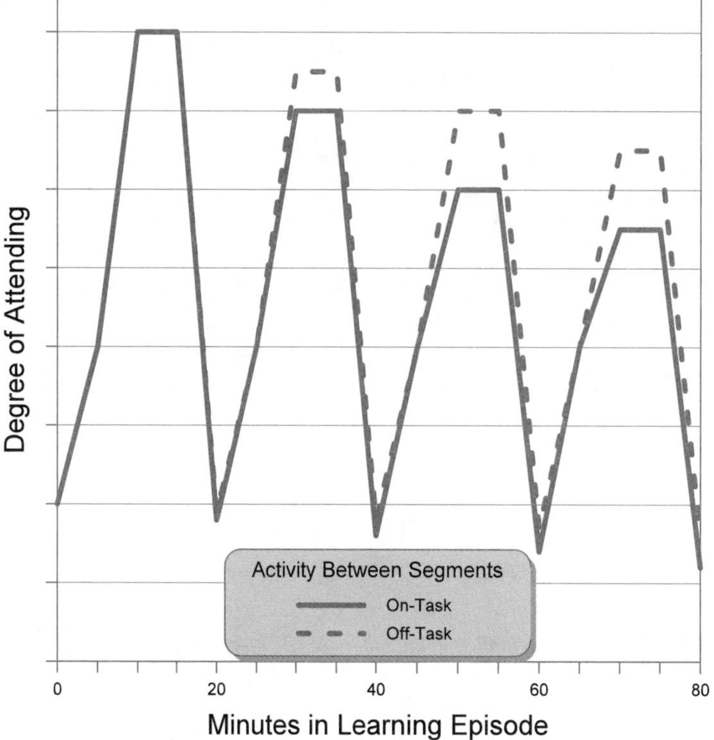

Figure 3.8 Compilation of 18 action research studies in secondary school classrooms comparing the degree of attending (focus) to on-task and off-task behavior between lesson segments of a block period.

the lesson segments if they go off-task *between* the segments. Granted, this is not a scientifically controlled study, but the results are not surprising given the higher novelty-seeking behavior of today's students. Teachers in nonblock classes (i.e., 40 to 45 minutes in length) who take an off-task break about half-way through the period have reported similar results.

Retention Varies With Teaching Method

The learner's ability to retain information is also dependent on the type of teaching method used. Some methods result in more retention of learning than others. The learning pyramid shown in Figure 3.9, devised in the 1960s by the National Training Laboratories of Bethel, Maine (now the NTL Institute of Alexandria, Virginia), comes from studies on retention of learning after students were exposed to different teaching methods. The pyramid shows the percentage of new learning that students can recall after 24 hours as a result of being taught *primarily* by the teaching method indicated. (Note: As discussed earlier, information recalled after 24 hours is presumed to be in long-term storage.) Although this study was conducted four decades ago, more recent studies on the factors affecting retention of learning generally support the original results. It is possible that the percentages may have changed somewhat over the years. For example, Moore (2005) reports studies showing that retention after three days is 10 percent from lecturing and 20 percent from demonstration.

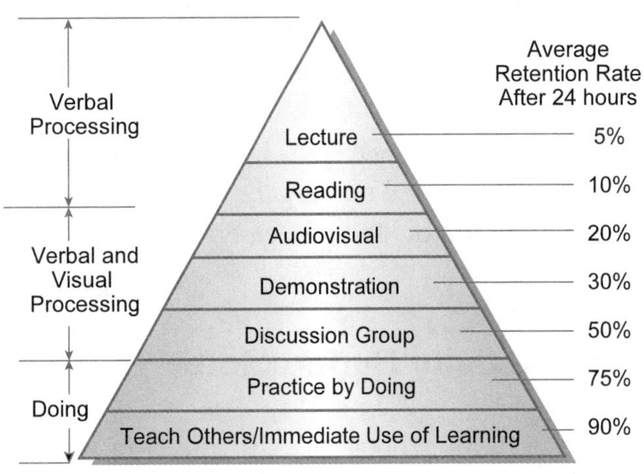

Figure 3.9 The diagram shows the average percentage of retention of material after 24 hours for each of the instructional methods.

The percentages (from the original study) are rounded to the nearest 5 percent and are not additive. At the top of the pyramid is lecture—the teaching method that results in an average retention of only 5 percent of learning after 24 hours. This is not surprising because lecture involves verbal processing with little student active participation or mental rehearsal. In this format, the teacher is telling and the students are listening just enough to convert the teacher's auditory output into written notes. Rote rehearsal predominates as auditory information moves onto the notebook paper. Elaborative rehearsal is minimal or nonexistent. Despite the impressive amount of evidence about how little students retain from lecture, it continues to be the most prevalent method of teaching, especially in secondary and higher education. No one doubts that the lecture method allows a lot of information to be presented in a short period of time. But the question is not what is presented, but what is learned.

Moving down the pyramid, input changes to verbal and visual processing as students become more involved in the learning process, and retention increases. The methods at the bottom of the pyramid involve having the students doing something through practice, and teaching others or using the new learning immediately. This results in from 75 to 90 percent retention after 24 hours. We have known for a long time that the best way to learn something is to prepare to teach it. In other words, whoever explains, learns. This is one of the major components of cooperative learning groups and helps to explain the effectiveness of this instructional technique.

> ***Lecture continues to be the most prevalent teaching method in secondary and higher education, despite evidence that it produces the lowest degree of retention for most learners.***

No One Teaching Method Is Best. No one teaching method exists that is best for all students all the time. Sometimes, lecture is the appropriate method when a lot of information needs to be given in a short period of time. But neither lecture, nor any other method for that matter, should be used almost all the time. Successful teachers use a variety of methods, keeping in mind that students are more likely to retain and achieve whenever they are actively engaged in the learning.

LEARNING MOTOR SKILLS

Scanning studies show that a person uses the frontal lobe, motor cortex, and cerebellum while learning a new physical skill. Learning a motor skill involves following a set of procedures and can be eventually carried out largely without conscious attention. In fact, too much conscious attention directed to a motor skill while performing it can diminish the quality of its execution.

Brain Activity During Motor Skill Acquisition

When first learning the skill, attention and awareness are obviously required. The frontal lobe is engaged because working memory is needed, and the motor cortex of the cerebrum (located across the top of the brain) interacts with the cerebellum to control muscle movement. As practice continues, the activated areas of the motor cortex become larger as nearby neurons are recruited into the new skill network. However, the memory of the skill is not established (i.e., stored) until after practice stops. It takes about 4 to 12 hours for this consolidation to take place in the cerebellum, and most of it occurs during deep sleep. Once the skill is mastered, brain activity shifts to the cerebellum, which organizes and coordinates the movements and the timing to perform the task. Procedural memory is the mechanism, and the brain no longer needs to use its higher-order processes as the performance of the skill becomes automatic (Penhume & Doyon, 2005; Press, Casement, Pascual-Leone, & Robertson, 2005; Shadmehr & Holcomb, 1997; Walker, Stickgold, Alsop, Gaab, & Schlaug, 2005).

Continued practice of the skill changes the brain structurally, and the younger the learner is, the easier it is for these changes to occur. Most music and sports prodigies began practicing their skills very early in life. Because their brains were most sensitive to the structural changes needed to acquire the skills, they can perform them masterfully. These skills become so much a part of the individual that they are difficult to change later in life. In the 1990s, Michael Jordan tried to become a major league baseball player at the age of 31 after a stellar career as a lead basketball scorer for the Chicago Bulls. Despite much effort, his attempt at baseball failed. Jordan had started playing basketball at the age of 8 and had developed a finely tuned set of motor skills in procedural memory that allowed him to be an expert basketball player. Trying to learn a new set of motor and perceptual skills to be a successful baseball player in a short period of time was just not possible.

The Problem of Learning Two Similar Skills

A surprising finding from these studies was that if the person practiced a very similar skill during the 4- to 12-hour down-time, the second skill interfered with the consolidation and mastery of the first skill—and vice versa. Consequently, the person was not able to perform either skill well (Oberauer & Kliegl, 2004; Witney, 2004). This appears to be evidence that negative transfer (see Chapter 4) can occur during the learning of motor

> ***Learning two skills that are too similar at the same time causes memory interference so that the student learns neither skill well.***

skills as well as during the learning of cognitive concepts. Think of the implications that this has for teaching, wherein similarity is one of the major criteria we use to decide the sequence for presenting information and skills. See the **Practitioner's Corner** on p. 117 on how similarity can interfere with new motor skill learning.

Test Question No. 5: Two very similar concepts or motor skills should be taught at the same time.

Answer: False. Teaching two very similar concepts or skills at the same time can cause interference so that the student learns neither.

Does Practice Make Perfect?

Practice refers to learners repeating a skill over time. It begins with the rehearsal of the new skill in working memory, the motor cortex, and the cerebellum. Later, the skill memory is recalled and additional practice follows. The quality of the practice and the learner's knowledge base will largely determine the outcome of each practice session.

Over the long term, repeated practice causes the brain to assign extra neurons to the task, much as a computer assigns more memory for a complex program. The assignment of these additional neurons is more or less on a permanent basis. Professional keyboard and string musicians, for example, have larger portions of the motor cortex devoted to controlling finger and hand movements. Furthermore, the earlier their training started, the bigger the motor cortex (Schlaug, Jancke, Huang, & Steinmetz, 1995). If practice is stopped altogether, the neurons that are no longer being used are eventually assigned to other tasks and skill mastery will decline (Amunts et al., 1997). In other words, use it or lose it!

The old adage that "practice makes perfect" is rarely true. It is very possible to practice the same skill repeatedly with no increase in achievement or accuracy of application. Think of the people you know who have been driving, cooking, or even teaching for many years with no improvement in their skills. I am a self-taught bowler, and although I have been bowling for 25 years, I do not improve. My bowling scores are embarrassingly low and remain there despite years of repeated bowling. Why is this?

Practice does not make perfect. Practice makes permanent.

How is it possible for one to continuously practice a skill with no resulting improvement in performance?

Conditions for Successful Practice

For practice to *improve* performance, four conditions must be met (Hunter, 2004):

1. The learner must be sufficiently motivated to *want* to improve performance.
2. The learner must have all the knowledge necessary to understand the different ways that the new knowledge or skill can be applied.
3. The learner must understand how to apply the knowledge to deal with a particular situation.
4. The learner must be able to analyze the results of that application and know what needs to be changed to improve performance in the future.

Teachers help learners meet these conditions when they do the following:

- Start by selecting the smallest amount of material that will have maximum meaning for the learner.
- Model the application process step-by-step. Studies show that the brain also uses observation as a means for determining the spatial learning needed to master a motor skill (Petrosini et al., 2003).
- Insist that the practice occur in their presence over a short period of time while the student is focused on the learning.
- Watch the practice and provide the students with prompt and specific feedback on what variable needs to be altered to correct and enhance the performance. Feedback seems to be particularly important during the learning of complex motor skills (Wulf, Shea, & Matschiner, 1998).

Guided Practice, Independent Practice, and Feedback

Practice does make permanent, thereby aiding in the retention of learning. Consequently, we want to ensure that students practice the new learning correctly from the beginning. This early practice (referred to as *guided practice),* then, is done in the presence of the teacher, who can now offer corrective feedback to help students analyze and improve their practice. When the practice is correct, the teacher can then assign *independent practice,* in which the students can rehearse the skill on their own to enhance retention.

Avoid giving students independent practice before guided practice.

This strategy leads to perfect practice, and, as Vince Lombardi said, "Perfect practice makes perfect." In my case, I go bowling every few months to be with the same close friends, who are very busy professionals. Bowling is simply the means that allows us to catch up on our lives, and our scores are of little importance. Thus, I have no *motivation* to improve—and, believe me, I don't.

Teachers should avoid giving students independent practice before guided practice. Because practice makes permanent, allowing students to rehearse something for the first time while away from the teacher is very risky. If they unknowingly practice the skill incorrectly, then they will learn the incorrect method well! This will present serious problems for both the teacher and learner later on because it is very difficult to change a skill that has been practiced and remembered, even if it is not correct.

Unlearning and Relearning a Skill. If a learner practices a skill incorrectly but well, unlearning and relearning that skill correctly is very difficult. The degree to which the unlearning and relearning processes are successful will depend on the

- Age of the learner (i.e., the younger, the easier to relearn)
- Length of time the skill has been practiced incorrectly (i.e., the longer, the more difficult to change)
- Degree of motivation to relearn (i.e., the greater the desire for change, the more effort that will be used to bring about change).

Sometimes, students who are young, and who have practiced the skill wrong for only a brief time, are so annoyed at having wasted their time with the incorrect practice that they lose motivation to learn the skill correctly.

Practice and Rehearsal Over Time Increases Retention

Hunter (2004) suggested that teachers use two different types of practice over time, massed and distributed. (Here, Hunter uses practice to include rehearsal.) Practicing a new learning during time periods that are very close together is called massed practice. This produces fast learning, as when you may mentally rehearse a new telephone number if you are unable to write it down. Immediate memory is involved here and the information can fade in seconds if it is not rehearsed quickly.

Teachers provide massed practice when they allow students to try different examples of applying new learning in a short period of time. Cramming for an exam is an example of massed practice. Material can be quickly chunked into working memory but can also be quickly dropped or forgotten if more sustained practice does not follow soon. This happens because the material has no further meaning, and thus the need for long-term retention disappears. Sustained practice over time, called distributed practice, is the key to retention. If you want to remember that new telephone number later on, you will need to use it repeatedly over time. Thus, practice that is distributed over longer periods of time sustains meaning and consolidates the learnings into long-term storage in a form that will ensure accurate recall and applications in the future. The graph in Figure 3.10 shows that recall after periodic review improves over time. This is the rationale behind the idea of the spiral

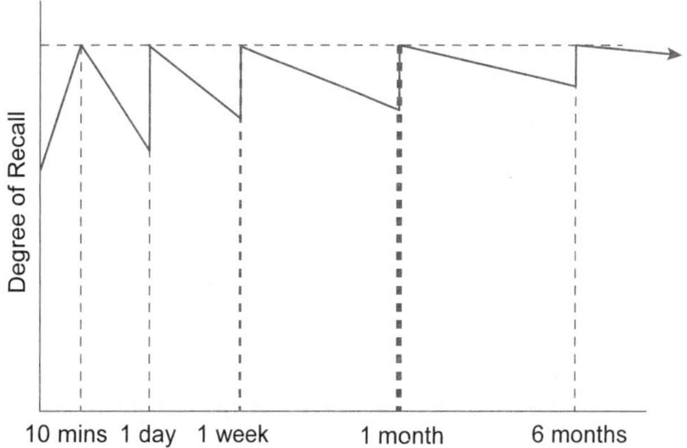

Figure 3.10 Practicing learnings over time (distributed practice) increases their degree of recall.

curriculum, whereby critical information and skills are reviewed at regular intervals within and over several grade levels.

Effective practice, then, starts with massed practice for fast learning and proceeds to distributed practice later for retention. As a result, the student is continually practicing previously learned skills throughout the year(s). Each test should not only test new material but also allow students to practice important older learnings. This method not only helps in retention but reminds students that the learnings will be useful for the future, not just for the time when they were first learned and tested.

DAILY BIOLOGICAL RHYTHMS AFFECT TEACHING AND LEARNING

Circadian Rhythms

Many of our body functions and their components, such as temperature, breathing, digestion, hormone concentrations, etc., go through daily cycles of peaks and valleys. These daily cycles are called circadian (from the Latin, "about a day") rhythms. The timing of these cycles is determined by the brain's exposure to daylight. Thus, some of the rhythms are related to the sleep-wake cycle and are controlled by a pair of small clusters of just 10,000 neurons in a tiny region of the brain located in the front part of the limbic area. These clusters are called the *suprachiasmatic nuclei* because they sit immediately above (supra) the optic chiasm—the area where the optic nerves from the left and right eye meet on their way to the brain.

One of these circadian rhythms regulates our ability to focus on incoming information with intent to learn. It can be referred to as the *psychological-cognitive cycle*. This cycle has drawn the attention of several research studies on the awake-and-asleep cycles of students (Carskadon, Acebo, Wolfson, Tzischinsky, & Darley, 1997; Millman, 2005). The findings show that the cognitive rhythm is about the same for a preadolescent and an adult, but starts later in an adolescent. This is because the onset of puberty shifts this particular cycle roughly an hour later than in the preadolescent. It returns to its previous level when the adolescent enters adulthood around the age of 22 to 24 years.

Figure 3.11 shows a comparison of the pre-/postadolescent, and adolescent cycles. Note the trough that occurs for both groups just past the middle of the day. This is a low point of focus.

Learning can still occur during this 20- to 60-minute period, but it will require more *effort*. I refer to the trough as the "dark hole of learning." Some cultures refer to it as the "siesta," having recognized long ago how difficult it is to accomplish much learning during this time.

Note that the adolescent cycle has shifted and that these students don't reach their peak until about an hour later. Note, too, that the second peak is flatter than for the other groups. This graph explains why adolescents are sleepier in the morning and tend to stay up later at night.

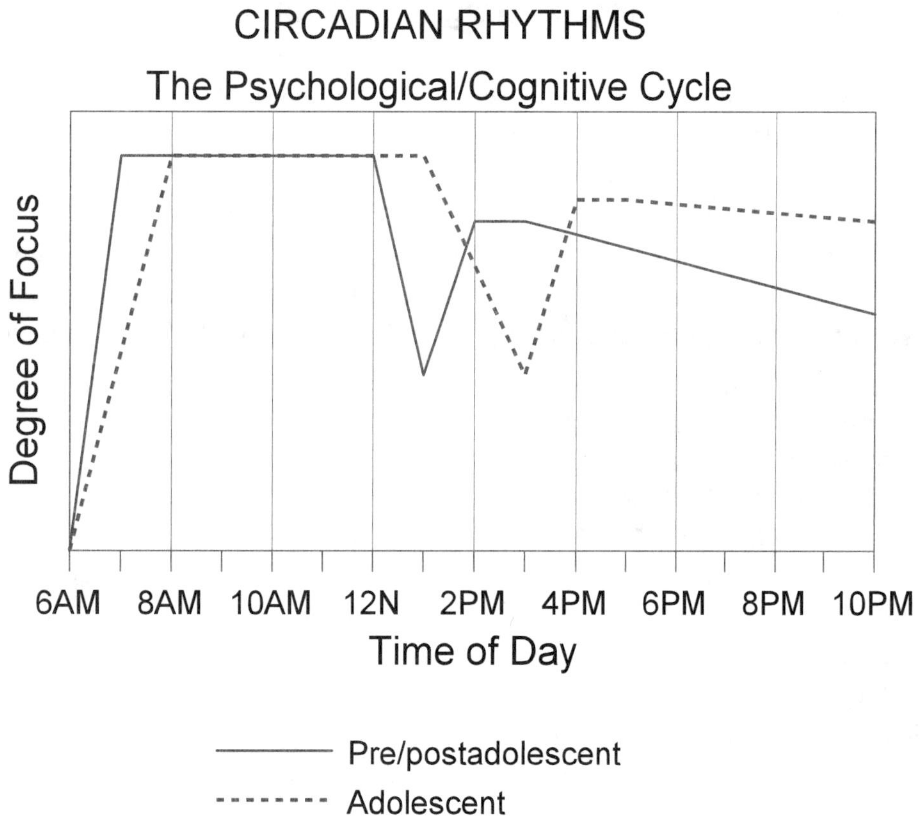

CIRCADIAN RHYTHMS

The Psychological/Cognitive Cycle

Degree of Focus

6AM 8AM 10AM 12N 2PM 4PM 6PM 8PM 10PM

Time of Day

——— Pre/postadolescent

-------- Adolescent

Figure 3.11 A comparison of the typical pre/postadolescent and adolescent cognitive cycles during the day. Note the trough that develops just past the middle of the day. This is a time when teaching and learning require more effort.

What Are the Implications? The different rhythms among preadolescents, adolescents, and their teachers have several implications. For example,

- How do the start times at elementary and secondary schools compare to the times when the students they serve are at their cognitive peak?
- Can the performance of students on standardized tests be affected when we test the whole K–12 population of students at the same time—usually in the morning?
- Can classroom climate in high schools be affected in the early afternoon when the teacher is in the trough and the students still at their peak?
- Can starting high schools later in the morning when students are more apt to be attentive result in lowering the drop-out rate?
- Would alternative high schools be more successful if they started in the afternoon?

See the **Practitioner's Corner** on p. 127 on the impact of circadian rhythms on schools and classrooms at the end of this chapter.

The Importance of Sleep in Learning and Memory

The encoding of information into the long-term memory sites occurs during sleep, more specifically, during the rapid-eye movement (REM) stage. This is a slow process that can flow more easily when the brain is not preoccupied with external stimuli. When we sleep, the brain reviews the events and tasks of the day, storing them more securely than at the time we originally processed them. What we think and talk about while awake very likely influences the nature and shape of the memory consolidation that occurs during sleep (Tuma, 2005). This may explain why people who review important information before going to sleep are likely to remember that information the next day during a test. Why not share this information with students?

Teenagers are not getting enough sleep. This sleep deprivation affects their ability to store information, increases irritability, and leads to fatigue which can cause accidents.

Adequate sleep is vital to the memory storage process, especially for young learners. Most teenagers need about nine hours of sleep each night. Many teenagers are not getting enough sleep. Several factors are responsible for eroding sleep time. In the morning, high schools start earlier, teens spend more time grooming, and some travel long distances to school. At the end of the day, there are athletic and social events, part-time jobs, homework, television, and video games. Add to this the shift in teens' body clocks that tends to keep them up later, and the average sleep time is more like five to six hours.

Delayed Sleep Phase Disorder

This problem is becoming so prevalent in middle and high schools that some neuroscientists and psychiatrists are convinced that it is a chronic disorder of the adolescent population. Called Delayed Sleep Phase Disorder (DSPD), it is characterized by a persistent pattern that includes difficulty falling asleep at night and getting up in the morning, fatigue during the day, and alertness at night. Caused mainly by the shift in the adolescent's circadian rhythm (Figure 3.11), DSPD is aggravated by other conditions.

Figure 3.12 shows the stages and cycles of sleep for teenagers and adults. Most of the encoding of information and skills into long-term storage is believed to occur during the rapid-eye movement (REM) phases. During the normal sleep time of eight to nine hours, five REM cycles occur. Adolescents getting just five to six hours of sleep lose out on the last two REM cycles, thereby reducing the amount of time the brain has to consolidate information and skills into long-term storage. This sleep deprivation not only disturbs the memory storage process but can lead to other problems as well. Students may nod off in class or become irritable. Worse, their decreased alertness due to fatigue can lead to accidents in school and in their cars (Acebo, Wolfson, & Carskadon,1997; Millman, 2005; Schacter, 1996).

Some studies show that students who get less sleep are more likely to get poorer grades in school than students who sleep longer. Sleep-deprived students also had more daytime sleepiness and depressed moods (Wolfson & Carskadon, 1998). It is important to remind students of the

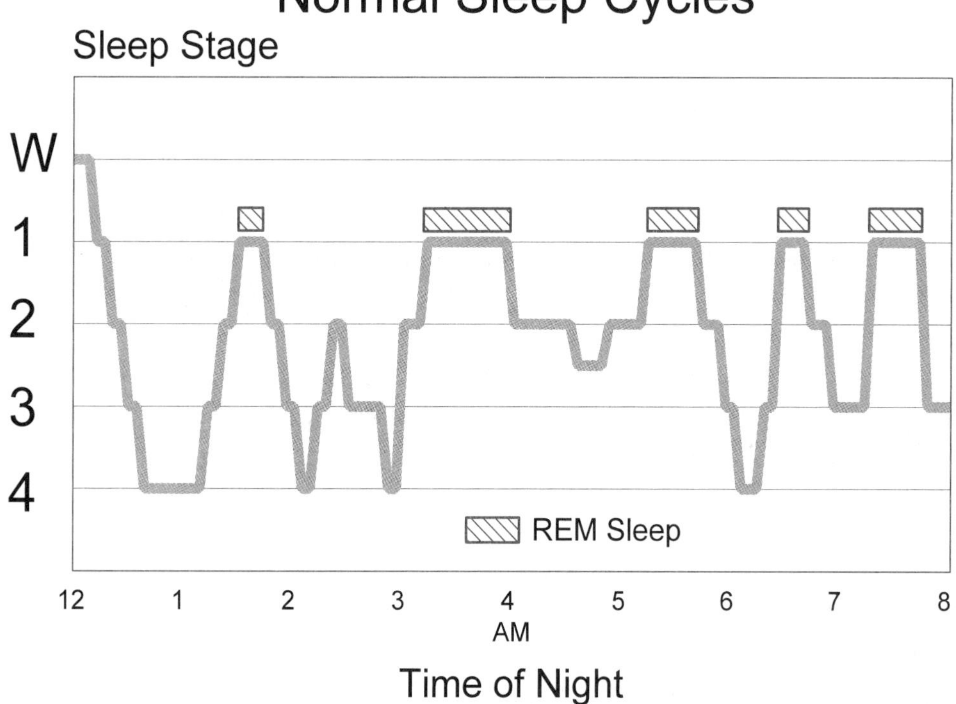

Figure 3.12 The chart shows the cycles of sleep from Waking through Stage 1 (Transitional), Stage 2 (Light Sleep), and Stages 3 to 4 (Deep Sleep). Long-term storage occurs during the rapid-eye movement (REM) phase.

significance of sleep to their mental and physical health and to encourage them to reexamine their daily activities to provide for adequate sleep. It should be noted that REM sleep is not required for *all* memory consolidation. Subsequent memory consolidation can occur when awake, especially the encoding of declarative memories, which seem to be less dependent on REM sleep.

INTELLIGENCE AND RETRIEVAL

Intelligence

Our modern notion of what constitutes human intelligence is growing increasingly complex. At the very least, it represents a combination of varied abilities and skills. For many years psychologists referred to a general mental ability, called the *g* factor. People who scored high on tests of general mental ability (i.e., I.Q. tests) were smarter than those who scored lower. The study of human intelligence took a major leap in the 1980s when psychologists Howard Gardner and Robert Sternberg proposed separate models of different types and patterns of intelligence. Their work changed our concept of intelligence from a singular entity to a multifaceted aptitude that varies even within the same person. Many educators have been using the ideas of Gardner and Sternberg in their curriculum, teaching, and school organization.

Different Views of Intelligence

Howard Gardner. In 1983, Howard Gardner defined intelligence as an individual's ability to use a learned skill, create products, or solve problems in a way that is valued by the society of that individual. This approach expands our understanding of intelligence to include divergent thinking and interpersonal expertise. Gardner differentiates between the terms *intelligence* and *creativity,* and suggested that in everyday life people can display intelligent originality in any of seven (now eight) intelligences. They are: musical, logical-mathematical, spatial, bodily-kinesthetic, linguistic, interpersonal, intrapersonal, and naturalist (Gardner, 1993).

Gardner made clear that intelligence is not just how a person thinks, but it also includes the materials and the values of the situation where and when the thinking occurs. The availability of appropriate materials and the values of any particular context or culture will thus have a significant impact on the degree to which specific intelligences will be activated, developed, or discouraged. A person's combined intellectual capability, then, is the result of innate tendencies (the genetic contribution) and the society in which that individual develops (the environmental contribution).

This theory suggests that at the core of each intelligence is an information-processing system (similar perhaps to that in Chapter 2) unique to that intelligence. The intelligence of an athlete is different from that of a musician or physicist. He also suggests that each intelligence is semi-autonomous. A person who has abilities in athletics but who does poorly in music has enhanced athletic intelligence. The presence or absence of music capabilities exists separately from the individual's athletic prowess.

Richard Sternberg. Two years after Gardner's work appeared, Robert Sternberg (1985) at Yale proposed a theory that distinguishes three patterns of intelligence: analytical, creative, and practical. People with analytical intelligence (the analyzers) have abilities in analyzing, critiquing, and evaluating. Those who are creatively intelligent (the creators) are particularly good at discovering, inventing, and creating. By contrast, the practically intelligent (the practitioners) excel at applying, utilizing, and implementing.

In this model, intelligence is defined by these three patterns of behavior, and intelligence refers to the ability to perform the skills in one or more of these areas with accuracy and efficiency. According to Sternberg, various combinations of these three areas produce different patterns of intelligence. This concept was tested in several studies conducted by Sternberg and his colleagues. Students were assessed for their memory as well as their analytical, creative, and practical achievement. The results showed that those students who were taught in ways that best matched their achievement patterns outperformed those whose method of instruction was not a good fit for their pattern of abilities (Sternberg, Ferrari, Clinkenbeard, & Grigorenko, 1996; Sternberg, et al., 2000).

Jeff Hawkins. In 2004, Jeff Hawkins, the inventor of the PalmPilot and a major researcher in artificial intelligence, described human intelligence as being measured by the capacity to remember and predict patterns in the world, including mathematics, language, social situations, and the properties of objects. The brain receives patterns from the outside world through experience, stores them as memories, and makes predictions by combining what it has seen before to what is happening now. In other words, to Hawkins, prediction, not behavior, is the proof of intelligence (Hawkins & Blakeslee, 2004).

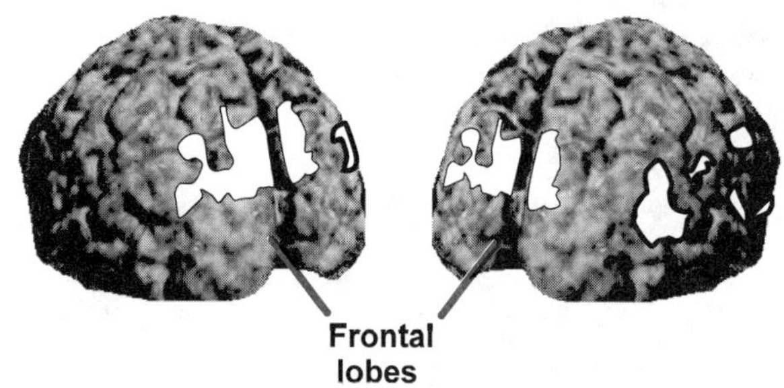

Figure 3.13 This composite MRI shows the key areas in the frontal lobes and left hemisphere where people with higher IQ scores had more gray matter than those with lower scores (Adapted from Haier et al., 2004).

It is clear that no agreement exists about what intelligence is, and major efforts to define intelligence are not likely to be advanced significantly by brain imaging anytime in the near future. PET scans and fMRIs do show some localization of brain activity for certain tasks. However, there is no scientific basis for equating the task with a particular type or pattern of intelligence. For example, visual stimuli are processed first in the visual cortex at the rear of the brain, and then in other parts of the brain for spatial perception and recognition. If anything, recent brain scans and case studies are revealing how remarkably integrated brain activity is when performing even the simplest task. Although most neuroscientists agree that there are areas that are specialized for certain tasks, areas rarely, if ever, work in isolation in the normal brain (See more about brain specialization in Chapter 5). Some researchers suggest that it is better to think of the brain as having a number of cerebral systems that are primarily responsible for processing the specific contents associated with each intelligence. For example, the motor cortex and cerebellum would take the lead in processing new skills associated with the bodily-kinesthetic area.

One interesting discovery is that general intelligence (that *g* factor) is closely linked to the amount of gray matter in key areas of the frontal lobes (Figure 3.13). People with more gray matter in their frontal lobes tend to score higher on tests of intelligence (Haier, Jung, Yeo, Head, & Alkire, 2004). The unanswered chicken-and-egg question is: Does the early development of more gray matter make a person more intelligent, or do challenging learning experiences result in the production of more gray matter? No one knows.

PET scans and EEGs also depict that people who score high on tests of reasoning and intelligence show less cerebral activity than people who score lower. These results imply that intelligence may be primarily a matter of *neural efficiency*, whereby the brain eventually learns to use fewer neurons or networks to accomplish a repetitive task (Neubauer, Grabner, Freudenthaler, Beckmann, & Guthke, 2004; Restak, 2003). If so, think of the implications this concept has for altering the way we allocate learning time as well as design and deliver lessons. It suggests, at the very least, that we should vary learning time to accommodate the task at hand and move learners to intensive practice as soon as comprehension is established. This approach is one of the basic components of differentiated instruction.

It is clear that no agreement exists about what intelligence is, and major efforts to define intelligence are not likely to be advanced significantly by brain imaging anytime in the near future.

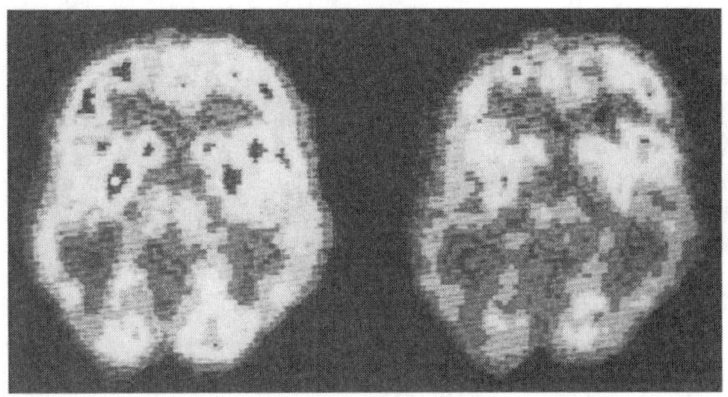

Figure 3.14 These PET images show the level of brain activity while playing a computer game. With the light colored areas indicating high levels of activity, the scans indicate that the expert player (right) uses significantly less energy than the novice player (left), an example of increased neural efficiency.

Further evidence of neural efficiency exists in PET scans taken of the brain while playing a computer game. When first learning the game there is a large amount of neural activity. As the player masters the game, the amount of brain activity diminishes significantly (Figure 3.14). Further, the higher the I.Q. of the player, the more quickly the neural activity drops while learning the game. Future research may describe these systems in greater detail and provide a neurological framework for better interpreting how data from the neurosciences support the notion of multiple intelligences.

For now, these current notions continue to move us away from the traditional model of intelligence as a singular entity, fixed at birth, and best measured by vocabulary and reading. They help us understand that the environment can have significant impact on intelligence, and that human beings can be smart in different ways.

Perhaps the next step is to realize that each of the intelligences described by Gardner, Sternberg, and others has many skills contained within it, and thus, there are *innumerable* ways that each brain can manipulate information and skills during the learning process. Expanding our view beyond separate intelligences to an integrated wealth of intelligences is supported by neuroscience, and it also reduces the chances that we will label kids as "word smart" or "music dumb." Rather, we can accept that the best teaching and learning occurs when we use the greatest variety of techniques, thereby making it more likely that all learners will succeed (Shearer, 2004).

Retrieval

It takes less than 50 milliseconds (a millisecond is 1/1,000th of a second) to retrieve an item from working memory. Retrieving a memory from long-term storage, however, can be complicated and comparatively time-consuming. One curious finding in recent years is that encoding information into memory involves the left hemisphere more than the right, and retrieval involves the right hemisphere more than the left. Although both processes involve the frontal lobes, it appears that encoding and retrieval activate separate neural systems.

The brain uses two methods to retrieve information from the long-term storage sites, *recognition* and *recall*. Recognition matches an outside stimulus with stored information. For example, the questions on a multiple-choice test involve recognizing the correct answer (assuming the learner stored it originally) among the choices. This method helps explain why even poor students almost always do better than expected on multiple-choice tests. Recall is quite different and more difficult. It describes the process whereby cues or hints are sent to long-term memory, which must search and retrieve information from the long-term storage sites, then consolidate and decode it back into working memory.

Both methods require the firing of neurons along the neural pathways to the storage site(s) and back again to working memory. The more frequently we access a pathway, the less likely it is to be obscured by other pathways. Information we use frequently, such as our name and telephone number, are quickly retrieved because the neural impulses to and from those storage sites keep the pathways clear. When the information is moved into working memory, we reprocess it to determine its validity and, in effect, relearn it.

> ***Whenever we retrieve something from long-term storage into working memory, we relearn it.***

Factors Affecting Retrieval

The rate at which the retrieval occurs depends on a number of factors.

- **Adequacy of the Cues.** The cue used to stimulate the retrieval of a memory may prompt a fully accurate recall or an ambiguous one. Since memory is not a videocassette recorder, the rememberer must reconstruct the memory based on the information retrieved by that cue. Having a strong memory does not seem to be as important as the retrieval cues (Schacter, 1996).
- **Mood of the Retriever.** Studies show that people in a sad mood more easily remember negative experiences, while those in a happy mood tend to recall pleasant experiences.
- **Context of the Retrieval.** Accurate recall is more likely to occur if the context during retrieval is very similar to the context of the period during which it was learned. Thus, testing for information in the same location in which it was learned is likely to result in better retrieval.
- **System of Storage.** Declarative memories get stored across brain structures, most likely in the areas that perceive and process incoming stimuli. Thus, the interests and past experiences of the learner will influence the type of cerebral networks that are constructed to contain the memory.

Students store the same item of information in different networks, depending on how they link the information to their past learnings. These storage decisions affect the amount of time it will take to retrieve the information later. This explains why some students need more time than others to retrieve the same information. When teachers call on the first hands that go up, they inadvertently signal to the slower retrievers to stop the retrieval process. This is an unfortunate strategy for two reasons: First, the slower retrieving students feel that they are not getting teacher recognition, thereby lowering their self-concept. Second, by not retrieving the information into working memory, they miss an opportunity to relearn it.

> ***Calling on the first hands that go up signals the slower retrievers to stop the retrieval process.***

Rates of Learning and Retrieval

It is no secret that some people learn a particular item faster or slower than others. The amount of time it takes someone to learn cognitive information with sufficient confidence that it will be consolidated into long-term memory is called the *rate of learning.* The rate of learning can vary within the same individual because it can be affected by motivation, emotional mood, degree of focus, and the context in which the learning occurs.

In the information processing model in Chapter 2, the rate of learning is represented by the data arrows flowing from left to right, from the senses through the sensory register to immediate memory and into working memory. The *rate of retrieval* is represented by the recall arrow moving information from right to left, from long-term storage to working memory. *These two rates are independent of each other.* This notion is quite different from classic doctrine which holds that the retrieval rate is strongly related to the rate of learning and, thus, anchored in genetic inheritance. The doctrine is further fueled in our society by timed tests and quiz programs that use the speed of retrieving answers as the main criterion for judging success and intelligence. The disclosure that the rate of retrieval is linked to the nature of the learner's storage method—a learned skill—rather than to the rate of learning is indeed significant. Because it is a *learned* skill, it can be taught. There is now great promise that techniques can be developed for helping us refine our long-term storage methods for faster and more accurate retrieval. (See the **Practitioner's Corners** on retention on pp. 118 and 130–132 at the end of this chapter.)

> ***The rate of learning and the rate of retrieval are independent of each other.***

Because the rate of learning and the rate of retrieval are independent, individuals can be fast or slow learners, fast or slow retrievers, and every combination in between. Although most people tend to fall midrange, some are at the extremes. Actually, not only have we had experience with learners possessing the extreme combinations of these two rates, but we have also (perhaps unwittingly) made up labels to describe them. An individual who is a fast learner and a fast retriever we call *gifted* or a *genius.* Such students retrieve answers quickly. Their hands go up first. Their responses are almost always correct, and they get reputations as "brains." Teachers call on them when they want to keep the lesson moving.

A student who is a fast learner but slow retriever we call an *underachiever.* Teachers say to these students, "Come on, John, I know you know this . . . keep trying." We often run out of patience and admonish them for not studying enough. A slow learner and fast retriever, we call an *overachiever.* These students respond quickly, but their answers may be incorrect. Teachers sometimes mistakenly view them as trying too hard to learn something that may be beyond them.

Test Question No. 6: The rate at which a learner retrieves information from memory is closely related to intelligence.

Answer: False. The rate of retrieval is independent of intelligence. It is more closely tied to how and where the information was stored originally.

For the student who is a slow learner and slow retriever, we have a whole list of uncomplimentary labels. More regrettable is that too often we interpret "slow learner" to mean "unable to learn." What being a slow learner really means is that the student is unable to learn something in the amount of time we have arbitrarily assigned for that learning. All these labels are unfortunate because they perpetuate the mistaken notion that the major factors promoting successful learning are beyond the control of the learner and teacher.

> ***Too often we interpret "slow learner" to mean "unable to learn".***

Teachers can help students improve their rate of retrieval by using instructional strategies that assist the learners' brain in deciding how and where to consolidate the new learning in long-term memory. One strategy deals with chunking, and is the next topic of discussion. The other involves identifying the critical attributes and is discussed in Chapter 4.

Chunking

There are three limits to our power of reasoning and thinking: our limited attention span, working memory, and long-term memory. Is it possible to consciously increase the number of items that working memory can handle at one time? The answer is yes, through a process called *chunking*. Chunking occurs when working memory perceives a set of data as a single item, much as we perceive *information* as one word (and, therefore, one item) even though it is composed of 11 separate letters. Going back to the number exercise in Chapter 2, some people may have indeed remembered all 10 digits in the right sequence. These may be people who spend a lot of time on the telephone. When they see a 10-digit number, their experience helps them to group it by area code, prefix, and extension. Thus, they see the second number, 4915082637, as (491) 508-2637, which is now three chunks, not 10. Since three are within the working memory's functional capacity, the digits can be remembered accurately.

Some researchers suggest that chunking occurs in two ways (Gobet et al., 2001). In one situation, chunking is a deliberate, goal-oriented process initiated and controlled by the learner. For example, in learning a poem, we are likely to rehearse the first line, then the first two lines, then three lines, and so on, gradually increasing the size of the chunk until we know the whole poem. The other mechanism is more subtle, automatic, continuous, and linked to perceptual processes. This occurs, for instance, when we learn to read. The brain gradually expands the number of words it processes at one time from a single word to two words, to a phrase, and so on. During this process, fMRIs show increased activity in the frontal lobes as working memory encodes the learning content into higher capacity chunks (Bor, Duncan, Wiseman, & Owen, 2003).

Chunking allows us to deal with a few large blocks of information rather than many small fragments. Problem solving involves the ability to access large amounts of relevant knowledge from long-term memory for use in working memory. The key to that skill is chunking. The more a person is able to chunk in a particular area, the more expert the person becomes. These experts have the ability to use their experiences to group or chunk all kinds of information into discernable patterns. Chunking is also a valuable strategy when learning a complicated procedure, especially if the learners are reading aloud the procedures while carrying them out (Duggan & Payne, 2001). Chunking is also a valuable strategy for learning a new language, especially when the chunking is combined with imagery (Carter, Hardy, & Hardy, 2001).

This ability to chunk is much more a reflection of how the expert's knowledge base is organized rather than a superior perceptual ability. Experience has changed the experts' brains so that they can encode relevant information in greater detail and more fully than the nonexperts. As they gain experience, more patterns are chunked and linked and the expertise becomes less conscious and more intuitive. Here are some examples:

- An experienced physician takes much less time to diagnose a medical condition than an intern.
- Expert waiters remember meal combinations rather than single menu items.
- Expert musicians recall long passages, not single notes.
- Chess masters recall board layouts as functional clusters rather than separate pieces.
- Expert readers take in phrases, not individual words.

Test Question No. 7: The amount of information a learner can deal with at one time is genetically linked.

Answer: False. The amount of information a learner can deal with at one time is linked to the learner's ability to add more items to the chunks in working memory—a learned skill.

Effect of Past Experiences on Chunking

Let's show how past experiences affect chunking. First, look at the following sentence:

Grandma is buying an apple.

This sentence has 22 letters, but only five chunks (or words) of information. Because the sentence is one complete thought, most people treat it as just one item in working memory. In this example, 22 bits of data (letters) become one chunk (complete thought). In addition, visual learners probably formed a mental image of a grandmother buying that apple.

Now let's add more information to working memory. Stare at the next sentence below for about 10 seconds. Now close your eyes and try recalling the two sentences.

Hte plpae si edr.

Having trouble with the second? That's because the words make no sense, and working memory is treating each of the 13 letters and three spaces as 16 individual items (plus the first sentence as 1 item, for a total of 17). The 5- to 9-item functional capacity range of working memory is quickly exceeded.

Let's rearrange the letters in each word of the second sentence to read as follows:

The apple is red.

Stare at this sentence for 10 seconds. Now close your eyes again and try to remember the first sentence and this sentence. Most people will remember both sentences because they are now just 2 items instead of 17 and their meanings are related. Experience, once again, helps the working memory decide how to chunk items.

Here's a frequently used example of how experience can help in chunking information and improving achievement. Get the pencil and paper again. Now stare at the letters below for 10 seconds. Then look away from the page and write them down in the correct sequence and groupings. Ready? Go.

LSDN BCT VF BIU SA

Check your results. Did you get all the letters in the correct sequence and groupings? Probably not, but that's OK. Most people would not get 100 percent by staring at the letters in such a short period of time.

Let's try it again. Same rules: Stare at the letters below for 10 seconds and write the letters down. Ready? Go.

LSD NBC TV FBI USA

How did you do this time? Most people do much better on this example. Now compare the two examples. Note that the letters in both examples are *identical and in the same sequence*! The only difference is that the letters in the second example are grouped—or chunked—in a way that allows past experience to help working memory process and hold the items. Working memory usually sees the first example as 14 letters plus 4 spaces (i.e., the grouping is important) or 18 items—much more than its functional capacity. But the second example is quickly seen as only 5 understandable items (the spaces no longer matter) and, thus, within the limits of working memory's capacity. Some people may even pair NBC with TV, and FBI with USA, so that they actually deal with just 3 chunks. These examples show the power of past experience in remembering—a principle of learning called *transfer,* which we will discuss in the next chapter.

Chunking is an effective way of enlarging working memory's capacity and for helping the learner make associations that establish meaning.

Chunking is a very effective way of enlarging working memory's capacity. It can be used to memorize a long string of numbers or words. Most of us learned the alphabet in chunks—for some it may have been *abcd*, *efg*, *hijk*, *lmnop*, *qrs*, *tuv*, *wxyz*. Chunking reduced the 26 letters to a smaller number of items that working memory could handle. Even people can be chunked, such as couples (for example, Romeo and Juliet, Gilbert and Sullivan, Bonnie and Clyde), in which recalling the name of one immediately suggests the name of the other. Although working memory has a functional capacity limit as to the number of chunks it can process at one time, there appears to be no limit to the number of items that can be combined into a chunk. Teaching students (and yourself) how to chunk can greatly increase learning and remembering.

Test Question No. 8: It is usually not possible to increase the amount of information that the working memory can deal with at one time.

Answer: False. By increasing the number of items in a chunk, we can increase the amount of information that our working memory can process simultaneously.

Cramming Is Chunking

Cramming for a test or interview is another example of chunking. The learner loads into working memory as many items as can be identified as needed. Varying degrees of temporary associations are made among the items. With sufficient effort and meaning, the items can be carried in working memory, even for days, until needed. If the source of the crammed items was outside the learner, that is, from texts or class notes, then it is possible for none of the crammed items to be transferred to long-term storage. This practice (which many of us have experienced) explains how a learner can be conversant and outwardly competent in the items tested on one day (while the items were in working memory) and have little or no understanding of them several days later after they drop out of working memory into oblivion. We cannot recall later what we have not stored. Is there anything teachers can do about this? See the **Practitioner's Corner** on p. 70 of Chapter 2 on "Testing Whether Information Is in Long-Term Storage."

Forgetting

Ask teachers how long they want their students to remember what they were taught, and the answer is a resounding, "forever." Yet, that is not usually the case. Much of what is taught in school is forgotten over time, sometimes within a few days. Forgetting is often viewed as the enemy of learning. But, on the contrary, forgetting plays an important role in promoting learning and facilitating recall.

The human brain processes an enormous amount of incoming information every day. Much of that information remains in temporary memory sites and soon fades. For example, the name of a person that one has just met may remain in memory for just a few minutes. Yet the name of one's best friend is turned into a long-term memory and lasts a lifetime. Why do we forget so much and preserve so little? Forgetting manifests itself in two major ways: the process of discarding newly acquired information, and the decay that occurs with memories already in long-term storage.

Forgetting New Information

The first major studies on forgetting were conducted by Hermann Ebbinghaus (1850 - 1909), a German psychologist, whose work led to the development of a forgetting curve. The curve was a mathematical representation of how quickly new experiences were forgotten. Subsequent studies have somewhat modified his findings. When the brain is exposed to new information, the greatest amount of forgetting occurs shortly after the learning task is completed, and continues rapidly throughout the first day. Items that do not make sense to the learner are usually forgotten first. Conversely, traumatic and vivid experiences are rarely forgotten, although what we recall of them may change over time. But for most information, forgetting slows down after two weeks when there is not much left to forget.

Forgetting new material can occur as a result of interference from earlier learning. This is a component of a process called transfer, which will be discussed in greater detail in Chapter 4. Even *how* one acquires new learning can affect forgetting. For most people, it is easier to forget what is heard than what is read. When listening to new information, extraneous sounds can divert the brain's attention. But reading is a much more focused activity, thereby reducing the effect of distractions (see Figure 3.9). Stress and lack of sleep also contribute to forgetting.

Forgetting has some definite advantages. When the brain is presented with a large amount of information, forgetting prevents irrelevant information from interfering with the acquisition, remembering, and recall of relevant information. By screening out the unimportant, the essential data and experiences have a chance to be fully consolidated into long-term memories. Forgetting may be frustrating, but it is most likely a survival adaptation of memory. There is little value in remembering everything that has happened to us. Forgetting the trivial leaves room for the more important and meaningful experiences that shape who we are and establish our individuality.

> ***By forgetting the trivial, we leave room for the more important and meaningful experiences that shape who we are and establish our individuality.***

Teachers, of course, believe that the material they present in class is relevant. Why doesn't the student's brain perceive it that way, too? We already answered that question in Chapter 2. You will recall that sense and meaning (relevancy) are key factors that affect whether new information will be remembered or forgotten.

Forgetting Past Memories

Imagine if the brain remembered everything for a lifetime. Just trying to recall the name of a childhood friend would be a significant challenge. The brain would have to search though thousands of names scattered among the long-term memory sites. At best, the name would take a long time to find; at worst, the result could be confusion, resulting in the recall of the wrong name. By gradually forgetting the names that are not important, the recall process becomes more efficient.

Forgetting also helps to update obsolete information. As one changes jobs and relocates, for example, new data, such as addresses and telephone numbers, overwrite the old data. The old data may still reside in long-term memory, but if it is not recalled and rehearsed, it will eventually become less accessible.

Exactly what happens in the brain to old memories over time is still an open question. Some researchers suggest that memory loss of a specific experience can occur if the memory has not been recalled for a long time. They believe that this leads to the slow but steady disassociation of the network of brain cells that form the memory, making retrieval increasingly difficult. Eventually, the integrity of the network fails and the memory is lost, perhaps forever. Such a process, the researchers say, frees up memory resources so that they become available for new information (Wixted, 2004).

Other researchers contend that old memories remain intact, though other factors somehow block access to them. These factors can include medications, drugs, vivid new experiences, stroke, and Alzheimer's disease. Recent studies have also found that some people can voluntarily block an unwanted past experience with such persistence that it results in forgetting (Fleck, Berch, Shear, & Strakowski, 2001). Does it make any difference whether forgetting is the deterioration of the memory sites or losing the pathways? Is not the result the same, the inability to recall the memory? Sure, the result is the same, but since our understanding of the storage process has changed, so has the method for trying to recall it. We can use a therapy that helps us to find the original pathway, or an alternate pathway, to the memory sites.

Here is an example. Suppose you try to recall the name of the teacher you had when you were in second grade. Unless you have thought recently about that teacher, the pathway to that name has not been used for a long time. It is blocked by newer pathways, and you will have difficulty finding it. The name is still there, but it may take you as long as several days to find it. It will probably come to you when you least expect it.

Another example: Suppose you start thinking about finding an old sweater that you have not seen in several years. If you believe you gave it away, you will not even begin to look for it. That is the same as if you believe that your forgotten memory has been destroyed over time; you will not even try to recall it. On the other hand, if you are convinced that the sweater is somewhere in that big attic, then it is just a matter of time before your hunt pays off and you find it. You'll probably start by thinking of the last time you wore it. This is the same process of memory therapy that is used with brain-damaged individuals. The therapy helps the patient seek other neural connections to find the original or an alternate pathway to the memory sites (Rose, 2005; Schacter, 2001).

Implications for Teaching. More research is needed before scientists can draw any conclusions about the mechanisms that result in the forgetting of old memories. Meanwhile, teachers can take advantage of what *is* known. Namely, that important information that students have already learned is more likely to be accurately and firmly consolidated in long-term memory if it is recalled and rehearsed periodically as the students progress through grade levels. Too often, information deemed important is taught just once, and the students are expected to remember it for a lifetime. They may even be tested on it years after they initially learned it. Something worth remembering is worth repeating. If important information is purposefully revisited throughout a student's entire school experience, then firmly consolidated and robust memories will be available for a long time to come.

Confabulation

Have you ever been discussing an experience with someone who had shared it with you and started arguing over some of the details? As described earlier, long-term memory is the process of searching, locating, retrieving, and transferring information to working memory. Rote recall, especially of frequently used information, such as your name and address, is actually simple. These pathways are clear and retrieval time is very short. Retrieving more complex and less frequently used concepts is much more complicated. It requires signaling multiple storage sites through elaborate, cluttered pathways for intermediate consolidation and ultimate decoding into working memory. It is less accurate. First, most of us do not retain 100 percent of elaborate experiences, such as an extensive vacation. Second, we store parts of the experience in many storage areas.

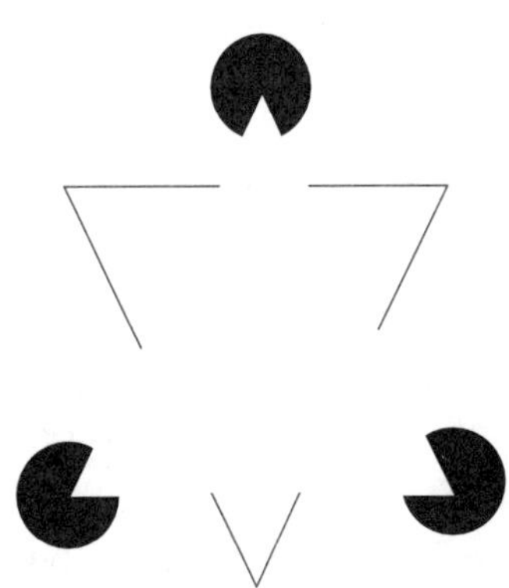

Figure 3.14 The white triangle you may see does not exist. It is a result of confabulation.

When retrieving such an experience, the long-term memory may not be able to locate all the events being requested, either because of insufficient time or because they were never retained. Moreover, older memories can be modified or distorted by the acquisition of newer information. During the retrieval process, memory can unconsciously fabricate the missing or incomplete information by selecting the next closest item it can recall. This process is called *confabulation* and occurs because the brain is always active and creative, and seems to abhor incompleteness. Confabulation is not unlike the way the brain completes visual patterns that do not exist, as in optical illusions. Take a look at Figure 3.14. Although you may see a white triangle in the diagram, it does not exist. It is the result of confabulation as the brain seeks to make sense of the pattern.

Confabulation is *not* lying, because it is an unconscious rather than a deliberate process, and the individual believes the fabricated information to be true. This explains why two people who participated in the same experience will later recall slightly—or even significantly—different versions of the same event. Neither individual stored 100 percent of the experience. If each stored 90 percent, it would not be the *same* 90 percent for both. Their missing and different 10 percent will be fabricated and will cause each to question the accuracy of the other's memory. The less of the experience remembered, the more the brain must fabricate. Over time, the fabricated parts are consolidated into the memory network. As we systematically recall this memory, minor alterations may continue to be made through confabulation. Gradually the original memory is transformed and encoded into a considerably different one that we believe to be true and accurate. Although we all fall victim to confabulation at one time or another, damage to certain brain areas can cause chronic and extreme confabulation where the recalled memories deviate significantly from

Our brain fabricates information and experiences that we believe to be true.

reality (Shallice, 1999). The left hemisphere seems to be the driving force behind confabulation. Experiments show that the left hemisphere is so intent on looking for order that it will find it even when there is none (Gazzaniga, 1998a). See more about this in Chapter 5.

Implications for Teaching. Confabulation also happens in the classroom. When recalling a complex learning, the learner is unaware of which parts are missing and, thus, fabricated. The younger the learner, the more inconsistent the fabricated parts can be. The teacher may react by thinking the student is inventing answers intentionally and may discipline accordingly. In another situation, a list of similar words or concepts may induce the confabulation of words or concepts *not* on the list. Studies show that this is a common phenomenon (Roediger & McDermott, 1995). In these cases, the teacher should be aware of confabulation as a possibility, identify the fabricated parts, and provide the feedback needed to help the student correct the inaccurate material. Through practice, the learner will incorporate the corrected material and transfer it to long-term memory.

Confabulation has implications for the justice system. This tendency for the brain to fabricate information rather than admit its absence can have serious consequences in court trials where eyewitnesses, under the pressure of testifying, feel compelled to provide complete information. Confabulation also raises questions about the accuracy of witnesses recalling very old memories of unpleasant events, such as a childhood accident or abuse. Experiments have shown how easy it is to distort a person's recollection of even recent events, or to "implant" memories. In the absence of independent verification, it is impossible to decide what events in the recalled "repressed memory" actually occurred and which are the result of confabulation (Loftus, 1997).

What's Coming Up?

One of the most important goals of education is to teach students how to apply what they learned to future situations they will encounter—what is known as the transfer of learning. Transfer affects old learning, new learning, memory, and recall. The nature and power of transfer as well as how it can help or hinder teaching and learning are unveiled in the next chapter.

PRACTITIONER'S CORNER

Avoid Teaching Two Very Similar Motor Skills

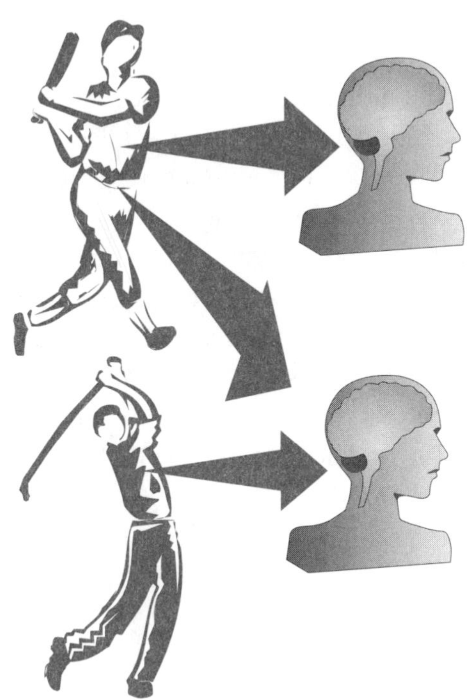

When a learner practices a new skill (in this example, swinging a baseball bat), the motor cortex (across the top of the cerebrum) coordinates with the cerebellum to establish the pathways that will consolidate the movements to perform the skill. After the learner stops the practice, it takes about 4 to 12 hours (down-time) for this consolidation to occur. Further memory pathways are established as the learner sleeps. Practicing the skill the next day will be much easier and more accurate.

If, during the 4- to 12-hour down-time, the learner practices a second skill (in this example, swinging a golf club) that is very similar to the first skill, the pathways for the two skills get confounded. As a result, the learner is able to perform *neither* skill well.

Implications for Practice:

- Avoid teaching two motor skills that are very similar to each other in the same day. When in doubt, make a list of their similarities and differences. If the similarities far outweigh the differences, it is best not to teach them together.

- When the time comes to teach the second skill, teach the *differences* first. This ensures that the differences are recognized during prime-time-1, which is the most powerful position for remembering.

PRACTITIONER'S CORNER

Using Rehearsal to Enhance Retention

Rehearsal refers to the learner's reprocessing of new information in an attempt to determine sense and meaning. It occurs in two forms. Some information items have value only if they are remembered *exactly* as presented, such as the letters and sequence of the alphabet, spelling, poetry, telephone numbers, notes and lyrics of a song, and the multiplication tables. This is called *rote rehearsal.* Sense and meaning are established quickly, and the likelihood of long-term retention is high. Most of us can recall poems and telephone numbers that we learned years ago.

More complex concepts require the learner to make connections and to form associations and other relationships in order to establish sense and meaning. Thus, the information may need to be reprocessed several times as new links are found. This is called *elaborative rehearsal.* The more senses that are used in this elaborative rehearsal, the more reliable the associations. Thus, when visual, auditory, and kinesthetic activities assist the learner during this rehearsal, the probability of long-term storage rises dramatically. That is why it is important for students to talk about what they are learning *while* they are learning it, and to have visual models as well.

Rehearsal is teacher initiated and teacher directed. Recognizing that rehearsal is a necessary ingredient for retention of learning, teachers should consider the following when designing and presenting their lessons:

Rote Rehearsal Strategies

- **Simple Repetition.** For remembering short items (telephone numbers, names, and dates), simply repeat aloud a set of items over and over until it can be recalled in correct sequence.

- **Cumulative Repetition.** For longer sets of items (song, poem, list of battles) the learner rehearses the first few items. Then the next set of items in the sequence is added to the first set and rehearsed, and so on. For example, to remember a poem of four stanzas, the learner starts by rehearsing the first stanza, then rehearsing the second stanza alone, followed by the first two stanzas together. With those in place, the learner rehearses the third stanza and then the three stanzas together. The process is repeated by rehearsing the fourth stanza alone, and finally, all four stanzas together.

Elaborative Rehearsal Strategies

- **Paraphrasing.** Students orally restate ideas in their own words, which then become familiar cues for later storage. Using auditory modality helps the learner attach sense, making retention more likely.

- **Selecting and Note Taking.** Students review texts, illustrations, and lectures, deciding which portions are critical and important. They make these decisions on the basis of criteria from the teacher, authors, or other students. Students then paraphrase the idea and write it into their notes. Adding the kinesthetic exercise of writing furthers retention.

- **Predicting.** After studying a section of content, the students predict the material to follow or what questions the teacher might ask about that content. Prediction keeps students focused on the new content, adds interest, and helps them apply prior learnings to new situations, thus aiding retention.

- **Questioning.** After studying content, students generate questions about the content. To be effective, the questions should range from lower-level thinking of recall, comprehension, and application to higher-level thinking of analysis, evaluation, and synthesis (see Bloom's Taxonomy in Chapter 7). When designing questions of varying complexity, students engage in deeper cognitive processing, clarify concepts, and predict meaning and associations—all contributors to retention.

- **Summarizing.** Students reflect on and summarize in their heads the important material or skills learned in the lesson. This is often the last and critical stage where students can attach sense and meaning to the new learning. Summarizing rehearsal is also called *closure* (see the **Practitioner's Corner** on closure on p. 69 in Chapter 2 for further explanation).

General Guidelines

If the retention of new information or skills beyond the immediate lesson is an important expectation, then rehearsal must be a crucial part of the learner's processing. The following considerations should be incorporated into decisions about using rehearsal.

- **Teach** students rehearsal activities and strategies. As soon as they recognize the differences between rote and elaborative rehearsal, they can understand the importance of selecting the appropriate type for each learning objective. With practice, they should quickly realize that fact and data acquisition require rote rehearsal, whereas analysis and evaluation of concepts require elaborative rehearsal.

- **Remind** students to continuously practice rehearsal strategies until they become regular parts of their study and learning habits.

- **Keep** rehearsal relevant. Effective elaborative rehearsal relies more on making personally meaningful associations to prior learning than on time-consuming efforts that lack these student-centered connections. Any associations that focus on the teacher's experiences may not be relevant to students.

- **Remember** that time alone is not a trustworthy indicator of the effectiveness of rehearsal. The degree of meaning associated with the new learning is much more significant than the time allotted.

- **Have** learners verbalize their rehearsal to peers or teachers while they are learning new material, as this increases the likelihood of retention.

- **Provide** more visual and contextual clues to make rehearsal meaningful and successful. Students with limited verbal competence will focus on visual and concrete lesson components to assist in their rehearsal. This will be particularly true of students whose first language is not English.

- **Vary** the rehearsal strategies that you initiate to ensure that there is plenty of novelty in the process. Students will bore quickly if the same method of rehearsal (e.g., sharing with the same partner) is used all the time.

PRACTITIONER'S CORNER

Using the Primacy-Recency Effect in the Classroom

The primacy-recency effect describes the phenomenon whereby, during a learning episode, we tend to remember best that which comes first (prime-time-1), second best that which comes last (prime-time-2), and least that which comes just past the middle (down-time). Proper use of this effect can lead to lessons that are more likely to be remembered.

Below is a sketch of two lessons. One is taught by Mr. Blue and the other by Mr. Green. Study their lesson sequences and look for any application of the primacy-recency effect.

Mr. Blue	Lesson Sequence	Mr. Green
"Get ready to tell me the two causes of the Civil War we discussed yesterday." After getting this he then says, "Today we will learn the third and most important cause as we are still living with its aftereffects 140 years later." "Before I tell you, let me give back some homework, collect today's homework, collect the notes from Bill and Mary who were absent yesterday, take attendance, and read a brief announcement."	Prime-time-1	"Get ready to tell me the two causes of World War I we discussed yesterday." After getting this he then says, "Today we will learn the third and most important cause as it set the stage for another world war just 30 years later." "And here is the third cause!" (He presents third cause, gives examples, and relates it to yesterday's two causes.)
"Here is the third cause." (He presents third cause, gives examples, and relates it to yesterday's two causes.)	Down-time	"Go into your discussion groups and discuss this third cause. Not only tie it to the two causes we learned yesterday but also to other wars we have learned so far. What are the similarities and differences?"
"OK, we've got only 5 minutes to the end of the period. You've listened attentively so you can do anything you want as long as you are quiet."	Prime-time-2	"Take 2 minutes to review quietly to yourself what you learned about this third cause. Be prepared to share your thoughts with the class."

If these sequences are representative of what happens most of the time in these two teachers' classes, whose students are more likely to remember what they have learned over time? Why? What are some other implications of using the primacy-recency effect in the classroom?

Here are some other considerations for using this effect in the classroom.

- **Teach the new material first** (after getting the students' focus) during prime-time-1. This is the time of greatest retention. Alternatively, this would also be a good time to **reteach** any concept that students may be having difficulty understanding.

- **Avoid asking students** at the beginning of the lesson if they know anything about a *new* topic being introduced. If it is a new topic, the assumption is that most students do not know it. However, there are always some students ready to take a guess—no matter how unrelated. Because this is the time of greatest retention, almost anything that is said, including incorrect information, is likely to be remembered. Give the information and examples yourself to ensure that they are correct.

- **Avoid using precious prime-time** periods for classroom management tasks, such as collecting absence notes or taking attendance. Do these before you get focus, or during the down-time.

- **Use the down-time** portion to have students practice the new learning or to discuss it by relating it to past learnings. Remember that retention of learning does occur during the down-time, but it just takes more effort and concentration.

- **Do closure during prime-time-2.** This is the learner's last opportunity to attach sense and meaning to the new learning, to make decisions about it, and to determine where and how it will be transferred to long-term storage. It is important, then, that the student's brain do the work at this time. If you wish to do a review, then do it *before* closure to increase the chances that the closure experience is accurate. Doing review *instead* of closure is of little value to retention.

- **Try to package lesson objectives** (or sublearnings) in teaching episodes of about 20 minutes. Link the sublearnings according to the total time period available (for example, two 20-minute lessons for a 40-minute teaching period, three for an hour period, and so on).

PRACTITIONER'S CORNER

Strategies for Block Scheduling

More high schools (and some middle schools, too) are converting from the standard 40- to 45-minute daily period to a block schedule consisting of longer teaching periods, usually 80 to 90 minutes. Although there are various formats for the blocks, the main goal of this change is to allow more time for student participation in the learning process.

The benefits of this approach are many: There is less fragmentation to the school day, more time to dig into concepts and allow for transfer to occur, and more time to develop hands-on activities, such as projects. It also allows for more performance-based assessments of student learning, reducing the reliance on paper-and-pencil tests.

The block experience is likely to be more successful if the teacher recognizes the value and need for novelty, and resists the temptation to be the focus of the block during the entire time period. Here are some suggestions for a brain-compatible block lesson.

- **Remember the primacy-recency effect.** Teaching a 90-minute episode as one continuous lesson will mean a down-time of about 35 minutes. Plan for four 20-minute learning segments and your down-time is reduced substantially to about 10 minutes. This down-time can also be productive if the students are engaged in discussions about the new learning.

- **Be in direct control of just one segment.** You may wish to do some direct instruction during one of the lesson segments. If so, use the first segment for this, and then shift the work burden to the students for the other segments. Remember that the brain that does the work is the brain that learns.

- **Go off-task between segments.** Figure 3.8 (p. 94) shows how going off-task between the lesson segments can increase the degree of focus when the students return to task. This is because of the novelty effect. If you prefer to stay on-task, however, then use a joke, story, or cartoon that is related to the learning. You still get the novelty effect without losing focus.

- **Eliminate the unnecessary.** Block scheduling is designed to give students a chance to dig deeper into concepts. To get the time to do this, scrap less important topics that sneak into the curriculum over time. We all know that everything in the curriculum is not of equal importance. Perform this selective abandonment on a regular basis.

- **Work with your colleagues.** Block activities offer an excellent opportunity for teachers to work together in planning the longer lessons. This collegial process can be very productive and interesting, especially when teachers deliver lessons together. Such planning can be within or across subject areas.

- **Vary the blocks.** Novelty means finding ways to make each of the segments different and multisensory. Here are just a few examples of block activities that you can use for the lesson segments:

Teacher talk	Guest speakers
Research	Videos, movies, slides
Cooperative learning groups	Audiotapes
Reading	Reflection time
Student peer coaching	Jigsaw combinations
Laboratory experiences	Discussion groups
Computer work	Role-playing and simulations
Journal writing	Instructional games and puzzles

- **Vary the assessment techniques.** Block scheduling offers students opportunities to explore content in many different ways. Thus, assessment techniques should also be varied to allow students different methods of showing what they have learned. Here are a few examples of assessment techniques to consider:

Written tests	Interviews
Questionnaires	Journals
Portfolios	Presentations
Exhibitions	Video production
Demonstrations	Dioramas
Modeling	Music and dance

PRACTITIONER'S CORNER

Using Practice Effectively

Practice does not make perfect, it makes ***permanent.*** Practice allows the learner to use the newly learned skill in a new situation with sufficient accuracy so that it will be correctly remembered. Before students begin practice, the teacher should model the thinking process involved and guide the class through each step of the new learning's application.

Since practice makes permanent, the teacher should monitor the students' early practice to ensure that it is accurate and to provide timely feedback and correction if it is not. This guided practice helps eliminate initial errors and alerts students to the critical steps in applying new skills. Here are some suggestions by Hunter (2004) for guiding initial practice:

- **Amount of Material to Practice.** Practice should be limited to the smallest amount of material or skill that has the most relevancy for the students. This allows for sense and meaning to be consolidated as the learner uses the new learning.

- **Amount of Time to Practice.** Practice should take place in short, intense periods of time when the student's working memory is running on prime- time. When the practice period is short, students are more likely to be intent on learning what they are practicing.

- **Frequency of Practice.** New learning should be practiced frequently at first so that it is quickly organized. This is called *massed practice.* If we expect students to retain the information in active storage and to remember how to use it accurately, it should continue to be practiced over increasingly longer time intervals. This is called *distributed practice*, and it is the real key to accurate retention and application of information and mastery of skills over time.

- **Accuracy of Practice.** As students perform guided practice, the teacher should give prompt and specific feedback on whether the practice is correct or incorrect and why. This process gives the teacher valuable information about the degree of student understanding and whether it makes sense to move on or reteach portions that may be difficult for some students.

PRACTITIONER'S CORNER

Relearning Through Recall

Every time we recall information from long-term storage into working memory, we relearn it. Therefore, teachers should use classroom strategies that encourage students to recall previously learned information regularly so they will relearn it. One strategy for doing this is to maintain learner participation throughout the lesson. Called *active participation*, this principle of learning attempts to keep the mind of the student consistently focused on what is being learned or recalled through covert and overt activities.

The covert activity involves the teacher asking the students to recall previously learned information and to process it in some way. It could be, "Think of the conditions that existed in America just after the Civil War that we learned yesterday, and be prepared to discuss them in a few minutes." This statement informs the students that they will be held accountable for their recall. This accountability increases the likelihood that the students will recall the desired item and, thus, relearn it. It also alleviates the need for the teacher to call on every student to determine if the recall has occurred. After sufficient wait time (see the **Practitioner's Corner** on wait-time, p. 129), overt activities are used to determine the quality of the covert recall.

Some suggestions follow on how to use active participation strategies effectively:

- **State the question** and allow thinking time *before* calling on a student for response. This holds all students accountable for recalling the answer until you pick your first respondent.

- **Give clear and specific directions** as to what the students should recall. Focus on the lesson objectives and not on the activities unless they were a crucial part of the learning. Repeat the question using different words and phraseology. This increases the number of cues that the learners have during their retrieval search.

- **Avoid predictable patterns** when calling on students, such as alphabetical order, up and down rows, or raised hands. These patterns signal the students *when* they will be held accountable, thereby allowing them to go off-task before and after their turns.

PRACTITIONER'S CORNER

Impact of Circadian Rhythms on Schools and Classrooms

This chapter explained the differences in circadian rhythms of adolescents compared to pre/postadolescents (Figure 3.11, p. 101). The adolescent rhythm is about an hour later, and these differences have implications for elementary and secondary schools. For example:

- **Planning Elementary School Lessons.** Remember that both the teacher and elementary school students are in the trough together. The tendency here would be for all to just take a nap! That's probably not an option, so we have to decide how to deal with the trough. Here are two things to consider:

  (1) Many elementary teachers can decide what time of day to teach certain subjects. Avoid teaching the same subject every day during the trough time. Because of low focus levels, it is boring for the students and tedious for the teacher. Varying the subject taught in the trough provides novelty and interest.

  (2) Keep assignments short, and frequently hold the students accountable for what they are learning. For example, instead of assigning 30 minutes of silent reading (a common practice during the trough time), assign just five minutes for the class to read two pages and give a specific assignment related to the reading. You might say: "After five minutes to read pages 12 and 13, decide what other choices the main character could have made, and why. I will call on some of you for your answers." Repeating this process results in four or five mini-lessons that will be more productive than trying to attempt a single 30-minute lesson.

- **School Start Times.** Because of this shift in rhythm, teenagers are sleepier in the morning and tend to stay up later at night. They come to school sleep deprived (i.e., many suffer from Delayed Sleep Phase Disorder), and often with an inadequate breakfast (i.e., lacking glucose, the brain's fuel). Meanwhile, students often face a long bus ride to get to high schools that are starting earlier. District leaders should consider realigning opening times and course schedules more closely with the students' biological rhythms to increase the chances of successful learning. School districts that have adopted later starting times for their high schools are reporting positive results. These same positive results apply to elementary schools that start earlier than the traditional time of 9:00 a.m.

- **Classroom Lighting.** Adolescents with Delayed Sleep Phase Disorder have a high amount of melatonin (the hormone that induces sleep) in their bodies. One of the best ways to reduce melatonin levels is with bright light. Keep classroom lights on, open blinds, lift shades, and look for ways to get the students into outdoor light, especially in the morning (Kripke, Youngstedt, & Elliot, 1997).

- **Testing.** School districts usually give standardized tests to all students in the morning. However, high school students tend to perform better in problem-solving and memory tasks later in the day rather than earlier. It is probable that a number of high school students do not do as well on these tests as they could because of the testing times. Some school districts have reported that testing high school students later in the morning and early afternoon improved their performance and scores.

- **Classroom Climate.** Classroom climate problems can arise in high schools if the teacher is in the postnoon trough while the students are still at their pretrough peak. The teacher is likely to be irritable, and minor discipline annoyances can easily escalate into major confrontations. High school administrators in charge of discipline often report a marked rise in student referrals in the early afternoon. One way to deal with this is for high school teachers to plan student-directed activities during this time, such as computer work, simulations, cooperative learning groups, and research projects. These strategies redirect student energy to productive tasks. Meanwhile, the teacher needs to walk around the room, not only to monitor student work, but also to overcome the lower energy levels experienced during the trough.

PRACTITIONER'S CORNER

Using Wait-Time to Increase Student Participation

Wait-time is the period of teacher silence that follows the posing of a question before the first student is called on for a response. Studies first conducted by Mary Budd Rowe (1974) and others indicate that high school teachers had an average wait-time of just over one second. Elementary teachers waited an average of three seconds. Although no major studies have been done in recent years, one can speculate that these wait-times have not increased, given the large amount of curriculum content that needs to be covered and the increased emphasis that many schools have placed on preparing for high-stakes tests. If anything, the times now may be even shorter.

One to three seconds is hardly enough time for slower retrievers, many of whom may know the correct answer, to locate that answer in long-term storage and retrieve it into working memory. And as soon as the teacher calls on the first student, the remaining students **stop the retrieval process** and lose the opportunity to relearn the information. Rowe found that the following happened when teachers extended the wait-time to at least **five** seconds or more:

- The length and quality of student responses increased.
- There was greater participation by slower learners.
- Students used more evidence to support inferences.
- There were more higher-order responses.

These results occurred at all grade levels and in all subjects.

Rowe also noted positive changes in the behavior of teachers who consistently used longer wait-times. Specifically, she observed that these teachers

- Used more higher-order questioning
- Demonstrated greater flexibility in evaluating responses
- Improved their expectations for the performance of slower learners

One effective method for using wait-time is Think-Pair-Share. In this strategy, the teacher asks the students to think about a question. After adequate wait-time, the students form pairs and exchange the results of their thinking. Some students then share their ideas with the entire class.

PRACTITIONER'S CORNER

Using Chunking to Enhance Retention

Chunking is the process whereby the brain perceives several items of information as a single item. Words are common examples of chunks. *Elephant* is composed of eight letters, but the brain perceives them as one item of information. The more items we can put into a chunk, the more information we can process in working memory and remember at one time. Chunking is a learned skill and, thus, can also be taught. There are different types of chunking.

Pattern Chunking: This is most easily accomplished whenever we can find patterns in the material to be retained.

- Say we wanted to remember the number 3421941621776. Without a pattern, these 13 digits are treated as separate items and exceed working memory's functional capacity of about seven items. But we could arrange the numbers in groups that have meaning. For example, 342 (my house number), 1941 (when the U.S. entered World War II), 62 (my father's age), and 1776 (the Declaration of Independence). Now the number is only four chunks with meaning: 342 1941 62 1776.

- The following example, admittedly contrived, shows how chunking can work at different levels. The task is to memorize the following string of words:

COW GRASS FIELD TENNIS NET SODA DOG LAKE FISH

We need a method to remember the sequence, because nine is more than the typical functional capacity of seven. We can chunk the sequence of items by using a simple story. First, we see a **cow** eating **grass** in a **field.** Also in the field are two people playing **tennis**. One player hits the ball way over the **net**. They are drinking **soda** while their **dog** runs after the ball that went into the **lake.** The dog's splashing frightens the **fish**.

- Learning a step-by-step procedure for tying a shoelace or copying a computer file from a CD-ROM to a hard disk are examples of pattern chunking. We group the items in a sequence and rehearse it mentally until it becomes one or a few chunks. Practicing the procedure further enhances the formation of chunks, and subsequent performance requires little conscious attention.

Categorical Chunking: This is a more sophisticated chunking process in that the learner establishes various types of categories to help classify large amounts of information. The learner reviews the information looking for criteria that will group complex material into simpler categories or arrays. The different types of categories can include the following:

- **Advantages and Disadvantages.** The information is categorized according to the pros and cons of the concept. Examples include energy use, global warming, genetically altered crops, abortion, and capital punishment.

- **Similarities and Differences.** The learner compares two or more concepts using attributes that make them similar and different. Examples are comparing the Articles of Confederation to the Bill of Rights, mass to weight, mitosis to meiosis, and the U.S. Civil War to the Vietnam War.

- **Structure and Function.** These categories are helpful with concepts that have parts with different functions, such as identifying the parts of an animal cell, a short story, or the human digestive system.

- **Taxonomies.** This system sorts information into hierarchical levels according to certain common characteristics. Examples are biological taxonomies (kingdom, phylum, class, etc.), taxonomies of learning (cognitive, affective, and psychomotor), and governmental bureaucracies.

- **Arrays.** These are less ordered than taxonomies in that the criteria for establishing the array are not always logical, but are more likely based on observable features. Human beings are classified, for example, by learning style and personality type. Dogs can be grouped by size, shape, or fur length. Clothing can be divided by material, season, and gender.

PRACTITIONER'S CORNER

Using Mnemonics to Help Retention

Mnemonics (from the Greek "to remember") are very useful devices for remembering unrelated information, patterns, or rules. They were developed by the ancient Greeks to help them remember dialogue in plays and for passing information to others when writing was impractical. There are many types of mnemonic schemes. The good news is that ordinary people can greatly improve their memory performance with appropriate strategies and practice (Ericsson, 2003). Here are two strategies that can be easily used in the classroom. Work with students to develop schemes appropriate for the content.

- **Rhyming Mnemonics.** Rhymes are simple yet effective ways to remember rules and patterns. They work because if you forget part of the rhyme or get part of it wrong, the words lose their rhyme or rhythm and signal the error. To retrieve the missing or incorrect part, you start the rhyme over again, and this helps you to relearn it. Have you ever tried to remember the fifth line of a song or poem without starting at the beginning? It is very difficult to do because each line serves as the auditory cue for the next line.

Common examples of rhymes we have learned are "*I* before *e*, except after *c* . . .," "Thirty days hath September . . . ," and "Columbus sailed the ocean blue . . . ". Here are some rhymes that can help students learn information in other areas:

The Spanish Armada met its fate
In fifteen hundred and eighty-eight.

Divorced, beheaded, died;
Divorced, beheaded, survived.
(the fate of Henry VIII's six wives, in chronological order)

The number you are dividing by,
Turn upside down and multiply.
(rule for dividing by fractions)

This may seem like a clumsy system, but it works. Make up your own rhyme, alone or with the class, to help you and your students remember more information faster.

- **Reduction Mnemonics:** In this scheme, you reduce a large body of information to a shorter form and use a letter to represent each shortened piece. The letters are either combined to form a real or artificial word or are used to construct a simple sentence. For example, the real word **HOMES** can help us remember the names of the great lakes (Huron, Ontario, Michigan, Erie, and Superior). **BOY FANS** gives us the coordinating conjunctions in English (but, or, yet, for, and, nor, and so). The name **ROY G BIV** aids in remembering the seven colors of the spectrum (red, orange, yellow, green, blue, indigo, and violet). The artificial word **NATO** recalls North Atlantic Treaty Organization. The sentence **My Very Earnest Mother Just Served Us Nine Pizzas** can help us remember the nine planets of the solar system in order from the sun (Mercury, Venus, Earth, Mars, Jupiter, Saturn, Uranus, Neptune, and Pluto). Here are other examples:

Please Excuse My Dear Aunt Sally.
(the order for solving algebraic equations: Parenthesis, Exponents, Multiplication, Division, Addition, Subtraction)

Frederick Charles Goes Down And Ends Battle.
(F, C, G, D, A, E, B: the order that sharps are entered in key signatures; reverse the order for flats)

In Poland, Men Are Tall.
(the stages of cell division in mitosis: Interphase, Prophase, Metaphase, Anaphase, and Telophase)

King Phillip Came Over From Greece Sailing Vessels.
(the descending order of zoological classifications: Kingdom, Phylum, Class, Order, Family, Genus, Species, Variety)

King Henry Doesn't Mind Drinking Cold Milk.
(the descending order of metric prefixes: Kilo, Hecto, Deca, (measure), Deci, Centi, and Milli)

Sober Physicists Don't Find Giraffes In Kitchens.
(the order of names for orbital electrons: s, p, d, f, g, i, and k)

Chapter 3—Memory, Retention, and Learning

Key Points to Ponder

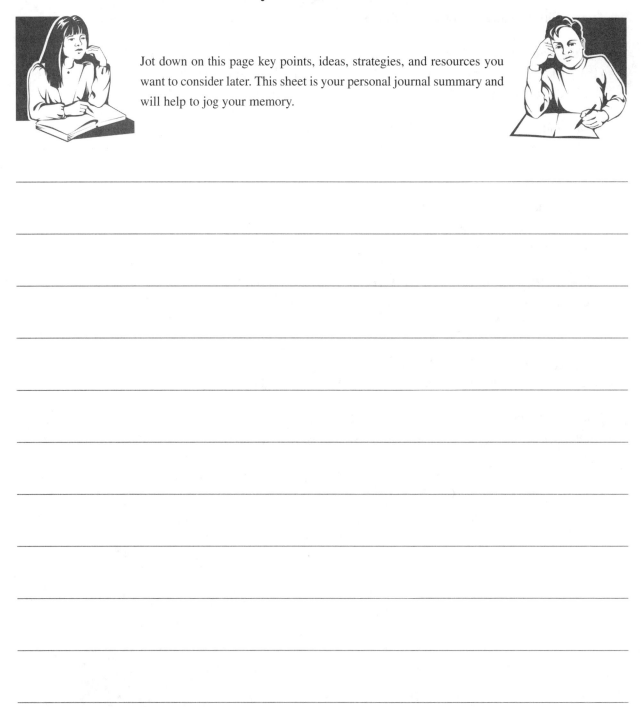

Jot down on this page key points, ideas, strategies, and resources you want to consider later. This sheet is your personal journal summary and will help to jog your memory.

Chapter 4

The Power of Transfer

Transfer is the basis of all creativity, problem solving and the making of satisfying decisions.

—Madeline Hunter,
Mastery Teaching

Chapter Highlights: This chapter explains the components of the most powerful principle of learning, transfer. It examines the factors that affect transfer and how teachers can use past learnings effectively to enhance present and future learning.

The brain is a dynamic creation that is constantly organizing and reorganizing itself when it receives new stimuli. More networks are formed as raw items merge into new patterns. Just as musicians in an orchestra join the individual sounds of their instruments in new and melodious ways, so does the brain unite disconnected ideas with wonderful harmony. We can add beauty and clarity, and forge isolated ideas into spectacular visions.

Transfer is one process that allows this amazing inventiveness to unfold. It encompasses the ability to learn in one situation and then use that learning, possibly in a modified or generalized form, in other situations. Transfer is the core of problem solving, creative thinking, and all other higher mental processes, inventions, and artistic products. It is also one of the ultimate goals of teaching and learning.

WHAT IS TRANSFER?

The principle of learning, called *transfer*, describes a two-part process:

(1) **Transfer *during* learning.** This refers to the effect that past learning has on the processing and acquisition of new learning.

(2) **Transfer *of* learning.** This refers to the degree to which the new learning is applied by the learner in future situations. Some researchers further separate this type of transfer into near and far transfer. Near transfer describes using the new learning in very similar and closely related settings. Far transfer includes the ability to use the new learning in a similar setting as well as the ability to solve novel problems that are not very similar but do share common elements with the learning that was initially acquired (Mestre, 2002).

Transfer During Learning

The process goes something like this: Whenever new learning moves into working memory, long-term memory (most likely stimulated by a signal from the hippocampus) simultaneously searches the long-term storage sites for any past learnings that are similar to, or associated with, the new learning. If the experiences exist, the memory networks are activated and the associated memories are reconsolidated in working memory (Hunter, 2004; Perkins & Salomon, 1988).

How much past learning affects the learner's ability to acquire new knowledge or skills in another context describes one phase of the powerful phenomenon called transfer. In other words, the information processing system depends on past learnings to associate with, make sense of, and treat new information. This recycling of past information into the flow not only reinforces and provides additional rehearsal for already-stored information but also aids in assigning meaning to new information. The degree of meaning attributed to new learning will determine the connections that are made between it and other information in long-term storage. Consider the following pieces of information:

1. There are seven days in the week.
2. Force = mass **X** acceleration.
3. North Korea is an evil country.
4. . . . They also serve who only stand and wait.
5. Jesus is the son of God.
6. There's a sucker born every minute.

In each instance, the meaning of the information depends on the experience, education, and state of mind of the reader. The third and last statements can arouse passionate agreement or disavowal. The second and fourth statements would be meaningless to a second grader, but not the first statement. The fifth could provoke an endless debate among adherents of different religions.

Meaning often depends on context. The transfer process not only provides interpretation of words, but often includes nuances and shadings that can result in very different meanings. "He is a piece of work!" can be either a compliment or a sarcastic comment, depending on tone and context.

These connections and associations give the learner more options to cope with new situations in the future (Figure 4.1).

Types of Transfer

Positive Transfer. When past learning *helps* the learner deal with new learning, it is called *positive transfer.* Suppose a violin player and a trombone player both want to learn to play the viola, an instrument similar to the violin. Who will learn the new instrument more easily? The violin player already possesses the skills and knowledge that will help in learning the viola. The trombone player, on the other hand, may be a very accomplished trombonist but possesses few skills that will help to play the viola. Similarly, Michelangelo, DaVinci, and Edison were able to transfer a great deal of their knowledge and skills to create magnificent works of art and invention. Their prior learnings made greater achievement possible.

Negative Transfer. Sometimes past learning *interferes* with the learner's understanding of new learning, resulting in confusion or errors. This process is called *negative transfer.* If, for example, you have been driving cars with only automatic shift, you will have quite a surprise the first time you drive a standard-shift car. You were accustomed to keeping your left foot idle or using it to brake (not recommended). In either case, the left foot has a very different function in a standard-shift car. If it keeps doing its automatic-shift functions (or does nothing), you will have great difficulty driving the standard-shift car. In other words, the skills that the driver's brain assigned to the left foot for the automatic-shift car are not the skills it needs to cope with the standard-shift car. The skill it used before is now interfering with the skill needed in the new situation, an example of negative transfer.

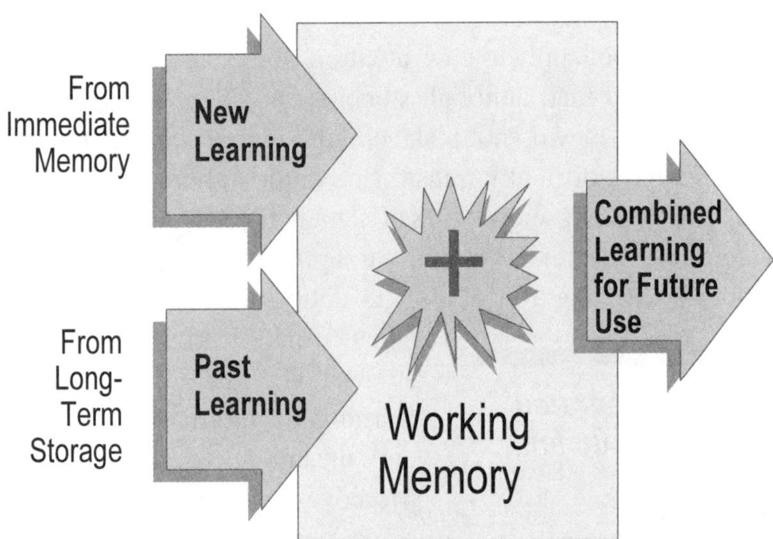

Figure 4.1 New learning and past learning coming together in working memory is one part of transfer. The learner's understanding of how the combined learning can be used in the future is the other part of transfer.

During a lesson, students are dealing continually with transfer as they process and practice new information and skills. Because students' experiences vary, the extent of what transfers also varies. Whether that transfer aids or impedes the acquisition of new learning is a major factor in determining the degree of success each student has in accomplishing the lesson objective.

> ***Never underestimate the power of transfer. Past learning always influences the acquisition of new learning.***

For example, teachers who teach Romance languages to native English speakers are frequently helped by positive transfer and plagued by negative transfer. Words like *rouge* in French and *mucho* in Spanish help to teach *red* and *much,* respectively, but when students see the French *librairie* and are told it is a place where books are found, experience prompts them to think that it means "library." It really means "bookstore." Never underestimate the power of transfer. Past learning *always* influences the acquisition of new learning.

Transfer of Learning

A review of any curriculum reveals that transfer is an integral component and expectation of the learning process. Every day, teachers deliberately or intuitively refer to past learning to make new learning more understandable and meaningful. For the long term, students are expected to transfer the knowledge and skills they learn in school to their daily routines, jobs, and ventures outside the school. Writing and speaking skills should help them communicate with others, scientific knowledge should inform their decisions on environmental and health issues, and their understanding of history should guide their responses to contemporary problems at personal, social, and cultural levels. Obviously, the more information students can transfer from their schooling to the context of everyday life, the greater the probability that they will be good communicators, informed citizens, critical thinkers, and successful problem solvers.

Yet studies continue to show that students are not successful in recognizing how the skills and knowledge they learned in school apply to new situations they encounter in other classes or outside school. One recent study found that, although students can spontaneously make inferences from one curriculum area to another, they do not make enough inferences to support fully fledged transfer and, thus, for example, have difficulty transferring computational skills they learned in mathematics class to solving problems in science class (Blanchette & Dunbar, 2002).

These studies suggest that the students' ability to apply knowledge to new situations is limited. Apparently, we are not doing enough in schools to deliberately make the transfer connections to enhance new learning. The more connections that students can make between past learning and new learning, the more likely they are to determine sense and meaning and thus retain the new learning. Moreover, when these connections can be extended across curriculum areas, they establish a framework of associative networks that will be recalled for future problem solving.

> ***Thematic units and an integrated curriculum enhance the transfer process.***

Successful transfer can be enhanced by educators who advocate thematic units and an integrated curriculum. This approach provides more stimulating experiences for students, and helps them see the commonalities among diverse topics, while reinforcing understanding and meaning for future applications. Thematic units, for instance, could focus on the environment (global warming, recycling, air quality), history (the Civil War, exploring the West, Black history month), science (sources of electrical power, space exploration, ecosystems), or language arts (tall tales, realistic fiction, poetry) (Roberts & Kellough, 2003). Integrated thematic units cut across curriculum areas. The Internet is an excellent source of ideas for integrated units (see Internet sites in the **Resources** section). Figure 4.2 is an example of an integrated thematic unit that could be adapted for elementary and secondary grade levels. Beyond restructuring curriculum, the question now becomes: How can we select teaching that will ensure transfer?

TEACHING FOR TRANSFER

Transfer is more frequently provoked by the environment than consciously by the learner. Have you ever heard a song that brings back a flood of memories? You could not really control that recall unless something else in the present environment now demanded your immediate attention, such as your crying baby or a ringing fire alarm. So who represents a large portion of the environment for students in school? Yes, the teachers! Teachers are the instruments of transfer for students. If teachers are not aware of that, they can inadvertently provoke negative transfer during learning situations just as easily as they can provoke positive transfer.

> ***Teachers are frequently the provokers of transfer for their students.***

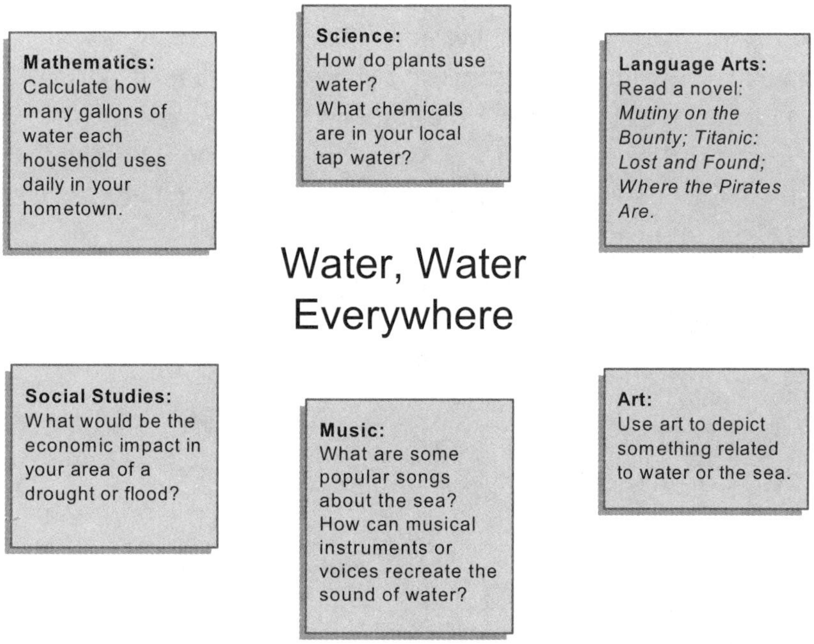

Mathematics:
Calculate how many gallons of water each household uses daily in your hometown.

Science:
How do plants use water?
What chemicals are in your local tap water?

Language Arts:
Read a novel: *Mutiny on the Bounty; Titanic: Lost and Found; Where the Pirates Are.*

Water, Water Everywhere

Social Studies:
What would be the economic impact in your area of a drought or flood?

Music:
What are some popular songs about the sea?
How can musical instruments or voices recreate the sound of water?

Art:
Use art to depict something related to water or the sea.

Figure 4.2 Here is an example of an integrated thematic unit on water. Students have opportunities to gain a deeper understanding of how water directly affects their daily lives. This approach increases the chances of transfer of learning to future situations.

Test Question No. 9: Most of the time, the transfer of information from long-term storage is under the conscious control of the learner.

Answer: False. The transfer process is more often provoked by the learner's present environment.

Example of Transfer in a Literature Class. The following anecdote illustrates how transfer can impede or promote a lesson objective. I once observed a senior class in British literature in a large urban high school. It was late April, and as the students entered the class, they were discussing the upcoming final examinations, the prom, and preparations for graduation. After the opening bell rang, the teacher admonished the students to pay attention and said, "Today, we are going to start another play by William Shakespeare." The moans and groans were deafening and abated only after the teacher used every threat short of ripping up their forthcoming diplomas. Judging from their reactions and unsolicited comments, the students' perceptions of past experiences with Shakespeare were hardly positive. Without realizing it, the teacher's brief introduction had provoked negative transfer; getting the students to focus constructively on the new play now would not be easy.

Later that afternoon, I found myself in a different teacher's British literature class. A large television monitor and a videocassette recorder in the front of the classroom got the students' attention as they entered. The teacher asked the students to "watch a videotape and be prepared to discuss what they saw." What unfolded over the next 15 minutes was a cleverly edited collection of scenes from the movie *West Side Story*. There was enough story to get the plot and enough music to maintain interest. The students were captivated; some even sang along. As the showdown between Tony and Maria's brother came on the screen, the teacher stopped the tape. The students complained, wanting to see who won the fight. The teacher noted that this was really an old story set in modern times, and that she had the script of the original play. The characters' names and the location were different, but the plot was the same. While the students were discussing what they had seen, she distributed Shakespeare's *Romeo and Juliet*. Many students eagerly flipped through the pages trying to find the outcome of the fight scene! The teacher's understanding of positive transfer was evident, and she had used it magnificently.

To use transfer effectively, teachers need to purposefully identify factors that facilitate learning (positive transfer) while minimizing or eliminating factors that can cause interference (negative transfer).

Factors Affecting Transfer

How quickly transfer occurs during a learning situation depends on the rate of retrieval. As noted earlier, the rate of retrieval is largely dependent on the storage system that the learner has created and how the learning was originally stored. Designing the filing system in long-term storage is a *learned* skill and can run the gamut from very loose connections to a highly organized series of networks. Working memory uses a sensory cue that it encodes with the material and files it in a network containing similar items.

The cue helps long-term memory locate, identify, and select the material for later retrieval, similar to the way the label on a file folder helps to locate and identify what is in the file. If the learner is recalling a complex concept, information has to come from various storage areas to the frontal lobes for assembly, verification, and decoding into working memory. Many factors in a learning system affect the nature of this transfer process. Researchers have identified four of these: the context and degree of original learning, similarity, critical attributes, and association. No factor is more important than the others, and they often work together (Hunter, 2004).

Context and Degree of Original Learning

The quality of transfer that occurs during new learning is largely dependent on the quality of the original learning. Most of us can recall easily our Social Security number or even a poem we learned in our early school years. If the original learning was well learned and accurate, its influence on new learning will be more constructive and help the student toward greater achievement. Students who did not learn the scientific method well, for example, will not be very effective in laboratory analysis, and they will not be able to transfer this learning to future success.

If something is worth teaching, it is worth teaching well. Rote learning does not tend to facilitate transfer, but learning with understanding does. Thus, trying to learn too many concepts too quickly may hinder transfer because the learner is simply memorizing isolated facts with little opportunity to organize the material in a meaningful fashion and link it to prior related knowledge.

Rote learning does not tend to facilitate transfer.

If we teach students to be conscious of both the new learning and the context into which it fits, we are helping them forge strong associations for future recall. If the new learning is too tightly bound to the context, then learners may fail to transfer that knowledge or skill to different contexts. When students perceive, for example, that grammatical correctness matters only in English class, then their writing in other classes gets careless.

In another example, a major study found that students who learned to solve arithmetic progression problems in algebra class were able to transfer the method they learned to solve similar physics problems involving velocity and distance in their science classes. On the other hand, students who learned to solve the physics problems first were unable to transfer the method to solve similar arithmetic progression problems in their algebra class (Bassok & Holyoak, 1989). The transfer of learning from physics to arithmetic was apparently blocked because the physics equations were embedded within the specific subject area context, thereby preventing the students from seeing their application to another context—algebra.

Not surprisingly, one study revealed that when students were required to process information more thoroughly for meaning, there was a high degree of transfer to new situations. The researchers found that students who did more thorough processing used the underlying conceptual information when they were asked to generate analogies, but they used superficial information when asked to do simple rote recall of similar information (Blanchette & Dunbar, 2000).

We discussed in the previous chapter that information is more likely to be remembered if the learner has multiple opportunities to rehearse and use it. But too often, we have time enough only to study a topic until the students reach some low level of mastery and then move on to the next topic. But research on transfer suggests that transfer is improved when students visit important topics often rather than just one intense exposure.

Today's learning is tomorrow's transfer. Therefore, if something is worth teaching, it is worth teaching well.

When using transfer, we ask students to bring learnings from their past forward to today. If the past learning was taught well, it should help the students acquire today's learning. What is taught today becomes past learning tomorrow. If it is taught well today, the positive transfer will enhance tomorrow's learning, and so forth. In other words, today's learning is tomorrow's transfer.

Similarity

Transfer can be generated by the similarity of the situation in which something is being learned and the situation to which that learning may transfer. Thus, skills learned in one environment tend to transfer to other environments that are similar. For example, commercial jet pilots are first trained in flight simulators before they sit in the cockpit of the actual plane. All the training and learnings they acquired in the simulator, an exact replica of the actual plane, will transfer to the real flying situation. This positive transfer helps the pilot get accustomed quickly to the actual plane, and it reduces errors. If you have ever rented a car, you realize that it does not take you very long to get accustomed to it and drive away. The environment is similar to your own car, and most of the important components are in familiar places. You may need a few moments, however, to locate the windshield wiper and light switches.

Teachers often use similarity when introducing new material. They may have students learn words with similar spelling patterns, such as *beat, heat, meat,* and *neat.* Students may use their skills at finding locations on a road map to help place ordered numbers on a graph grid. However, as we shall discuss shortly, presenting two items of information at the same time that are *too* similar can cause problems during retention. Other examples of using similarity are fire and tornado drills. Even giving students major tests in the room where they learned the material being tested uses similarity of the environment for positive transfer.

Similarity of sensory modalities is another form of transfer. Using the color red to represent danger can alert us to traffic lights, the location of fire alarm boxes, or hazardous areas. Sensory similarity can also cause error. Students may confuse *there, their,* and *they're* because they sound alike, or they may not be able to pronounce *read* until they know the word's context.

The more specific the cue that working memory attaches to a new learning, the easier it is for long-term memory to identify the item being sought. This process leads to an interesting phenomenon regarding long-term storage and retrieval: We store by similarity, but we retrieve by difference. That is, long-term memory most often stores new learnings into a network that contains learnings with similar characteristics or associations, as perceived by the learner. This network identification is one

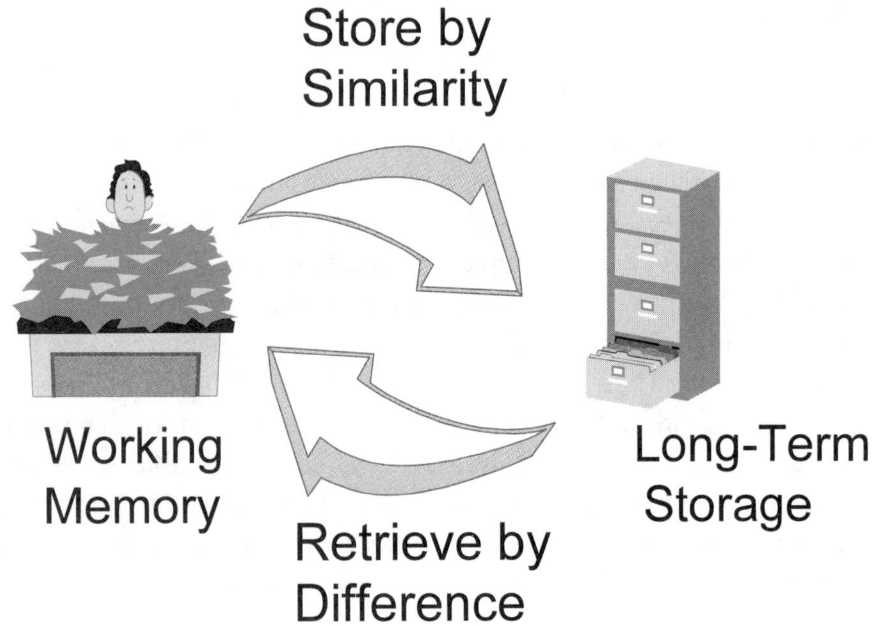

Figure 4.3 We tend to store information in networks by similarity, but retrieve it back into working memory by difference.

of the connections made in working memory during rehearsal and closure. To retrieve an item, long-term memory identifies how it is *different* from all the other items in that network (Figure 4.3).

For example: How would you recognize your best friend in a crowd? It is not because he has two arms, two legs, a head, and a torso. These characteristics make him *similar* to all the others. Rather, it is his more subtle *differences,* such as facial features, walk, and voice, that allow you to distinguish him from everyone else. His unique characteristics are called his *critical attributes.* If your friend is an identical twin, however, you might have difficulty picking him out from his brother if both are in the crowd. Similarly, the high degree of similarity between two concepts, coupled with few differences, makes it difficult for the learner to tell them apart.

Take, for example, the concepts of latitude and longitude. The similarities between these two ideas far outweigh their differences. Both use identical units of measure, deal with all four compass points, are imaginary lines, locate points on the Earth's surface, and are similar in sound and spelling. Their only real difference is their orientation in space. Teaching them together can be very difficult because their many similarities obscure their singular difference. The problem of similarity can be pervasive because curriculums are often written with the most alike concepts taught together. In fact, a useful task for a committee rewriting a curriculum is to list those concepts that students find the most difficult. Then determine if the difficulty is that two very similar concepts or motor skills are taught together, resulting in confusion. See the **Practitioner's Corner** at the end of this chapter, p. 151, for precisely when this can be a problem and how to deal with it.

> ***Two concepts that are very similar to each other ordinarily should not be taught at the same time.***

Critical Attributes

Transfer is sometimes generated when a special property, called a *critical attribute,* is recalled. Critical attributes, characteristics that make one idea unique from all others, are the cues of *difference* that learners can use as part of their storage process. Statements like *Amphibians live both on land and in water, Homonyms are words that sound alike but have different spellings and meanings*, and *To produce sound, something must vibrate* are examples of identifying a concept's critical attributes.

Identifying the critical attributes of a concept is a powerful memory tool, but it is not an easy task. We live in a culture driven by a quest for equality for all. This culture places a higher value on similarities than on differences. Thus, our cerebral networks are organized around similarity from an early age, and teachers frequently use similarity in the classroom to introduce new ideas. Successful retrieval from mental storage areas is accomplished by identifying differences among concepts. Consequently, teachers can help learners process new learnings accurately by having them identify the unique characteristics that make one concept different from all others. For example, what are the critical attributes of an explorer? Will these attributes help to separate Vasco da Gama from Napoleon Bonaparte? Students can use critical attributes to sort concepts so that they are stored in logical networks with appropriate cues. This will facilitate long-term memory's searches and increase the probability that it will accurately identify and retrieve the concept being sought.

Another useful task for a committee that is updating curriculum is to identify the critical attributes of all the major concepts that will be taught. If the committee members have difficulty agreeing on the critical attributes of a particular topic, imagine the challenge this will pose for the learner. See the **Practitioner's Corner** at the end of this chapter, p. 153, on how to identify critical attributes.

Association

Whenever two events, actions, or feelings are learned together, they are said to be *associated,* or bonded, so that the recall of one prompts the spontaneous recall of the other. The word *Romeo* elicits *Juliet,* and *Batman* gets *Robin.* A song you hear being played at a mall may elicit memories of some event that are associated with that song. The odor of a cologne once worn by a close friend from the past triggers the emotions of that relationship. Trademarks and product symbols, such as McDonald's golden arches, are designed to recall the product. Although there is no similarity between the two items, they were learned together and are, therefore, recalled together.

Here is a simple example of transfer. Look at the words listed below. On the lines to the right, write one or two words that come to mind as you read each word in the list.

Monday	______________	______________
dentist	______________	______________
Mom	______________	______________
vacation	______________	______________
babies	______________	______________
emergency	______________	______________

money ______________ ______________

Sunday ______________ ______________

What you wrote down represents thoughts that you have associated with each word in the list. Here are some responses that others have written for Monday: *work, blues, quarterback, beginning.* For Mom, others have written: *love, apple pie, caring, important, security, dad.* Were your words anything like these? Maybe they were, or maybe not. Show the list to your family and friends and note their responses. Each of us makes different connections with concepts based on our unique experiences; this activity points out the variety of associations that different people can make with the same thought.

The more we learn and retain, the more we can learn.

Making associations expands the brain's ability to retain information. New connections are formed between neurons and new insights are encoded. Much like a tree growing new branches, everything we remember becomes another set of branches to which memories can be attached. The more we learn and retain, the more we *can* learn and retain.

Emotions Associated With Learning. Association is particularly powerful when feelings or emotions are associated with a learning. We mentioned earlier that the brain's amygdala encodes emotional messages when they are strong and bonds them to learnings for long-term storage. We also noted that emotions usually have a higher priority than cognitive processing for commanding our attention. Words like *abortion, Holocaust,* and *capital punishment* often evoke strong feelings. Math anxiety is an example of a strong feeling (probably failure) associated with mathematics. Some students will avoid new situations involving learning mathematics to avoid the negative feelings that are recalled with the content. On the other hand, people devote hours to their hobbies because they associate feelings of pleasure and success with these activities. Thus, teachers should strive to bond positive feelings to new learnings so that students feel competent and can enjoy the process. Positive emotions can be associated with learning whenever teachers do the following:

- Use humor (not sarcasm) as an integral part of the lesson.
- Design and tell stories that enhance understanding of the concepts. Studies show that stories engage all parts of the brain because they touch on the learner's experiences, feelings, and actions (Schank, 1990; Scott-Simmons, Barker, & Cherry, 2003).
- Incorporate real-world examples and activities that have meaning for the learners.
- Demonstrate that they really *care* about their students' success. This means spending less time on the class rules and test schedule, and more time on asking "How do *you* learn? What teaching strategies work best for you?" A 2004 Gallup poll of students indicated that they respond best to teachers who have plenty of latitude to be highly creative, to build strong relationships, and to tailor the learning process to the needs of each individual student (Gallup, 2004b).
- Learning new concepts is rarely a smooth-flowing linear progression. Rather, it is a dynamic with fits and starts, successes generating positive emotions and failures leading to negative feelings. When learning stalls, the teacher helps the student overcome negative emotions associated with failure by providing the support that leads the student to success—no matter how small that success is.

Teaching Methods

Teachers should not assume that transfer will automatically occur after students acquire a sufficient base of information. Significant and efficient transfer occurs only if we teach to achieve it. Hunter (2004), Mestre (2002), Perkins and Salomon (1988), and others have suggested that when teachers understand the factors that affect transfer, they can plan lessons that use the power of positive transfer to help students learn faster, solve problems, and generate creative and artistic products that enrich the learning experience.

To teach for transfer, we need to consider two major factors: The time sequence and the complexity of the transfer link between the learnings. The time sequence refers to the way the teacher will use time and transfer in the learning situation. Transfer can occur from past to present or from present to future.

Transfer From Past to Present

Past Learning ——➤ **Helps in** ——➤ **Present Learning**

In this, the teacher links something from the learner's past that helps add sense and meaning to the new learning. It is important to select an experience that is clear, unambiguous, and closely relevant (not just related) to the new learning. Some examples are as follows:

- An English teacher uses *West Side Story* to introduce *Romeo and Juliet* so that students transfer their knowledge about street gangs and feuds to help them understand Shakespeare's plot.
- A science teacher asks students to recall what they have learned about plant cells to study the similarities and differences in animal cells.
- A social studies teacher asks students to think of the causes of the U.S. Civil War to see if they can also explain the causes of the Vietnam War.

Transfer From Present to Future

Present Learning ——➤ **Helps in** ——➤ **Future Learning**

The teacher makes the present learning situation as similar as possible to a future situation to which the new learning should transfer. For the transfer to be successful, students must attain a high degree of original (current) learning and be able to recognize the critical attributes and concepts that make the situations similar and different. For example,

- Students learn the critical attributes of fact and opinion so they can transfer that learning in the future when evaluating advertising, news reports, election campaigns, and the like.

- Students learn how to read graphs, pie charts, and tables so that in the future they can evaluate data presented to them for analysis and action.
- Students learn safe personal and interpersonal hygiene practices to protect their health throughout their lives.

Teaching techniques, such as *bridging* and *hugging*, are designed to help students make transfer links from past to present, and present to future. They can be used in all subject areas and for learning both cognitive concepts and psychomotor skills. Examples of these techniques are found in the **Practitioner's Corners** at the end of this chapter on pp. 157 and 159.

Complexity of the Link Between Learnings

The way that transfer occurs during a learning situation can range from a very superficial similarity to a sophisticated, abstract association. For example, when renting a car, it takes just a few minutes to get accustomed to the model, find the windshield wiper and light controls, and drive off. Interpreting a pie chart in the school budget requires the recall of graph analysis skills from a prior mathematics course. The new learning environments are perceived as being *similar* to others that the learner has practiced, and that similarity automatically triggers the same learned behaviors.

Metaphors can convey meaning of abstract material as well and as rapidly as literal language.

Metaphor, Analogy, and Simile. The transfer connection can also be much more complex, requiring the learner to make an abstract application of knowledge and skills to the new situation. Metaphors, analogies, and similes are useful devices for promoting abstract transfer. The *metaphor* is the application of a word or phrase to an object or concept that it does not literally denote to suggest a comparison with another object or concept. A person may say "It's raining cats and dogs outside. I'm drowned!" Obviously, it is not raining animals and the person did not drown. He is speaking figuratively and the metaphor compares things that are essentially dissimilar. An *analogy* compares partial similarity between two things, such as comparing a heart to a pump. The *simile* compares two unlike things: *She is like a rose.*

Metaphors can often convey meaning of abstract material as well and as rapidly as literal language. Metaphors help to explain complex concepts or processes. A geologist explains the movement of glaciers as flowing like batter on a griddle, and that the glacier was like an enormous plow upon the land. Comparing life to taking a long trip also is a metaphor. We ask the learner to reflect on how the situations encountered on the road compare to those encountered in life. How can the meaning of bumps, detours, road signs and billboards, places we have visited, passed through, or stayed in for a while all compare to life situations? Complex transfer patterns can reach back to the past: *How does the thinking strategy I used when I encountered a major detour help me to decide what course to choose in life now?* They can also transfer to the future: *The planning I used in preparing for the trip should help me prepare for other major decisions I need to make in my life that require extensive planning.*

These strategies are rich in imagery and enhance the thinking process by encouraging students to seek out associations and connections that they would not ordinarily make. They gain insights into relationships among ideas that help to forge a more thorough understanding of new learning. See more on imagery in Chapter 5; see also the **Practitioner's Corner** on p. 161 on using metaphors to enhance transfer.

Journal Writing for Transfer

Transfer is more likely to occur when students have an opportunity to reflect on their new learning. This reflection time can occur during closure, and is more likely to take place if the student is given a specific task. Journal writing is a very useful technique for closure because the specific steps help students to make connections to previous knowledge and organize concepts into networks for eventual storage. The strategy takes but a few minutes, but it can have enormous payback in terms of increased understanding and retention of learning. See the **Practitioner's Corner** on p. 163 for the specific steps that are likely to make this a successful effort.

> ***Journal writing is a highly effective strategy for closure and transfer.***

Transfer and Constructivism

The proper and frequent use of transfer greatly enhances the constructivist approach to learning. Constructivist teachers (Brooks & Brooks, 1999) are those who:

- Use student responses to alter their instructional strategies and content
- Foster student dialogue
- Question student understanding before sharing their own
- Encourage students to elaborate on their initial responses
- Allow students time to construct relationships and create metaphors

All these strategies have been discussed here and in previous chapters and are characteristic of teachers who are proficient in using transfer deliberately throughout their lessons.

Additional Thoughts About Transfer

Transfer can be referred to as the "so what?" phase of learning. The context in which students learn information and skills is often different from the context where they will apply that learning. If students do not perceive how the information or skill can be used for the future, they will tend to pay little attention and exert even less effort. The cognitive research supports the notion that transfer occurs easier if students have processed the initial learning in ways that promote deep, abstract understanding of the material, rather than emphasizing the rote application of superficial similarities. Teachers help students achieve deep, abstract understandings when they involve students in multiple examples that illustrate the critical attributes in as wide a variety as possible.

Of course, there are times when some rote memorization is needed to facilitate transfer. In fact, research in areas such as reading and early mathematical development suggests that both conceptual learning and rote activities (e.g., decoding skills for reading, number facts for early mathematics) are important (Mestre, 2002).

Teaching strategies mentioned elsewhere in this book can enhance transfer. For example, using music and songs, or performing some physical movements when learning a particular concept allows students to associate these activities with the concept and assist in recall at some future time.

Transfer and High Stakes Testing. The recent attention to accountability and high stakes testing may actually work against efforts to increase the transfer of learnings. Teaching to the high stakes test might emphasize rote activities in place of strategies that foster the deep understandings needed for transfer. We need to devise tests that assess transfer of knowledge. Computer programs, for instance, can aid in devising assessments that look at deep conceptual processing. Assessments that focus on preparedness for future learning (e.g., solving a relatively complex novel problem) may be more revealing of transfer than those focused strictly on solving superficial problems in an isolated subject area.

What's Coming Up?

One of the most interesting discoveries about the brain in the last 40 years is the research evidence showing that each hemisphere specializes in performing certain functions. Subsequent studies have given researchers fascinating insights into how the brain is organized and clues about a broad range of cognitive processes. Brain specialization has also spawned some myths and stories that endure to this day. What are the facts and fallacies about the left and right sides of the brain? Why is this information so important for teachers and parents? The answers to these and other intriguing questions about brain specialization are found in the next chapter.

PRACTITIONER'S CORNER

Strategies for Connecting to Past Learnings

Transfer helps students make connections between what they already know and the new learning. It is important to remember that the connections are of value only if they are relevant to the *students'* past, not necessarily the teacher's. This process also helps the teacher find out what the students already know about the new material. If students already have knowledge of what is planned for the new lesson, then teachers should make some adjustments and move on. (The curriculum is notably cluttered with too much repetition at every grade level and in every subject area.) This method also alerts the teacher to any prior knowledge that may interfere with new learning (negative transfer). Here are a few suggestions to discover what students already know so that prior learnings can help facilitate new learning (positive transfer). Note that the activities use novelty and shift the task burden to the student. Choose those that are grade-level appropriate.

- **Short Story.** Students write short stories to describe what they already know about a given topic. This can be used in any subject area because writing is a skill that should be continually practiced. (Note: This activity is not journal writing, which serves a different purpose.)

- **Interviews.** In a think-pair-share format, students interview their partners to determine their knowledge levels.

- **Graphic Organizers.** Students select an appropriate graphic organizer to explain and relate their past learning.

- **Mural or Collage.** Students make a mural or collage to communicate their current knowledge.

- **Music Activity.** Students write a song that tells of their prior knowledge.

- **Models.** Students build or draw models to express what they know.

- **Student Ideas.** Students may suggest other ways of showing what they know, such as writing a poem, painting a picture, creating a quiz show, etc.

PRACTITIONER'S CORNER

Avoid Teaching Concepts That Are Very Similar

Teachers often use similarity to introduce new topics. They say, "You already learned something about this topic when we . . . " This helps students to use positive transfer by recalling similar items from long-term storage that can assist in learning new information. But as we saw in the Chapter 3 discussion on learning motor skills, similarity can also be a problem.

Whenever two concepts have many more similarities than differences, such as latitude and longitude, mitosis and meiosis, or simile and metaphor, there is a high risk that the learner cannot tell them apart. In effect, the similarities overwhelm the differences, resulting in the learner attaching the same retrieval cues to both concepts. Thus, when the learner uses that cue later to retrieve information, it could produce either or both concepts and the learner may not recognize which is correct.

How to Deal With This Problem. When planning a lesson with two very similar concepts, list their similarities and differences. If the number of similarities and differences is about the same, there is less chance the students will be confused, but if the number of similarities is far greater than the differences, confusion is likely. In that case, try the following:

- **Teach the Two Concepts at Different Times.** Teach the first concept. Make sure that the students thoroughly understand it and can practice it correctly. Then teach a related concept to give the first concept time to be consolidated accurately and fully into long-term storage. Teach the second concept a few weeks later. Now information from the first concept acts for positive transfer in learning the second concept.

- **Teach the Difference(s) First.** Another option is to start by teaching the difference(s) between the two concepts. This works better with older students because they have enough prior learnings to recognize subtle differences. For example, teach that the only real difference between latitude and longitude is their orientation in space, and that this can cause confusion when labeling a location. Focusing on and practicing the difference gives learners the warnings and the cues they need to separate the two similar concepts and identify them correctly in the future.

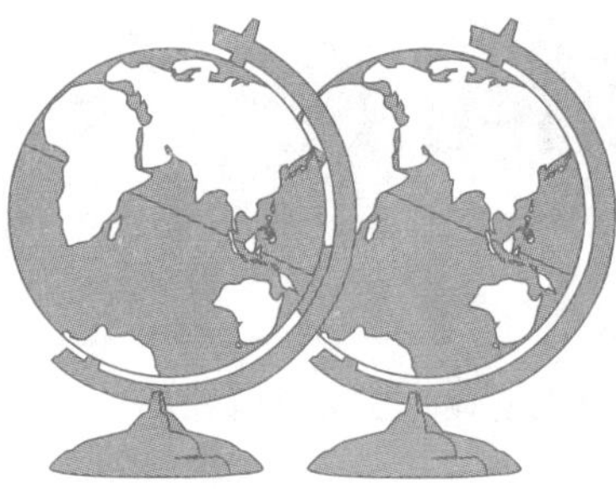

It seems so logical that two concepts that have many similarities should be taught at the same time. And so, for years, teachers have struggled with introducing concepts like the following in the same lesson: latitude and longitude; mitosis and meiosis; simile, analogy, and metaphor; complementary and supplementary angles; monarchy, oligarchy, plutocracy; writing lower-case b, d, p, and q, and many others. But the very fact that they are *so* similar can lead to retrieval problems.

To see how similarity may affect your work, try this activity:

A. Think about and list two or more concepts that are so similar they could cause confusion.

____

B. How could these concepts be presented to minimize confusion?

____

PRACTITIONER'S CORNER

Identifying Critical Attributes for Accurate Transfer

Critical attributes are characteristics that make one concept *unique* among all others. Teachers need to help students identify these attributes so students can use them for eventual and accurate retrieval. Hunter (2004) suggested a five-step process:

1. **Identify the Critical Attributes.** Suppose the learning objective is for the students to understand how mammals are different from all other animals. The two critical attributes of mammals are that (a) they nurse their young through mammary glands, and (b) they have hair.

2. **Teacher Gives Simple Examples.** The teacher offers some simple examples, such as the human being, cat, dog, and gerbil, to establish the concept. The teacher gives the examples at this point, not the students. Because this new learning is occurring in prime-time-1 when retention is highest, the examples must be correct. Be sure to match the example to the two critical attributes.

3. **Teacher Gives Complex Examples.** Now the teacher gives more complex examples, such as the porpoise and whale, which, unlike most mammals, live in water. It is important here to show again how the critical attributes apply.

4. **Students Give Examples.** Here the teacher checks for student understanding to ensure that the critical attributes are used correctly and that the concept is firmly in place. The students must also prove that the attributes apply to their examples.

5. **Teach the Limits of the Critical Attributes.** The learner must recognize that critical attributes may have limits and not apply in every instance. In this lesson, these attributes will accurately identify all mammals, but may incorrectly identify some nonmammals. There is a small group of animals called *platypuses*, that exhibit not only mammalian characteristics but also those of amphibians and birds. They are in a separate classification.

Take each major concept you teach and use the five-step process above to identify its critical attributes. These attributes help students clearly recognize what makes this concept *different* from all others. These attributes become valuable cues for accuracy and later retrieval.

By identifying the critical attributes, the student learns how one concept is different from all other similar concepts. This leads to clearer understanding, concept attainment, the ability to relate the new concept properly to others, and the likelihood that it will be stored, remembered, and recalled accurately. All subject areas have major concepts whose critical attributes should be clearly identified. Here are a few simple examples:

Social Studies

Law	Rule made by a government entity that is used for the control of behavior, is policed, and carries a penalty if broken.
Culture	The common behavior of a large group of people who can be identified by specific foods, clothing, art, religion, and music.
Democracy	A system of government in which the citizens have power through their elected representatives.

Science

Atom	The smallest part of an element that still retains the properties of that element.
Mammal	An animal that has hair and mammary glands.
Planet	A natural heavenly body that revolves around a star, rotates on its axis, and does not produce its own light.

Mathematics

Triangle	A two-dimensional figure that is closed and three-sided.
Prime	An integer with a value greater than 1 whose only positive factors are itself and 1.
Histogram	A bar graph that shows how many data values fall into a certain interval.

Language Arts

Sonnet	A poem of 14 lines, written in iambic pentameter with a specific rhyming pattern.
Simile	A figure of speech that compares two unlike things.
Hyperbole	An intentional exaggeration not intended to be taken literally.

Try the activity on the next page to help identify the critical attributes of important concepts from your own teaching or learning experiences.

A. Work with a partner to complete the worksheet on the next page, *Identifying Unique and Unvarying Elements*. Begin by using the Analogy Map below to help you decide on the differences between two similar concepts.

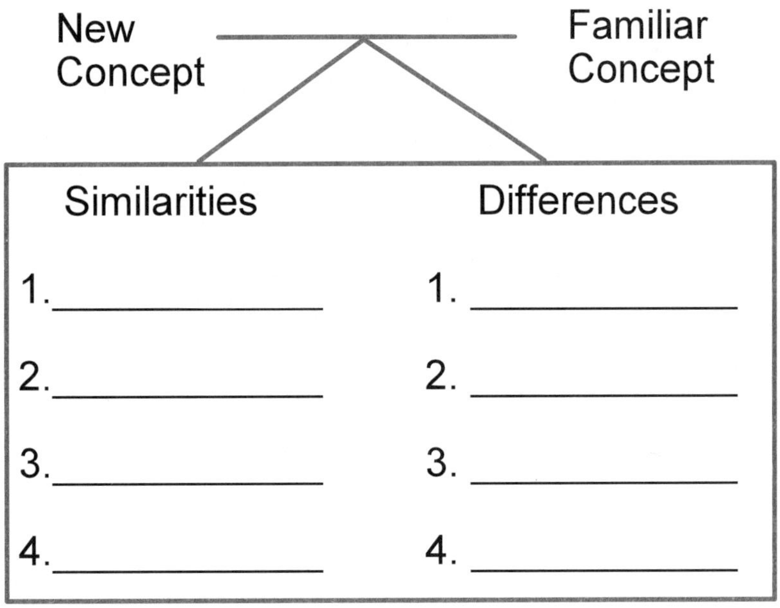

New Concept ____________ Familiar Concept

Similarities	Differences
1.____________	1. ____________
2.____________	2. ____________
3.____________	3. ____________
4.____________	4. ____________

B. After completing the worksheet, decide what benefits are provided to the learner by identifying the unique and unvarying elements/critical attributes.

C. List here some concepts in your curriculum that would be good candidates for this strategy.

Worksheet on Identifying Unique and Unvarying Elements (Critical Attributes)

Identify a major concept and decide on its unique and unvarying elements (critical attributes).

Concept:____

1. Its unique and unvarying elements (critical attributes) are

____

____

2. Simple examples are

____

____

3. Complex example(s) are

____

____

4. Student examples could be

____

____

5. Limits of the unique and unvarying elements (if any) are

____

____

PRACTITIONER'S CORNER

Teaching for Transfer: Bridging

Perkins and Salomon (1988), among others, have suggested various techniques for teachers to use to achieve positive transfer. In the technique called *bridging,* the teacher invokes transfer by helping students see the connection and abstraction from what the learner knows to other new learnings and contexts. There are many ways this can be accomplished. Here are a few:

- **Brainstorming.** When introducing a new topic, ask students to brainstorm ways this new learning can be applied in other situations. For example, can students use the skills they have just learned in analyzing charts, tables, and graphs? How else can they use their understandings about the law of supply and demand? What future value is there in knowing about nuclear power generation and alternative energy sources?

- **Analogies.** After learning a topic, use an analogy to examine the similarities and differences between one system and another. For example, ask students to make comparisons: How was the post-Vietnam War period in Vietnam similar to and different from the post-U.S. Civil War period in the United States? How is the post-Soviet Union period in Russia today similar to and different from the United States post-Revolutionary War period?

- **Metacognition.** When solving problems, ask students to investigate ways of approaching the solutions and discuss the advantages and disadvantages of each. For example, what solutions are there to meet the increased demand for electrical power in a densely populated area? What power sources could be used and which would be safest, most economical, most practical, etc.? What are the ways in which governments could regionalize to improve their effectiveness and economy of services? What impact might this have on local government and the democratic process? After applying their solutions, the students discuss how well their approaches worked and how they might change their approaches next time to improve their success.

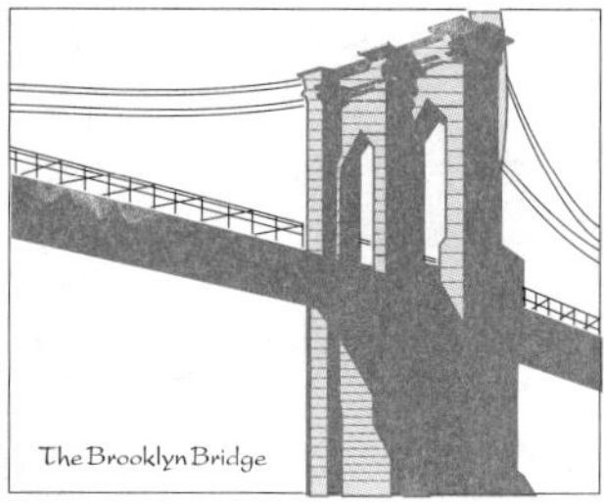

Bridging: Invoking transfer by connecting what the learner knows to other new learning and contexts. Select a concept (e.g., energy, democracy, equilibrium, allegory) and use the strategies below to link that concept to the learner's past knowledge. Look at the **Practitioner's Corner** on concept mapping in Chapter 5, p. 200 for help with this task.

Brainstorming (applying new learning in other situations):

____

____

Analogies (examining similarities and differences):

The Analogy Map could help here (see p. 202).

____

____

____

Metacognition (solving problems by investigating advantages and disadvantages of alternative solutions):

Advantages	Disadvantages

PRACTITIONER'S CORNER

Teaching for Transfer: Hugging

Hugging, suggested by Perkins and Salomon (1988), uses similarity to make the new learning situation more like future situations to which transfer is desired. This is a lower form of transfer and relies on an almost automatic response from the learner when the new situation is encountered. Teachers should ensure that the similarity of a situation actually involves the student using the skill or knowledge to be transferred. When students use a word search puzzle to identify certain French verbs written forward or backward, this does not mean that they will be able to understand these verbs in written or spoken French. *Hugging* means keeping the new instruction as close as possible to the environment and requirements that the students will encounter in the future. Here are a few ways to design hugging:

- **Simulation Games.** These are useful in helping students practice new roles in diverse situations. Debates, mock trials, and investigating labor disputes are ways that students can experiment with various approaches to solving complex legal and social issues.

- **Mental Practice.** When a student is unable to replicate an upcoming situation, it is very useful for the student to mentally practice what that situation could be like. The student reviews potential variations of the situation and devises mental strategies for dealing with different scenarios. Suppose a student is to interview a political candidate for the school newspaper. In addition to the prepared questions, what other questions could the student ask, depending on the candidate's response? What if the candidate is reticent or changes the course of the questioning?

- **Contingency Learning.** Here the learner asks what other information or skill must be acquired to solve a problem, and then learns it. For example, if the student is building a model to demonstrate gas laws, what else must the student learn in order to design and construct the apparatus at a reasonable cost so that it shows the desired gas relationships effectively?

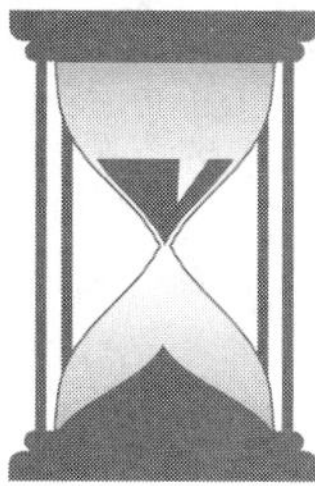

Hugging: Invoking transfer by making the new learning situation more like future situations to which transfer is desired. Select a concept (or the same one you chose in Bridging) and use the strategies that follow to show how the concept can be useful in future circumstances.

Simulation games (practicing new roles in diverse situations):

Be prepared to present the simulation to the group.

Mental practice (devising mental strategies for dealing with different scenarios):

Contingency learning (secondary learnings needed to accomplish primary learning):

PRACTITIONER'S CORNER

Using Metaphors to Enhance Transfer

Metaphors can convey meaning as well and as rapidly as literal language. They are usually rich in imagery, are useful bridging strategies, and can apply to both content and skill learnings. West, Farmer, and Wolff (1991) suggest a seven-step process for using metaphors in lesson design.

1. **Select the Metaphor.** The criteria for selecting the appropriate metaphor center on goodness of fit (how well the metaphor explains the target concept or process), degree or richness of imagery, familiarity that the students will have with it, and its novelty.

2. **Emphasize the Metaphor.** The metaphor must be emphasized consistently throughout the lesson. Students should be alerted to interpret the metaphor figuratively and not literally.

3. **Establish Context.** Proper interpretation of the metaphor requires that the teacher establish the context for its use. Metaphors should not be used in isolation, especially if the students lack the background to understand them.

4. **Provide Instructions for Imagery.** Provide students with the instructions they will need to benefit from the rich imagery usually present in metaphors. "Form a mental picture of this" is good advice (See the **Practitioner's Corner** on imagery in Chapter 6, p. 237).

5. **Emphasize Similarities and Differences.** Because the metaphor juxtaposes the similarities of one known object or procedure with another, teachers should emphasize the similarities and differences between the metaphor and the new learning.

6. **Provide Opportunities for Rehearsal.** Use rote and elaborate rehearsal strategies to help students recognize the similarities and differences between the metaphor and the new learning, and to enhance their depth of understanding and types of associations.

7. **Beware Mixed Metaphors.** Because metaphors are such powerful learning devices, make sure you choose them carefully. Mixed metaphors cause confusion and lead to inaccuracy.

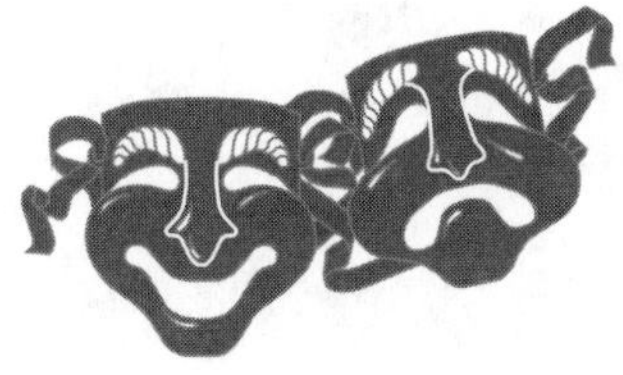

We used metaphors in designing the Information Processing Model (See the **Practitioner's Corner** in Chapter 2 on redesigning the model, p. 56) to help remember the important stages in the process. Now, let's practice it with a different concept.

Directions: Working with a partner, select a concept and decide what metaphor(s) would help you or your students remember it.

Concept:______________________________

Metaphor(s):

____

____

____

____

____

____

____

____

____

PRACTITIONER'S CORNER

Using Journal Writing to Promote Transfer and Retention

Journal writing can be a very effective strategy to promote positive transfer and increase retention. It can be done in nearly all grade levels and subject areas and is particularly effective when used as a closure activity.

Teachers may be reluctant to use this technique because they believe it takes up too much class time while adding more papers for them to evaluate. However, this strategy takes just three to five minutes, two or three times a week. That is, the teacher only spot checks journals periodically. The gain in student understanding and retention will be well worth the small amount of time invested. Here are some suggestions for using journal writing for maximum effectiveness:

- Students should keep a different journal for each class or subject area.
- To use this as a closure activity, ask students to write down their responses to these three questions:
    1. "**What did we learn today about** . . . (insert here the *specific* learning objective)?" Avoid questions like, "Write down what we did today," because younger students are likely to focus on activities rather than on the learning. This question helps to establish *sense*.
    2. "**How does this connect or relate to what we already know about** . . . (insert here some past learning that will help students with positive transfer)?" It is permissible to give hints to guide student thinking. After all, we want to facilitate accuracy. This question can help the learner *chunk* new learning into existing networks.
    3. "**How can this help us, or how can we use this information/skill in the future?**" Give hints if necessary. This question aids in finding *meaning*.
- You can use one day's journal entry as a prefocus activity for the following day, provided the new day's lesson is related.

Chapter 4—The Power of Transfer

Key Points to Ponder

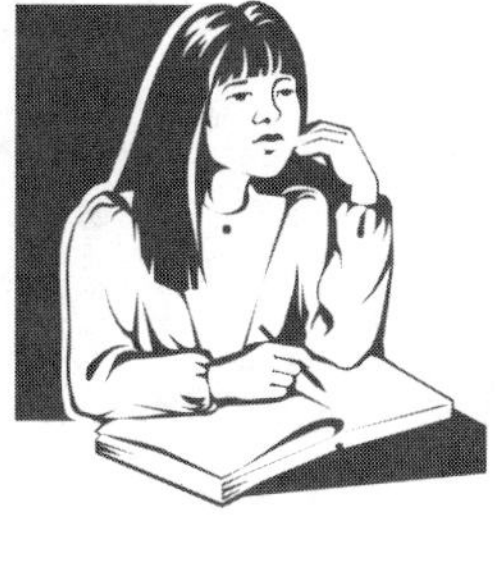

Jot down on this page key points, ideas, strategies, and resources you want to consider later. This sheet is your personal journal summary and will help to jog your memory.

Chapter 5

Brain Specialization and Learning

Despite myriad exceptions, the bulk of split-brain research has revealed an enormous degree of lateralization—that is, specialization in each of the hemispheres.

—Michael Gazzaniga,
The Split Brain Revisited

Chapter Highlights: This chapter explores the research on how the brain is specialized to perform certain tasks. It examines hemispheric specialization, debunks some myths, and allows you to determine your hemispheric preference. The chapter also examines how we learn to speak and read, and the implications of this research for classroom instruction and for the curriculum and structure of schools.

It may seem strange at a point this late in the book to introduce another chapter that focuses on brain function—in this case, how brain areas are specialized. But this functional specialization has led to the development of traits that are uniquely human, such as different learning styles and sophisticated spoken and written languages. These remarkable traits rely heavily on memory systems and transfer. Thus, I thought a review of how memory and transfer work was needed first in order to understand better the nature and impact of brain specialization on learning.

BRAIN LATERALIZATION

One of the intriguing characteristics of the human brain is its ability to integrate disparate and seemingly disconnected activities going on in specialized areas of the brain into a unified whole. Brain scans reveal how certain areas of the brain get involved in processing and performing specific tasks. For example, the auditory cortex responds to sound input, the frontal lobe to cognitive rehearsal, and sections of the left hemisphere to spoken language. The ability of certain areas of the brain to perform unique functions is known as cerebral *specialization.* If the activity is mainly limited to one hemisphere, it is called cerebral *lateralization.*

As evidence continues to accumulate regarding specialized brain areas, neuroscientists have had to modify their theories of brain organization accordingly. Researchers are now endorsing the idea that the brain is a set of modular units that carry out specific tasks. According to this *modular model*, the brain is a collection of units that supports the mind's information-processing requirements (e.g., a speech module, a numerical computation module, a face recognition module, etc.) and not a singular unit whose every part is capable of any function (Gazzaniga,1998a; Gazzaniga et al., 2002; Pinker, 1994; Rose, 2005).

The first indications of brain lateralization were discovered long before scanning technologies were developed. During the late 1950s, neurosurgeons decided that the best way to help patients with severe epileptic seizures was to sever the *corpus callosum* (Figure 1.2), the thick cable of 200 million nerve fibers that connects the two cerebral hemispheres. This last-ditch approach isolated the hemispheres so that seizures in the damaged hemisphere would not travel to the other side. The surgery had been tried on monkeys with epilepsy, and the results were encouraging. By the early 1960s, surgeons were ready to try the technique on human beings. One of the pioneers was Dr. Roger Sperry of the California Institute of Technology. Between 1961 and 1969, surgeons Joseph Bogen and Phillip Vogel successfully performed several operations under Sperry's guidance.

Although the operations resulted in a substantial reduction or elimination of the seizures, no one was sure what effect cutting this bridge between the hemispheres would have on the "split-brain" patients. Sperry and his student Michael Gazzaniga conducted experiments with these patients and made a remarkable discovery. Splitting the brain seemed to result in two separate domains of awareness. When a pencil was placed in the left hand (controlled by the right hemisphere) of a blindfolded patient, the patient could not name it. When the pencil was shifted to the right hand, however, the patient named it instantly. Neither hemisphere seemed to know what the other was doing and they acted, as Sperry said, "each with its own memory and will, competing for control."

As the tests progressed, Sperry charted the characteristics each hemisphere displayed. He concluded that each hemisphere seems to have its own separate and private sensations; its own perceptions; and its own impulses to act. This research showed that the right and left hemispheres have distinctly different functions that are not readily interchangeable. It also solved the mystery of the corpus callosum. Its purpose is largely to unify awareness and allow the two hemispheres to share memory and learning. Sperry won the 1981 Nobel Prize in medicine in part for this work.

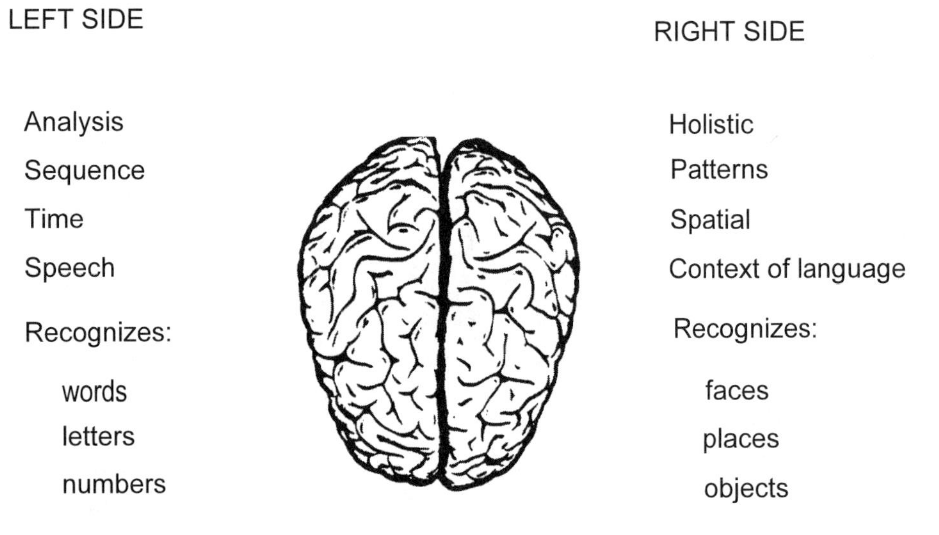

Figure 5.1 The left and right hemispheres of the brain are specialized and process information differently. However, in complex tasks, both hemispheres are engaged.

Left and Right Hemisphere Processing (Laterality)

Continued testing of split-brain patients and brain scans of normal (whole-brained) individuals have revealed considerable consistency in the different ways the two halves of the brain store and process information. This cerebral separation of tasks was earlier called *hemisphericity,* but is now more widely referred to as *laterality.* The results of numerous studies on laterality continue to provide more insights into the kind of processing done by each hemisphere and expand our understanding of this remarkable division of labor. Figure 5.1 summarizes and Table 5.1 shows more specifically the functions that the hemispheres carry out as they deal with the vast amount of new and past information that must be assessed every second.

Left Hemisphere

The left brain monitors the areas for speech. It understands the literal interpretation of words, and recognizes words, letters, and numbers written as words. It is analytical, evaluates factual material in a rational way, and detects time and sequence. It also performs simple arithmetic computations. Arousing attention to deal with outside stimuli is another specialty of the left hemisphere.

Right Hemisphere

The right brain gathers information more from images than from words, and looks for patterns. It interprets language through context—body language, emotional content, and tone of voice—rather

Table 5.1 Functions of the Left and Right Cerebral Hemispheres

Left Hemisphere Functions	CORPUS CALLOSUM	Right Hemisphere Functions
Connected to right side of the body		Connected to the left side of the body
Processes input in a sequential and analytical manner		Processes input more holistically and abstractly
Time-sensitive		Space-sensitive
Generates spoken language		Interprets language through gestures, facial movements, emotions, and body language
Does invariable and arithmetic operations		Does relational and mathematical operations
Specializes in recognizing words and numbers (as words)		Specializes in recognizing faces, places, objects, and music
Active in constructing false memories		More truthful in recall
Seeks explanations for why events occur		Puts events in spatial patterns
Better at arousing attention to deal with outside stimuli		Better at internal processing

Sources: Carter (1998); Gazzaniga (1998a,1998b); Gazzaniga, Ivry, & Mangun (2002)

than through literal meanings. It specializes in spatial perception, recognizes places, faces, and objects, and focuses on relational and mathematical operations, such as geometry and trigonometry.

What Causes Specialization?

No one knows exactly why the brain is specialized, although it does seem that such a capacity enables it to deal with a great amount of sensory data without going on overload. Why would we need two speech centers or face recognition areas? It would seem that as soon as one area of the brain acquired a specialization, there would be no need for it to be duplicated in the other hemisphere. How it *becomes* specialized is another question. The key to answering this may lie in the brain's structure and wiring. There is general agreement among neuroscientists now that the brain is hardwired for certain functions, such as spoken language, and that this hardwiring is localized.

Another possibility may center around the time it takes for signals to move in the brain. James Ringo and his colleagues (Ringo, Doty, Demeter, & Simard, 1994) used a neural network model that offered an possible explanation for hemispheric specialization. The researchers pointed out that nerve fibers within a hemisphere are shorter than the nerve fibers in the corpus callosum that run between hemispheres. As a result, nerve signals move faster *within* a hemisphere than *between* hemispheres. It would seem, then, that the brain has developed so that each hemisphere can have rapid access to information within itself, but a slower and more limited response to tasks that require communication back and forth across the corpus callosum. The time delays associated with communication between the hemispheres can limit the degree of their cooperation and encourage the development of hemispheric specialization.

Another factor may be that left and right hemispheres are physically different. The hemispheres are made up of the cortex (the thin but tough surface) called *gray matter* and the support tissue below it called *white matter*. The left hemisphere has more gray matter, while the right has more white. The left hemisphere's more tightly-packed neurons are better able to handle intense, detailed work. The right hemisphere's white matter contains neurons with longer axons that can connect with modules farther away. These long-range connections help the right to come up with broad but rather vague concepts. The information from each hemisphere is then pooled by sending signals across the corpus callosum (Carter, 1998).

Specialization Does Not Mean Exclusivity

The research data support the notion that each hemisphere has its own set of functions in information processing and thinking. However, these functions are rarely *exclusive* to only one hemisphere, and in even some simple tasks, it is possible for both hemispheres to be involved. Many tasks can be performed by either hemisphere, although one may be better at it than the other.

Although each hemisphere has specialized functions, both usually work together when learning.

In a typical individual, the results of the separate processing are exchanged with the opposite hemisphere through the corpus callosum. There is harmony in the goals of each, and they complement one another in almost all activities. Thus, the individual benefits from the integration of the processing done by both hemispheres and is afforded greater comprehension of whatever situation initiated the processing. For example,

- Logic is not confined to the left hemisphere. Some patients with right-brain damage fail to see the lack of logic in their thinking when they propose to take a walk even though they are completely paralyzed.
- Creativity or intuition is not solely in the right hemisphere. Creativity can remain, though diminished, even after extensive right-hemisphere damage.
- Because the two hemispheres do not function independently in a normal brain, it is impossible to educate only one hemisphere.
- Specialization does not mean **exclusivity**. There is no evidence that people are purely left or right brained. One hemisphere may be more active in most people, but only in varying degrees.
- Both hemispheres are capable of synthesis, that is, putting pieces of information together into a meaningful whole.

Hemispheric Preference: A Question of Learning Style

Since the work of Sperry, case studies and additional testing procedures have enabled researchers to understand more about the functions of each hemisphere. These tests include anesthetizing one hemisphere, PET imaging scans, electroencephalographs (which record electrical impulses), and hemisphere-specific vision and hearing tests. The research shows that most people have a preferred (or dominant) hemisphere, and that this preference affects personality, abilities, and learning style. Why this preference? No one knows for sure, any more than we know what causes handedness. It may be that if one hemisphere is more efficient than the other at developing within-hemisphere networks and processing, then that hemisphere contributes more during cognitive processing. As a result, hemispheric preference emerges.

Most people have a preferred hemisphere. This preference affects their personality, abilities, and learning style.

Hemispheric preference is largely a matter of processing style. Just as some people prefer more visual than auditory information when learning, people with strong but opposite hemispheric preferences will interact and interpret their worlds differently. Hemispheric preference runs the gamut from neutral (no preference) to strongly left or right. Those who are left-hemisphere preferred tend to be more verbal, analytical, and able to solve problems. Right-hemisphere-preferred individuals paint and draw well, are good at math, and deal with the visual world more easily than with the verbal (Springer & Deutsch, 1998).

Once again, the preference for either hemisphere does not mean that we do not use both hemispheres. In doing a simple task, we use more the hemisphere which specializes in that task. When we are faced with a task that is more complex, the preferred hemisphere will take the lead, although the nonpreferred hemisphere will likely get involved as well, contributing in its specialized manner (Weisman & Banich, 2000).

Preference and Consciousness

One of the more fascinating revelations from the continued studies of split-brain patients is the realization that their left and right hemispheres can give different answers to questions about themselves. It is as though they have a distinct consciousness residing in each hemisphere. For example, the inventive left hemisphere's consciousness surpasses that of the right. But the mind-boggling suggestion here is that even though our consciousness reflects that of the preferred hemisphere, another—and perhaps very different—consciousness lurks hidden in the nonpreferred hemisphere (Gazzaniga, 1998b). Sperry, himself, suspected as much of his split-brain patients. He wrote, "Everything we have seen indicates that the surgery has left these people with two separate minds . . . that is, two separate spheres of consciousness" (Sperry, 1966).

Examples of Preference

Suppose you are right-handed. A pen is on the table just next to your left hand, and someone asks you to pass the pen. Because this is a simple task, you will pick up the pen with your left hand in a smooth motion and pass it. You are not likely to stretch your right hand across your body or twist your torso to hand it over. If the person asks you to throw the pen, however, you will probably use your right hand because this task is more difficult.

During learning, both hemispheres are engaged, processing the information or skill according to their specializations and exchanging the results with the opposite hemisphere through the corpus callosum. So if someone were to toss a pen to you, your likelihood of successfully catching it would increase greatly if you used *both* hands, not just the right (dominant) hand.

Knowing the difference between how the left and right hemispheres process information explains why we succeed with some tasks but not with others, especially when we are trying to do them simultaneously. For instance, most of us can carry on a conversation (left-hemisphere activity) while driving a car (right-hemisphere and cerebellar activity). In this case, each task is controlled by different hemispheres. However, trying to carry on a conversation on the telephone while talking to someone in the room at the same time is very difficult because these are functions of the same (left) hemisphere and can interfere with each other.

Implications of Preference for Teachers

Hemispheric preference is just one component of learning style. Because teachers tend to teach the way they learn, they need to know as much about their own learning style as possible. Besides telling them something about themselves, this knowledge also helps them to understand learners with very different styles. To determine your hemispheric preference, see the **Practitioner's Corner** at the end of this chapter on p. 191.

So What? Cautions About Interpreting Hemispheric Preference

Perhaps no single piece of brain research has received so much attention and controversy as the notion that the two hemispheres of the brain process information differently. Although a substantial body of evidence suggests that each hemisphere has its specialized abilities, we should not jump to the conclusion that normal people have two brains or are functioning with only half a brain. The differences are not all-or-nothing. Quite the contrary, normal people have one integrated and magnificently differentiated brain that generates a single mind and self.

Unfortunately, some people have misused this research, referring to themselves, or worse, to students as "too left-brained" or "too right-brained." What is important to remember is that the two hemispheres work together as an integrated whole, sharing their different stimuli through the corpus callosum. Nevertheless, misinformation about the specialization of the hemispheres and several popular myths persist.

Some Myths About Hemispheric Preference

Several myths connecting hemispheric preference to other variables have evolved and endured during the past two decades. The myths have obscured the benefit of this research and undermined its value to the teaching and learning process. Here are two common myths we can debunk.

Handedness (lateral preference). Because the hemispheres of the brain control the opposite sides of the body, many have speculated that hemispheric preference is directly connected to handedness, or lateral preference. There is evidence that more right-hemisphere-preferred individuals are left-handed than right-handed. Scanning evidence also shows that most right-handers (about 93 to 95 percent) have left-hemisphere language preference (Knecht et al., 2000), whereas only 70 percent of left-handers have left-hemisphere language preference; the other 30 percent have language preference in the right or in both hemispheres (Carter, 1998). However, no direct cause-and-effect connection between handedness and hemispheric preference has been established. Thus, it is incorrect to assume that most right-handed people are left-hemisphere preferred and vice versa.

Handedness is established in the fetus by the fifteenth week of gestation. Despite all the sophisticated brain research of modern times, the cause of handedness has still escaped explanation. With nearly 90 percent of people right-handed, this would seem to be the outcome of the logical left hemisphere's control. Is left-handedness, then, pathological? Explanations run from simple genetic determination to some pre-natal disturbance that may have upset the left-brain/right-hand connection, such as unusually high testosterone levels. The mystery continues.

Intelligence. There is no research to support the notion that those with one hemispheric preference are any more or less intelligent than those with the opposite preference. Individuals who are strongly and oppositely preferred will exhibit vastly different personalities and learning styles, but this has no connection to intelligence or the ability to learn.

The Gender Connection

Scientists have known for years that there are structural and developmental (Table 5.2) as well as performance differences (Table 5.3) between male and female brains. Studies begun in the early 1970s and subsequent studies by other researchers have shown some gender differences in brain characteristics and capabilities. PET scans and fMRIs, for instance, indicate that males and females use different areas of their brains when accomplishing similar tasks (Cahill, 2005; Diamond & Hopson, 1998; Kimura, 1992; Yegger, 2002). Let's see what those differences are before we discuss what they mean. Keep in mind that research studies deal with groups of males and females. It is not always valid to assign characteristics to a specific person because individuals vary widely from one to another.

Structural and Developmental Differences

- Males have a higher percentage of gray matter (the thin cortex layer containing mostly dendrites) in the left hemisphere than females. In females, the percentage of gray matter is the same in both hemispheres. However, females have a higher percentage of total gray matter, whereas males have a higher percentage of white matter (mainly myelinated axons below the cortex layer) and cerebral spinal fluid. The corpus callosum (cable connecting the hemispheres) is proportionately larger and thicker in females than in males (Gazzaniga et al., 2002; Gur et al, 1999). All of these differences could be further evidence to support the idea that female brains are better at communicating between hemispheres and male brains within those hemispheres.

- For most males and females, the language areas are in the left hemisphere. But females also have an active language processor in the right hemisphere (Figure 5.2). Females possess a greater density of neurons in the language areas than males (Gazzaniza et al., 2002; Gur et al., 2000; Shaywitz, 2003; Shaywitz, Shaywitz, & Gore, 1995).
- The amygdala (which responds to emotional stimulation), loaded with testosterone receptors, grows more rapidly in teenage boys than in teenage girls, and

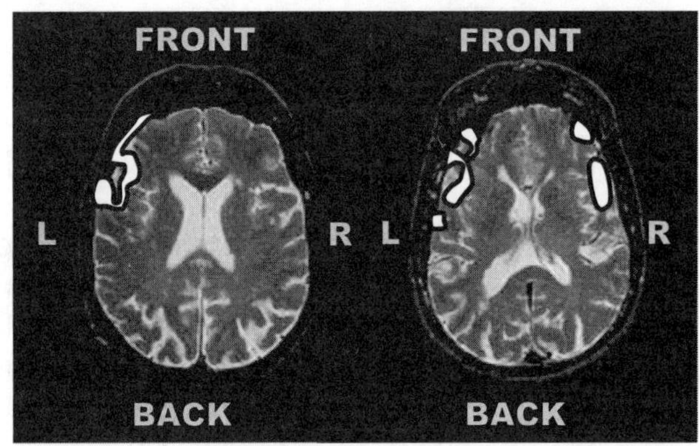

Figure 5.2 While processing language, fMRI scans show that male brains (left) use left hemisphere regions and that female brains activate regions in both hemispheres (white areas).

Table 5.2 Structural and Developmental Differences Between Female and Male Brains

	Females	Males	Sources
Gray matter	Higher percentage than males, with same amount in both hemispheres.	Lower percentage than females, with more in left hemisphere than right.	Gur et al., 1999
White matter	Lower percentage than males.	Higher percentage than females, with same amount in both hemispheres	Gur et al., 1999
Cerebral spinal fluid	Lower percentage than men, with same amount in both hemispheres	Higher percentage than females, with more in right hemisphere than left	Gur et al., 1999
Corpus callosum	Larger and thicker than in males	Smaller and thinner than in females	Gazzaniga et al., 2002; Gur et al, 1999
Language areas	Main areas in left hemisphere, with additional processing areas in right hemisphere. Density of neurons in language areas greater than in males.	Located almost exclusively in left hemisphere. Density of neurons in language areas less than in females.	Cahill, 2005; Gazzaniga et al., 2002; Gur et al., 2000; Shaywitz, 2003
Amygdala	Grows slower in teenage girls than in boys, and final size is smaller than in males. Only left amygdala activated by emotional stimulation.	Grows faster in teenage boys than in girls, and final size is larger than in females. Only right amygdala activated by emotional stimulation.	Cahill, 2005; Kreeger, 2002
Hippocampus	Grows faster in teenage girls than in boys, and final size is larger than in males	Grows slower in teenage boys than in girls, and final size is smaller than in females	Kregger, 2002

Table 5.3 Performance Differences Between Female and Male Brains

	Females	Males	Sources
Testing	No different from males in overall cognitive performance, but better than males on tests of perceptual speed, verbal fluency, determining the placement of objects (sequence), identifying specific attributes of objects, precision manual tasks, and arithmetic calculations.	No different from females in overall cognitive performance, but better than females on spatial tasks, such as mentally rotating three-dimensional objects, at target-directed motor skills, at spotting shapes embedded in complex diagrams, and in mathematical reasoning.	Cahill, 2005; Gazzaniga et al., 2002; Gur et al., 2000; Kimura, 1997; Njemanze, 2005
Facial recognition and expressions	Use more of their left hemisphere	Use more of their right hemisphere	Baron-Cohen, 2003; Everhart, Shucard, Quatrin, & Shucard, 2001

its final size is larger in men than in women. This is at least a partial explanation of why males tend to demonstrate more overt aggressive behavior than females. PET scans reveal that during emotional stimulation, females tend to activate only the amygdala in the left hemisphere while males tend to activate the amygdala only in the right hemisphere. Follow-up studies noted that females remembered the details of an emotional event (a typical left hemisphere function) better than males, whereas the males remembered better the central aspects, or gist, of the situation (Cahill, 2005; Kreeger, 2002).

- Meanwhile, the hippocampus (responsible for memory formation and consolidation), filled with estrogen receptors, grows more rapidly in girls than boys during adolescence (Kreeger, 2002). This could explain why preadolescent girls are generally better at language, arithmetic computations, and tasks involving sequence because all these depend on efficient memory processing.

Performance Differences

- There is no significant difference in overall cognitive performance between the sexes. However, on specific skills, more females perform better on tests of perceptual speed, verbal fluency, determining the placement of objects (sequence), identifying specific attributes of objects, precision manual tasks, and arithmetic calculations. More males perform better on spatial tasks, such as mentally rotating three-dimensional objects, at target-directed motor skills, at spotting shapes embedded in complex diagrams, and in mathematical reasoning

(Cahill, 2005; Gazzaniga et al., 2002; Gur et al., 2000; Neubauer, Grabner, Fink, & Neuper, 2005; Njemanze, 2005).

- When recalling emotions, females use a larger portion of their limbic system than do males. Females are also better at recognizing different types of emotions in others (Baron-Cohen, 2003).
- In face recognition and expression tasks, boys use more of their right brain while girls use more of their left (Everhart, Shucard, Quatrin, & Shucard, 2001).

The results of these and other studies further indicate that more females are left-hemisphere preferred and more males are right-hemisphere preferred. Why is this so? To what extent do nature (genetic makeup) and nurture (environment) contribute to these structural and performance differences? Although no one knows for sure, the research evidence suggests that the influence of prenatal hormones, natural selection, and environment could explain these results.

Possible Causes of Gender Differences

The Effects of Hormones. One possibility is that hormones, such as testosterone and androgen, influence brain development differently in the sexes. As they bathe the fetal brain, these substances direct the wiring and organization of the brain and stimulate the growth and density of neurons in specific areas. Testosterone, for instance, seems to delay the development of the left hemisphere in boys. Thus, girls get a head start in using the left hemisphere; boys are forced to rely more on their right hemisphere (this might also explain why more males are left-handed than females). The early exposure to these hormones seems to alter other brain functions (such as language acquisition and spatial perception) permanently for the individual. The resurgence of hormones with the onset of puberty may further reconfigure the mental organization of teens, especially as new social pressures emerge with their accompanying emotional shifts (Cahill, 2005; Kimura, 1992, 1997; Lutchmaya, Baron-Cohen, & Raggatt, 2002).

The Effects of Natural Selection. A related explanation is that natural selection affected our brain characteristics as we evolved. For thousands of years, the division of labor between the sexes was distinct. In prehistoric times, men were responsible for hunting large game over long distances, making weapons, and defending the group from predators, animal and otherwise. Women took care of the home and the children, prepared food, and made clothing. Such specialization required different cerebral operations from men and women. Men needed more route-finding and spatial abilities and better targeting skills. Women needed more fine-motor and timing skills to maintain the household and language skills to pass on the native language to their offspring. The individual males and females who could perform their respective tasks well survived long enough to pass their genes on to their children. Moreover, any new genetic combinations eventually led to structural changes in the brain—and other parts of the body—that were specific to each gender.

The Impact of the Environment. Another prevailing explanation looks to a combination of the different ways the sexes develop and interact with their environment. First, studies of infant boys and girls demonstrate that the acuity of senses does not develop identically in both genders. That is, hearing and touch (left-hemisphere controlled) develop more quickly in girls. Spatial vision (right-hemisphere controlled), however, develops more rapidly in boys. Second, parents tend to treat baby boys differently from baby girls. And third, boys and girls between the ages of 6 and 12 typically spend their out-of-school time quite differently as they are growing up. Girls are more likely to spend their free time indoors. In this structured environment, girls are exposed to more language through radio and television, and they are more conscious of time because of clocks, media, and other family members who may be coming home. This environment, psychologists argue, enhances left-hemisphere processes. On the other hand, more boys spend their free time outdoors. In this unstructured environment, boys rely more on space (location) than time, design their own games, use more visual than verbal skills during play, and use little language and only in context to accomplish a task. This behavior enhances right-hemisphere processes.

The Empathizing Female and Systemizing Male. Simon Baron-Cohen (2003) has summarized the essential laterality differences by proposing that female brains are predominantly wired for empathy, and that male brains are predominantly wired for systemizing, that is, understanding and building systems. According to his intriguing theory, a person (whether female or male) can be one of three brain types. An individual who is stronger at empathizing than systemizing is Type E. Those who are stronger at systemizing are Type S, and those who are equally strong at both are Type B (for balanced). Baron-Cohen believes that the effects of hormones during prenatal and early postnatal development are largely responsible for these sex differences. He does, however, admit that genetic traits and the environment also exert their influence.

The brains of males and females organize differently from very early in their development through their formative years, leading to different preferences in learning.

Baron-Cohen rightly points out something we should all remember as we study differences in the human brain: sex does not solely determine how an individual's brain is organized. Some males will have brains organized more like females, and some females will have brains organized more like males. Individuals of any brain type can be successful in any endeavor.

The evidence suggests that we no longer think in terms of nature versus nurture. Rather, we should see the relationship of these forces as more circular. Genes influence behavior, and behavior can influence how genes function as a child grows and develops. Thus, a combination of nature and nurture factors causes the brains of males and females to organize differently from very early in their development through their formative years, leading, among other things, to different preferences in learning and how they interact with their world.

More girls than boys are left-hemisphere preferred; more boys than girls are right-hemisphere preferred. The reasons are not as important as our response.

However, during the past decade, technology, such as video games and computers, has had significant impact on how and where children occupy their spare time. It is possible that this impact has already begun to narrow the current differences in the hemispheric preferences of the genders and will continue to do so in the coming years.

Regardless of the source of these preferences, **we should avoid using hemispheric preference to stereotype individuals**, to assume that one preference is better than another, or that persons cannot accomplish certain tasks because of their preference. The cause of hemispheric preference, for all practical purposes, is not relevant. It is our response that really matters. We can use this research to understand better how hemispheric preference affects learning and what teachers can do about it in their classrooms.

Schools and Hemispheric Preference

Recognizing that hemispheric preference is a contributor to learning style, the question arises as to whether school climate and classroom instruction are designed to embrace different styles so that all learners can succeed. Is it possible that schools may be designed inadvertently to favor one type of learning style over another?

Left-Hemisphere Schools?

Take a moment to think about the entire schooling process that takes place from kindergarten through grade 12. During this mental review, look again at the list of left- and right-hemisphere functions. Is K–12 schooling best described by the characteristics listed for the left hemisphere, the right hemisphere, or both equally? Most educators readily admit that schools are predominantly left-hemisphere oriented, especially in the elementary grades. Schools are structured environments that run according to time schedules, favor facts and rules over patterns, and offer predominantly verbal instruction, especially at the secondary level.

This means that left-hemisphere preferred learners (mainly girls) feel more comfortable in this environment. The stronger the left-hemisphere preference, the more successful these learners can be. Conversely, right-hemisphere preferred learners (mainly boys) are not comfortable; the stronger the right-hemisphere preference, the more hostile the learning environment seems. This could explain why most teachers admit that they have many more discipline problems with boys than with girls. Maybe what this research is saying is that boys (more accurately, right-hemisphere-preferred learners) are not born with a "mean gene," but are too often placed in uncomfortable learning environments where they react rebelliously. This might also partially explain why over twice as many boys as girls are in remedial and special education programs nationally. Curiously, there are over 11 percent more girls than boys enrolled in gifted and talented programs (USDOE, 2000).

Most K–12 public schooling inadvertently favors left-hemisphere-preferred learners.

The currently popular notion of differentiating instruction should recognize that young female and male brains do not mature at the same time. More boys, then, may succeed in schools that recognize different learning styles and individualize instruction accordingly. All students will achieve more when teachers purposefully plan strategies that teach to the whole brain by addressing the strengths and weaknesses of both genders. See the **Practitioner's Corner** at the end of this chapter on strategies for teaching to the whole brain, starting on page 194.

Impact on Mathematics and Science Programs

A major storm erupted in 2005 when the president of Harvard University suggested that males may have more intrinsic aptitude for science (and presumably higher mathematics) than females. Male and female brains deal differently with numbers and computation. However, scanning studies indicate that gender differences in computational processing are more pronounced in preadolescence and become much less important when the brain encounters higher mathematics (Dehaene, Spelke, Pinel, Stanescu, & Tsivkin, 1999). In other words, the genetic (nature) component is less significant than we once thought. It seems more likely that social and cultural forces have had greater influence. Boys in secondary schools are encouraged by their parents and teachers to take more mathematics and science, their experiences in such classes are more compatible with their hemispheric preferences, and they thus score better on tests in these areas. Girls, on the other hand, often encounter a stereotype that presumes females are poor performers in mathematics. One study showed that female performance on mathematics tests was lower than males just because of the existence of this stereotype, and that female performance improved once the stereotype threat was removed (Spencer, Steele, & Quinn, 1999).

The good news is that the gender gap is narrow. The percentage of girls taking various mathematics and science courses is close to or exceeds that of boys, and their test scores on a national average are only a few points lower and not statistically significant (NCES, 2003). This is an encouraging trend. In part, the explanation for this outcome may be the use of computers in the classroom. Both boys and girls are on a level playing field. Computer lessons are not closely linked with past successes or failures, representing a new set of skills that both boys and girls are learning at a very early age. Moreover, computers are patient and fun, contributing to novelty and the fulfillment of expectations of success.

Our job now is to ensure that educators and parents recognize that boys may have some different learning preferences from girls, but that both genders have similar *capabilities* to succeed in mathematics and science. To that end, we need to curb the cultural and social forces that would feed past stereotypes about whether students of a certain gender should take only certain subjects. There is plenty of evidence that when girls are encouraged and motivated, they can excel at science and mathematics. It is worth repeating here that scientific studies tell us about averages within groups and nothing about how any particular individual will succeed or fail in any subject area.

SPOKEN LANGUAGE SPECIALIZATION

Many animals have developed ways to communicate with other members of their species. Birds and apes bow and wave appendages; honeybees dance to map out the location of food; and even one-celled animals can signal neighbors by emitting an array of different chemicals. By contrast, human beings have developed an elaborate and complex means of spoken communication that many say is largely responsible for our place as the dominant species on this planet. Spoken language is truly

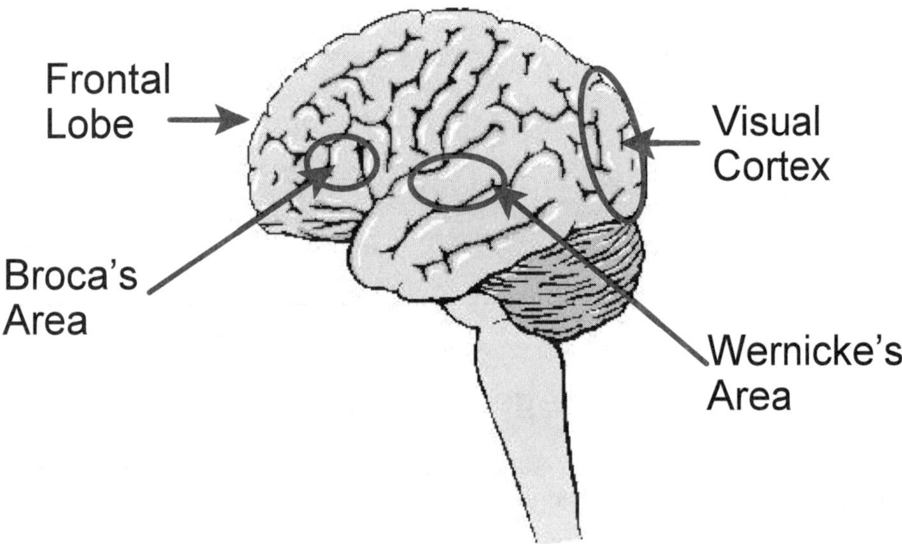

Figure 5.3 Broca's area and Wernicke's area, located in the left hemisphere, are the two major language processing centers of the brain. The visual cortex across the back of both hemispheres, processes visual stimuli, including reading.

a marvelous accomplishment for many reasons. At the very least, it gives form to our memories and words to express our thoughts. The human voice can pronounce all the vowel and consonant sounds that allow it to speak any of the estimated 6,500 languages that exist today. With practice, the voice becomes so fine-tuned that it makes only about one sound error per million sounds and one word error per million words (Pinker, 1994).

Long before the advent of scanning technologies, scientists explained how the brain produced spoken language on the basis of evidence from injured brains. In the 1860s, French surgeon Paul Broca noted that damage to the left frontal lobe induced language difficulties generally known as *aphasia,* wherein patients muttered sounds or lost speech completely. Broca's area (just behind the left temple) is about the size of a quarter. A person with damage to Broca's area (Figure 5.3) could understand language but could not speak fluently.

Later, in the 1870s, German neurologist Carl Wernicke described a different type of aphasia—one in which patients could not make sense out of words they spoke or heard. These patients had damage in the left temporal lobe. Wernicke's area (above the left ear) is about the size of a silver dollar. Those with damage to Wernicke's area could speak fluently, but what they said was quite meaningless. The inferences, then, were that Broca's area processed vocabulary, grammar, and probably syntax of one's native language, while Wernicke's area was the site of native language sense and meaning.

But more recent research, using scanners, indicates that spoken language production is a far more complex process than previously thought. When preparing to produce a spoken sentence, the brain uses not only Broca's and Wernicke's areas, but also calls on several other neural networks scattered

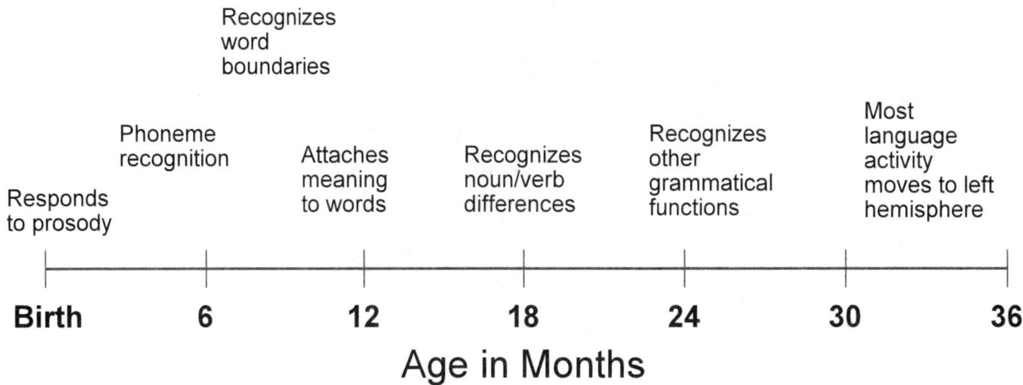

Figure 5.4 An average timeline of spoken language development during the child's first 3 years. There is considerable variation among individual children.

throughout the left hemisphere. Nouns are processed through one set of patterns; verbs are processed by separate neural networks. The more complex the sentence structure, the more areas that are activated, including the right hemisphere, although more so in females than in males.

Learning Spoken Language

Although early language learning begins in the home, schools are largely responsible for enhancing the spoken language of children and teaching them to read. How quickly and successfully the brain learns to read is greatly influenced by the spoken language competence the child has developed. Therefore, it is important to understand what cognitive neuroscience has revealed about how the brain acquires and processes spoken words. Figure 5.4 presents a general timeline for spoken language development during the first three years of growth. The chart is a rough approximation. Obviously, some children will progress faster or slower than the chart indicates. Nonetheless, it is a useful guide for parents and teachers to show the progression of skills acquired during the process of learning language (Sousa, 2005).

Learning Sounds Called Phonemes

The neurons in a baby's brain are capable of responding to the sounds of all the languages on this planet. At birth (some say even before birth) babies respond first to the *prosody*—the rhythm, cadence, and pitch—of their mothers' voice, not the words. Spoken language consists of minimal units of sound, called *phonemes*, which combine to form syllables. For example, in English, the consonant sound "t" and the vowel sound "o" are both phonemes that combine to form the syllable *to-* as in *tomato*. Different languages have different numbers of phonemes. It can be as few as 15 in some languages to well over 40 in English. The total number of phonemes in all the world's languages is around 90, which represents the maximum number of sounds that the human voice apparatus can create (Beatty, 2001).

> ***The neurons in a baby's brain are capable of responding to the sounds of all the languages on this planet.***

Although the infant's brain can perceive the entire range of phonemes, only those that are repeated get attention, as the neurons reacting to the unique sound patterns are continually stimulated and reinforced. By the age of 10 to 12 months, the toddler's brain has begun to distinguish and remember phonemes of the native language and to ignore foreign sounds. For example, one study showed that at the age of 6 months, American and Japanese babies are equally good at discriminating between the "l" and "r" sounds, even though Japanese has no "l" sound. However, by age 10 months, Japanese babies have a tougher time making the distinction, while American babies have become much better at it. During this and subsequent periods of growth, the ability to distinguish native sounds improves, while one's ability to distinguish nonnative speech sounds diminishes (Cheour et al., 1998).

From Phonemes to Words

The next step for the brain is to detect words from the stream of sounds it is processing. This is not an easy task because people don't pause between words when speaking. Yet the brain has to recognize differences between, say, *green house* and *greenhouse*. Remarkably, babies begin to distinguish word boundaries by the age of 8 months even though they don't know what the words mean (Van Petten & Bloom, 1999). Before they reach the age of 12 months, many babies can learn words in one context and understand them in another (Schafer, 2005). They begin to acquire new vocabulary words at the rate of about 8 to 10 a day. At the same time, memory and Wernicke's areas are becoming fully functional so the child can now attach meaning to words. Of course, learning words is one skill; putting them together to make sense is another, more complex skill.

Learning Grammar

In the 1950s, MIT linguist Noam Chomsky argued that all languages contain some common rules that dictate how sentences are constructed, and that the brain has preprogrammed circuits that respond to these rules. Modern linguists think that the brain may not be responding so much to basic language rules as to statistical regularities heard in the flow of the native tongue. They soon discern that some words describe objects while others describe actions. Toddlers detect patterns of word order—person, action, object—so they can soon say, "I want cookie." Other grammar features emerge, such as tense, and by the age of 3, over 90 percent of sentences uttered are grammatically correct. Errors are seldom random, but usually result from following perceived rules of grammar.

If "I batted the ball" makes sense, why shouldn't "I holded the bat" also make sense? Regrettably, the toddler has yet to learn that nearly 200 of the most commonly used verbs in English are irregularly conjugated (Pinker, 1994).

During the following years, practice in speaking and adult correction help the child decode some of the mysteries of grammar's irregularities and a sophisticated language system emerges from what once was babble. No one knows how much grammar a child learns just by listening, or how much is pre-wired. What is certain is that the more children are exposed to spoken language in the early years, the more quickly they can discriminate between phonemes and recognize word boundaries.

Although toddlers may be attracted to the rapidly changing sounds and images on a television, there is little or no language development in progress. Television may actually impair a toddler's brain development.

Just letting the toddler sit in front of a television does not seem to accomplish this goal, probably because the child's brain needs live human interaction to attach meaning to the words. Moreover, television talk is not the slow, expressive speech that parents use with their infants, which infants like and want to hear. Although toddlers may be attracted to the rapidly changing sounds and images on a television, little or no language development is in progress. There is further evidence that prolonged television watching can impair the growth of young brains. A recent longitudinal study indicated that the more television toddlers had watched before the age of 3 years, the lower their scores on later tests of reading achievement and number manipulation (Zimmerman & Christakis, 2005).

Language Delay

Most toddlers begin to speak words around the age of 10 to 12 months. In some children, there is a delay and they may not speak coherent words and phrases until nearly 2 years of age. There is evidence that this language delay to 2 years is inherited, and thus represents a distinct disorder not easily remedied by environmental interventions. This revelation diminishes the claim some people make that mainly environmental influences cause language delay (Dale et al., 1998).

Implications

Given the evidence that the brain's ability to acquire spoken language is at its peak in the early years, parents should create a rich environment that includes lots of communication activities, such as talking, singing, and reading. In schools, it means addressing any language-learning problems quickly to take advantage of the brain's ability to rewire improper connections during this important period of growth. It also means that parents and teachers should not assume that children with language-learning problems are going to be limited in cognitive thought processes as well.

Learning a Second Language

The power of a young child's brain to learn spoken languages is so immense that it can learn several languages at one time. But by the age of 10 to 12 months, the brain is already beginning to lose its ability to discriminate sounds between its native language and nonnative languages. The implication here is that if we wish children to acquire a second language, it makes sense to start that acquisition during the early years when the brain is actively creating phonemic sound and syntactic networks.

> ***Proficiency in learning a second language depends not on how long nonnatives have been speaking the language, but on how early in life they began learning it.***

Studies show that proficiency in learning a second language depends not on *how long* nonnatives have been speaking the language, but on *how early in life* they began learning it. Researchers Jacqueline Johnson and Elissa Newport found that immigrants who started speaking English at ages 3 to 7 spoke like natives and with no discernible accent. Those who started speaking between ages of 8 and 10 had about 80 percent of the proficiency of native speakers; those who started between ages 11 and 15 spoke with only half the proficiency, and those who started after age 17 had only about 15 percent of the proficiency of the average person born in America (Johnson & Newport, 1991). This indicates that the window of opportunity (see Chapter 1) for language acquisition slides down in the preteen years so that learning a second language later is certainly possible, but more difficult.

Why Is It More Difficult to Learn a Second Language Later?

For most people, the brain areas primarily involved in language acquisition are not very responsive to foreign sounds after the preteen years. Thus, additional areas of the brain must be programmed to recognize, distinguish, and respond to foreign phonemes. Furthermore, scanning studies using fMRIs show that second languages acquired in adulthood show some spatial separation in the brain from native languages. However, when acquired in the preteen years, native and second languages are represented in the same frontal areas (Broca's area). Hence, younger and older brains react to second language learning very differently (Kim, Relkin, Lee, & Hirsch, 1997; Perani & Abutalebi, 2005; Silverberg & Samuel, 2004).

> ***Although young brains are naturally adept at language learning, this research should not be interpreted to discourage adolescents and adults from pursuing second language study.***

Although it seems that younger brains are more adept at language learning, this research should not be interpreted to discourage adolescents and adults from pursuing second language study. Nor should it be assumed that youngsters will become fluent solely by studying a second language a few hours a week in the primary grades. Like learning any skill, continuous practice is needed for fluency. Further, the difficulties facing adults learning a second language are very different from those of children. For example, the phonemes, grammar, and syntax rules of the native language are likely to interfere somewhat (an example of negative transfer) with learning those of the second language (Iverson et al., 2003). If these difficulties are properly addressed, then learning a second language as an adult can be a rewarding experience, although it may require more focus, more effort, and greater motivation. See the **Practitioner's Corner** on p. 204 at the end of this chapter on acquiring a second language.

LEARNING TO READ

Let's take a little time now to discuss the one area where neuroscience has made its most important contribution to teaching and learning to date—understanding how the brain learns to read. The more scientists learn about the neural systems required for successful reading, the more they realize how complicated the process is and how much can go wrong. My purpose here is to present a quick description of how we believe the brain learns to read and to mention a few common reading problems. For a much more extensive discussion on reading and teaching strategies, see Sousa (2005) and Shaywitz (2003).

Is Reading a Natural Ability?

Not really. The brain's ability to acquire spoken language with amazing speed and accuracy is the result of genetic hardwiring and specialized cerebral areas that focus on this task. But there are no areas of the brain that specialize in reading. In fact, reading is probably the most difficult task we ask the young brain to undertake. Reading is a relatively new phenomenon in the development of humans. As far as we know, the genes have not incorporated reading into their coded structure, probably because reading—unlike spoken language—has not emerged over time as a survival skill.

Many cultures (but not all) do emphasize reading as an important form of communication and insist it be taught to their children. And so the struggle begins. To get that brain to read, here's what we are saying, for example, to the English-speaking child: "That language you have been speaking quite correctly for the past few years can be represented by abstract symbols we invented called letters of the alphabet. We are going to disrupt that sophisticated spoken language network you have already developed and ask you to reorganize it to accommodate these letters, which, by the way, are not very reliable. You see, although it takes more than about 44 different sounds to speak English, we have only 26 letters to represent them. That means some sounds have more than one letter and some letters stand for more than one sound. Seem like fun? Plus, there are lots of exceptions, but you'll just have to adjust." Female brains are already relishing the adventure while male brains are wondering how they ever got into this mess.

> ***There are no areas of the brain that specialize in reading. Reading is probably the most difficult task we ask the young brain to undertake.***

Once exposed to formal instruction, about 50 percent of children make the transition from spoken language to reading with relative ease. For the other 50 percent, reading is a much more formidable task, and for about 20 to 30 percent, it definitely becomes the most difficult cognitive task they will ever undertake in their lives.

Learning to read successfully requires three neural systems and the development of specific skills that will work together to help the brain decode abstract symbols into meaningful language. We will first look at the neural systems involved because that will help clarify what skills an individual needs to develop to learn to read.

Neural Systems Involved in Reading

Researchers using fMRIs are getting a clearer picture of the cerebral processes involved in reading. For successful reading to occur, three neural systems are required to work together. Figure 5.5 illustrates those systems. Visual processing begins when the eyes scan the letters of the printed word (in this example, *d-o-g*), and the visual signals travel to the visual cortex located in the occipital lobes at the rear of the brain (see also Figure 5.2). The word's signals are decoded in an area on the left side of the brain called the *angular gyrus*, which separates it into its basic sounds, or phonemes. This process activates the language areas of the brain located in the left hemisphere near and in the temporal lobe, where auditory processing also occurs. The auditory processing system sounds out the phonemes in the head, *duh-awh-guh*. Broca's and Wernicke's areas supply information about the word from their mental dictionaries, and the frontal lobe integrates all the information to provide meaning—a furry animal that barks.

The three systems can prompt each other for more information (represented by the double arrows). For instance, if auditory processing is having difficulty sounding out the word, it might prompt the visual system to rescan the print to ensure that it read the letters correctly. Similarly, the frontal lobe may prompt another visual scan or auditory rehearsal if it is having difficulty attaching meaning to the information. All this occurs in a fraction of a second. The actual process is a little more complicated than described here, but this is essentially what neuroscientists believe happens.

Although the process outlined in Figure 5.5 appears linear and singular, it is really bidirectional and parallel, with many phonemes being processed at the same time. That the brain learns to read at all attests to its remarkable ability to sift through seemingly confusing input and establish patterns and systems. For a few children, this process comes naturally, but most have to be taught.

Skills Involved in Reading

In order for this complex integration of neural systems to result in successful reading, an individual must develop specific skills and possess certain information. Specifically,

- **Phonological and phonemic awareness.** *Phonological awareness* is the recognition that oral language can be divided into smaller components, such as sentences into words, words into syllables and, ultimately, into individual sounds. This recognition includes identifying

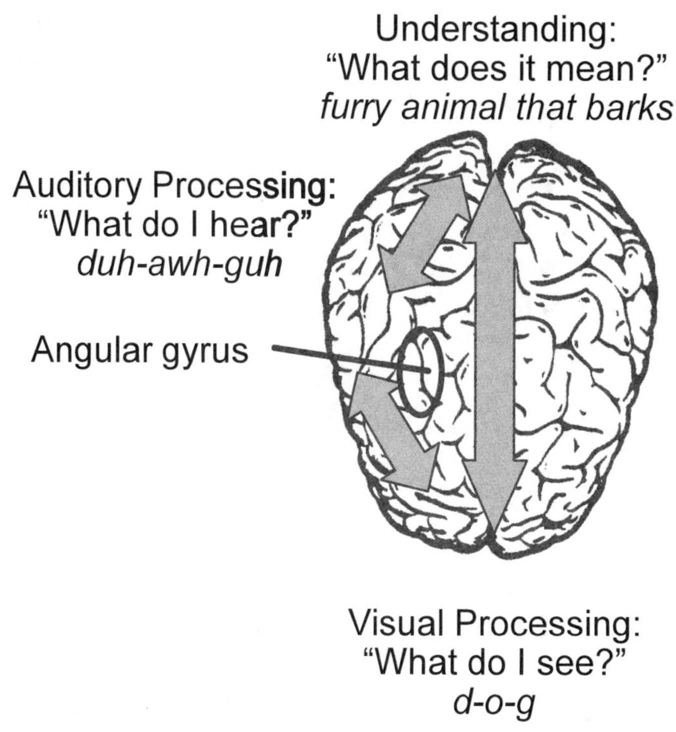

Figure 5.5 Three neural systems are involved in reading. The visual processing system scans the printed word, the auditory processing system sounds it out in the head, and the frontal lobe integrates the information to produce meaning. The angular gyrus helps decode the visual word recognition signals for further processing in the left hemisphere's language centers (Broca's and Wernicke's areas).

and manipulating onsets and rimes as well as having an awareness of alliteration, rhyming, syllabication, and intonation. Being phonologically aware means hearing the difference between *bat* and *pat* and between *bat* and *bet.* Before tackling the printed word, children need to be able to recognize that words are made up of individual sounds (phonemes) and that these sounds can be manipulated to create new words. This skill is called *phonemic awareness* (a subdivision of phonological awareness) and includes the ability to isolate a phoneme (first, middle, or last) from the rest of the word, to segment words into their component phonemes, and to delete a specific phoneme from a word.

- **Alphabetic principle and phonics.** The *alphabetic principle* describes the understanding that spoken words are made up of phonemes and that the phonemes are represented in written text as letters. This system of using letters to represent phonemes is very efficient in that a small number of letters can be used to write a very large number of words. Matching just a few letters on a page to their sounds in speech enables the reader to recognize many printed words. *Phonics* is an instructional approach that builds on the alphabetic principle and associates letters and sounds with *written* symbols. To demonstrate phonics knowledge, a child tells the teacher which letter is needed to change *cat* to *can.* Simply learning letter-sound relationships during phonics instruction does not necessarily lead to phonemic awareness.

- **Vocabulary.** Readers must usually posses a word in their mental dictionary in order to recognize it in print. Children learn the meanings of most words indirectly, through everyday experiences with oral and written language. These experiences include conversations with other people, listening to adults read to them, and reading on their own. They learn vocabulary words directly when they are explicitly taught individual words and word-learning strategies. Some vocabulary should be taught directly. Direct instruction is particularly effective for teaching difficult words representing complex concepts that are not part of the children's everyday experiences.
- **Fluency.** Fluency is the ability to read a text orally with speed, accuracy, and proper expression. Children who lack fluency read slowly and laboriously, often making it difficult for them to remember what has been read (recall the limited capacity of working memory) and to relate the ideas expressed in the text to their own experiences. Frequent practice in reading is one of the main contributors to developing fluency. Fluency bridges the gap between word recognition and comprehension. Because fluent readers do not need to spend much time decoding words, they can focus their attention on the meaning of the text. With practice, word recognition and comprehension occur almost simultaneously.
- **Text comprehension.** Comprehension is a complex interactive process that begins with identifying words by using knowledge outside the text, accessing word meaning in context, recognizing grammatical structures, drawing inferences, and monitoring oneself to ensure that the text is making sense. When confronted with several meanings for a word in a sentence, the brain needs to select the one that makes sense in context. Many English words have dozens of meanings, depending on their context. Thus, developing the ability to quickly block irrelevant meanings becomes a necessity for reading fluency and comprehension.

Some of these skills may begin to develop at home during the preschool years as parents read to their children and expose them to print materials. This allows them to hear word sounds, to practice pronunciation and speak more fluently, and to learn new words and their meanings. Thus, the degree to which children experience literacy at home will determine largely whether they begin school not just *able* to learn to read, but *ready* to learn to read. Children from low-income families are not often exposed to print materials and reading at home. Yet, studies show that when parents and school districts make the extra effort to provide these experiences, the acquisition of language and phonological skills for low-income preschool children is greatly enhanced (Poe, Burchinal, & Roberts, 2004).

The degree to which children experience literacy at home determines whether they begin school not just able to learn to read, but ready to learn to read.

Problems in Learning to Read

Reading is so complex that any little problem along the way can slow or interrupt the process. It is small wonder that children have more problems with reading than any other skill we ask them to learn. In recent years, researchers have made significant progress using fMRI scans to understand how the brain reads. Yet, despite these advancements, fMRI scans are not a practical tool at present for diagnosing reading problems in a single individual. That is because the results of fMRI studies are usually reported for groups rather than for individuals. Researchers have found some variations in the activated areas of the brain among individuals within both poor readers and control groups. More research is needed to clarify these differences before fMRI or any other imaging techniques can be used confidently for diagnostic purposes. Until that time, however, researchers can use the information gained from imaging studies to develop other kinds of diagnostic tests that more closely align with our new understanding of reading and reading problems.

For the moment, critical observation of a child's progress in learning to speak, and eventually in learning to read, remains our most effective tool for spotting potential problems. Most difficulties associated with reading do not go away with time. Therefore, the earlier that parents and teachers can detect reading problems in children, the better.

Most research studies on reading have focused primarily on developmental reading problems that scientists refer to as *developmental dyslexia.* In developmental dyslexia, the child experiences unexpected difficulty in learning to read despite adequate intelligence, environment, and normal senses. It is a spectrum disorder, varying from mild to severe. Neuroimaging studies have established that there are significant differences in the way normal and dyslexic brains respond to specific spoken and written language tasks. Furthermore, there is now strong evidence that these differences may weaken with appropriate instructional interventions (Shaywitz, 2003).

Scientists have long been searching for the causes of reading problems. This has not been an easy task because of the large number of sensory, motor, and cognitive systems that are involved in reading. Struggling readers may have impairments in any one or more of these systems, but not all struggling readers have dyslexia. Specifically, dyslexia seems to be caused by deficits in the neural regions responsible for language and phonological processing or by problems in nonlinguistic areas of the brain.

The following is a brief description of some of the causes of difficulties when learning to read. Most reading problems can be divided into linguistic and nonlinguistic causes. Parents and teachers should consult other resources, such as NAEYC (1998), Shaywitz (2003), and Sousa (2005), for an in-depth discussion of these problems and how to deal with them,.

Linguistic Causes

- **Phonological deficits.** The readers have difficulty sounding out the sounds of the phonemes in their heads.
- **Differences in auditory and visual processing speeds.** When learning to read, the visual and auditory processing systems work at similar speeds to decode letters into sounds. Research studies of poor readers have revealed that some of them have a slower than normal auditory processing speed. Consequently, the visual system may already be processing the third letter of a word while the auditory system is still processing the first letter's sound. As a result, the brain incorrectly associates the sound of the first letter with the symbol of the third letter. For example, in reading the word *dog,* the visual system may already be processing the *g,* but the slower auditory system is still processing the *duh* sound associated

with the letter *d*. This reader's brain, then, mistakenly associates the letter *g* with the sound *duh*.

- **Structural differences in the brain.** MRI studies have found that the brain of people diagnosed with dyslexia are structurally different from non-dyslexic brains. These differences could contribute to the deficits associated with dyslexia.
- **Phonological memory deficits.** Some poor readers have difficulty retaining phonemes in working memory and are thus unable to remember a sequence of words long enough to generate a sentence.
- **Genetics and gender.** There is a strong association between dyslexia and genetic mutations in twins and families. Dyslexia is a chronic problem and not just a "phase." The stereotype that nearly all dyslexics are boys is not true, although it probably persists because boys are more likely to show their frustration with reading by acting out. In fact, Shaywitz (2003) found that boys tend to be over-identified as having reading problems, while girls are often under-identified.
- **Brain lesions in the word processing areas.** PET scans have shown that some people with developmental dyslexia have lesions in the areas on the left side of the brain responsible for processing and decoding written words.
- **Word-blindness.** Word-blindness is the inability to read words even though the person's eyes are optically normal. It results from either a congenital defect or trauma to the word processing areas of the brain.

Nonlinguistic Causes

- **Perception of sequential sounds.** Some poor readers are unable to detect and discriminate sounds presented in rapid succession. This deficit is related to auditory processing in general, not just to distinguishing phonemes.
- **Sound-frequency discrimination.** Some individuals with reading disorders are impaired in their ability to hear differences in sound frequency. This auditory defect can affect the ability to discriminate tone and pitch in speech.
- **Detection of target sounds in noise.** The inability to detect tones within noise is another recently discovered nonlinguistic impairment. When added to the findings in the two deficits mentioned just above, this evidence suggests that auditory functions may play a much greater role in reading disorders than previously thought.
- **Motor coordination and the cerebellum.** Several imaging studies show that many dyslexic readers have processing deficits in the cerebellum of the brain. The cerebellum is located at the rear of the brain just below the occipital lobe. It is mainly responsible for coordinating learned motor skills. Deficiencies in this part of the brain could result, according to researchers, in problems with reading, writing, and spelling.
- **Attention-deficit hyperactivity disorder (ADHD).** Attention-deficit hyperactivity disorder (ADHD) is a developmental disorder characterized by difficulty in focusing and sustaining attention. Children with ADHD are often assumed to also have developmental reading problems. But that is not usually the case. ADHD and developmental dyslexia are separate disorders, and less than 25 percent of ADHD children also have dyslexia.

Several computer programs, including *Fast ForWord* (Scientific Learning Corp.) and *Earobics Literacy Launch* (Cognitive Concepts, Inc.), have had considerable success in helping struggling readers overcome some of these difficulties. See the **Resources** section for more information.

Implications for Teaching Reading

Teaching children to read is no easy task, especially in primary classrooms where teachers welcome children from an ever-increasing variety of home situations, culture, and native languages. Given these variables, successful teachers of reading are flexible rather than rigid in their approach, and they know through experience what they need to do to make learning to read exciting and meaningful. They also acknowledge that the findings of scientific studies are clear: effective reading programs must contain components that support phonemic awareness, the alphabetic principle, vocabulary building, comprehension, and fluency. Developmentally appropriate literature complements this process to provide relevant and enjoyable reading experiences. See the **Practitioner's Corner** on p. 207 for suggestions on teaching reading.

What's Coming Up?

In too many schools, budget constraints and anxiety over high-stakes testing are reducing the amount of time that students are exposed to the arts and physical education. Yet, scientific evidence continues to accumulate about the positive impact that music, visual arts, and movement have on brain growth and development. The next chapter discusses some of that evidence and argues why we must preserve the arts and physical education if schools are to be truly brain-compatible.

PRACTITIONER'S CORNER

Testing Your Hemispheric Preference

There are many instruments available to help individuals assess their hemispheric preference. The one below takes just a few minutes. The results are only an indication of your preference and are not conclusive. You should use additional instruments to collect more data before reaching any firm conclusion about your hemispheric preference.

Directions: From each pair below, circle A or B corresponding to the sentence that **best describes you.** Answer all questions. There are no right or wrong answers.

1. A. I prefer to find my own way of doing a new task.
B. I prefer to be told the best way to do a new task.

2. A. I have to make my own plans.
B. I can follow anyone's plans.

3. A. I am a very flexible and occasionally unpredictable person.
B. I am a very stable and consistent person.

4. A. I keep everything in a particular place.
B. Where I keep things depends on what I am doing.

5. A. I spread my work evenly over the time I have.
B. I prefer to do my work at the last minute.

6. A. I know I am right because I have good reasons.
B. I know when I am right, even without reasons.

7. A. I need a lot of variety and change in my life.
B. I need a well-planned and orderly life.

8. A. I sometimes have too many ideas in a new situation.
B. I sometimes don't have any ideas in a new situation.

9. A. I do easy things first and the important things last.
B. I do the important things first and the easy things last.

10. A. I choose what I **know** is right when making a hard decision.
B. I choose what I **feel** is right when making a hard decision.

11. A. I plan my time for doing my work.
B. I don't think about the time when I work.

12. A. I usually have good self-discipline.
B. I usually act on my feelings.

13. A. Other people don't understand how I organize things.
B. Other people think I organize things well.

14. A. I agree with new ideas before other people do.
B. I question new ideas more than other people do.

15. A. I tend to think more in **pictures.**
B. I tend to think more in **words.**

16. A. I try to find the one best way to solve a problem.
B. I try to find different ways to solve a problem.

17. A. I can usually **analyze** what is going to happen next.
B. I can usually **sense** what is going to happen next.

18. A. I am not very imaginative in my work.
B. I use my imagination in nearly everything I do.

19. A. I begin many jobs that I never finish.
B. I finish a job before starting a new one.

20. A. I look for new ways to do old jobs.
B. When one way works well, I don't change it.

21. A. It is fun to take risks.
B. I have fun without taking risks.

Scoring:

Count the number of "A" responses to questions 1, 3, 7, 8, 9, 13, 14, 15, 19, 20, and 21. Place that number on the line to the right. A.__________

Count the number of "B" responses to the remaining questions. Place that number on the line to the right. B.__________

Total the "A" and "B" responses you counted. Total________

The total indicates your hemispheric preference according to the following scale:

0–5	Strong left hemisphere preference
6–8	Moderate left hemisphere preference
9–12	Bilateral hemisphere balance (little or no preference)
13–15	Moderate right hemisphere preference
16–21	Strong right hemisphere preference

Reflection:

A. Did your score surprise you? Why or why not?

B. Describe here what your score may tell you about your teaching.

C. What implications do your answers in B above have for your students?

PRACTITIONER'S CORNER

Teaching to the Whole Brain: General Guidelines

Although the two hemispheres process information differently, we learn best when both are engaged in learning. Just as we would catch more balls with both hands, we catch more information with both hemispheres processing and integrating the learning. Teachers should design lessons that include activities directed at both hemispheres so that students can integrate the new learning into a meaningful whole. In doing so, students get opportunities to develop both their strong and weak learning style preferences. Here are some ways to do that in daily planning:

- **Deal With Concepts Verbally *and* Visually.** When teaching new concepts, alternate discussion with visual models. Write key words on the board that represent the critical attributes of the concept, then use a simple diagram to show relationships among the key ideas within and between concepts. This helps students attach both auditory and visual cues to the information, increasing the likelihood that sense and meaning will emerge, and that they will be able to accurately retrieve the information later. When using a video presentation, show the *smallest* segment with *maximum* meaning, then stop the tape and have students discuss what was shown.

- **Design Effective Visual Aids.** How we position information on a visual aid (e.g., overhead transparency, board, easel pad, video screen) indicates the relationships of concepts and ideas, which are processed by the right hemisphere. Vertical positioning implies a step or time sequence, or hierarchy. Thus, writing

  Delaware

  Pennsylvania

  New Jersey

  is appropriate to indicate the order of these states' admission into the Union (chronology). Writing them horizontally

  Delaware, Pennsylvania, New Jersey

  implies a parallel relationship that is appropriate to identify any three populous eastern states. Avoid writing information in visual aids in a haphazard way whenever a parallel or hierarchical relationship among the elements is important for students to remember.

- **Discuss Concepts Logically and Intuitively.** Concepts should be presented to students from different perspectives that encourage the use of both hemispheres. For example, if you are teaching about the Civil War, talk about the factual (logical) events, such as major causes, battles, and the economic and political impacts. When the students understand these, move on to more thought-provoking (intuitive) activities, such as asking what might have happened if Lincoln had not been assassinated, or what our country might be like now if the Confederate states had won the war.

  After teaching basic concepts in arithmetic, ask students to design a number system to a base other than 10. This is a simple and interesting process that helps students understand the scheme of our decimal number system. In literature, after reading part of a story or play, ask students to write a plausible ending using the facts already presented. In science, after giving some facts about the structure of the periodic table of the elements, ask students to explain how they would experiment with a new element to determine its place in the table.

- **Avoid Conflicting Messages.** Make sure that your words, tone, and pacing match your gestures, facial expressions, and body language. The left hemisphere interprets words literally, but the right hemisphere evaluates body language, tone, and content. If the two hemispheric interpretations are inconsistent, a conflicting message is generated. As a result, the student withdraws internally to resolve the conflict and is no longer focused on the learning.

- **Design Activities and Assessments for Both Hemispheres.** Students of different hemispheric preference express themselves in different ways. Give students options in testing and in completing assignments so they can select the option best suited to their learning styles. For example, after completing a major unit on the U.S. Civil War, students could write term papers on particular aspects of the war, draw pictures, create and present plays or write songs of important events, or construct models that represent battles, the surrender at Appomattox, and so on. Simulations, role-playing, designing computer programs, and building models are all effective assessment tools in addition to the tradition paper-and-pencil tests.

PRACTITIONER'S CORNER

Strategies for Teaching to the Whole Brain

Students learn best when teachers use strategies that engage the whole brain. Although current research shows that both hemispheres work together in many processing activities, it is still useful to know teaching strategies that involve the skills inherent in—but not necessarily limited to—each hemisphere. *Remember that we cannot educate just one hemisphere.* Rather, we are ensuring that our daily instruction includes activities that stimulate the whole brain. Here are some teaching strategies to consider (Key, 1991).

Teaching Strategies That Activate Left-Hemisphere Functions

- **Efficient Classroom Organization.** Have an efficient work area. Distribute the talkers around the room; they will spark discussions when needed.

- **Relevant Bulletin Boards.** Organize bulletin boards to be relevant to the current content and easily understood.

- **Clean the Board.** Make clean erasures on the board. This reduces the chance that previous and unrelated word cues will become associated with the new topic under discussion.

- **Use a Multisensory Approach.** Let students read, write, draw, and compute often in all subject areas.

- **Use Metaphors.** Create and analyze metaphors to enhance meaning and encourage higher-order thinking.

- **Encourage Punctuality.** Stress the importance of being on time. Encourage students to carry agendas.

- **Encourage Goal Setting.** Teach students to set study goals for themselves, stick to their goals, and reward themselves when they achieve them.

- **Stimulate Logical Thinking.** Ask "what if?" questions to encourage logical thinking as students consider all possibilities for solving problems.

Teaching Strategies That Activate Right-Hemisphere Functions

- **Give Students Some Options.** For example, allow them to do oral or written reports. Oral reports help students piece concepts together while requiring fewer mechanics than written work. Some students may prefer to present a short play or skit.

- **Use Visual Representations.** Use the board and overhead projector to show illustrations, cartoons, charts, timelines, and graphs that encourage students to visually organize information and relationships. Have students create or collect their own visual representations of the new concepts.

- **Help Students Make Connections.** Tying lessons together and using proper closure (Chapter 3) allow the brain to compare new information to what has already been learned.

- **Encourage Direct Experiences.** Facilitate direct experiences with new learning through solving authentic problems and involvement in real-world situations.

- **Allow for Student-to-Student Interaction.** Students need time to interact with each other as they discuss the new learnings. Remember, whoever explains, learns.

- **Teach for Transfer.** Teach students to use generalities and perceptions. Have them use metaphors and similes to make connections between unlike items. This is an important function for future transfer of learning.

- **Incorporate Hands-On Learning.** Provide frequent opportunities for experiential and hands-on learning. Students need to realize that they must discover and order relationships in the real world.

Use the chart below to decide what types of classroom strategies would work best with students whose hemisphere and sensory preferences are as indicated. Use the **bridging** and **hugging** strategies you learned in Chapter 4 to help you with this.

Modality	Left-Hemisphere Preference	Right-Hemisphere Preference
Visually Preferred 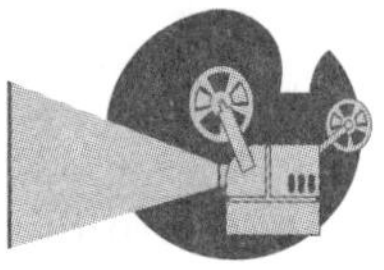		
Kinesthetically Preferred 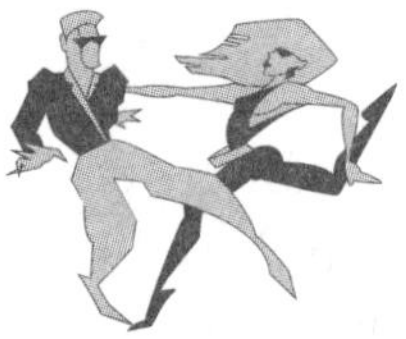		
Auditorily Preferred 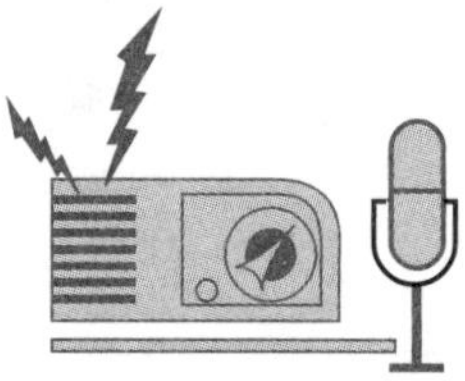		

Reflection:

A. What are your hemispheric and sensory preferences?

Hemispheric Preference:________________________________

Sensory Preference(s):________________________________

B. How did your preferences in A influence the strategies you designed in the chart for this activity? Jot down the results of your analysis here. Were there any surprises?

PRACTITIONER'S CORNER

Concept Mapping—General Guidelines

Concept mapping consists of extracting ideas and terms from curriculum content and plotting them visually to show and name the relationships among them. The learner establishes a visual representation of relations between concepts that might have been presented only verbally. Integrating visual and verbal activities enhances understanding of concepts whether they be abstract, concrete, verbal, or nonverbal. The key to concept mapping is the clear indication of the relationship that one item has to another. West et al. (1991) summarize nine types of cognitive relationships:

Name	Relationship	Example
1. Classification	A is an example of B	A cat is a mammal.
2. Defining/subsuming	A is a property of B	All mammals have hair.
3. Equivalence	A is identical to B	$2(a + b) = 2(b + a)$
4. Similarity	A is similar to B	A donkey is like a mule.
5. Difference	A is unlike B	A spider is not an insect.
6. Quantity	A is greater/less than B	A right angle is greater than an acute angle.
7. Time sequence	A occurs before/after B	In mitosis, prophase occurs before metaphase.
8. Causal	A causes B	Combustion produces heat.
9. Enabling	A enables/allows B	A person must be at least 18 years old to vote.

Concept mapping uses graphic diagrams to organize and represent the relationships between and among the components. These diagrams are also called *graphic* and *visual organizers*. Studies show that graphic organizers are particularly effective with students who have learning disabilities (Kim, Vaughn, Wanzek, & Wei, 2004) and with students who are English language learners (Chularut & DeBacker, 2004). Students should discuss these different types of relationships and give their own examples before attempting to select a concept map. There are dozens of possible organizers (Bromley, Irwin-DeVitis, & Modlo, 1995; Hyerle, 1996, 2004). Below are three common types. In each, the relationship between items is written as a legend (for a few examples) or next to the line connecting the items (when there are many examples).

- **Spider maps** best illustrate classification, similarity, and difference relationships.
- **Hierarchy maps** illustrate defining and/or subsuming, equivalence, and quantity relationships.
- **Chain maps** illustrate time sequence, causal, and enabling relationships.

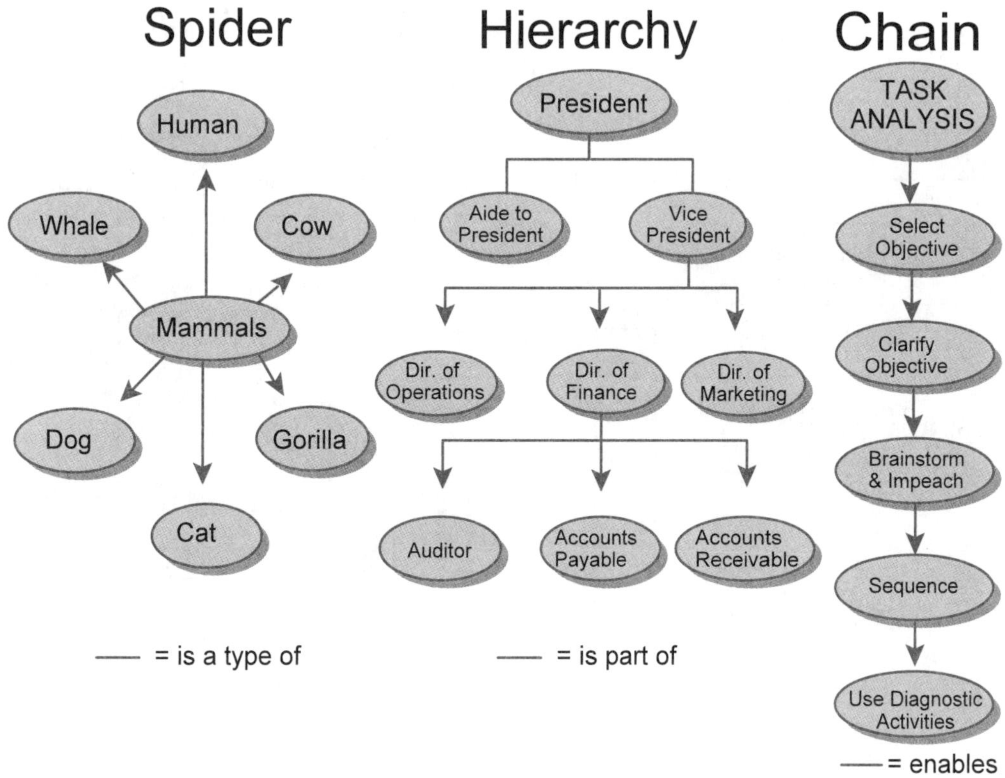

More types of concept maps:

- **Story maps** are useful for classifying main ideas with supporting events and information from the story. These are particularly helpful for readers who have difficulty finding the main idea in a piece of writing.
- **Analogy maps** illustrate similarities and differences between new and familiar concepts. This map can help teachers determine whether two concepts are too similar to each other and should, therefore, be taught at different times (see Chapter 4).
- **K-W-L maps** illustrate the degree of new learning that will be needed. The "K" is for what we already *know*; "W" is for what we *want* to know; and "L" is for what we *learned*. This map is a useful device for lesson closure (see Chapter 2).

More types of concept maps:

- **Venn diagrams** map the similarities and differences between two concepts. Like analogy maps, these help teachers determine if two concepts are too similar to each other to be taught in the same lesson.
- **Plot diagrams** are used to find the major parts of a novel.
- **A brace map** shows subsets of larger items.

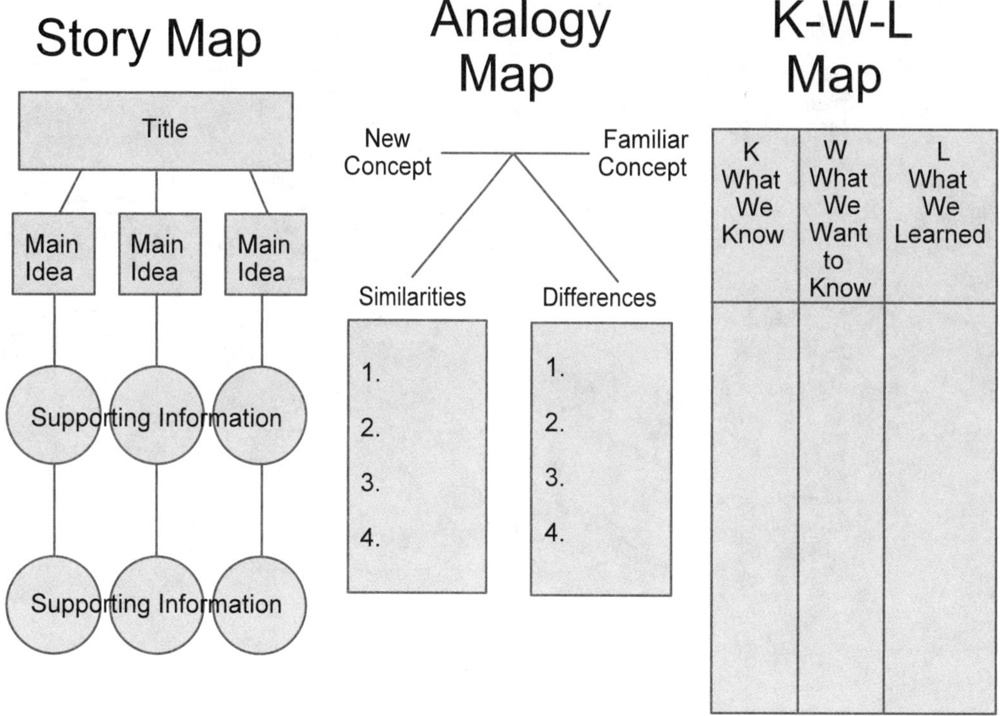
Story Map
Title
Main Idea
Main Idea
Main Idea
Supporting Information
Supporting Information
Analogy Map
New Concept
Familiar Concept
Similarities
Differences
1.
2.
3.
4.
1.
2.
3.
4.
K-W-L Map
K What We Know
W What We Want to Know
L What We Learned

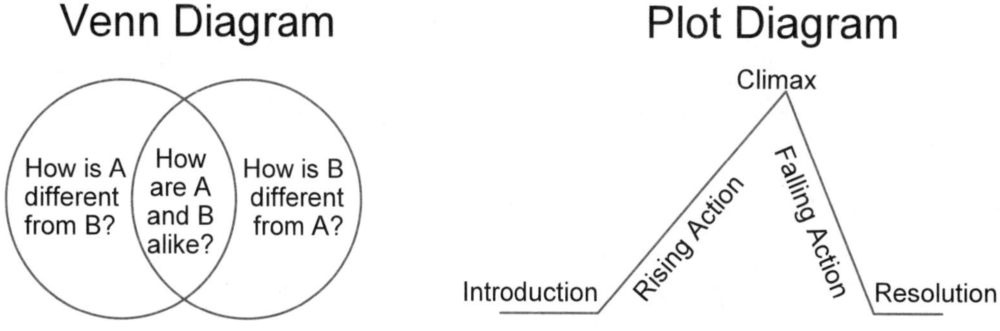
Venn Diagram
How is A different from B?
How are A and B alike?
How is B different from A?
Plot Diagram
Climax
Introduction
Rising Action
Falling Action
Resolution

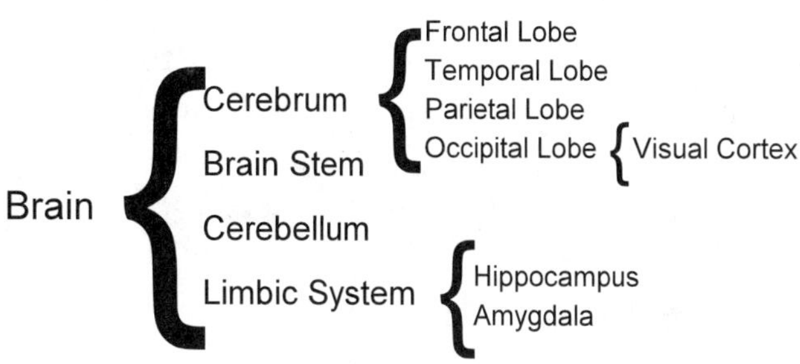
A Brace Map
Brain
Cerebrum
Brain Stem
Cerebellum
Limbic System
Frontal Lobe
Temporal Lobe
Parietal Lobe
Occipital Lobe
Visual Cortex
Hippocampus
Amygdala

Directions: Time for practice. Select a broad curriculum concept, such as energy, time, or forms of government. Draw an appropriate graphic organizer in the box below and fill it in with the major parts of the concept. Present your work to other participants.

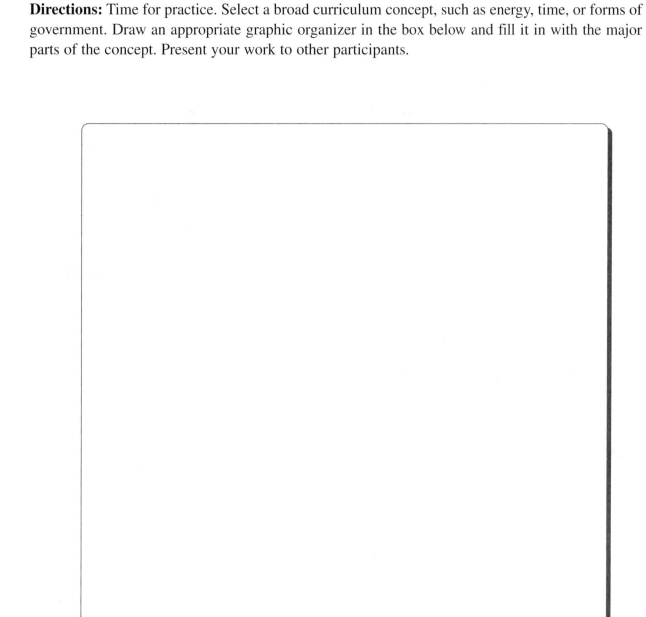

PRACTITIONER'S CORNER

Acquiring Another Language

When Should Children Learn Another Language? Although the brain maintains its ability to learn throughout life, it is quite clear from the research described earlier in this text that language learning occurs most easily during the first ten years or so. We should take advantage of this window of opportunity if we offer additional languages in schools.

Why Learn Another Language? In addition to knowing our native language, we benefit from learning another language as well. Language instruction should start as soon as possible. Here are some reasons for learning another language at an early age:

- Enriches and enhances a child's mental development.
- Gives students more flexibility in thinking, greater sensitivity to language, and a better ear for listening. (The brain learns to respond to phonemes that are different from the native language.)
- Improves understanding of a child's native language. (Unless a language or hearing difficulty exists, research does not support the claim that learning a second language early will interfere with learning the native language.)
- Gives a child the ability to communicate with people he or she would otherwise not have the chance to know.
- Opens the door to other cultures and helps a child understand and appreciate people from other countries. (This is important as our country becomes increasingly multicultural.)
- Gives a student a head start in language requirements for college.
- Increases job opportunities in many careers where knowing another language is a considerable asset.

What Are Barriers to Primary-Grade Second Language Programs? The two most common objections are that it is too expensive and that it might interfere with native language development. Primary-grade programs need not cost much at all. Volunteer parents can be the source of native speakers, and the materials come at low cost. As for interference, no research evidence supports this contention. Rather, several studies show that strategies used to acquire another language often help children understand and speak their native language better (DeHouwer, 1999).

What Are the Characteristics of an Effective K–6 Additional Language Program?

- **All students** have access to the program regardless of race/ethnic origin, learning styles, home language, or future academic goals.

- **Program goals** are consistent with the time devoted to additional language instruction. In the primary grades, the main goal is to hear the sounds, flow, and syntax of another language. There are different types of K–6 second language programs that achieve different levels of language proficiency and require different time commitments.

- **Sequence** of language instruction should be available through the K–12 school years. Acquisition of another language requires consistent practice, so a K–12 sequence is crucial to mastery. For this reason, instruction in other languages is often exempted from block scheduling formats that limit classes to one semester per year.

- **Systematic curriculum development** in content of another language is part of the school plan. Look for ways to include these language experiences across the curriculum.

- **Native speakers** must be used for the primary-grade instruction to ensure that the young brain hears authentic language sounds.

- **Connections between language and culture** are made explicit so that the learners understand the development of the additional language in the context of its culture.

Teaching Strategies for Acquiring Another Language

Teaching strategies for instruction in another language vary with the age of the learner who is beginning the study. Primary-grade teaching focus is mainly on recognizing, discriminating, and practicing the phonemes of the other language, as spoken by native speakers. Grammar is not taught per se, but implied through extensive student conversation. In the intermediate and later grades (including adult levels), the main goal is to develop communication competencies so that the student feels comfortable speaking, writing, and thinking the other language. Thus, teachers of other languages and of English Language Learners (ELL) should follow a sequence that begins with young learners. This sequence aims to do the following:

- **Develop Communication Competence.** One of the primary goals of learning another language is to gain competence in communication. This involves acquiring four major competencies, requiring integration of the verbal and nonverbal aspects of language as well as right- and left-hemisphere processing. Teachers should keep these four competencies in mind as they select their instructional strategies:

Grammatical Competence. The degree to which a student has mastered the formal linguistic code of the language including vocabulary, rules of punctuation, word formation, and sentence structure. This entails the analytic and sequential processing of the left hemisphere.

Sociolinguistic Competence. The ability to use grammatical forms appropriately in contexts that range from very informal to very formal styles. It includes varying the choice of verbal and nonverbal language to adapt the speech to a specific person or social context, and this requires sensitivity to individual and sociocultural differences. This is essentially the right hemisphere's ability to contextualize language.

Discourse Competence. The ability to combine form and thought into a coherent expression. It involves knowing how to use conjunctions, adverbs, and transitional phrases to achieve continuity of thought. This requires the integration of both hemispheres; the analytic ability of the left hemisphere to generate the grammatical features, and the use of the right hemisphere to synthesize them into meaningful, coherent wholes.

Strategic Competence. The ability to use verbal and nonverbal communication strategies, such as body language and circumlocution, to compensate for the user's imperfect knowledge of the language, and to negotiate meaning.

This research points out the need for teachers to ensure that the nonverbal form of intellect is not neglected in second language acquisition. In planning lessons, teachers should:

- Not rely heavily on grammar, vocabulary memorization, and mechanical translations, especially during the early stages of instruction.

- Do more with contextual language, trial and error, brainstorming of meaning, visual activities, and role-playing.

- Give students the opportunity to establish the contextual networking they need to grasp meaning, nuance, and idiomatic expressions.

When these skills are in place, shift to more work on enlarging students' vocabulary and knowledge of grammar.

PRACTITIONER'S CORNER

Considerations for Teaching Reading

Reading is the result of a complex process that relies heavily on previously acquired spoken language, but also requires the learning of specific skills that are not innate to the human brain. Because of the many steps involved in learning to read, challenges can occur anywhere along the way. Children often devise strategies to overcome problems but may need help in getting to the next step. As with learning any skill, reading requires practice.

The scientific research suggests that reading instruction include a balance between the development of phonemic awareness and the use of enriched texts to help learners with syntax and semantics. Here are some basic points to consider when teaching reading. For more specific teaching strategies, see NRP (2000), Shaywitz (2003), and Sousa (2005).

Basic Guidelines for a Balanced Approach.

- **No one reading program is best for all children.** Successful teachers of reading have developed activities that differentiate among their students according to their current level of readiness to read.

- **Developing phonemic awareness.** The brain reads by breaking words into sounds. Children first need to be taught the 44 basic sounds (phonemes) in the English language and be able to manipulate these sounds successfully. This is known as phonemic-awareness training. The more difficulty a learner has in beginning reading, the more likely the need for concentrated practice on phonemic awareness.

- **Mastering the Alphabetic Principle (Decoding).** Beginning readers need to be able to recognize the sounds represented by the letters of the alphabet. The better that a learner can *sound out* words, the faster the brain learns to match what it sees to what it hears. Therefore, readers should be taught to discern the individual sounds within words as they read them, and to say them aloud. *Dog* is "duh-awh-guh," and *bat* is "bah-ah-tuh." This practice helps the brain remember the decoding process of sight-to-sound so crucial to accurate and fast reading. However, problems develop when the reader's eyes move faster than the sound processing system can decode the phonemes. In this case, slow down the visual speed by having the student move a finger under each letter (grapheme). This also ensures that readers keep their eyes moving across the page, not fixating them into a stare, which also retards the reading process.

- **Phonics are important.** Phonics is the instructional approach that helps students master the alphabetic principle. It is an important component of learning to read but should not be taught as a separate unit through drill and rote memorization. Students lose interest and motivation to read. It is more effective to teach phonics as a means of developing spelling strategies and word analysis skills.

- **Practice for Comprehension.** Once the alphabetic principle is learned, practice in reading aloud is needed to develop speed and accuracy so that learners can comprehend what they are reading and get a sense of the language's syntax. This also helps teachers hear how accurately the student has matched the visual grapheme with the auditory phoneme.

- **Read With the Learners.** Teachers should read aloud as learners follow along in the text. This helps students with prosody—hearing the flow, rhythm, and tonal changes of the language. Have students move a finger under the words to show that they are correctly matching what they hear the teacher say with what they see on paper.

- **Read to the Learners.** Read literature slightly advanced for the learner while students listen, even with their eyes closed, to absorb the richness, rhythm, imagery, sound, and feeling of language in different contexts.

- **Introduce Literature.** Move on to interesting books and other forms of literature for practice and motivation to read. At this point, it is important to emphasize the contextual nature of the English language. Most meaning and pronunciation comes from *how* words are used in relation to all other words in the sentence (the context). Compare, for example, "The boy picked up the *lead* weight" to "The boy had a *lead* part in the school play."

- **Avoid** asking new readers to guess the sounds of words if they have not had phonemic-awareness training. Without the training, they have no clue how the word should sound, and mispronouncing the word will only reinforce the incorrect association between the grapheme and the phoneme. Remember that practice makes permanent, not necessarily perfect.

The chart on the next page is a reasonable hierarchy to be considered for teaching reading based on a deeper scientific understanding of the complexity of how the brain reads. In this hierarchy, emphasis is placed on ensuring accurate phonemic awareness at the very beginning of reading instruction. More evidence is emerging from brain scans of children reading that problems arise when there is poor phonemic awareness, thus confusing the decoding system.

<table>
<tr><th colspan="2">EXAMPLE OF A HIERARCHY FOR TEACHING READING</th></tr>
<tr><td colspan="2">Note: This procedure for teaching reading reflects the research on how the brain learns to read. It balances the early need for solid phonemic awareness with the later introduction of literary samples illustrating the more complex semantic and syntactic elements of language.</td></tr>
<tr><td>Semantic Level: The learners recognize that the meaning of words can change in different contexts. The teacher selects a variety of literature examples to illustrate contextual variations of language.</td><td rowspan="2">Students are likely to master these skills with literary texts that are rich with writing that contains syntactic and semantic variations.</td></tr>
<tr><td>Syntax Level: The learners create more complex sentences with correct grammatical structure. The teacher reads stories aloud to help learners develop a sense of syntax by listening to the phrasing and word positions in sentences. They recognize that in the sentences, “The dog chased the boy” and “The boy was chased by the dog,” the syntax has changed but not the meaning. Having students read aloud allows the teacher to check pronunciation.</td></tr>
<tr><td>Discourse Level: The learners construct and connect simple sentences in a logical sequence. Their spoken language has already developed some sentence patterns intuitively, such as subject-predicate-object, as in “I want a cookie” or “He throws the ball.” Prefixes and suffixes are introduced and practiced.</td><td rowspan="2">Students are likely to master these skills faster if they use texts with the words that contain the phonemes being taught. These are called decoded texts.</td></tr>
<tr><td>START HERE:

Phonological Level: This level focuses on developing phonological awareness and mastering the alphabetic principle. Learners are processing the basic sound elements of language. Students read aloud to ensure that the correct connections are made between the 44 English phoneme sounds and the 26 letters of the alphabet. Then practice with rhyming, word recognition, and meaning.</td></tr>
</table>

PRACTITIONER'S CORNER

Reading Guidelines for All Teachers

To some extent, all teachers are teachers of reading. Beyond the primary grades, students read to learn, and teachers place heavy reliance on their students' ability to acquire information through reading. Because this reliance increases substantially in the upper grades, reading ability is a major determinant of student success in high school. Reading in all subject areas is likely to be more successful when teachers help students use reading skills efficiently and effectively. Here are some strategies to consider (Sousa, 2005).

- **Use direct instruction** to clearly identify important concepts in the reading and explain why we are learning them. Ask students to summarize the main points you just made. This helps the students determine sense and meaning. The amount of reading assigned should be just enough to accomplish the task. Don't overwhelm students with non-essential reading, especially in subject areas where they lack confidence.

- **Conquer vocabulary** by defining any new words or words used in an unfamiliar context. This should be done *before* assigning the reading.

- **Help with comprehension** by advising students to scan for key words and phrases that aid in comprehension, and to ask themselves questions like: How much do I need to read in this sitting? Why am I reading this? What's the main point? Why is it important? What else is this like that I've already learned? Can I summarize in my own words what I just read?

- **Talk, Talk, and Talk Some More.** You will remember that talk is a very powerful learning and memory tool. When working together, students should ask each other questions about the text they are reading, summarize main points, and clarify anything they did not understand. Cooperative learning groups is an effective strategy to accomplish this sharing, especially in classes that have a wide range of student abilities, including reading.

- **Use Graphic Organizers.** Have students use or design their own graphic organizers and concept maps to help understand the major points in their reading. This is particularly useful in textbooks and nonfiction reading that is full of detail.

- **Add Novelty.** Add novelty (Chapter 3) so that students don't see reading as drudgery. For example, get students to speculate on what might happen next in a story, or have them write their own plausible endings. Consider giving them the option to write a song or a poem or a short skit to illustrate some of the story's main events or characters. Let them create their own stories, plays, or publications, which they can read or perform for other students.

- **Incorporate supplemental textbooks** that cover the same material as the course text but are written at a lower reading level. This may require several books because it is unlikely that one book will cover all the course content.

- **Establish in-class vertical files** of magazine and newspaper articles about subjects found in the course text. Update the files periodically and encourage students to contribute to the files when they come across an appropriate article.

- **Use audiovisual aids.** These are a great help to students who have reading problems. Many students have become acclimated to a multimedia environment. Whenever possible, use videotapes, audiotapes, computer programs, television, overhead transparencies, and other technology to supplement and accompany direct instruction.

Chapter 5—Brain Specialization and Learning

Key Points to Ponder

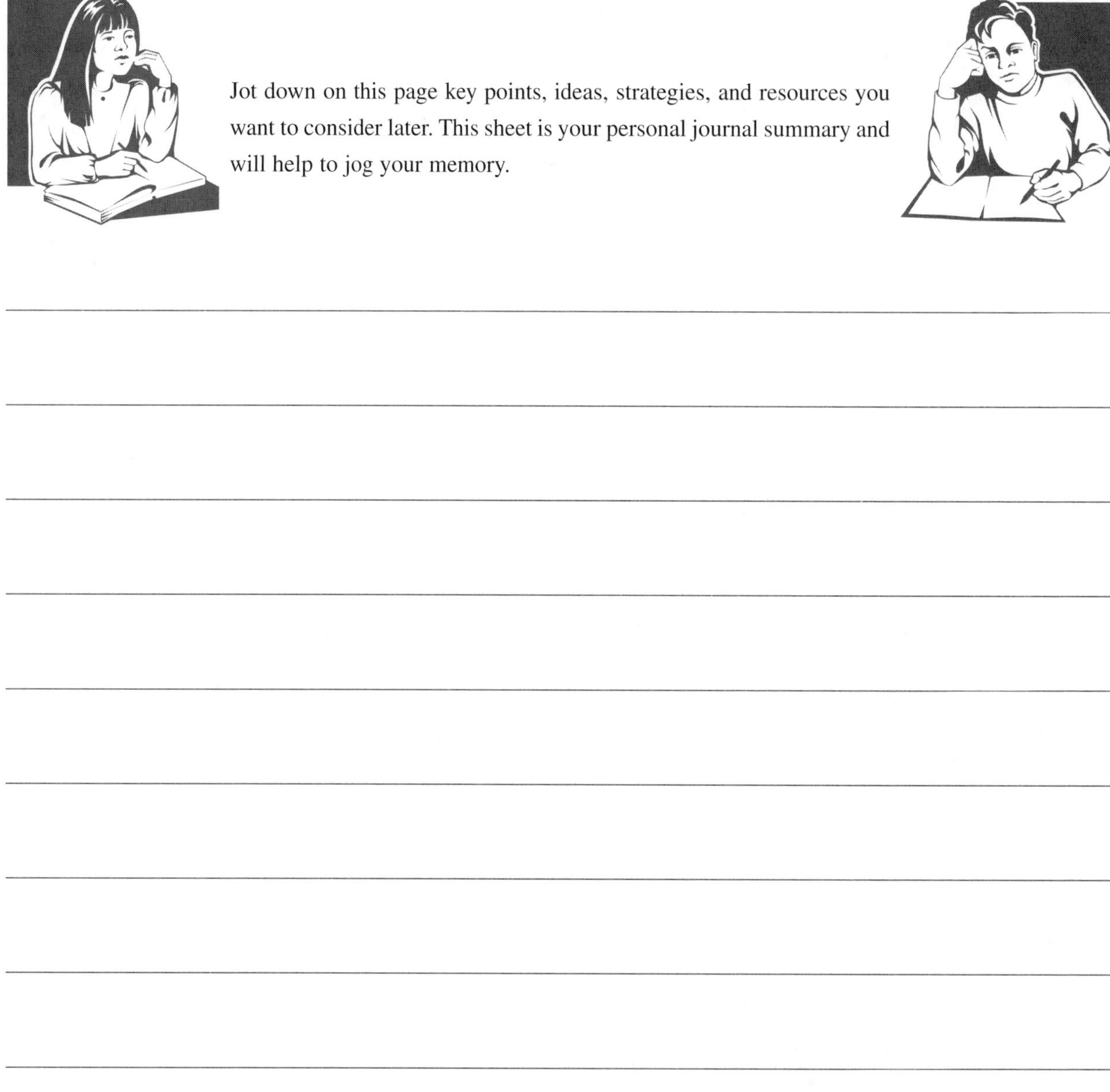

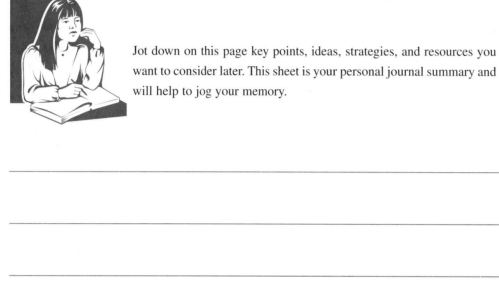

Jot down on this page key points, ideas, strategies, and resources you want to consider later. This sheet is your personal journal summary and will help to jog your memory.

Chapter 6

The Brain and the Arts

The quality of civilization can be measured through its music, dance, drama, architecture, visual art, and literature. We must give our children knowledge and understanding of civilization's most profound works.

—Ernest L. Boyer

Chapter Highlights: This chapter discusses how recent brain imaging studies are helping us understand the role and importance of music, the visual arts, and movement in brain growth and cognitive function. It suggests ways to incorporate artistic activities into lessons at all grade levels and in all subject areas.

We have never discovered a culture on this planet, past or present, that doesn't have art. Yet there have been a number of cultures—even today—that don't have reading and writing. Why is that? One likely explanation is that the activities represented by the arts—dance, music, drama, and visual arts—are basic to the human experience and necessary for survival. If they weren't, why would they have been part of every civilization from the Cro-Magnon cave dwellers to the urban citizens of the 21st century?

THE ARTS ARE BASIC TO THE HUMAN EXPERIENCE

As we learn more about the brain, we continue to find clues as to why the activities required for the arts are so fundamental to brain function. Music: It seems that certain structures in the auditory cortex respond only to musical tones. Dance: A portion of the cerebrum and most of the cerebellum are devoted to initiating and coordinating all kinds of movement, from intense running to the delicate sway of the arms. Drama: Specialized areas of the cerebrum focus on spoken language acquisition and call on the limbic system to provide the emotional component. Visual arts: The internal visual processing system can recall reality or create fantasy with the same ease.

> ***We have never discovered a culture on this planet—past or present—that doesn't have music, art, and dance.***

These cerebral talents did not develop by accident. They are the result of many centuries of interaction between humans and their environment, and the continued existence of these talents must indicate they contribute in some way to our survival. In those cultures that do not have reading and writing, the arts are the media through which that culture's history, mores, and values are transmitted to the younger generations and perpetuated. They also transmit more basic information necessary for the culture's survival, such as how and what to hunt for food and how to defend the village from predators.

Consequently, art is an important force behind group survival. For example, about 1,000 of the 6,500 languages on this planet are spoken in just one place—New Guinea! Each language is totally unrelated to any other known language in New Guinea (or elsewhere) and is spoken by a tribe of just a few thousand people living within a ten-mile radius. Even more astonishing is that each tribe has its own music, visual arts, and dance (Diamond, 1992).

In modern cultures, the arts are rarely thought of as survival skills, but rather as frills—the esthetic product of a wealthy society with lots of time to spare. In fact, people pay high ticket prices to see the arts performed professionally, leading to the belief that the arts are highly valued. This cultural support is often seen in high schools, which have their choruses, bands, drama classes, and an occasional dance troupe.

Yet seldom do public elementary schools enjoy this continuous support, precisely when the young brain is most adept at refining the skills needed to develop artistic talent (Several private school initiatives have been the exception, most notably the Montessori schools and the Waldorf schools). Furthermore, when school budgets get tight, elementary grade art and music programs are among the first to be reduced or eliminated. Now, pressure from the No Child Left Behind Act to improve reading and mathematics achievement is prompting elementary schools to trade off instruction in the arts for more classroom preparation for the Act's high-stakes testing.

WHY TEACH THE ARTS?

The basic arguments I make here are these:

- The arts play an important role in human development, enhancing the growth of cognitive, emotional, and psychomotor pathways.

- Schools have an obligation to expose children to the arts at the earliest possible time and to consider the arts as fundamental—not optional—curriculum areas.
- Learning the arts provides a higher quality of human experience throughout a person's lifetime.

The Arts and the Young Brain

In Chapter 1, we discuss the explosive growth of dendrites and synaptic connections during the brain's early years. Much of what young children do as play—singing, drawing, dancing—are natural forms of art. These activities engage all the senses and help wire the brain for successful learning. When children enter school, these art activities need to be continued and enhanced. The cognitive areas are developed as the child learns songs and rhymes, and creates drawings and finger paintings. The dancing and movements during play develop gross motor skills, and the sum of these activities enhances emotional well-being.

The arts also contribute to the education of young children by helping them realize the breadth of human experience, see the different ways humans express sentiments and convey meaning, and develop subtle and complex forms of thinking (Eisner, 2002a).

The Arts Develop Cognitive Growth

Although the arts are often thought of as separate subjects, like chemistry or algebra, they really are a collection of skills and thought processes that transcend all areas of human engagement. When taught well, the arts develop cognitive competencies that benefit learners in every aspect of their education and prepare them for the demands of the 21st century. Elliot Eisner (2002b) of Stanford University identifies these eight competencies:

- **The perception of relationships.** Creating a work in music, words, or any other art discipline helps students recognize how parts of a work influence each other and interact. For example, this is the kind of skill that enables an executive to appreciate the way a particular system affects every other subsystem in an organization.
- **An attention to nuance.** The arts teach students that small differences can have large effects. Great amounts of visual reasoning go into decisions about nuance, form, and color to make an art work satisfying. In writing, similarly, great attention to detail in use of language is needed to employ allusion, innuendo, and metaphor.
- **The perspective that problems can have multiple solutions, and questions can have multiple answers.** Good things can be done in different ways. Schools often emphasize learning focused on a single correct answer. In business and in life, most difficult problems require looking at multiple options with differing priorities.
- **The ability to shift goals in process.** Work in the arts helps students recognize and pursue goals that were not thought of at the beginning. Too often in schools, the relationship of means to ends is oversimplified. Arts help us see that ends can shift in process.

- **The permission to make decisions in the absence of a rule.** Arithmetic has rules and measurable results, but many other things lack that kind of rule-governed specificity. In the absence of rules, it is personal judgment that allows one to assess what feels right and to decide when a task is well done.
- **The use of imagination as the source of content.** Arts enhance the ability to visualize situations and use the mind's eye to determine the rightness of a planned action.
- **The acceptance of operating within constraints.** No system, whether linguistic, numerical, visual, or auditory covers every purpose. Arts give students a chance to use the constraints of a medium to invent ways to exploit those constraints productively.
- **The ability to see the world from an aesthetic perspective.** Arts help students frame the world in fresh ways—like seeing the Golden Gate Bridge from a design or poetic angle.

It is encouraging that more states have recently promoted the arts in their curriculum through policies, such as including the arts as part of high school graduation requirements, standards, and assessments. Although the extent of commitment varies, some states have developed more extensive programs in the arts for schools and created partnerships with state arts councils and local arts organizations. The Education Commission of the States is sponsoring a two-year initiative (2004 to 2006) to ensure that every child has the opportunity to learn about, enjoy, and participate in the arts.

My point is that the arts should be taught for the arts' sake, and one should not have to suggest that we teach the arts only because they enhance the learning of other academic subjects. Nonetheless, I am a realist, and I recognize that it is important, nonetheless, to document any spillover effects that learning the arts can have on learning other subjects. That is because of the risk that the arts will fall by the wayside as schools are held more accountable for improving achievement in language arts and mathematics, despite strong public support for arts programs.

The Sciences Need the Arts

Few people will argue against studying the natural sciences in the elementary and middle schools, and support remains strong for the sciences—including Advanced Placement courses—in high schools. When budgets get tight, some people even view music and other arts courses as a drain on the funds needed to preserve science and mathematics courses. Others often see science and the arts as polar opposites. The sciences are thought of as objective, logical, analytical, reproducible, and useful; the arts are supposed to be subjective, intuitive, sensual, unique, and frivolous. In the competition between the arts and sciences in U.S. society, the arts have frequently lost. Typically, more public and private funds are given to any single technical or scientific discipline than all the arts combined.

But scientists and mathematicians know that the arts are vital to their success and use skills borrowed from the arts as scientific tools. These include the ability to observe accurately, to think spatially (how does an object appear when I rotate it in my head?) and perceive kinesthetically (how does it move?). These skills are not usually taught as part of the science curriculum but are at home in writing, drama, painting, and music.

Indeed, the arts often inform the sciences (Root-Bernstein, 1997). For example:

- Buckminster Fuller's geodesic domes can describe soccer balls and architectural buildings, as well as the structure of viruses and some recently discovered complex and enormous molecules.
- NASA employs artists to design displays that present satellite data so that it is accurate, yet understandable.
- A biochemist looks at the fiber folds in her weaving cloth as another way of explaining protein folding.
- Computer engineers code messages to the frequencies of a specific song to prevent interception or blocking of the message, unless the decoder knows the song.
- Genetic researchers convert complex data into musical notation to facilitate analysis of the data, as for example, decoding the sequence of genes in a chromosome.

Thus, playing the piano, writing a poem, or creating a painting sharpen observations, hone details, and put things into context. These are the same tools needed by a good scientist. The study of the arts not only allows students to develop skills that will improve the quality of their lives but also sustains the same creative base from which scientists and engineers seek to develop their innovations and breakthroughs of the future.

IMPACT OF THE ARTS ON STUDENT LEARNING AND BEHAVIOR

Arts Education and Arts Integration

Numerous research studies show that well-designed arts experiences produce positive academic and social effects as well as assist in the development of critical academic skills, basic and advanced literacy, and numeracy. The studies look at both stand-alone arts programs as well as programs that integrate concepts and skills from the arts into the many areas of study. One intriguing and important revelation of these studies is that the most powerful effects are found in programs that *integrate* the arts with subjects in the core curriculum.

Researchers speculate that arts integration causes both students and teachers to rethink how they view the arts and generates conditions that educational researchers and cognitive scientists say are ideal for learning. The arts are not just expressive and affective, they are deeply cognitive. They develop essential thinking tools: pattern recognition and development; mental representations of what is observed or imagined; symbolic, allegorical, and metaphorical representations; careful observation of the world; and abstraction from complexity. Studies repeatedly show that in schools where arts are integrated into the core curriculum (Rabkin & Redmond, 2004):

- Students have a greater emotional investment in their classes
- Students work more diligently and learn from each other
- Cooperative learning groups turn classrooms into learning communities
- Parents become more involved
- Teachers collaborate more
- Art and music teachers become the center of multi-class projects
- Learning in all subjects becomes attainable through the arts
- Curriculum becomes more authentic, hands-on, and project-based
- Assessment is more thoughtful and varied
- Teachers' expectations for their students rise

The following research studies are but a few of the many that have accumulated in recent years about the effects of art instruction on student learning. They include results from both stand-alone and arts integration programs.

SAT Scores

The association between students taking arts courses and their SAT scores is one of the largest studies of its kind. It included over several years more than 10 million American high schoolers who responded to a questionnaire indicating the number of years of arts classes they took. The results were amazingly consistent (Vaughn & Winner, 2000).

- Students who took arts classes had higher math, verbal, and composite SAT scores than students who did not take arts classes.
- SAT scores increased linearly with the addition of more years of arts classes, that is, the more years of arts classes, the higher the SAT scores.
- The strongest relationship with SAT scores was found with students who took four or more years of arts classes.
- The correlations with mathematics scores were consistently smaller than those for verbal scores.
- Acting classes had the strongest correlation with verbal SAT scores. Acting classes and music history, theory, or appreciation had the strongest relationship with math SAT scores. However, all classifications of arts classes were found to have significant relationships with both verbal and math SAT scores.

It is important to note that although enrollment in arts courses is positively correlated with higher SAT verbal and mathematics scores, it does not prove that one caused the other. Perhaps there are other variables involved. Nonetheless, it is difficult to challenge the strength of this relationship, given the magnitude of the study.

Disaffected Students

The arts reach students who are not otherwise being reached. Arts sometimes provide the only reason that certain students stay in touch with school. Without the arts, these young people would be left with no access to a community of learners. A ten-year ongoing study in the Chicago public schools shows test scores rising faster on the Iowa Test of Basic Skills reading section than a matched population (for neighborhood, family income, and academic performance) of sixth graders in the regular schools. A study of the Minneapolis schools showed that arts integration had positive effects on all students, but much more so with disadvantaged students (Rabkin & Redmond, 2004). In Florida, 41 percent of potential dropout students said something about the arts kept them in school. Further, these students were more engaged in their art classes than in academic classes (Barry, Taylor, & Walls, 2002).

Different Learning Styles

Ample research evidence indicates that students learn in many different ways. This research also notes that some students can become behavior problems if conventional classroom practices are not engaging them. Success in the arts is often a bridge to successful learning in other areas, thereby raising a student's self-concept. Table 6.1 shows how students involved in arts-based youth organizations have a better self-concept than a standard student population. These numbers are particularly significant considering that students in the arts organizations are twice as likely to have stressful home situations involving parents getting a divorce, going on and off welfare, or losing a job. The students in this sample noted how the arts allowed them to express pent-up feelings and to gain some distance from these problems by talking about them, thinking, and listening (Fiske, 1999).

Table 6.1 Percentage of Students in Standard School Population and in Arts-Based Youth Organizations Reporting a Positive Perception of Self

	Standard School Population	**Arts-Based Youth Organizations**
Student feels good about him/herself.	76.2	92.3
Student feels s/he is a person of worth.	75.9	90.9
Student is able to do things as well as others.	76.2	88.8
Student, on the whole, is satisfied with self.	70.0	84.6

Source: Fiske (1999)

Personal and Interpersonal Connections

The arts connect students to themselves and each other. Creating art is a personal experience, as students draw upon their own resources to produce the result. This is a much deeper involvement than just reading text to get an answer. Studies indicate that the attitudes of young people toward one another improve through their arts learning experiences. For instance, more than 2,400 elementary and middle school students from 18 public schools participated in a study that showed students in arts-rich schools scoring higher in creativity and several measures of academic self-concept than students in schools without that level of arts instruction (Burton, Horowitz, & Abeles, 2000).

School and Classroom Climate

The arts transform the environment for learning. Schools become places of discovery when the arts are the focus of the learning environment. Arts change the school culture, break down barriers between curriculum areas, and can even improve the school's physical appearance. Because administrators and teachers determine a school's climate, a study of 29 arts-rich New York City schools compared some indicators of school climate to the remaining, non-arts schools. In the arts-rich schools, administrators encouraged teachers to take risks, broaden the curriculum, and learn new skills. The teachers had a significantly higher degree of innovation in their instruction, were more supportive of students, and had greater interest in their own professional development. Once again, the arts-rich program had a much greater impact on these results than did the students' socioeconomic status (Fiske, 1999).

Gifted and Talented Students

The arts provide new challenges for students already considered successful. Students who outgrow their learning environment usually get bored and complacent. The arts offer a chance for unlimited challenge. For instance, older students may teach and mentor younger ones who are learning to play musical instruments, and some advanced students may work with professional artists.

The World of Work

The arts connect learning experiences to the world of everyday work. The adult workplace has changed. The ability to generate ideas, bring ideas to life, and communicate them to others are keys to workplace success. Whether in a classroom or in a studio as an artist, the student is learning and practicing future workplace behaviors.

Let's take a look at the three major forms of artistic expression—music, visual arts, and dance and drama—and observe what brain research is telling us. What impact will these studies have on student learning and success?

MUSIC

Music exerts a powerful effect on the brain through intellectual and emotional stimulation. It can also affect our body by altering our heart rate, breathing, blood pressure, pain threshold, and muscle movements. These responses result from the activation of neural networks that include the frontal cortex, the amygdala, and other limbic areas involved in motivation and reward.

Is Music Inborn?

Many researchers now believe that the ability to perceive and enjoy music is an inborn human trait. But is there any credible evidence to support this biological basis of music? First of all, any behavior thought to have a biological foundation must be universal. Even though the uses of music may vary across past and current cultures, all cultures do sing and associate certain meanings and emotions with music.

> ***Compelling evidence suggests that the brain's response to music is innate and has strong biological roots.***

Second, biologically based behaviors should reveal themselves early in life. Researchers have shown that infants of just three months old can learn and remember to move an overhead crib mobile when a certain song is played. Thus, infants can use music as a retrieval cue. In addition, the memory of the specific song lasted more than seven days (Fagan et al., 1997). Babies can also differentiate between two adjacent musical tones and can recognize a melody when it is played in a different key (Weinberger, 2004). At the age of seven months, infants can categorize rhythmic and melodic patterns on the basis of underlying meter (Hannon & Johnson, 2005). Moreover, preschool children spontaneously use music in their communication and play.

Third, if music has a strong biological component, then it should exist in other animals. Monkeys, for example, can form musical abstractions, such as determining harmonic patterns. Although many animals use musical sounds to attract mates and signal danger, only humans have developed a sophisticated and unlimited musical repertoire.

Fourth, if music has biological roots, we might expect the brain to have specialized areas for music—and it does. For example, areas in the auditory cortex are organized to process pitch. Furthermore, the brain's ability to respond emotionally to music is connected to biology and culture. The biological aspect is supported by the fact that the brain has specialized areas that respond only to music, and these areas are able to stimulate the limbic system, provoking an emotional response. PET scans show that the neural areas stimulated depend on the type of music—melodic tunes stimulate areas that evoke pleasant feelings, whereas dissonant sounds activate other limbic areas that produce unpleasant emotions (Blood, Zatorre, Bermudez, & Evans, 1999; Menon & Levitin, 2005).

Effects of Listening to Music Versus Creating Instrumental Music

No one arts area has gained more notoriety in recent years than the impact of music on the brain. Numerous books are on the market touting the so-called "Mozart Effect" and promising that music can do all sorts of things from relieving pain, to increasing a child's IQ, to improving mathematics skills. To what degree are these claims backed by credible scientific evidence? As with most claims of this nature, there is a growing body of scientific data, followed by media attention and a lot of hype. Let's try to sort out what the research in music is saying so that we can reap its benefits while making informed decisions about the validity of the assertions.

> ***How the brain responds when listening to music is very different from how it responds when creating music.***

Research on the effects of music on the brain and body can be divided into the effects of *listening* to music, and the effects of *creating* or *producing* music on an instrument, especially an acoustic rather than an electronic one. The brain and body respond differently in these two situations. Unfortunately, not enough attention has been paid to this crucial distinction. Consequently, people have mistakenly assumed that the results of studies that involved creating music would be repeated when listening to music. If educators want to use the research on the effects of music to benefit students, then it is important that they differentiate the studies on listening from those on creating music.

How the Brain Listens to Music

The sounds of music are transmitted to the inner ear and are broken down according to the specific frequencies that make up the sounds (Figure 6.1). Different cells in the *cochlea* respond to different frequencies, and their signals are mapped out in the auditory cortex, especially in the right hemisphere in which perceptions of pitch, melody, timbre, and harmony emerge. This information is then transmitted to the frontal lobe where the music can be linked to emotion, thoughts, and past experiences. Over time, the auditory cortex is "retuned" by experience so that more cells become sensitive to important sounds and musical tones. This sets the stage for the processing of the more complex music patterns of melody, harmony, and rhythm.

Each hemisphere of the brain contains areas that respond to both music and language. But, as mentioned in Chapter 5, the left hemisphere also contains regions of specialization that respond only to language, and the right hemisphere has areas devoted exclusively to music perception. This explains why some people can be extraordinarily talented in language skills but have difficulty humming a melody. The reverse situation occurs in the brains of individuals with savant syndrome, who are talented musicians despite severe language retardation.

The discovery that the auditory cortex (located in the temporal lobes) in the right hemisphere has regions that respond only to music came from studies comparing patients who have damage to their left or right temporal lobes. Patients with right temporal lobe damage have lost the ability to

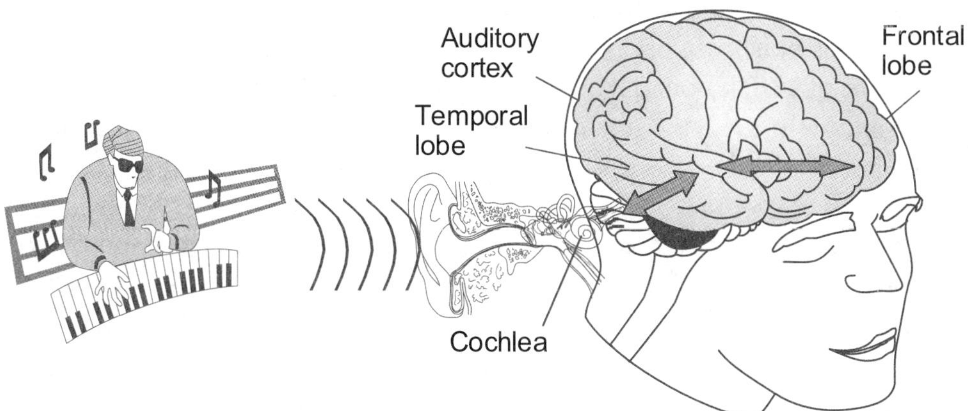

Figure 6.1 Sound entering the ear is converted into nerve impulses in the cochlea. These impulses are transmitted to the auditory cortex in the temporal lobe in which specialized regions, especially in the right hemisphere, analyze pitch and timbre. Information from the auditory cortex is transmitted to the frontal lobe, which associates the sound of music with thought and stimulates emotions and past experiences.

recognize familiar songs, a condition known as *amusia.* However, only the response to music is affected. The patients can still recognize human voices, traffic sounds, and other auditory information.

Music can also be imagined because people have stored representations of songs and the sounds of musical instruments in their long-term memory. When a song is imagined, the brain cells that are activated are identical to those used when a person actually hears music from the outside world. But when a song is imagined, brain scans show that the visual cortex is also stimulated so that visual patterns are imaged as well. The mechanism that triggers musical imagery is not yet understood, but it is not uncommon for people to have songs running through their heads when they get up in the morning.

The Benefits of Listening to Music

Therapeutic Benefits. For many years, medical researchers and practitioners have reported on the therapeutic effects of music to relieve stress, diminish pain, and treat other more severe disabilities, such as mental retardation, Parkinson's disease, Alzheimer's disease, and visual and hearing impairments. Other studies have shown that listening to music can boost immune function in children and that premature babies exposed to lullabies in the hospital went home earlier. The sheer volume of studies and positive results attest to music's therapeutic benefits.

How does music work this magic? That is still a mystery, but there are some important hints. Researchers have known for a long time that music can directly influence blood pressure, pulse, and the electric activity of muscles. Newer evidence shows that music may even help build and strengthen connections between brain cells in the cortex. This effect is important, and some doctors are already using music to help rehabilitate stroke patients. Some stroke patients who have lost their ability to speak retain their ability to sing. By getting patients to sing what they want to say, their fluency improves, and therapists can use existing pathways to retrain the speech centers of the brain.

Educational Benefits. The notion that music could affect cognitive performance catapulted from the research laboratory to the television talk shows in 1993 when Frances Rauscher and Gordon Shaw conducted a study using 84 college students. They reported that the students' spatial-temporal reasoning—the ability to form mental images from physical objects, or to see patterns in time and space—improved after listening to Mozart's Sonata for Two Pianos in D Major (K.448) for 10 minutes. But the students' improved abilities faded within an hour (Rauscher, Shaw, & Ky, 1993).

The results of this study, promptly dubbed "The Mozart Effect," were widely publicized and soon reinterpreted to incorrectly imply that listening to a Mozart sonata would enhance intelligence by raising IQ. In fact, the study reported that the music improved only spatial-temporal reasoning (one of many components of total IQ) and that the effect quickly faded. But the results did encourage the researchers to go further and test whether *creating* music would have a longer-lasting effect.

Shaw was convinced that listening to the complex melodic variations in Mozart's sonata (K.448) stimulated the frontal cortex more than simpler music. He and several colleagues tested this idea by having subjects take turns listening to Mozart's sonata (K.448), Beethoven's *Für Elise*, and popular piano music. The fMRIs showed that both the popular and the Beethoven piano music activated only the auditory cortex in all subjects. The Mozart sonata, however, activated the auditory as well as the frontal cortex in all of the subjects, leading Shaw to suggest that there *is* a neurological basis for the "Mozart Effect" (Muftuler, Bodner, Shaw, & Nalcioglu, 1999).

Recent studies confirm that the Mozart effect is real, and that it can occur with other kinds of music beside Mozart.

Subsequent studies confirm that listening to Mozart enhances various types of spatial and temporal reasoning tasks, especially problems requiring a sequence of mental images to correctly reassemble objects. The data suggest that the effect is real, yet it can occur with other kinds of music besides Mozart. However, researchers do not yet know conclusively *why* the effect occurs. Nonetheless, the effect is important to educators because it shows that passive listening to music appears to stimulate spatial thinking, and that neural networks normally associated with one kind of mental activity can readily share the cognitive processes involved in a different activity. So learning or thinking in one discipline may not be completely independent of another (Hetland, 2000a).

Several studies have shown that listening to certain music can stimulate the parts of the brain that are responsible for memory recall and visual imagery (Nakamura et al., 1999). Researchers have also found that listening to background music enhances the efficiency of those working with their hands. In a study of surgeons, for example, background music enhanced their alertness and concentration (Restak, 2003). This explains why background music in the classroom helps many students stay focused while completing certain

Listening to background music can enhance recall, visual imagery, attention, concentration, and dexterity.

learning tasks. However, one must exercise caution in selecting the *type* of background music. Several studies show that overly stimulating music serves more as a distraction and interferes with cognitive performance (Hallam, 2002). See the **Practitioner's Corner** on page 235 on using background music in the classroom.

Creating Music

Although passive listening to music does have some therapeutic and short-term educational benefits, the making of music seems to provide many more cerebral advantages. Learning to play a musical instrument challenges the brain in new ways. In addition to being able to discern different tone patterns and groupings, new motor skills must be learned and coordinated in order to play the instrument. These new learnings cause profound and seemingly permanent changes in brain structure. For example, the auditory cortex, the motor cortex, the cerebellum, and the corpus callosum are larger in musicians than in non-musicians.

This raises an interesting question: Are the brains of musicians different because of their training and practice in music, or did these differences exist before they learned music? The answer came when researchers trained non-musicians to listen for small changes in pitch and similar musical components. In just three weeks, their brains showed increased activation in the auditory cortex. This suggests that the brain differences in highly skilled musicians are more likely the result of training and not inherited (Restak, 2003). In support of this notion, another study compared 5- to 7-year-olds who were beginning piano or string lessons with a similar group not beginning instrument training. The researchers found no pre-existing neural, cognitive, motor, or musical differences between the two groups, and no correlations between music perceptual skills or visual-spatial measures. As in previous studies, correlations were found between music perceptual skills and phonemic awareness (Norton et al., 2005). No doubt some genetic traits enhance music learning, but it seems that most musicians are made, not born.

No doubt some genetic traits enhance music learning, but it seems that most musicians are made, not born.

Benefits of Creating Music

The effects of learning to play an instrument can begin at an early age. One major study involved 78 preschoolers from three California preschools, including one serving mostly poor, inner-city families. The children were divided into four groups. One group (Keyboard) took individual, 12- to 15-minute piano lessons twice a week along with singing instruction. Another group (Singing) took 30-minute singing lessons five days a week, and a third group (Computer) trained on computers. The fourth group received no special instruction. All students took tests before the lessons began to measure different types of spatial-reasoning skills.

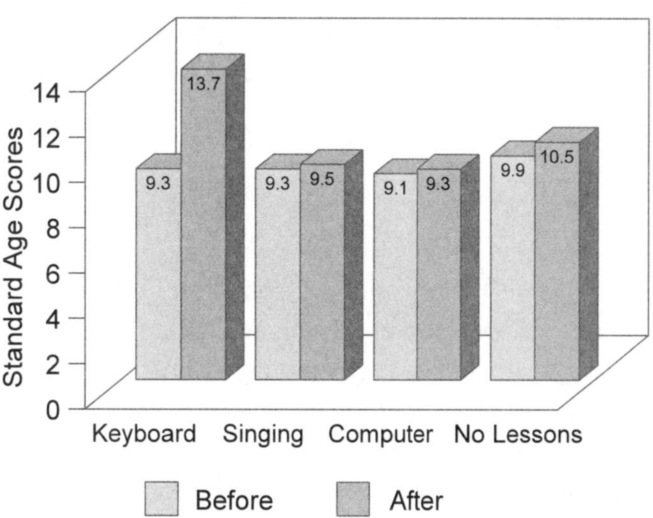

Figure 6.2 The graph shows the results of a spatial-temporal task performed by the preschool students before and after piano keyboard training, group singing, training on the computer, and no lessons. National standard age scores for all ages are 10, showing that these were average children before training.

After six months, the children who received six months of piano keyboard training had improved their scores by 34 percent on tests measuring spatial-temporal reasoning (Figure 6.2). On other tasks, there was no difference in scores. Furthermore, the enhancement lasted for days, indicating a substantial change in spatial-temporal function. The other three groups, in comparison, had only slight improvement on all tasks (Rauscher et al., 1997). Subsequent studies continue to show a strong relationship between creating music with keyboards and the enhancement of spatial reasoning in young children (Hetland, 2000b; Rauscher & Zupan, 2000).

Why did piano keyboard training improve test performance by 34 percent while the computer keyboard training didn't? Remember that the study measured spatial-temporal improvements only. As this and other studies show, music training seems to specifically influence neural pathways responsible for spatial-temporal reasoning, and that effect is more noticeable in the young brain. This may be due to the combination of tactile input from striking the piano keys, auditory input from the sounds of the notes, and the visual information of where one's hand is on the keyboard. This is a much more complex interaction than from the computer keyboard. Computers, of course, are very valuable teaching tools, but when it comes to developing the neural pathways responsible for spatial abilities, the piano keyboard is much more effective.

Creating Music Benefits Verbal Memory

Numerous studies have shown that musical training improves verbal memory. Researchers in one study administered memory tests to 90 boys between the ages of 6 and 15. Half belonged to their school's strings program for one to five years, while the other half had no musical training. The musically trained students had better verbal memory, but showed no differences in visual memory. Apparently, musical training's impact on the left temporal lobe seems to improve the ability of that region (where Broca's and Wernicke's areas are located) to handle verbal learning. Furthermore, the memory benefits of musical training are long-lasting. Students who dropped out of the music training group were tested a year later and found to retain the verbal memory advantage they had gained earlier (Ho, Cheung, & Chan, 2003).

Does Creating Music Affect Ability in Other Subjects?

Research studies continue to look for the impact that music instruction can have on learning in other subject areas. Two subject areas of particular interest are mathematics and reading.

Music and Mathematics

Of all the academic subjects, mathematics seems to be most closely connected to music. Music relies on fractions for tempo and on time divisions for pacing, octaves, and chord intervals. Here are some mathematical concepts that are basic to music.

- **Patterns.** Music is full of patterns of chords, notes, and key changes. Musicians learn to recognize these patterns and use them to vary melodies. Inverting patterns, called counterpoint, helps form different kinds of harmonies.
- **Counting.** Counting is fundamental to music because one must count beats, count rests, and count how long to hold notes.
- **Geometry.** Music students use geometry to remember the correct finger positions for notes or chords. Guitar players' fingers, for example, form triangular shapes on the neck of the guitar.
- **Ratios and Proportions, and Equivalent Fractions.** Reading music requires an understanding of ratios and proportions, that is, a whole note needs to be played twice as long as a half note, and four times as long as a quarter note. Because the amount of time allotted to one beat is a mathematical constant, the duration of all the notes in a musical piece are relative to one another on the basis of that constant. It is also important to understand the rhythmic difference between 3/4 and 4/4 time signatures.
- **Sequences.** Music and mathematics are related through sequences called intervals. A mathematical interval is the difference between two numbers; a musical interval is the ratio of their frequencies. Here's another sequence: Arithmetic progressions in music correspond to geometric progressions in mathematics.

Because of the many common mathematical concepts that underlie music, scientists have long wondered how these two abilities are processed in the brain. Several recent fMRI studies have shown that musical training activated the same areas of the brain (mainly the left frontal cortex) that are also activated during mathematical processing. It may be, then, that early musical training begins to build the very same neural networks that will later be used to complete numerical and mathematical tasks (Schmithhorst & Holland, 2004).

Keyboard Training. Motivated by the studies showing that music improved spatial-temporal reasoning, Gordon Shaw set out to determine whether this enhancement would help young students learn specific mathematics skills. He focused on proportional mathematics, which is particularly difficult for many elementary students, and which is usually taught with ratios, fractions, and comparative ratios. Shaw and his colleagues worked with 136 second-grade students from a

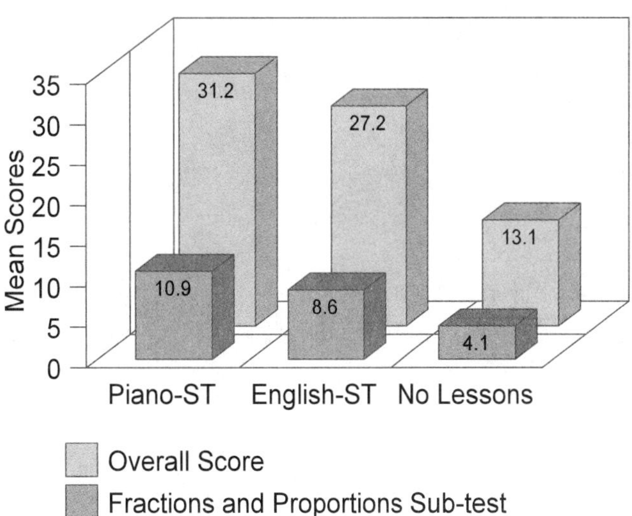

Figure 6.3 The mean overall, and fraction and proportions sub-test scores of the group that had piano and computer training with special software (Piano-ST), the group with computer and software (English-ST), and the group with no lessons.

low socioeconomic neighborhood in Los Angeles. One group (Piano-ST) was given four months of piano keyboard training, as well as computer training and time to play with a newly designed computer software to teach proportional mathematics. The second group (English-ST) was given computer training in English and time to play with the software; the third group (No Lessons) had neither music nor specific computer lessons, but did play with the computer software.

The Piano-ST group scored 27 percent higher on proportional math and fractions subtests than the English-ST students, and 166 percent higher than the No Lessons group (Figure 6.3). These findings are significant because proportional mathematics is not usually introduced until fifth or sixth grade, and because a grasp of proportional mathematics is essential to understanding science and mathematics at higher levels (Graziano, Peterson, & Shaw, 1999).

Strings Training. Begun in 2000, the Newark (NJ) Early Strings Program created a partnership with the New Jersey Symphony Orchestra to provide Suzuki-based string instruction to students in Newark's elementary schools, starting in second grade. A recent assessment showed that students in the program in grades two through four performed significantly better on standardized tests in language arts and mathematics than their peers. The program also had a positive effect on the students' self-esteem and self-discipline, and increased parent involvement in the schools (Abeles & Sanders, 2005).

A 1998 study showed how creating music can make a difference for students from low socioeconomic status. The low socioeconomic students who took music lessons from eighth through twelfth grade increased their test scores in mathematics and scored significantly higher than those low socioeconomic students who were not involved in music. Mathematics scores more than doubled, and history and geography scores increased by 40 percent (Catterall, Chapleau, & Iwanga, 1999).

The creating of instrumental music seems to provide the greatest cerebral advantages.

A subsequent review of studies involving more that 300,000 secondary school students confirmed the strong association between music instruction and achievement in mathematics. Of particular interest is an analysis of six experimental studies that revealed a causal relationship between music and mathematics performance, and that the relationship had grown stronger in recent years (Vaughn, 2000). Isn't this something that educators should consider in planning the core curriculum? If numeracy is so important, perhaps every student should learn to play a musical instrument.

Music and Reading

Several studies confirm a strong association between music instruction and standardized tests of reading ability. Although we cannot say that this is a causal association (that taking music instruction *caused* improvement in reading ability), this consistent finding in a large group of studies builds confidence that there is a strong relationship (Butzlaff, 2000). Researchers suggest that this strong relationship may result because of positive transfer occurring between language and reading. Their rationale is as follows:

- Although music and written language use highly differentiated symbol systems, both involve similar decoding and comprehension reading processes, such as reading from left to right, sequential ordering of content, etc.
- There are interesting parallels in the underlying concepts shared between music and language reading skills, such as sensitivity to phonological or tonal distinctions.
- Reading music involves the simultaneous incorporation and reading of written text with music.
- Learning in the context of a highly motivated social context, such as music ensembles, may lead to a greater desire for academic responsibility and performance that enhances reading achievement.

Studies done with 4- and 5-year-old children revealed that the more music skills children had, the greater their degree of phonological awareness and reading development. Apparently, music perception taps and enhances auditory areas that are related to reading (Anvari, Trainor, Woodside, & Levy, 2002).

THE VISUAL ARTS

The human brain has the incredible ability to form images and representations of the real world or sheer fantasy within its mind's eye. Solving the mystery of DNA's structure, for example, required Watson and Crick in the early 1950s to imagine numerous three-dimensional models until they hit on the only image that explained the molecule's peculiar behavior—the spiral helix. This was an incredible marriage of visual art and biology that changed the scientific world forever. Exactly how the brain performs the functions of imagination and meditation may be uncertain, but no one doubts the importance of these valuable talents, which have allowed human beings to develop advanced and sophisticated cultures.

Imagery

For most people, the left hemisphere specializes in coding information verbally whereas the right hemisphere codes information visually. Although teachers spend much time talking (and sometimes have their students talk) about the learning objective, little time is given to developing visual cues. This process, called *imagery*, is the mental visualization of objects, events, and arrays related to the new learning and represents a major way of storing information in the brain. Imagery can take place in two ways: *imaging* is the visualization in the mind's eye of something that the person has actually experienced; *imagining* depicts something the person has not yet experienced and, therefore, has no limits.

A mental image is a pictorial representation of something physical or of an experience. The more information an image contains, the richer it is. Some people are more capable of forming rich images than others, but the research evidence is clear: Individuals can be taught to search their minds for images and be guided through the process to select appropriate images that, through hemispheric integration, enhance learning and increase retention. When the brain creates images, the same parts of the visual cortex are activated as when the eyes process real world input. Thus, the powerful visual processing system is available even when the brain is creating internal pictures in the mind's eye (Kosslyn et al., 1999; Mazard, Laou, Joliot, & Mellet, 2005).

The human brain's ability to do imagery with such efficiency is likely due to the importance of imagery in survival. When confronted with a potentially life-threatening event—say, a car speeding toward you in the wrong traffic lane—the brain's visual processing system and the frontal lobes process several potential scenarios in a fraction of a second and initiate a reflex reaction that is most likely to keep you alive. As students today engage with electronic media that produce images, they are not getting adequate practice in generating their own imaging and imagining, skills that not only affect survival but also increase retention and, through creativity, improve the quality of life.

Imagery not only affects survival, but increases retention and improves the quality of life.

Training students in imagery encourages them to search long-term memory for appropriate images and to use them more like a movie than a photograph. For example, one recalls the house one lived in for many years. From the center hall with its gleaming chandelier, one mentally turns left and "walks" through the living room to the sun room beyond. To the right of the hall is the paneled dining room and then the kitchen with the avocado green appliances and oak cabinets. In the back, one sees the flagstone patio, the manicured lawn, and the garden with its variety of flowers. The richness of the image allows one to focus on just a portion of it and generate additional amounts of detail. In this image, one could mentally stop in any room and visualize the furniture and other decor. Imagery should become a regular part of classroom strategies as early as kindergarten. In the primary grades, the teacher should supply the images to ensure accuracy.

Imagery can be used in many classroom activities, including notetaking, cooperative learning groups, and alternative assessment options. Mindmapping is a specialized form of imagery that originated when the left-brain/right-brain research emerged in the 1970s. The process combines language with images to help show relationships between and among concepts, and how they connect to a key idea. Buzan (1989) and Hyerle (2004) illustrate different ways in which mind maps can be drawn.

Research on Visual Arts and Learning

A review of the research literature shows a serious lack of studies that examine the impact of the visual arts and imagery on learning. One reason is the difficulty in determining which aspects of visual arts training (apart from imagery) are at work in programs that integrate visual art into core curriculum subjects.

Most studies in this area relate to imagery in sports. Coaches have known for a long time that athletes who use imagery to mentally rehearse what they intend to do perform better than if they do not use imagery. Studies reveal that the more time and intensity devoted to imagery, the better the athletic performance (Cumming & Hall, 2002; Harwood, Cumming, & Hall, 2003).

Apart from sports, one meta-analysis did look at imagery and creativity. Data from nine studies involving nearly 1,500 students were analyzed and showed a statistically significant association between imagery and creativity. Not surprisingly, students who used more imagery during learning displayed more creativity in their discussions, modeling, and assessments (LeBoutillier & Marks, 2003).

MOVEMENT

The mainstream educational community has often regarded thinking and movement as separate functions, assigning them different priorities. Activities involving movement, such as dance, theater, and occasionally sports, are often reduced or eliminated when school budgets get tight. But as brain studies probe deeper into the relationship between body and mind, the importance of movement to cognitive learning becomes very apparent.

Movement and the Brain

A New Role for the Cerebellum

In earlier chapters, we discussed the long-known role of the cerebellum in coordinating the performance of motor skills. For several decades, neuroscientists assumed that the cerebellum carried out its coordinating role by communicating exclusively with the cerebrum's motor cortex. But this view did not explain why some patients with damage to the cerebellum also showed impaired cognitive function. Recent research using scans centered on the cerebellum shows that its nerve fibers communicate with other areas of the cerebrum as well.

Studies have found that the cerebellum plays an important role in attention, long-term memory, spatial perception, impulse control, and the frontal lobe's cognitive functions—the same areas that are stimulated during learning (Bower & Parsons, 2003). It seems that the more we study the cerebellum, the more we realize that movement is inescapably linked to learning and memory (Figure 6.4).

Autism and ADHD. Further evidence of the link between the cerebellum and cognitive function has come from some studies of autism. Brain images show that many autistic children have

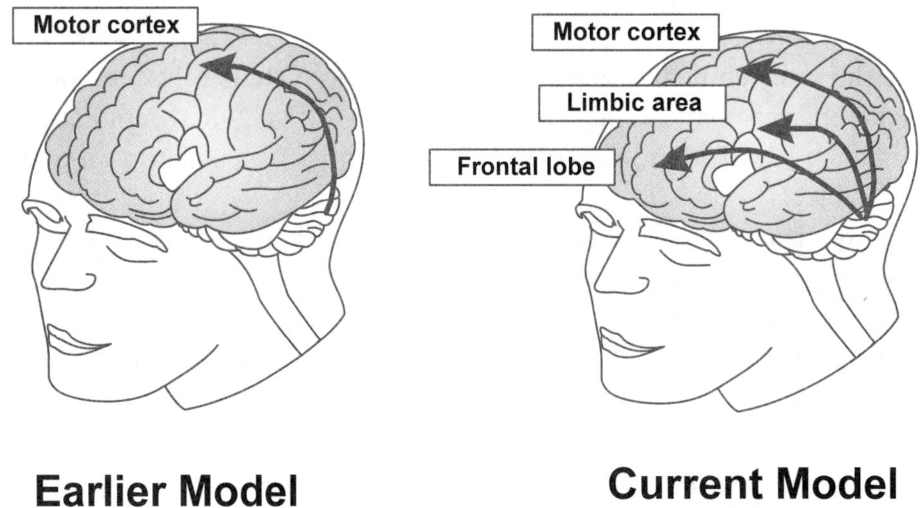

Figure 6.4 Researchers earlier thought that the cerebellum's role was limited to coordinating movement with the motor cortex. Recent studies indicate that the cerebellum also acts to support limbic functions (such as attention and impulse control) and cognitive processes in the frontal lobe.

> ***The more we study the role of the cerebellum, the more we realize that movement and learning are inescapably linked.***

smaller brain stems and cerebellums and fewer cerebellar neurons. This cerebellar deficit may explain the impaired cognitive and motor functions seen in autism (Courchesne, 1999; Rodier, 2000). Using movement and other intense sensory experiences, therapy centers working with autistic children and those with attention-deficit hyperactivity disorder (ADHD) are reporting remarkable improvement in their ability to focus their attention to complete a task, as well as an increased ability to listen quietly when others share ideas.

Physical Exercise Improves Brain Performance

Even short, moderate physical exercise can improve brain performance. Studies indicate that physical activity increases the number of capillaries in the brain thus facilitating blood transport. It also increases the amount of oxygen in the blood, which the brain needs for fuel. The concentration of oxygen affects the brain's ability to carry out its tasks. Studies confirm that higher concentrations of oxygen in the blood significantly enhanced cognitive performance in healthy young adults. They were able to recall more words from a list and perform visual and spatial tasks faster. Moreover, their cognitive abilities varied directly with the amount of oxygen in the brain (Chung et al., 2004; Scholey et al., 1999).

Despite the realization that physical activity enhances brain function and learning, secondary students spend most of their classroom time sitting. Although enrollment in high school daily physical education classes has risen slightly in recent years, it is only about 25 percent.

Implications for Schools

Armed with the knowledge that movement is connected to cognitive learning, teachers and administrators need to encourage more movement in all classrooms at all grade levels. At some point in every lesson, students should be up and moving about, preferably talking about their new learning. Not only does the movement increase cognitive function, but it also helps students use up some kinesthetic energy—the "wiggles," if you will—so they can settle down and concentrate better later. Mild exercise before a test also makes sense. So does teaching dance to all students in K–8 classrooms. Dance techniques help students become more aware of their physical presence, spatial relationships, breathing, and of timing and rhythm in movement.

> ***At some point in most lessons, students should be up and moving around, talking about the new learning.***

Summarizing the research on the interplay of motion and the cognitive functions of the brain, we should consider using movement activities (Patterson, 1997) because they

- Involve more sensory input, which is likely to hold the students' attention for a longer period of time.
- More closely resemble what students would be doing outside of school. Many students are involved with interesting kinesthetic activities after school. Doing these types of activities in school awakens and maintains that interest.
- Engage other cerebral aptitudes, such as music or visual-spatial skills, thus enhancing integration of sensory perception. This process will help students make connections between new and past learnings.
- Are more likely to lead to long-term recall. You can easily recall that time you participated in the school play or other public performance. Your memory is clear because this experience activated your kinesthetic sensory system.
- Stimulate the right hemisphere and help the student perceive concepts in their totality, rather than in the traditional language patterns (left hemisphere) that are so common.

Teachers can find many ways to weave movement into all lessons: act out a social studies lesson; walk through a map of the world or plot out a geometric formula on the gymnasium floor; use a dance to show the motion of molecules in the different states of matter or the planets in the solar system. See **Practitioner's Corner** on pp. 240–241 for some additional suggestions.

What's Coming Up?

Solving the environmental, social, and economic problems of the 21st century will require plenty of creative thinking and imagination. Are schools doing enough to teach students how to analyze problems, judge competing solutions, and create new answers to old problems? Is the strong emphasis on high-stakes testing really advancing the level of thinking or is it merely stressing the acquisition of more facts? How to foster a classroom that genuinely encourages higher-order thinking, while trying to do everything else, is the subject of the next chapter.

PRACTITIONER'S CORNER

Including the Arts in All Lessons

Including arts activities in any subject and at any grade level can be simple and fun. It doesn't need to be additional work and may substitute for some other activity you usually do.

- **Visual Arts.** Are there components of the lesson that students can draw, sketch, color, or paint? Would a visual arts project be acceptable as an alternative assessment to measure student understanding?
  Example: A science teacher has a student draw a chart to illustrate the important steps in an experiment.

- **Music.** Is there an appropriate song or other musical composition that could be incorporated into the lesson or unit? Remember that music is a very effective memory device. Is there a familiar tune that would help students remember important facts about the unit?
  Example: A social studies teacher has students put important facts about the Revolutionary War to a familiar melody.

- **Literary Device.** Could students write a poem, limerick, or play to illustrate major points in the unit? Rhyming is also an excellent memory tool: "In fourteen hundred ninety-two, Columbus sailed the ocean blue . . ."
  Example: A mathematics teachers has students devise limericks to help them remember the mathematical order of operations.

- **Dance and Theater.** Is there a dance that could help students remember some critical events or information? Can students act out a play that other students wrote?
  Example: An English teacher has students write and act out a different but plausible ending to Shakespeare's *Romeo and Juliet.*

- **Community Artists.** Are there community artists who can demonstrate their skills in the classroom? Teachers working with artists receive on-the-job training, and learn techniques that they can use later on their own.

PRACTITIONER'S CORNER

Using Music in the Classroom

Listening to music in the classroom can promote student focus and productivity at all grade levels. Remember that no one musical selection, nor the volume at which it is played, will please *everyone*. Just ensure that the music played enhances rather than interferes with the situation or task. Here are a few guidelines to consider when planning to use music:

- **When to Play the Music.** Music can be played at different times during the learning episode. Be sure to choose the appropriate music for the particular activity. Music can be played:
  - Before class begins (choose music that sets the emotional mood)
  - When students are up and moving about (choose an upbeat tune)
  - When the students are busy doing seat work, either alone or in groups (choose music that facilitates the learning task)
  - At the end of the class (students leave on a positive note, looking forward to returning)

It is *not* advisable to play music when you are doing direct instruction (unless the music is part of the lesson) because it can be a distraction.

- **Be Aware of Beats Per Minute.** Because music can affect a person's heart rate, blood pressure, and emotional mood, the number of beats per minute in the music is very important. If you are using the music as background to facilitate student work, choose music that plays at about 60 beats per minute (the average heartbeat rate). If the music is accompanying a fast-paced activity, then choose 80 to 90 beats per minute. To calm down a noisy group as, say, in the school cafeteria or commons area, choose music at 40 to 50 beats per minute.

- **With or Without Lyrics?** Using music with or without lyrics depends on the purpose of playing the music. Music played at the beginning or end of class can contain lyrics because the main purpose is to set a mood, not get focus. But if students are working on a learning task, lyrics become a distraction. Some students will try to listen to the lyrics, and others may discuss them—in both instances, they are off the task.

- **Select Familiar or Unfamiliar Music?** Once again, this depends on the music's purpose. Familiar music is fine when setting a mood. However, when working on a specific assignment, you may wish to use music that is unfamiliar. If the students know the background music, some will sing or hum along, causing a distraction. Choose unfamiliar music, such as classical or new age music, and have enough different selections so that they are each played infrequently. Avoid the nature sounds selections as background music because they can be the source of much discussion and controversy. Of course, nature sounds could be used to stimulate discussion in appropriate lesson contexts.

- **Student Input.** Students may ask to bring in their own selections. To maintain a positive classroom climate, tell them that they *can* bring in their music, *provided the selections meet the above criteria.* Explain to them why this is necessary. Some kinds of student music would be appropriate in certain contexts as, for example, to facilitate a student discussion on interpreting music or another art form. In some cases, music may provide just the amount of meaning needed to enhance learning and retention.

- **Suggestions** (from teachers who have tried these, and reported success):

Beginning and end of class:
Vivaldi – *The Four Seasons*
Kenny G – Any selection
Bach – *Brandenburg Concertos*
Yanni – Most selections
The Beach Boys
Chopin – Most selections

Fast-paced activity:
Rock
Disco
Reggae
Hits from the 1950s
Hits from the 1960s
Marches (e.g., Sousa)

Reflection or processing activity:
Beethoven – *Moonlight Sonata*
Pachebel – *Canon in D major*
Mozart – Piano concertos
Enya (New Age) – Most selections
Ray Lynch (New Age) – Any selection
George Winston – *Seasons*
Gary Lamb (Original) – Any selection

Happy listening!

PRACTITIONER'S CORNER

Using Imagery

Imagery runs the gamut from simple concrete pictures to complex motor learning and multistep procedures. Because imagery is still not a common instructional strategy, it should be implemented early and gradually. These guidelines are adapted from Parrott (1986) and West et al. (1991) for using imagery as a powerful aid to understanding and retention.

- **Prompting.** Use prompts for telling students to form mental images of the content being learned. They can be as simple as "form a picture in your mind of . . ." to more complex directions. Prompts should be specific to the content or task and should be accompanied by relevant photographs, charts, or arrays, especially for younger children.

- **Modeling.** Model imagery by describing your own image to the class and explaining how that image helps your recall and use of the current learning. Also, model a procedure and have the students mentally practice the steps.

- **Interaction.** Strive for rich, vivid images where items interact. The richer the image, the more information it can include. If there are two or more items in the images, they should be visualized as acting on each other. If the recall is a ball and a bat, for example, imagine the bat hitting the ball.

- **Reinforcement.** Have students talk about the images they formed and how it helped their learning. Ensure that they get ample feedback from others on the accuracy and vividness of the images.

- **Add Context.** Whenever possible, add context to the interaction to increase retention and recall. For example, if the task is to recall prefixes and suffixes, the context could be a parade with the prefixes in front urging the suffixes in the rear to catch up.

- **Avoid Overloading the Image.** Although good images are complete representations of what is to be remembered, they should not overload the working memory's capacity in older students of about seven items.

PRACTITIONER'S CORNER

Visualized Notetaking

Visualized notetaking is a strategy that encourages students to associate language with visual imagery. It combines on paper sequential verbal information with symbols and holistic visual patterns. Teachers should encourage students to link verbal notes with images and symbols that show sequence, patterns, or relationships. Here are a few examples:

- **Stickperson.** Use the stickperson symbol to remember information about a person or group of people. The student attaches notes about a person in eight areas to the appropriate spot on the stick figure: ideas to the brain; hopes/vision to the eyes; words to the mouth; actions to the hands; feelings to the heart; movement to the feet; weaknesses to the Achilles tendon; and strengths to the arm muscle.

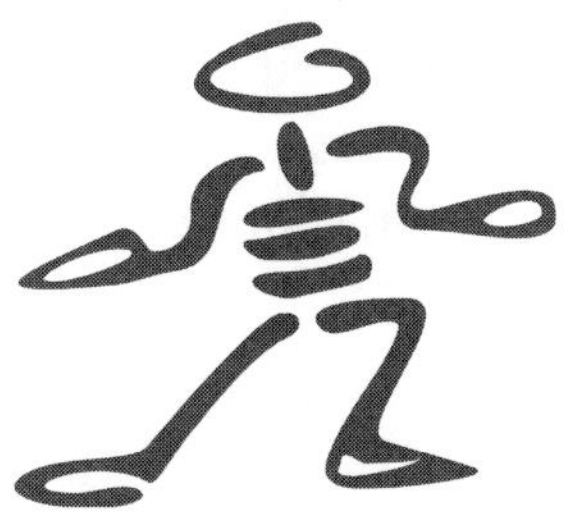

- **Expository Visuals.** These take many forms. Use a set of flow boxes to help students collect and visualize the cause-effect interrelationships for an event. Causes are written in the boxes on the left, the event in the center box, and effects in the boxes on the right. Creating different designs to visualize other topics is a valuable imaging activity.

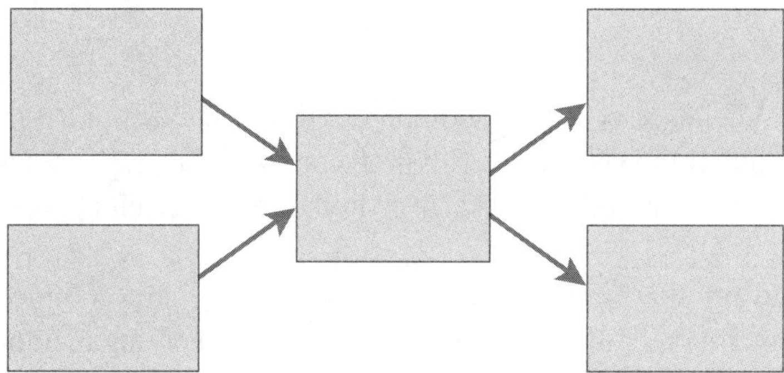

- **Notebook Design.** Even the design of the notebook page can call imagery into play to enhance learning and retention. One variation involves dividing the notebook page into sections for topics, vocabulary, important questions, things to remember, next homework assignment, and next test (see example below). Positioning each area on the page acts as a visual organizer that promotes the use of appropriate symbols.

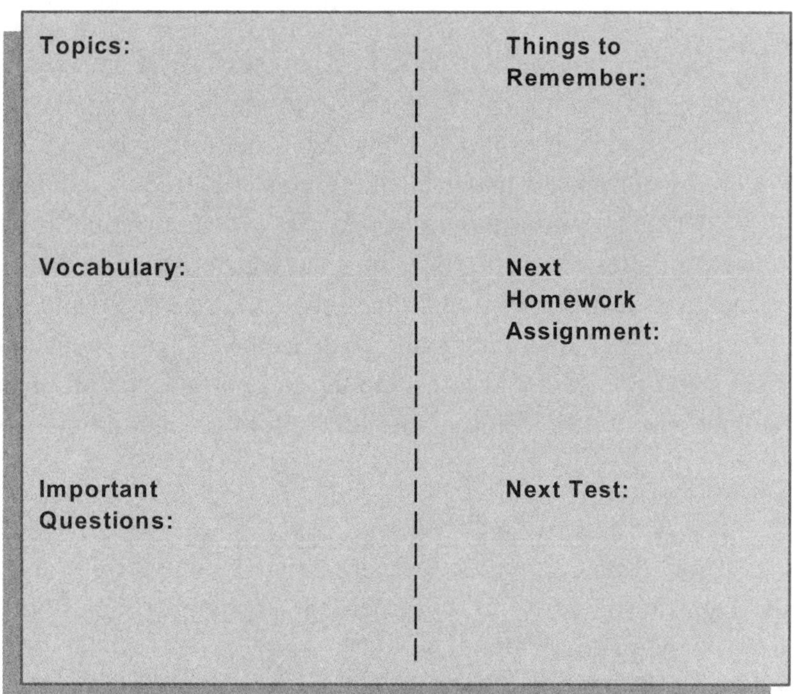

Notebook Pages

- **Mindmapping.** Mind maps are powerful visual tools for remembering relationships between and among parts of a key idea. Using a mind map for notes helps the student see relationships unfolding during the notetaking process. The maps also allow students to look beyond the obvious, make inferences, and discover new knowledge not otherwise possible in the traditional lecture notetaking format. See Buzan (1989) and Hyerle (1996, 2004) for lots of ideas on different ways to draw and use mind maps.

PRACTITIONER'S CORNER

Strategies for Using Movement

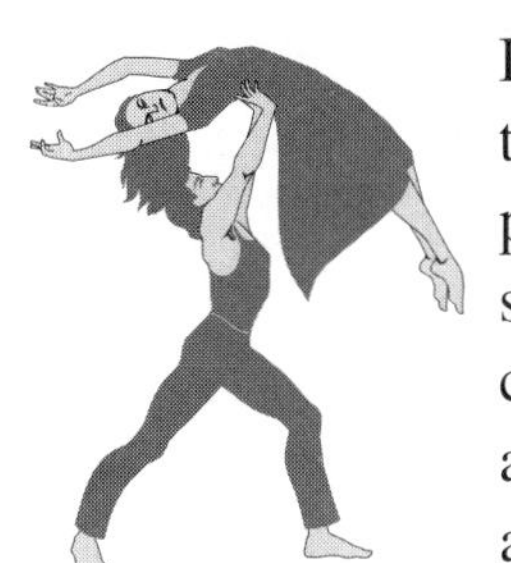

Incorporating movement activities into lessons is interesting and fun for the teacher and the students. Although moving around in class is common in the primary grades, it drops dramatically at the secondary level. Middle and high school teachers are understandably concerned about having adequate time to cover the enormous amount of material in the curriculum. But because trading a few minutes of teacher talk for a movement activity can actually increase the amount of learning retained, it could be a very worthwhile investment of time.

Remember that not many students participate in the physical education program. Yet physical activity is essential to promoting the normal growth of mental function, to generating positive emotions, and in learning and remembering cognitive material. Some suggestions are as follows:

- **Energizers.** Use movement activities to energize students who are at low points in their energy levels (e.g., during early morning periods for high school students or during that downtime just past the middle of the day). For example,

  "Measure the room's length in hand spans."
  "Touch seven objects in the room that are the same color."
  "Go to four different sources of information in this room."
  "In your group, make a poster-sized mind map of this unit."
  "Use ball toss games for review, storytelling, and vocabulary building.

- **Acting Out Key Concepts.** This strategy uses the body in a physical way to learn and remember a difficult concept. If the lesson objective is to learn the continents, try this: Stand in front of a world map. Say the continent and point to the assigned body part (Chapman & King, 2000).

  North America = left hand   Europe = forehead
  Asia = right hand   Africa = waist
  South America = left knee   Australia = right knee
  Antarctica = a point on the floor between the feet

Allow time for practice, then remove the map and repeat the activity.
Is there a difficult concept that you teach that could be acted out?

- **Role-Playing.** Do role-plays on a regular basis. For example, students can organize extemporaneous pantomime or play charades to dramatize major points in a unit. Have them develop and act out short commercials advertising upcoming units or to review previously learned material.

- **Vocabulary Building: Act Out the Word**. Look for vocabulary words that lend themselves to a physical movement. Then,

  a. Say the word
  b. Read the meaning
  c. Do the movement (the movement acts out the meaning of the word).

  For example,

  a. *oppugn*
  b. "to oppose or attack"
  c. make body gestures that indicate "opposing" or "attacking."

  Do the three parts (a, b, and c) three times. This places the information in working memory. Now continue rehearsing the word, and use it in context so that it transfers to long-term memory (Chapman, 1993).

- **Verbal to Physical Tug-of-War.** In this activity, students choose a partner and a topic from the unit they have been learning. Each student forms an opinion about the topic and has 30 seconds to convince a partner why his or her own topic is more important (the verbal tug-of-war). After this debate, the partners separate to opposite sides for a physical tug-of-war with a rope.

Chapter 6—The Brain and the Arts

Key Points to Ponder

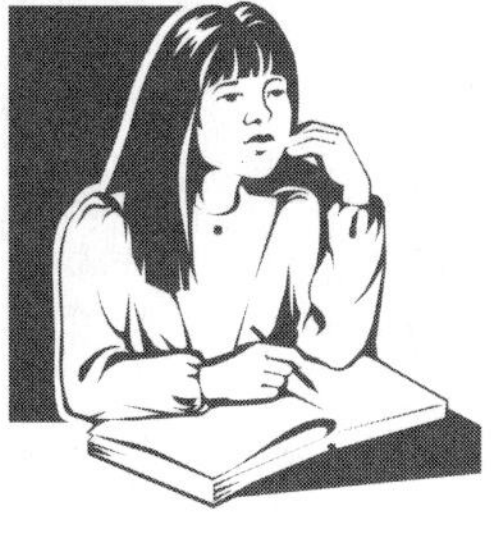

Jot down on this page key points, ideas, strategies, and resources you want to consider later. This sheet is your personal journal summary and will help to jog your memory.

Chapter 7

Thinking Skills and Learning

Too often children are given answers to remember rather than problems to solve.

—Robert Lewin

Chapter Highlights. This chapter discusses some of the characteristics and dimensions of human thinking. It examines the revised Bloom's Taxonomy, notes its continuing compatibility with current research on higher-order thinking, and explains its relationship to difficulty, complexity, and intelligence.

How can something as tangible as the human brain create such phantom things as ideas? How does it create Beethoven's symphonies, Michelangelo's sculptures, and Einstein's universe? What processes translate the countless neuron firings into thoughts and then into products of magnificent beauty or weapons of destruction? The human brain collects information about the world and organizes it to form a representation of that world. This representation, or mental model, describes *thinking,* a process that an individual human uses to function in that world.

CHARACTERISTICS OF HUMAN THINKING

Thinking is easier to describe than to define. Its characteristics include the daily routine of reasoning where one is at the moment, where one's destination is, and how to get there. It includes developing concepts, using words, solving problems, abstracting, intuiting, and anticipating the future. Other aspects of thinking include learning, memory, creativity, communication, logic, and generalization. How and when we use these aspects often determine the success or failure of our many interactions with our environment. This chapter discusses thinking, explores strategies that attempt to describe the characteristics of various types of thinking, and suggests how they can be used in the classroom to promote higher-order thinking and learning.

Types of Thinking

Can you answer these questions?

- Who was the second president of the United States?
- What are the similarities and differences between the post-Civil War and post-Vietnam War periods?
- Defend why we should or should not have capital punishment.

Each of these questions requires you to think, but the type of thinking involved is not the same. The first question requires you to simply refer to a listing you have in long-term memory that recalls the sequence of presidents. Dealing with the second question is quite different. You must first recall what you have stored about both wars, separate these items into lists, then analyze them to determine which events were similar and which were different. The third question requires the retrieval and processing of large amounts of information about capital punishment, its impact on society, and its effectiveness as a deterrent to crime. Then you need to form a judgment about whether you believe criminals will be influenced by a capital punishment penalty. These three questions require different and increasingly complex thought processes to arrive at acceptable answers. Thus, some thinking is more complex than other thinking. Brain scans indicate that different parts of the brain, particularly in the frontal cortex, are involved as the problem-solving task becomes more complicated (Goldberg, 2001; Jausovec & Jausovec, 2000).

Brain scans show that different parts of the brain are involved as the problem-solving task becomes more complicated.

The brain has evolved different mechanisms for dealing with various situations. Logic is one of those. It recognizes, for example, that if A is equal to B, and B is equal to C, then A must be equal to C. There are other mechanisms, too. Rationality, pattern identification, image making, and approximation are all forms of thinking that serve to help the individual deal with a concept, a problem, or a decision.

Thinking as a Representational System

Although the file cabinets and their ordered system are useful metaphors for explaining the operation of long-term storage in the information processing model (Chapter 2), they do not explain all the situations one encounters when the brain behaves as a representational system. Sometimes we cannot recognize a person's face, but we remember the name and the events that surrounded our first meeting with this person. And just thinking of the word *beach* evokes a complex series of mental events that corresponds to the internal representation we have of all the beaches we have ever encountered. Beaches gleam in the sun, are often hot, create a shoreline, merge with water, are dotted with umbrellas, and recall memories of holiday fun. The word itself is not actually a beach, but it brings forth many associations having to do with beaches. This is an example of a representational system, and it illustrates the diversity of patterns in human thinking. It is this recognition of diversity that has led to the notion of multiple intelligences. That is, an individual's thinking patterns vary when encountering different challenges, and these semiautonomous variations in thinking result in different degrees of success in learning.

Thinking and Emotion

Emotions play an important role in the thinking process. In Chapter 2, we discussed the amygdala's role in encoding emotional messages into long-term memory. We also noted that emotions often take precedence during cerebral processing and can impede or assist cognitive learning. If we like what we are learning, we are more likely to maintain attention and interest and move to higher-level thinking. We tend to probe and ask those "what if?" kinds of questions. When we dislike the learning, we usually spend the least amount of time with it and stay at minimal levels of processing. That's why the classroom's emotional climate is so important.

Students sometimes feel neutral about a new learning topic. Challenging them with activities that require higher-order thinking often sparks an interest that brings forth positive feelings. Recent studies reaffirm that as learners generate positive emotions, their scope of attention broadens and their critical thinking skills are enhanced. Neutral and negative emotions, on the other hand, narrow the scope of attention and thinking (Fredrickson & Branigan, 2005). When students recognize the power of their own thinking, they use their skills more and solve problems for themselves rather than just waiting to be told the answers.

THE DIMENSIONS OF HUMAN THINKING

Designing Models

Cognitive psychologists have been designing models for decades in an effort to describe the dimensions of thinking and the levels of complexity of human thought. The models have generally divided thought into two categories, *convergent* or lower-order thinking and *divergent* or higher-order thinking. Other multidimensional frameworks have appeared that attempt to describe all aspects of thinking in detail. Of course, a model is only as good as its potential for achieving a desired goal (in this case, encouraging higher-order thinking in students) and the likelihood that teachers feel sufficiently comfortable with the model to make it a regular part of their classroom practice. In examining the models that describe the dimensions of thinking, most include the following major areas:

- **Basic processes** are the tools we use to transform and evaluate information, such as:
  Observing: includes recognizing and recalling.
  Finding patterns and generalizing: includes classifying, comparing and contrasting, and identifying relevant and irrelevant information.
  Forming conclusions based on patterns: includes hypothesizing, predicting, inferring, and applying.
  Assessing conclusions based on observations: includes checking consistency, identifying biases and stereotypes, identifying unstated assumptions, recognizing over- and under-generalizations, and confirming conclusions with facts.

The consistency with which these basic processes appear in most models results from the recognition that they allow us to make sense of our world by pulling together bits of information into understandable and coherent patterns. Further, these processes support the notion that conclusions should be based on evidence. From these conclusions, we form patterns that help us to hypothesize, infer, and predict.

- **Domain-specific knowledge** refers to the knowledge in a particular content area that one must possess in order to carry out the basic processes described above.
- **Critical thinking** is a complex process that is based on objective standards and consistency. It includes making judgments using objective criteria and offering opinions with reasons.
- **Creative thinking** involves putting together information to arrive at a whole new concept, idea, or understanding. It often involves four stages that include preparation (gathering and examining the needed information), incubation (mulling over the idea and making connections to other experiences), illumination (the "Aha!" when the new idea comes to light), and verification (methods for testing the idea).
- **Metacognition** is the awareness one has of one's own thinking processes. It means that students should know when and why they are using the basic processes, and how these functions relate to the content they are learning. Metacognition consists of two processes occurring simultaneously: monitoring progress while learning, and making appropriate changes when problems occur during learning.

Are We Teaching Thinking Skills?

The ordinary experience of thinking about that sunny beach raises intriguing questions about how the brain is organized to think with increasing complexity. What skills does the human brain need to maneuver through simple and complex thoughts? Can these skills be learned and, if so, how and when should they be taught?

Most humans are born with a brain that has all the sensory components and neural organization necessary to survive successfully in its environment. The neural organization changes dramatically, of course, as the child grows and learns, resulting in the expansion of some networks and the elimination of others. Even the most superficial look at human information processing reveals a vast system of magnificent neural networks that can learn language, recognize one face among thousands, and infer an outcome by rapidly analyzing data. Every bit of evidence available suggests that the human brain is *designed* for a broad range of thinking patterns. So if the brain is capable of higher-order thinking, why do we see so little of it in the normal course of student discussion and performance?

It just may be that the reason our students are not thinking critically is that we have not exposed them consistently to models or situations in school that require them to do so. Schooling, for the most part, still demands little more than several levels of convergent thinking. Its practices and testing focus on content acquisition through rote rehearsal, rather than the processes of thinking for analysis and synthesis. Even those teachers who have worked conscientiously to include activities requiring higher-order thinking are confronted with the realities of preparing students for high stakes testing that usually focuses on recall and application. Repeating the answer becomes more important than the process used to get the answer. Consequently, students and teachers frequently deal with learning at the lower levels of complexity.

> ***We do not teach the brain to think. We can, however, help learners to organize content to facilitate more complex processing.***

What we are trying to do now is recognize these limitations, rewrite curriculum, retrain teachers, and encourage students to use their innate thinking abilities to process learning at higher levels of complexity. In other words, we need to work harder at teaching them *how to organize content in such a way that it facilitates and promotes higher-order thinking.*

Modeling Thinking Skills in the Classroom

Teachers serve as valuable and authentic role models when they use creative and critical reflection to improve their practice. Students are more likely to learn thinking skills in classrooms where teachers nurture a love for learning and establish a setting that is conducive to creative and critical thought. Such a positive learning climate emerges when teachers:

- Exhibit genuine interest and commitment to learning
- Analyze their own thinking processes and classroom practices and explain what they do
- Change their own positions when the evidence warrants it
- Are willing to admit a mistake
- Allow students to participate in setting rules and making decisions related to learning and assessment

- Encourage students to follow their own thinking and not just repeat the teacher's views
- Allow students to select assignments and activities from a range of appropriate choices
- Prepare and present lessons that require higher-order thinking to achieve learning objectives

Having established a classroom environment that fosters higher-level thinking, the teacher's next task is to select a practical and easily understood model for teaching students the skills they need for creative, critical, and divergent thinking. Of all the current models available, let's look at a very workable and effective design that has stood the test of time—Bloom's Taxonomy.

REVISITING BLOOM'S TAXONOMY OF THE COGNITIVE DOMAIN

What model can teachers use that, when properly implemented, promotes thinking, has been successful in the past, and holds the promise of success for the future? My suggestion is to start with the taxonomy of the cognitive domain developed about 50 years ago by Benjamin Bloom, and see if we can adapt it to the needs of the modern era. Some readers may be thinking "Oh, no, not Bloom again!" Perhaps some newer teachers are asking, "Who's Bloom?" Regardless of your response, I hope you will bear with me to learn why this model may continue to form the basis for successful classroom activities that promote higher-order thinking.

Why do I continue to propose this type of model? In recent years, I have seen the spread of state-adopted curriculum standards, the mandates of the No Child Left Behind Act, a greater emphasis on state and national testing, and an intense public insistence that school and teacher accountability be measured in test scores. Consequently, teachers who are under pressure to teach to the test are not likely to implement overly complicated, multi-level thinking skills programs. That is why I am comfortable proposing that we reexamine this familiar model and decide how, with some adjustments, it can still serve our needs. My aim is to convince you of its value in aiding less able students experience the excitement of higher-order thinking and the exhilaration of greater achievement.

Why Start With This Model?

One of the more enduring and useful models for enhancing thinking was developed by Benjamin Bloom and his colleagues in the 1950s. Bloom's system of classification, or taxonomy, identifies six levels of complexity of human thought (Bloom, Engelhart, Furst, Hill, & Krathwohl, 1956). I believe that with some revisions, this framework can upgrade the quality of teacher instruction and student learning for the following reasons:

- It is familiar to many prospective and practicing teachers.
- It is user-friendly and simple when compared to other models.
- It provides a common language about learning objectives that cuts across subject matter and grade levels.

- It requires only modest retraining for teachers to understand the relationship between the difficulty and complexity components.
- It helps teachers recognize the difference between difficulty and complexity, so they can help slower learners improve their thinking and achievement significantly.
- It can be implemented in every classroom immediately without waiting for major reform or restructuring.
- It is inexpensive in that teachers need only a few supplementary materials to use with the current curriculum.
- It motivates teachers because they see their students learning better, thinking more profoundly, and showing more interest.
- With revisions, it can reflect fairly well the latest research on brain functions.

I know that Bloom's Taxonomy has been standard fare in preservice and inservice teacher training for many years. Yet I suspect, as Bloom himself had conjectured, that the taxonomy's value as a model for moving all students to higher levels of thinking has not been fully explored. In fact, my experience recently has been that, although most teachers remember this model, they have little enthusiasm for it in the current atmosphere that emphasizes preparing students for high stakes tests at the expense of promoting higher-order thinking and learning. Moreover, as we will discuss later, the taxonomy's connection to student ability has been largely misunderstood and misapplied. This situation is regrettable because the model is easy to understand and, when used correctly, can accelerate learning and elevate student interest and achievement, especially for slower learners.

> ***With revisions, Bloom's Taxonomy can still be a useful tool for moving students, especially slower learners, to higher levels of thinking.***

The Model's Structure and Revision

Bloom's original taxonomy contained six levels that many readers can no doubt recite from memory. Moving from the least to the most complex, they are: knowledge, comprehension, application, analysis, synthesis, and evaluation (Figure 7.1). From 1995 through 2000, a group of educators worked to revise the original taxonomy based on more recent understandings about learning. The group published the results of their work in 2001 and the basic revision is shown in Figure 7.2 (Anderson et al., 2001).

Revising the taxonomy provided the opportunity to rename three categories and interchange two of them, as well as change the names of all levels to the

Levels of Bloom's Taxonomy

Original Version (1956)

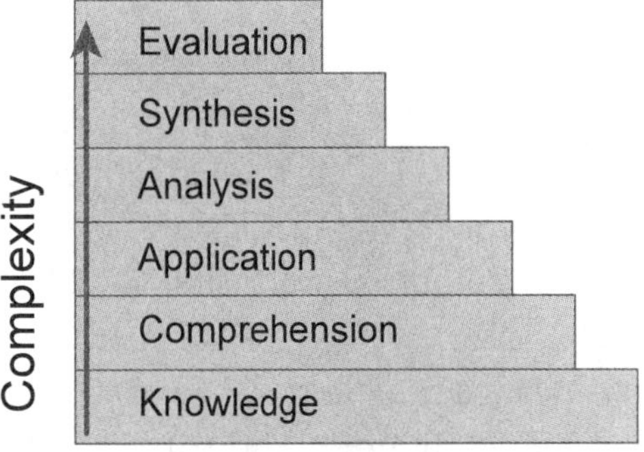

Figure 7.1 Bloom's original taxonomy had six levels from knowledge (lowest complexity) to evaluation (highest complexity).

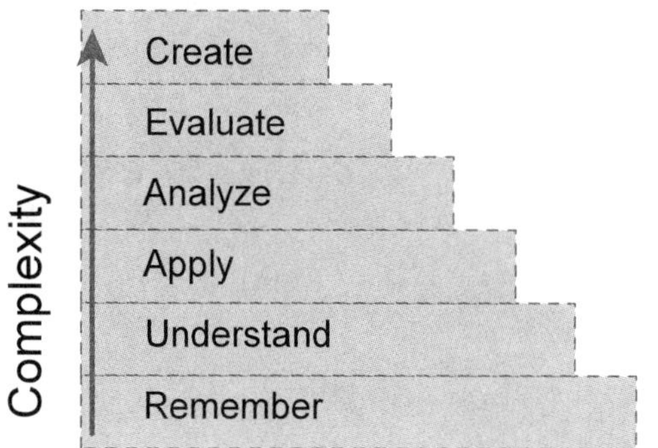

Figure 7.2 The revised taxonomy retains the six levels but changes the labels to verb form, renames three levels, and interchanges the top two levels. The dotted outline suggests a more open and fluid model, recognizing that an individual may move among the levels during extended processing.

verb form to fit the way they are used in learning objectives. The original *Knowledge* level was renamed *Remember* because it more accurately describes the recall process occurring at this level. Also, knowledge can be acquired at *all* levels. *Comprehension* was renamed *Understand* because that is the term most commonly used when teachers discuss this level. *Application, Analysis,* and *Evaluation* were changed to the verbs *Apply, Analyze,* and *Evaluate.*

Synthesis changed places with *Evaluation* and was renamed *Create.* This exchange was made because the researchers felt that recent studies in cognitive neuroscience suggest that generating, planning, and producing an original product demands more complex thinking than making judgments based on accepted criteria (Table 7.1). Although there are still six separate levels, the hierarchy of complexity is not as rigid, and it recognizes that an individual may move easily among the levels during extended processing.

Below is a review of each level using the story of *Goldilocks* and the bombing of Pearl Harbor as examples of how two differing concepts can be taken through the taxonomy.

Remember. Remember refers to the mere rote recall and recognition of previously learned material, from specific facts to a definition or a complete theory. All that is required is bringing it forth from long-term memory in the form in which it was learned. This is recall of semantic memory. It represents the lowest level of learning in the cognitive domain because there is no presumption that the learner understands what is being recalled. Students in first grade recite the Pledge of Allegiance daily. Do they all comprehend what they are saying? If so, would one fine, patriotic boy have started his pledge with, *I led the pigeons to the flag of the United . . .* ?

Examples: What did Goldilocks do in the three bears' house?
What was the date of the bombing of Pearl Harbor?

Understand. This level describes the ability to make sense of the material. Understanding may occur by converting the material from one form to another (words to numbers), by interpreting the material (summarizing a story), or by estimating future trends (predicting the consequences or effects). The learning goes beyond mere rote recall and represents the lowest level of comprehension. When a student understands the material, rather than merely recalling it, the material becomes available for future use to solve problems and to make decisions. Questions at this level attempt to determine if the students comprehend the information in a sensible way. When this happens, students may say, "Now I get it."

Table 7.1 Revision of Bloom's Taxonomy of the Cognitive Domain

Below are the levels in decreasing order of complexity with terms and sample activities that illustrate the thought processes at each level.

Level	Terms	Sample Activities
Create	imagine compose design infer	Pretend you were a participant in the Boston Tea Party and write a diary entry that tells what happened. Rewrite *Little Red Riding Hood* as a news story. Design a different way of solving this problem. Formulate a hypothesis that might explain the results of these three experiments.
Evaluate	appraise assess judge critique	Which of the two main characters in the story would you rather have as a friend? Why? Is violence ever justified in correcting injustices? Why or why not? Which of the environments we've studied seems like the best place for you to live? Defend your answer. Critique these two products and defend which one you would recommend to the consumer.
Analyze	analyze contrast distinguish deduce	Which events in the story are fantasy and which really happened? Compare and contrast the post–Civil War period with the post–Vietnam War period. Sort this collection of rocks into three categories. Which of these words are Latin derivatives and which are Greek?
Apply	practice calculate apply execute	Use each vocabulary word in a new sentence. Calculate the area of your classroom. Think of three situations in which we would use this mathematics operation. Use the parts to reassemble this motor correctly.
Understand	summarize discuss explain outline	Summarize the paragraph in your own words. Why are symbols used on maps? Write a paragraph explaining the duties of the mayor. Outline the steps for completing this experiment.
Remember	define label recall recognize	What is the definition of a verb? Label the three symbols on this map. What are the three branches of government? Which object in the picture is a xylophone?

Source: Adapted from Anderson et al., 2001

Examples: Why did Goldilocks like the baby bear's things best?
Why did the Japanese bomb Pearl Harbor?

Apply. This level refers to the ability to use learned material in new situations with a minimum of direction. It includes the application of such things as rules, concepts, methods, and theories to solve problems. The learner activates procedural memory and uses convergent thinking to select, transfer, and apply data to complete a new task. Practice is essential at this level.

Examples: If Goldilocks came to your house today, what things might she do? If you had been responsible for the defense of the Hawaiian Islands, what preparation would you have made against an attack?

Analyze. This is the ability to break material into its component parts so that its structure may be understood. It includes identifying parts, examining the relationships of the parts to each other and to the whole, and recognizing the organizational principles involved. The learner must be able to organize and reorganize information into categories. The brain's frontal lobes are working hard at this level. This stage is more complex because the learner is aware of the thought process in use (metacognition) and understands both the content and structure of the material.

Examples: What things in the Goldilocks story could have really happened?
What lesson did our country learn from Pearl Harbor?

Evaluate. This level deals with the ability to judge the value of material based on specific criteria and standards. The learner may determine the criteria or be given them. The learner examines criteria from several categories and selects those that are the most relevant to the situation. Activities at this level almost always have multiple and equally acceptable solutions. This is a high level of cognitive thought because it contains elements of many other levels, plus conscious judgments based on definite criteria. At this level, learners tend to consolidate their thinking and become more receptive to other points of view.

Examples: Do you think it was right for Goldilocks to go into the bears' house without having been invited? Why or why not?
Do you feel that the bombing of Pearl Harbor has any effect on Japanese-American relations today? Why or why not?

Create. This refers to the ability to put parts together to form a plan that is new to the learner. It may involve the production of a unique communication (essay or speech), a plan of operations (research proposal), or a scheme for classifying information. This level stresses creativity, with major emphasis on forming *new* patterns or structures. This is the level where learners use divergent thinking to get an *Aha!* experience. It indicates that being creative requires a great deal of information, understanding, and application to produce a tangible product. Michelangelo could never have created the *David* or the *Pietà* without a thorough comprehension of human anatomy and types of marble, as well as the ability to use polishing compounds and tools with accuracy. His artistry comes from the mastery with which he used his knowledge and skill to carve magnificent pieces. Although most often associated with the arts, this process can occur in all areas of the curriculum (see Chapter 6).

Examples: Retell the story as *Goldilocks and the Three Fishes.*
Retell the story of Pearl Harbor assuming the U.S. armed forces had been ready for the attack.

Test Question No. 10: Bloom's Taxonomy has not changed over the years.

Answer: False. In 2001, a team of researchers and psychologists published a revision of Bloom's Taxonomy that aligned it more closely with current research and usage.

Important Characteristics of the Revised Model

Several points need to be made here about the revision, especially in light of recent discoveries in how the brain processes information.

Loosening of the Hierarchy

Bloom's original model held that the six levels were cumulative, that is, each level above the lowest required all the skills of lesser complexity. To Bloom, a learner could not comprehend material without mentally possessing it. Similarly, one could not correctly apply a learning to new situations without understanding it. However, because the 2001 revision gives much greater weight to teacher choice and usage, the strict hierarchy has been loosened to allow levels to overlap one another. For example, certain forms of explaining, usually associated with *Understand,* might be more complex than executing, which is associated with *Apply.*

Moreover, this loosening is more consistent with recent evidence from brain research showing that different brain areas are used to solve different types of problems. One study using PET scans found that problems requiring deductive reasoning activated areas in the right hemisphere while problems involving inductive reasoning stimulated areas in the left hemisphere (Parsons & Osherson, 2001). Another study using EEG found that different cerebral regions were involved in solving problems of logic and sequence rather than in solving open-ended problems with multiple answers (Jausovec & Jausovec, 2000). This evidence tends to weaken Bloom's basic notion that one type of thinking is dependent on the prior activation of lower level thinking. But cognitive psychologists have long suspected that thinking skills at the upper levels were a lot more fluid than Bloom's rigid hierarchy suggested. Nonetheless, the experimental findings support the notion that there are different types of thinking which the revised taxonomy accurately describes.

Cognitive and Emotional Thinking

It is important to remember that this is a model to describe the *cognitive* processing of information that poses no immediate danger to the learner. It is *not* intended to describe *emotional* thinking, which often occurs without cognitive input. For example, when a stranger walks near you on a dark street, the amygdala in your brain immediately evaluates the environmental stimuli to determine if a threat exists. The amygdala reacts to a threatening voice or menacing look, often triggering a fight-or-flight reaction. In this situation, the individual's brain is evaluating without the benefit of conscious thought. There is no time for remembering, understanding, applying, or analyzing. Let's just get out of here! The taxonomy is not appropriate here because it addresses conscious and deliberate cognitive thought, not survival behavior.

Other Ways to View the Levels

To align the revised taxonomy more with recent studies on cognitive processing, it is helpful to look at other ways of describing the levels. For example, the lower three levels (*Remember, Understand,* and *Apply*) describe a *convergent* thinking process whereby the learner recalls and focuses what is known and comprehended to solve a problem through application. The upper three levels (*Analyze, Evaluate,* and *Create*) describe a *divergent* thinking process, because the learner's processing results in new insights and discoveries that were not part of the original information. When the learner is thinking at these upper levels, thought flows naturally from one to the other and the boundaries disappear.

Another approach is to view *Remember* and *Understand* as skills designed to acquire and understand information and *Apply* and *Analyze* as skills for changing and transforming information through deduction and inference. The skills at *Evaluate* and *Create* generate new information by appraising, critiquing, and imagining. Even here, one must remember that the levels are fluid and overlap.

Testing Your Understanding of the Taxonomy

To determine if you understand the revised taxonomy's six different levels, complete the activity below. Then, look at the answers and explanation following the activity.

Directions. Identify the highest level (remember, the levels are cumulative) of the taxonomy indicated in these learning objectives.

1. Given a ruler to measure the room, find how long the room is.
2. What is the Sixth Amendment to the U.S. Constitution?
3. Given copies of the Articles of Confederation and the Bill of Rights, the learner will write a comparison of the two documents and discuss similarities and differences.
4. Identify and write a question for each level of the taxonomy.
5. Use your own words to explain the moral at the end of the fable.
6. Given two ways to solve the problem, the learner will make a choice of which to use and give reasons.
7. Write your own fairy tale including all the characteristics of a fairy tale.

Answers:

1. *Apply.* The learner must know the measuring system, comprehend the meaning of length, and use the ruler correctly.
2. *Remember.* The learner simply recalls that the Sixth Amendment deals with the rights of the accused.
3. *Analyze.* The learner must separate both documents into their component parts and compare and contrast them for relationships that describe their similarities and differences.
4. *Apply.* The learner knows each level, comprehends its definition, then uses this information to write the question for each level.
5. *Understand.* The learner shows comprehension by explaining the fable's moral.
6. *Evaluate.* The learner chooses between two feasible options and explains the reasons for the choice.
7. *Create.* Using the general characteristics of fairy tales, the learner creates a new one.

The Taxonomy and the Dimensions of Thinking

To what extent does the revision of Bloom's taxonomy address the major areas mentioned earlier that are included within most of the current models describing the dimensions of thinking?

Basic Processes. The six levels of the revised taxonomy cover all the skills included under these processes. *Observing* is contained in the levels of *Remember* and *Understand. Finding patterns* and *generalizing* are skills in the levels of *Remember, Understand,* and *Analyze.* Forming conclusions based on patterns is in *Analyze* and *Create.* Finally, *assessing conclusions* is a characteristic of the taxonomy's *Evaluate* level.

Domain-Specific Knowledge. The revised taxonomy recognizes that the acquisition of knowledge occurs at all levels. It specifically separates this domain into four types of knowledge: factual (names, dates), conceptual (ideas, patterns), procedural (steps, sequences), and metacognitive (reflections on thought processes).

Critical Thinking. The upper levels of the taxonomy require critical thinking in order to analyze, contrast, criticize, and assess information.

Creative Thinking. Students working diligently at the *Create* level are using all the skills associated with creative thinking.

Metacognition. This is the one area that is not explicitly cited in any one of the six levels. Nonetheless, when analyzing or discussing the rationale for selecting from among equally viable choices at the *Evaluate* level, the learner has to reflect on the processes used to arrive at the selection and gather data to defend the choice. This self-awareness of the thinking process used is the essence of metacognition. The other components, such as having a respect for self-monitoring as a valued skill, a positive and personal attitude toward learning, and an attention to learning through introspection and practice, are very likely to result from the accurate, frequent, and systematic use of the taxonomy's upper levels.

The Critical Difference Between Complexity and Difficulty

Complexity and difficulty describe different mental operations, but are often used synonymously. This error, resulting in the two factors being treated as one, limits the use of the taxonomy to enhance the thinking of all students. By recognizing how these concepts are different, the teacher can gain valuable insight into the connection between the taxonomy and student ability. *Complexity* describes the *thought process* that the brain uses to deal with information. In the revision of Bloom's Taxonomy (Table 7.1), it can be described by any of the six words representing the six levels. For example, the question, "What is the capital of Rhode Island?" is at the *Remember* level, while the question "Tell me in your own words what is meant by a state capital" is at the *Understand* level. The second question is more *complex* than the first because it is at a higher level in the taxonomy.

Difficulty, on the other hand, refers to the *amount of effort* that the learner must expend *within* a level of complexity to accomplish a learning objective. It is possible for a learning activity to become increasingly difficult without becoming more complex. For example, the task "Name the states of the Union" is at the *Remember* level of complexity because it involves simple recall (semantic memory) for most students. Similarly, the task "Name the states of the Union and their capitals" is also at the *Remember* level, but is more difficult than the prior question because it involves more effort to recall additional information. Similarly, the task "Name the states and their capitals in order of their admission to the Union" is still at the *Remember* level, but it is considerably more difficult than the first two. It requires gathering more information and then sequencing it in chronological order.

Teachers are more likely to increase difficulty, rather than complexity, when attempting to raise student thinking.

These are examples of how students can exert great effort to achieve a learning task while processing at the lowest level of thinking. When seeking to challenge students, classroom teachers are more likely (perhaps unwittingly) to increase difficulty rather than complexity as the challenge mode. This may be because they do not recognize the difference between these concepts or that they believe that difficulty is the method for achieving higher-order thinking (Figure 7.3).

Connecting Complexity and Difficulty to Ability

When teachers are asked whether complexity or difficulty is more closely linked to student ability, they more often choose complexity. Some explain their belief that only students of higher ability can carry out the processes indicated in the *Analyze, Evaluate,* and *Create* levels. Others say that whenever they have tried to bring slower students up the taxonomy, the lesson got bogged down. But the real connection to ability is difficulty, not complexity.

The mistaken link between complexity and ability is the result of an unintended but very real self-fulfilling prophesy. Here's how it works. Teachers allot a certain amount of *time* for the class to learn a concept, usually based on how long they think it will take the *average* student to learn it

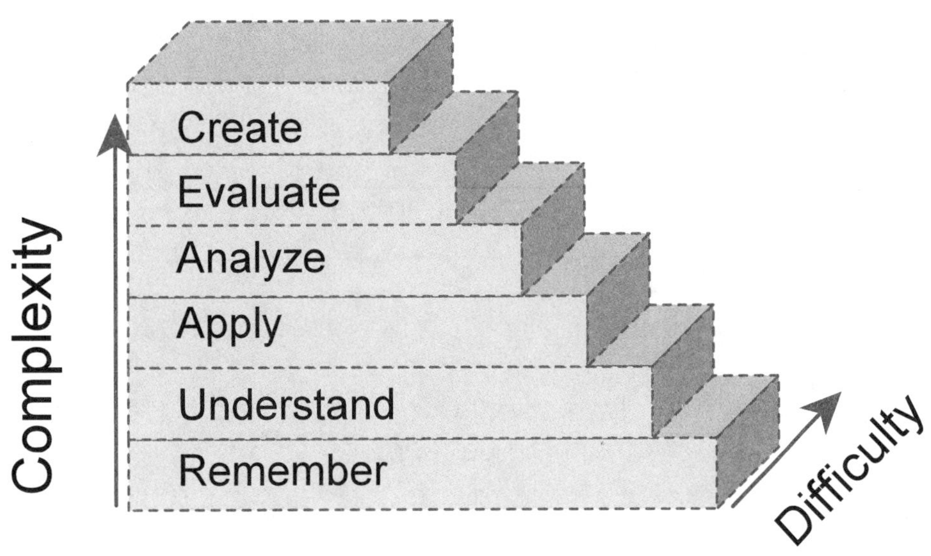

Figure 7.3 Complexity and difficulty are different. Complexity establishes the level of thought while difficulty determines the amount of effort required within each level.

(Figure 7.4). The fast learners learn the concept in less than the allotted time. During the remaining time, their brains often sort the concept's sublearnings into important and unimportant categories, that is, they select the critical attributes for storage and discard what they decide is unimportant. This explains why fast learners are usually fast retrievers: They have not cluttered their memory networks with trivia.

Meanwhile, the slower learners need more than the allotted time to learn the concept. If that time is not given to them, not only do they lose part of the sublearnings but they also do not have time to do any sorting. If the teacher attempts to move up the taxonomy, the fast learners have the concept's more important attributes in working memory to use appropriately and successfully at the higher levels of complexity. The slow learners, on the other hand, have not had time to sort, have cluttered their working memory with all the sublearnings (important and unimportant), and do not recognize the parts needed for more complex processing. For them, it is like taking five big suitcases on an overnight trip, whereas the fast learners have taken just a small bag packed with the essentials. As a result, teachers become convinced that higher-order thinking is for the fast learners and that ability is linked to complexity.

> ***With guidance and practice, slower learners can regularly reach the higher levels of Bloom's revised taxonomy.***

Bloom reported on studies that included slower students for whom the unimportant material was not even taught. The curriculum was sorted from the start, and the focus was on

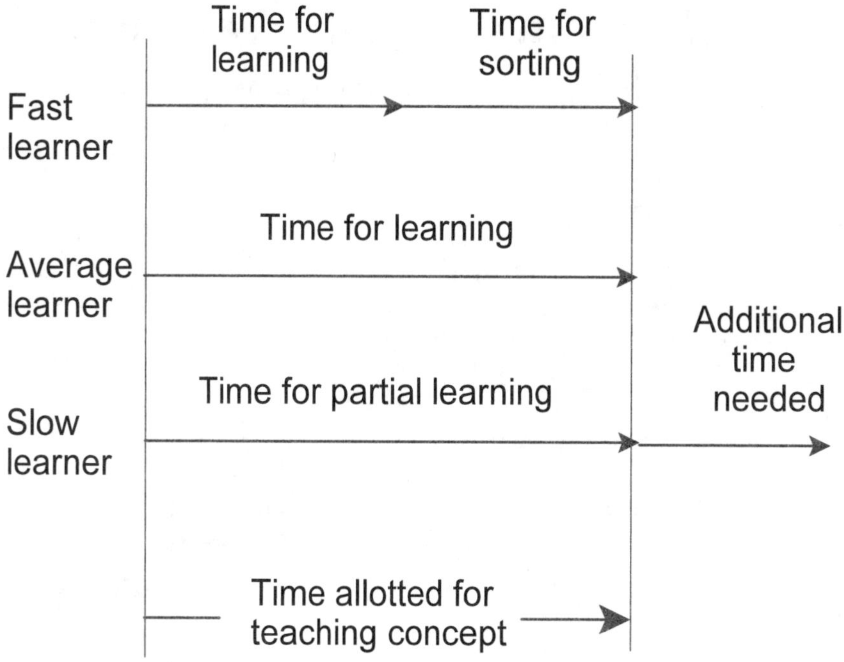

Figure 7.4 The time allotted to learn a concept is usually fixed even though students learn at different rates.

critical attributes and other vital information. When the teacher moved up the taxonomy, these students in some cases demonstrated better achievement than the control groups (Bloom, 1976). When teachers differentiate between complexity and difficulty, a new view of Bloom's Taxonomy emerges, one which promises more success for more students.

The Taxonomy and Constructivism

In their description of the characteristics of constructivist teachers, Brooks and Brooks (1993) noted that these teachers ask open-ended questions and continually encourage students to analyze, evaluate, and create. From this description, it seems evident that teachers who constantly use the upper levels of Bloom's revised taxonomy are demonstrating, among other things, constructivist behaviors.

Curriculum Changes to Accommodate the Taxonomy

The implications from these studies are very significant in that they suggest two important things about using the taxonomy.

- If teachers avoid the self-fulfilling prophecy snare, they can get slower learners to do higher-order thinking successfully and often.

- One way to accomplish this is to review the curriculum and remove the topics of least importance in order to gain the time needed for practice at the higher levels. An effective method for doing this pruning is to list among all the concepts in a curriculum in order of most important to least. Delete the least important bottom 20 to 25 percent, and use the time gained by this sorting and paring to move all students up the taxonomy. Finally, take advantage of the power of positive transfer by integrating these concepts with previously taught material and connecting them to appropriate concepts in other curriculum areas.

Higher-Order Thinking Increases Understanding and Retention

The number of neurons in our brains declines as we age, but our ability to learn, remember, and recall is dependent largely on the number of connections between neurons. The stability and permanency of these connections reflect the nature of the thinking process and the type and degree of rehearsal that occurred during the learning episode.

> ***Our students would make a quantum leap to higher-order thinking if every teacher in every classroom correctly and regularly used a model such as Bloom's revised taxonomy.***

As mentioned earlier, PET scans show that elaborative rehearsal, involving higher-order thinking skills, engages the brain's frontal lobe. This engagement helps learners make connections between past and new learning, creates new pathways, strengthens existing pathways, and increases the likelihood that the new learning will be consolidated and stored for future retrieval.

Many teachers recognize the need to do more activities that require elaborate thinking rather than just rote rehearsal. They admit that when they move up through higher levels of Bloom's Taxonomy (or any other thinking skills framework) students demonstrate a much greater depth of understanding. However, they also admit that there are barriers to using this approach regularly because it takes more time. Examples of the barriers they cite are the pressures to cover an ever-expanding curriculum and the tyranny of quick-answer testing of all types. These obstacles will not be overcome easily, but teachers can work toward a compromise—finding ways to engage the novel brain with challenging activities and developing alternative assessment strategies.

Other Thinking Skills Programs

Other thinking skills programs and models exist, and new ones are appearing regularly. My analysis of them is that they can be very useful after extensive teacher training, substantial curricular reform, and sizable investments for new curriculum materials. Some programs assert that even Bloom's revised taxonomy is too restrictive and does not include other important thinking skills. Yet in reviewing these programs, I have not found one thinking skill that cannot be associated with at least one level of the revised taxonomy. In most of these programs, the difference is in how the skills are labeled and organized. Consequently, I am convinced that if every teacher correctly used the revised taxonomy in every classroom and in every subject area, our students would make a quantum leap forward in their ability to do higher-order thinking. And they can do this now while waiting for more comprehensive reform efforts to become reality.

What's Coming Up?

Now that we have looked at important aspects of how the brain learns and remembers, the next step is to consolidate this information into a workable design for planning lessons. What components should be included in a lesson? What questions should teachers be asking when considering content and strategies for instruction? How do teachers get the support they need in their school to try out new techniques and to keep abreast of what we are learning about learning? The answers to these vital questions are coming up in the next chapter.

PRACTITIONER'S CORNER

Understanding Bloom's Revised Taxonomy

Directions: With a partner, explain verbally what the pictorial view below is all about. Then fill in the chart on the next page, using the explanation of the pictures to describe your thought processing at each level of the taxonomy.

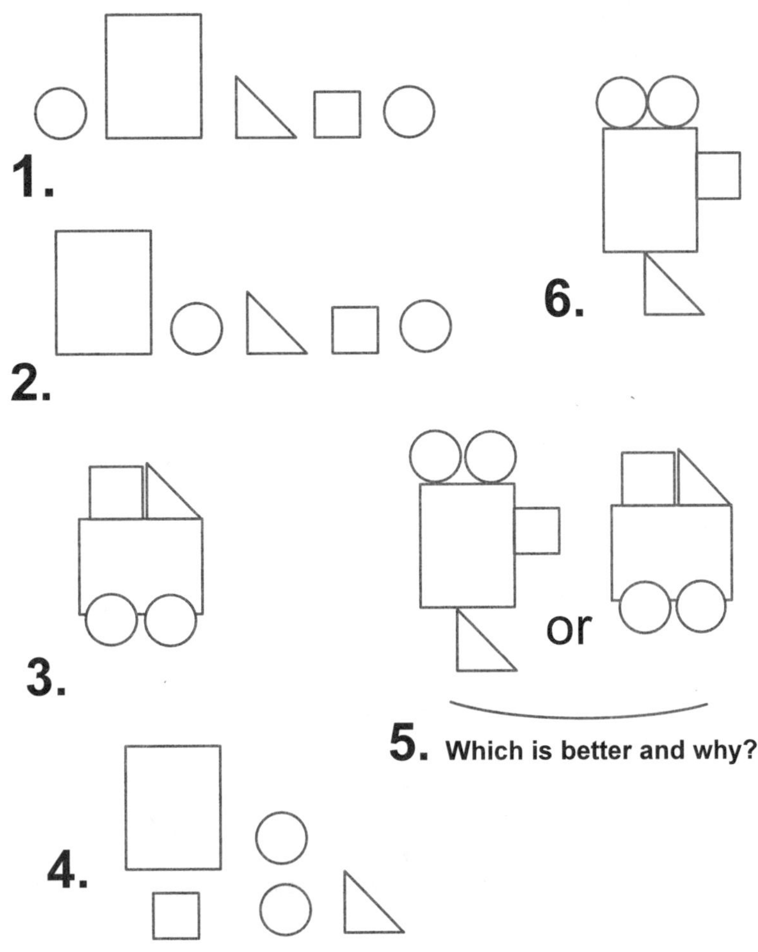

Directions: Write on the lines below the six levels of the revised Bloom's Taxonomy, starting with the least complex at the bottom. Then write a few words next to each level that explain the type of processing that occurs when describing the various pictures on the previous page.

LEVEL	DESCRIPTION of PROCESSING
6.	
5.	
4.	
3.	
2.	
1.	

PRACTITIONER'S CORNER

Take a Concept/Situation Up the Taxonomy!

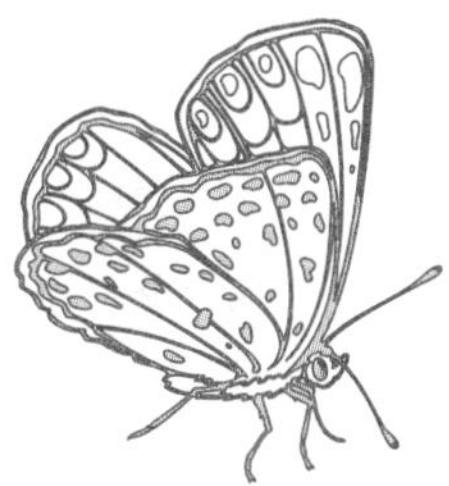

Directions: Think of a task that you need to accomplish with your own child, parent, colleague, or spouse (e.g., how to use the washing machine with different types of clothes, planning a vacation) and describe questions or activities that move the task up Bloom's revised taxonomy.

CONCEPT/SITUATION:___________________________________

Create (putting ideas together to form a new whole):

Evaluate (judging material using certain criteria):

Analyze (breaking down a concept and looking for relationships):

Apply (using a concept or principle in a new situation):

Understand (translating the material to achieve comprehension):

START HERE: Remember (rote remembering of information):

PRACTITIONER'S CORNER

Tips on Using Bloom's Revised Taxonomy

- **Watch the Behavior of the Learner.** The learner's behavior reveals the level of complexity where processing is taking place. Whenever the brain has the option of solving a problem at two levels of complexity, it generally chooses the less complex level. Teachers can inadvertently design activities that they believe are at one level of complexity that students actually accomplish at a different (usually lower) level.

- **Provide Sufficient Practice at the Lower Levels.** In most instances, students should deal with the new learnings thoroughly and successfully at lower levels before moving to upper levels. It is very difficult to create a product without a solid knowledge base and sufficient practice in applying the learnings.

- **Beware of Mimicry.** Sometimes students seem to be applying their learning to a new situation (*Apply* level) when they are just mimicking the teacher's behavior. Mimicry is usually the *Remember* level. For students to be really at the *Apply* level, they must understand and explain why they are using a particular process to solve *new* problems.

- **Discuss Core Concepts at the Higher Levels.** Not all topics are suitable for processing at the upper levels. There are some areas in which creativity is not desired (e.g., basic arithmetic, spelling, the rules of grammar), but consider taking to the upper levels every concept that is identified as a core learning. This helps students to attach meaning and make connections to past learnings, thereby significantly increasing retention.

- **Choose Complexity Over Difficulty.** Give novel, multisensory tasks to move students progressively up the taxonomy. Limit the exposure to trivial information and discourage students from memorizing it, a process that many find monotonous and meaningless. Instead, give them divergent activities in *Analyze, Evaluate,* and *Create* that are more interesting and more likely to result in a deeper understanding and retention of the learning objectives. For example, Raths (2002) suggests that a discussion of tourists, migrants, and immigrants could ask students to *analyze* these concepts in the context of rights and obligations of nonresidents and noncitizens, *evaluate* proposals for dealing with social problems such as illegal immigrants, and *create* policies that solve specific social problems without causing other problems (e.g., dealing with immigrants without negatively affecting tourism).

PRACTITIONER'S CORNER

Bloom's Taxonomy: Increasing Complexity

Examples become more complex from bottom to top, and more difficult from left to right.

	BLOOM'S LEVEL	INCREASING LEVEL OF DIFFICULTY ⟶	
↑ INCREASING COMPLEXITY	CREATE	Rewrite the story from the point of view of the dog.	Rewrite the story from the points of view of the dog *and of the cat.*
	EVALUATE	Compare the *two* main characters in the story. Which would you rather have as a friend and why?	Compare the *four* main characters in the story. Which would you rather have as a friend and why?
	ANALYZE	What were the similarities and differences between this story and the one we read about the Civil War hero?	What were the similarities and differences between this story, the one we read about the Civil War hero, *and the one about the Great Depression*?
	APPLY	Think of another situation that could have caused the main character to behave that way.	Think of at least *three* other situations that could have caused the main character to behave that way.
	UNDERSTAND	Write a paragraph that describes the childhood of any one of the main characters.	Write a paragraph that describes the childhood of each of the *four* main characters.
	REMEMBER	Name the major characters in this story.	Name the major characters and the *four locations* in this story.

PRACTITIONER'S CORNER

Understanding the Difference Between Complexity and Difficulty

First, let's try a real-life application.

1. Select a partner and decide who is Partner A and who is Partner B.
2. Each partner performs, in turn, the activities for each situation in the Table X below.
3. When both partners have completed the three situations, discuss whether complexity or difficulty was changed **in each situation** when moving from A's to B's activity.

Table X. Deciding Whether Complexity or Difficulty Is Increased

Situation	Partner A's Activity	Partner B's Activity	Complexity or Difficulty Changed? How?
1	Tell your partner the month of your birth and the city and state where you were born.	Tell your partner the make of your current automobile.	
2	Roll a piece of paper into a ball. Stand 10 feet from your partner. Ask your partner to stand and to form his/her arms into a ring in front (as though to hug someone). Now toss the ball five times and try to get all five tosses through the ring formed by your partner's arms.	Repeat what your partner just did, except stand facing away from your partner and toss the paper ball over your head five times, still aiming for your partner's ringed arms.	
3	Fanfold a piece of paper. Then explain to your partner three uses for the folded paper.	After listening to your partner's explanation of the uses, choose one you think is best and explain why.	

Now, let's try a school situation. Examine how each teacher in Table Y below changes Activity A to Activity B. Then decide if the teacher has increased that activity's level of complexity or difficulty.

Table Y. Deciding Whether Complexity or Difficulty Is Increased			
Teacher	**Activity A**	**Activity B**	**Increased Complexity or Difficulty?**
1	Make an outline of the story you just read.	Make an outline of the last two stories you read.	
2	Compare and contrast the personalities of Julius Caesar and Macbeth.	After reading three acts of *Macbeth*, write a plausible ending.	
3	Choose one character in the story you would like to be and explain your choice.	Choose two characters in the story you would like to be and explain why.	
4	Name the three most common chemical elements on Earth.	Describe in your own words what is meant by a chemical element.	

Reflections:

Is complexity or difficulty more closely related to intelligence?

How will understanding that difference affect my teaching?

Summary: Increasing the *difficulty* of a task adds to the students' efforts without increasing the level of their thinking processes. Think of it as moving *horizontally* within a level of the revised Bloom's Taxonomy. Strategies such as repetition and drill tend to increase difficulty. Jot down below some other strategies that increase difficulty. For what types of learning would it be important to use strategies to increase difficulty?

Increasing the *complexity* of a task causes the students to change the way they mentally process the task. Think of it as moving *vertically* up the taxonomy from one level to a higher one. Strategies that cause students to compare and contrast, or to choose among options and defend their choice, are examples of increasing complexity. Jot down below some other strategies that increase complexity. For what types of learning would it be important to use strategies to increase complexity?

PRACTITIONER'S CORNER

Questions to Stimulate Higher-Order Thinking

Incorporate these questions into lesson plans to stimulate higher-order thinking. Be sure to read the guidelines for using the Bloom's revised taxonomy to ensure the maximum effectiveness of these questions. Remember to provide adequate wait-time. Students should become accustomed to this type of questioning in every study assignment.

What would you have done? Why do you think this is the best choice?

What are some of the things you wondered about while this was happening?

Could this ever really happen? What might happen next?

What do you think might happen if . . . ? What do you think caused this?

How is it different from . . . ? Can you give an example?

Where do we go next? Where could we go for help on this?

Have we left out anything important?

Can we trust the source of this material?

In what other ways could this be done? How can you test this theory?

How many ways can you think of to use . . . ?

Do you agree with this author/speaker? Why or why not?

Can you isolate the most important idea?

How could you modify this? How would changing the sequence affect the outcome?

How can you tell the difference between . . . and . . . ?

PRACTITIONER'S CORNER

Activities to Stimulate Higher-Order Thinking

The following activities help teachers encourage higher-order thinking in their classrooms:

- Encourage students to use analogies and metaphors when describing and comparing new concepts, theories, and principles.

- Have students attempt to solve real life problems (e.g., energy crisis, environmental pollution) where there is a possibility of more than one adequate solution.

- Ask questions that foster higher-order thinking, such as those with multiple answers or several equally correct answers.

- Involve students in debates and discussions that tackle more than one side of an issue, and require students to support their arguments with evidence.

- Get students in role plays or simulations of historical events where people held conflicting views (e.g., drafting the U.S. Constitution, women's right to vote).

- Supplement regular textbooks with additional materials (including audio/visual content) that provide a wider variety of perspectives about a particular idea.

- Encourage students to watch television programs, attend community meetings, and read newspaper articles that express different viewpoints. Follow this with an analysis of the relative strengths and weaknesses of the arguments, including an analysis of the possible motives underlying the various positions.

- Have students analyze the content of popular media (e.g., television, movies, music) for their accuracy and completeness of its portrayals of everyday life. For example, do commercials glorifying the acquisition of expensive personal goods balance with the existence of poverty in the community. Do the media perpetuate stereotypes?

- Explore with students the methods used to develop knowledge in a particular field. For example: What technologies help us look inside the living human brain?

Chapter 7—Thinking Skills and Learning

Key Points to Ponder

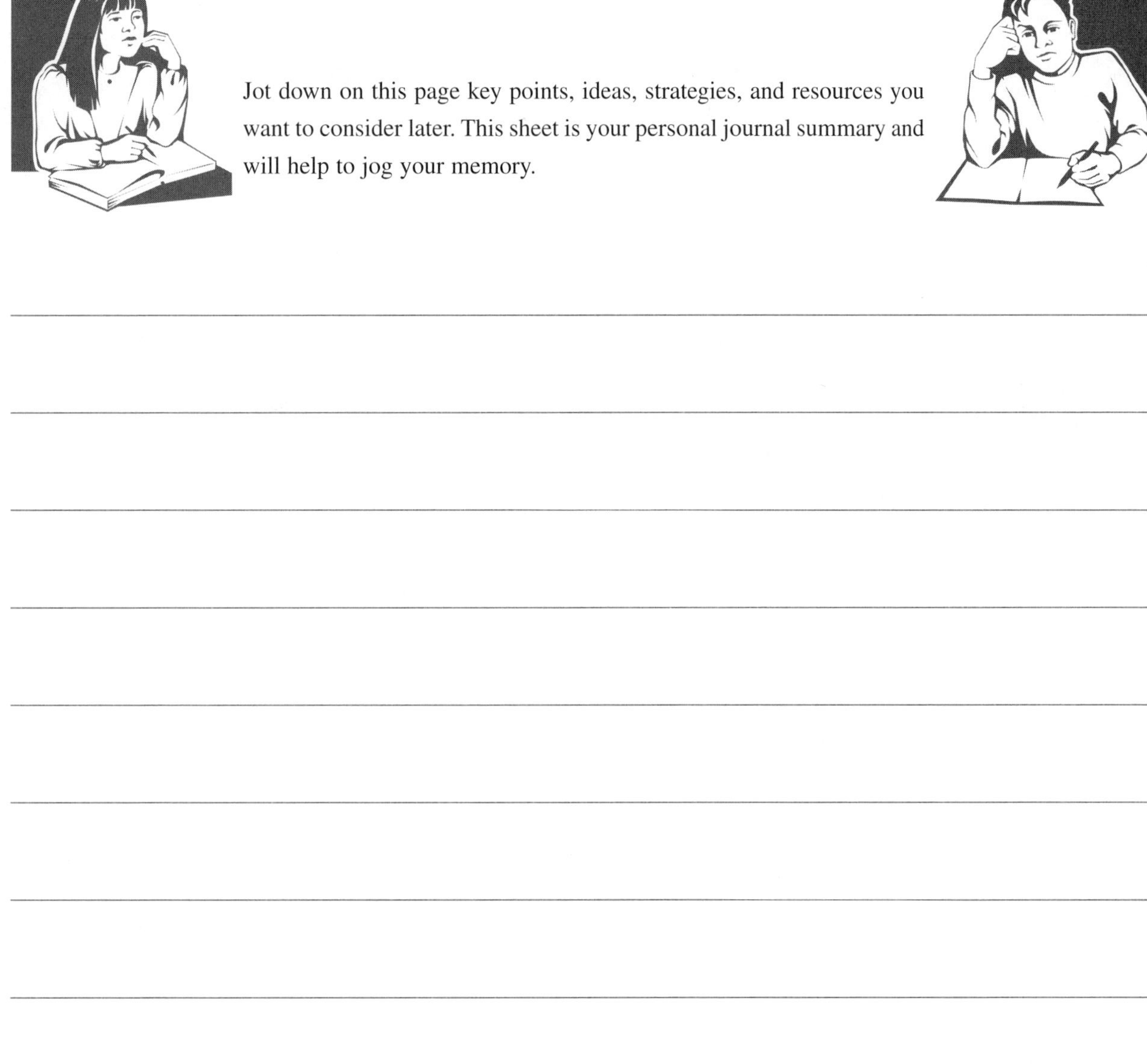

Jot down on this page key points, ideas, strategies, and resources you want to consider later. This sheet is your personal journal summary and will help to jog your memory.

Chapter 8

Putting It All Together

In the world of the future, the new illiterate will be the person who has not learned to learn.

—Alvin Toffler

Chapter Highlights. This chapter focuses on how to use the research presented in this book to plan daily lessons. It suggests guidelines and a format for lesson design, and mentions support systems to maintain expertise in the techniques and continuous professional growth.

The preceding chapters discussed some of the major strides that research is making in exploring how the brain processes information and learns. Suggestions are offered in each chapter's **Practitioner's Corners** on how to translate these new discoveries into practical classroom strategies that can improve the efficacy of teaching and learning. But this information is of value to students only if teachers can incorporate it into their classroom practice so that it becomes part of their daily instructional behavior. The question now is: How do we use this large amount of information when planning our daily lessons?

DAILY PLANNING

General Guidelines

Start by keeping the following general thoughts in mind while planning:

- Learning engages the entire person (cognitive, affective, and psychomotor domains).
- The human brain seeks patterns in its search for meaning.
- Emotions affect all aspects of learning, retention, and recall.
- Past experience always affects new learning.
- The brain's working memory has a limited capacity.
- Lecture usually results in the lowest degree of retention.
- Rehearsal is essential for retention.
- Practice does not make perfect.
- Each brain is unique.

Daily Lesson Design

To use this research in daily planning, we need a lesson plan model as a framework. The type of lesson plan that a teacher uses depends to a large degree on the instructional method the teacher decides to use. The following are examples of some instructional methods (Moore, 2005):

- **Direct Teaching.** The teacher lectures, does much of the work, and can present a great deal of information in a short period of time. Extent of student participation varies from none to considerable. Still the most common teaching method in secondary schools and higher education.
- **Demonstration.** Teacher shows something, tells what is happening, and asks the students to discuss the demonstration.
- **Concept Attainment.** Students figure out the attributes of a group or category (provided by the teacher) by comparing and contrasting examples that possess the attributes and examples that do not. Through discussion, students develop a definition or hypothesis about the concept (lesson objective).
- **Socratic Method.** This lesson draws information from students through a series of carefully designed questions that eventually help students achieve the lesson objective.
- **Cooperative Learning.** Students work together in heterogeneous groups to accomplish a specific task.
- **Simulations and Games.** The lesson centers around a problem situation that represents reality. Role-playing is used to help students understand the motives and behaviors of people. Educational games involve students in decision-making roles.
- **Individualized Instruction.** These methods include differentiated instruction, mastery learning, and independent study.
- **Drill and Practice.** This lesson specifically targets the recall and improvement of certain skills to enhance accuracy and speed.

No single lesson plan format fully addresses every aspect of every possible teaching method. But I do think one comes very close. The format I propose evolved from Madeline Hunter's (2004) work at UCLA in the 1970s. Hunter was a clinical psychologist who was a pioneer in recognizing the need to include strategies from cognitive science in teaching. Despite its age, the format is based on sound principles of brain-compatible learning while being flexible enough to use with a variety of instructional methods.

I have made minor modifications to Hunter's original format by expanding it to include some of the more recent strategies. The nine components of the design are:

1. *Anticipatory Set.* This strategy captures the students' focus. Almost any technique to get their initial attention can be valuable. Vary the initial attention-getter to provide novelty, and remember the power of humor in getting attention and setting a positive emotional climate for the lesson to follow. Once you get their initial attention, the rest of the set is most effective when it

   (a) allows students to remember an experience that will help them acquire the new learning (positive transfer from past to present)
   (b) involves active student participation (while avoiding "guessing" games during prime-time-1),
   (c) is relevant to the learning objective.

2. *Learning Objective.* This is a clear statement of what the students are expected to accomplish during the learning episode, including the levels of difficulty and complexity, and should include

   (a) a specific statement of the learning,
   (b) the overt behavior that demonstrates whether the learning has occurred, and whether the appropriate level of complexity has been attained.

When the teacher states the learning objective explicitly at the beginning of the lesson, it is called an *expository* lesson—that is, the objective is now "exposed." Sometimes, we prefer to have the students discover the lesson objective on their own. This is obviously called a *discovery* lesson. Discovery lessons require more careful planning and guidance to ensure that the students actually get to the intended objective. If the learner doesn't know where the lesson is going, *any* place will do.

3. *Purpose.* This states *why* the students should accomplish the learning objective. Whenever possible, it should refer to how the new learning is related to the students' prior and future learnings to facilitate positive transfer and meaning.

4. *Input.* This is the information and the procedures (skills) that students will need to acquire in order to achieve the learning objective. It can take many forms, including reading, lecture, cooperative learning groups, audiovisual presentations, the Internet, and so on.

5. *Modeling.* Clear and correct models help students make sense of the new learning and establish meaning. Models must be given first by the teacher and be accurate, unambiguous, and non-controversial. Nonexemplars could be included later to show contrast.

6. *Check for Understanding.* This refers to the strategies the teacher will use during the learning episode to verify that the students are accomplishing the learning objective. The check could be in the form of oral discussion, questioning, written quiz, think-pair-share, or any other overt format that yields the necessary data. Depending on the results of these checks, the teacher may decide to provide more opportunities for input, reteach, or move on to new material.

7. *Guided Practice.* During this time, the student is applying the new learning in the presence of the teacher who provides immediate and specific feedback on the accuracy of the learner's practice. Later, the teacher checks any corrections that the student made as a result of feedback.

8. *Closure.* This is the time when the mind of the learner can summarize for itself its perception of what has been learned. The teacher gives specific directions for what the learner should mentally process and provides adequate time to accomplish it. This is usually the last opportunity the learner has to attach sense and meaning to the new learning, both of which are critical requirements for retention. Daily closure activities can take many forms, such as using synergy strategies or journal writing. Closure activities for the end of a unit might include writing plays, singing songs, reciting poetry, playing quiz games, and so on.

> ***Closure is usually the last opportunity the learner has to attach sense and meaning to new learning.***

9. *Independent Practice.* After the teacher believes that the learners have accomplished the objective at the correct level of difficulty and complexity, students try the new learning on their own to enhance retention and develop fluency.

Important Note. Not every lesson needs to include every component. However, the teacher should consider each component and choose those that are relevant to the learning objective and teaching method. For example, when introducing a new major unit of study, the lesson may focus primarily on *objectives* (What do we hope to accomplish?) and *purpose* (Why are we studying this?). On the other hand, a review lesson before a major test might include more ways of *checking for understanding* and for *guided practice*.

> ***Not every lesson needs every component. The teacher should consider each component and choose those that are relevant to the learning objective and teaching method.***

Table 8.1 shows the lesson components that could be used with each teaching method. Table 8.2 shows the lesson components, their purpose, their relationship to the research, and an example from a lesson on teaching the characteristics of suffixes.

Twenty-One Questions to Ask During Lesson Planning

Table 8.3 contains some important questions that teachers should ask while planning lessons. The questions relate to information and strategies included in previous chapters. Following each question is the rationale for considering it and the chapter number where its main reference can be found.

Table 8.1 Lesson Components for Different Teaching Methods

	Direct Teaching	Demon-station	Concept Attain	Socratic Method	Coop. Learning	Simul. & Games	Indepen. Instruc.	Drill & Practice
Antic. Set	X	X	X	X	X	X		
Lesson Objective	X	X	X		X	X		X
Purpose	X	X	X		X	X	X	X
Input	X		X	X	X		X	X
Modeling	X	X	X	X	X			X
Check for Under.	X	X	X	X	X	X	X	X
Guided Practice	X		X				X	X
Closure	X	X	X	X	X	X	X	X
Indepen. Practice	X					X	X	X

Table 8.2 Components to Consider in Designing Lessons

Lesson Component	Purpose	Relationship To Research	Example
Anticipatory Set	Focuses students on the learning objective.	Establishes relevance and fosters positive transfer during prime-time-1.	"Think of what we learned yesterday about prefixes and be prepared to discuss them."
Learning Objective	Identifies what is to be learned by the end of the lesson.	Students know what they should learn and how they will know they have learned it.	"Today we will learn about suffixes, and you will make up words with them."
Purpose	Explains why it is important to accomplish this objective.	Knowing the purpose for learning something builds interest and establishes meaning.	"Learning about suffixes will help us understand more vocabulary and give us greater creativity in our writing."
Input	Gives students the information, sources, and skills they will need to accomplish the objective	Bloom's **remember** level. Helps identify critical attributes	"Suffixes are letters placed after words to change their meanings."

(Continued)

Table 8.2 (Continued)

Lesson Component	Purpose	Relationship To Research	Example
Modeling	Shows the process or product of what students are learning.	Modeling enhances sense and meaning to help retention	"Examples are: -*less*, as in helpless; -*able*, as in drinkable; and -*ful*, as in doubtful."
Check for Understanding	Allows instructor to verify if students understand what they are learning.	Bloom's **understand** level.	"I'll ask some of you to tell me what you learned so far about the meaning and use of suffixes."
Guided Practice	Allows the students to try the new learning under teacher guidance.	Bloom's **apply** level. Practice provides for fast learning.	"Here are 10 words. Add an appropriate suffix to each and explain their new meanings."
Closure	Allows students time to mentally summarize and internalize the new learning.	Last chance to attach sense and meaning, thus improving retention.	"I'll be quiet now while you think about the attributes and uses of suffixes."
Independent Practice	Students try new learning on their own to develop fluency.	This practice helps make the new learning permanent.	"For homework, add suffixes to the words on page 121 to change their meanings."

UNIT PLANNING

Teacher's Work Sample

Federal and state initiatives to ensure that teachers are highly qualified has prompted some teacher training institutions to develop designs that assist beginning teachers in planning instructional units. Called the Teacher Work Sample, the design can also be used for daily lessons, and some of its components parallel the modified Hunter model discussed earlier. One sample, developed by the Renaissance Partnership for Improving Teacher Quality, contains the following elements:

- **Contextual Factors.** The teacher lists information about the community, school, and characteristics of students, including their prior learning and learning styles.
- **Learning Goals.** The teacher sets significant and challenging learning objectives that are clear, appropriate for the specific student population, and consistent with national, state, and local standards.

Table 8.3 Questions to Ask When Planning Lessons

Question	Rationale	Chapter
1. What tactics am I using to help students attach meaning to the learning?	Meaning helps retention.	2
2. How will I use humor in this lesson?	Humor is an excellent focus device and adds novelty.	2
3. Have I divided the learning episode into mini-lessons of about 20 minutes each?	Short lesson segments have proportionally less down-time than longer ones.	3
4. What motivation and novelty strategies am using?	Motivation and novelty increase interest and accountability.	1 & 2
5. Which type of rehearsal should be used with this learning, and when?	Rote and elaborative rehearsal serve different purposes.	3
6. Am I using the prime-times to the best advantage?	Maximum retention occurs during the prime-times.	3
7. What will the students be doing during down-time?	Minimum retention occurs during down-time.	3
8. Does my plan allow for enough wait-time when asking questions?	Wait-time is critical to allow for student recall to occur.	3
9. What chunking strategies are appropriate for this objective?	Chunking increases the number of items working memory can handle at one time.	3
10. What related prior learning should be included for distributed practice?	Distributed practice increases long-term retention.	3
11. How will I maximize positive transfer and minimize negative transfer?	Positive transfer assists learning; negative transfer interferes.	4
12. Have I identified the critical attributes of this concept?	Critical attributes help distinguish one concept from all others.	4
13. Are the concepts or skills too similar to each other?	Concepts and skills that are too similar should not be taught together.	4
14. How will I show students how they can use (transfer) this learning in the future?	The prospect of future transfer increases motivation and meaning.	4
15. Is it appropriate to use a metaphor with this objective?	Metaphors enhance transfer, hemispheric integration, and retention.	4
16. Have I included activities that are multisensory?	Using many senses increases retention.	5
17. Would a concept map help here?	Concept maps help hemispheric integration and retention.	5
18. Am I using strategies that promote imaging and imagining?	Imaging and imagining help establish meaning, promote novelty, and increase retention.	6
19. Would some music be appropriate? If so, what kind and when?	Some music assists processing and cooperative learning activities.	6
20. How will I move this objective up Bloom's Taxonomy?	The taxonomy's upper levels involve higher-order thinking and are more interesting.	7
21. What emotions (affective domain) need to be considered or avoided in learning this objective?	Emotions play a key role in student acceptance and retention of learning.	7

- **Assessment Plan.** The teacher indicates the technically sound multiple assessments to determine student learning before, during, and after instruction.
- **Design for Instruction.** The teacher designs the unit's lesson plans that use a variety of instructional methods, activities, assignments, and resources, including technology.
- **Instructional Decision-Making.** The teacher uses ongoing analysis of student progress to make instructional decisions, and ensure that any adjustments to instruction are consistent with the learning objectives.
- **Analysis of Student Learning.** The teacher uses assessment data to profile student learning by using graphs to compare the pre-assessment and assessment results for individuals and for the class.
- **Reflection and Self-Evaluation.** The teacher reflects on the instruction to determine what went well and why, what needs to be changed and why, and what implications there are for future decisions on teaching practice and assessment.

Teacher work samples are particularly helpful in assisting novice and veteran teachers in assessing their skills, refining their craft, and improving their classroom presentations. They also serve to measure the training outcomes of professional development initiatives and to validate new teaching practices.

MAINTAINING SKILLS FOR THE FUTURE

This book suggests strategies that teachers can try in order to enhance the effectiveness of the teaching-learning process. The strategies have been derived from the current research on how we learn. Teachers who try these strategies for the first time may need support and feedback on the effectiveness of their implementation. The school-based support system is very important to maintaining teacher interest and commitment, especially if the new strategies don't produce the desired results in the classroom right away.

The Building Principal's Role

Building principals and head teachers play a vital role in establishing a school climate and culture that are receptive to new instructional strategies and in maintaining the support systems necessary for continuing teacher development. Providing opportunities for teachers to master an expanded repertoire of research-based instructional techniques is an effective way for principals to foster collaboration, establish their role as an instructional leader, and enhance the teaching staff's pursuit of professional inquiry. Such opportunities can include peer coaching, in-building study groups, action research projects, and workshops that keep the staff abreast of continuing discoveries about the teaching-learning process (Sousa, 2003).

Types of Support Systems

Peer Coaching

This structure pairs two teachers who periodically observe each other in class. During the lesson, the observing teacher is looking for the use of a particular strategy or technique that was identified in a preobservation conference. After the lesson, the observing teacher provides feedback on the results of the implementation of the strategy. The non-threatening and supportive nature of this peer relationship encourages teachers to take risks and try new techniques that they might otherwise avoid for fear of failure or administrative scrutiny. Peer coaches undergo initial training in how to set the observation goal at the preconference and on different methods for collecting information during the observation.

Study Groups

Forming small groups of teachers and administrators to study a particular topic further is an effective means of expanding understanding and methods of applying new strategies. The group members seek out new research on the topic and exchange and discuss information, data, and experiences in the group setting. Each group focuses on one or two topics, such as wait-time, transfer, and retention techniques. Groups within a school or district can use cooperative learning techniques as a means of sharing information across groups.

Action Research

As discussed more fully in the Introduction, conducting small research studies in a class or school can provide teachers with the validation they may need to incorporate new strategies permanently into their repertoire. Action research gives the practitioner a chance to be a researcher and to investigate specific problems that affect teaching and learning.

For example, deliberately changing the length of the wait-time after posing questions yields data on how the amount and quality of student responses vary with the wait-time. If several teachers carry out this research and exchange data, they will have the evidence to support the continued use of longer wait-time as an effective strategy. Action research on the use of humor and music in the classroom can help teachers determine the value of these strategies on student performance. Teachers can then share their results with colleagues at faculty meetings or study group sessions. This format also advances the notion that teachers should be involved in research projects as part of their professional growth.

Workshops on New Research

Periodic workshops that focus on new research findings in the teaching and learning process are valuable for updating teachers' knowledge base. Areas such as the transfer and transformation of learnings, reflection, memory, and concept development are the targets of extensive research at this time and should be monitored to determine if new findings are appropriate for district and school workshops.

When educators encourage ongoing staff development activities, such as study groups and action research, they are recognizing that our understanding of the teaching-learning process is in continual change as the research yields more data on how the amazing brain learns. True professionals are committed to updating their knowledge base constantly, and they recognize individual professional development as a personal and lifelong responsibility that will enhance their effectiveness.

CONCLUSION

The potential contributions of neuroscience to educational practice continue to accumulate. The very fact that neuroscientists and educators are meeting and talking to each other regularly is evidence that we have crossed a new frontier in our profession. There are, of course, no magic answers that make the complex processes of teaching and learning successful all the time. Educators recognize that numerous variables affect this dynamic interaction, many of which are beyond the teacher's influence or control. What teachers *can* control is their own behavior. Although a few students can learn on their own, most of them rely heavily on the instructional talents of their teachers to learn information and skills. For them, the quality of their learning rarely exceeds the quality of teaching. My hope is that this book provides teachers with some new information, strategies, and insights that will increase their chances of success with more students.

The quality of learning rarely exceeds the quality of teaching

HAPPY TEACHING AND LEARNING!

PRACTITIONER'S CORNER

Reflections on Lesson Design

Here's a sample lesson design using the information processing model in Chapter 2.

Objective: The learner will be able to describe verbally the major parts of the brain processing model in the text *How the Brain Learns*.

Anticipatory Set: "Take a moment to think about whether it is important for teachers to know how we believe the brain selects and processes information. Then discuss your thoughts with your partner."

Purpose: "The purpose of this lesson is to give you some of the latest research we have on how we think the brain processes information so that you can be more successful in choosing those teacher actions that are more likely to result in learning."

Input: The teacher describes major steps in the process, including uptake by senses, interplay of the perceptual register and short-term memory, working memory, long-term storage, the cognitive belief system, and self-concept. Emphasizes the importance of sense and meaning, as well as of past experiences, throughout the entire process.

Modeling: Teacher explains the four metaphors (venetian blinds, clipboard, work table, and filing cabinets). Uses examples of working memory capacity, uses hands as model, and shows the model brain.

Check for Understanding: Teacher has students fill in the function sheet after several parts of the model are covered, and has them use the synergy strategy to discuss with their partners.

Guided Practice: Teacher gives examples of sense and meaning differences, and of positive and negative self-concept differences, to determine the extent of application of the model.

Closure: "Take a few minutes to quietly summarize in your mind the major parts of the brain processing model, and be prepared to explain them."

Chapter 8—Putting It All Together

Key Points to Ponder

Jot down on this page key points, ideas, strategies, and resources you want to consider later. This sheet is your personal journal summary and will help to jog your memory.

Glossary

Action research. A systematic process for evaluating the effectiveness of classroom practices using the techniques of research.

Alphabetic principle. The understanding that spoken words can be broken down into phonemes, and that written letters represent the phonemes of spoken language.

Amygdala. The almond-shaped structure in the brain's limbic system that encodes emotional messages to long-term storage.

Angular gyrus. A brain structure that decodes visual information about words so they can be matched to their meanings.

Apoptosis. The genetically programmed process that destroys unneeded or unhealthy brain cells.

Associative learning. A learning situation whereby a response gets linked to a specific stimulus.

Axon. The neuron's long and unbranched fiber that carries impulses from the cell to the next neuron.

Brain stem. One of the major parts of the brain, it receives sensory input and monitors vital functions such as heartbeat, body temperature, and digestion.

Cerebellum. One of the major parts of the brain, it coordinates muscle movement.

Cerebrum. The largest of the major parts of the brain, it controls sensory interpretation, thinking, and memory.

Chunking. The ability of the brain to perceive a coherent group of items as a single item or chunk.

Circadian rhythm. The daily cycle of body functions, such as breathing and body temperature.

Closure. The teaching strategy that allows learners quiet time in class to mentally reprocess what they have learned during a lesson.

Cognitive belief system. The unique construct one uses to interpret how the world works, on the basis of experience.

Computerized tomography (CT, formerly CAT) scanner. An instrument that uses X-rays and computer processing to produce a detailed cross-section of brain structure.

Confabulation. The brain's replacement of a gap in long-term memory by a falsification which the individual believes to be correct.

Constructivism. A theory of learning stating that active learners use past experiences and chunking to construct sense and meaning from new learning, thereby building larger conceptual schemes.

Corpus callosum. The bridge of nerve fibers that connects the left and right cerebral hemispheres and allows communication between them.

Cortex. The thin but tough layer of cells covering the cerebrum that contains all the neurons used for cognitive and motor processing.

Critical attribute. A characteristic that makes one concept different from all others.

Declarative memory. Knowledge of events and facts to which we have conscious access.

Delayed sleep phase disorder. A chronic condition caused mainly by a shift in an adolescent's sleep cycle that results in difficulty falling asleep at night and waking up in the morning.

Dendrite. The branched extension from the cell body of a neuron that receives impulses from nearby neurons through synaptic contacts.

Distributed practice. The repetition of a skill over increasingly longer periods of time to improve performance.

Electroencephalograph (EEG). An instrument that charts fluctuations in the brain's electrical activity via electrodes attached to the scalp.

Emotional memory. The retention of the emotional components of an experience.

Endorphins. Opiate-like chemicals in the body that lessen pain and produce pleasant and euphoric feelings.

Engram. The permanent memory trace that results when brain tissue is anatomically altered by an experience.

Episodic memory. Knowledge of events in our personal history to which we have conscious access.

Flashbulb memory. A vivid memory of the circumstances surrounding a shocking or emotionally charged experience.

Frontal lobe. The front part of the brain that monitors higher-order thinking, directs problem solving, and regulates the excesses of the emotional (limbic) system.

Functional magnetic resonance imaging (fMRI). An instrument that measures blood flow to the brain to record areas of high and low neuronal activity.

Glial cells. Special "glue" cells in the brain that surround each neuron providing support, protection, and nourishment.

Gray matter. The thin but tough covering of the brain's cerebrum also known as the cerebral cortex.

Guided practice. The repetition of a skill in the presence of the teacher who can give immediate and specific feedback.

Hippocampus. A brain structure that compares new learning to past learning and encodes information from working memory to long-term storage.

Hypothalamus. A small brain structure at the base of the limbic area that regulates body functions in response to internal and external stimuli.

Imagery. The mental visualization of objects, events, and arrays.

Immediate memory. A temporary memory where information is processed briefly (in seconds) and subconsciously, then either blocked or passed on to working memory.

Independent practice. The repetition of a skill on one's own outside the presence of the teacher.

Laterality (also Hemisphericity). The notion that the two cerebral hemispheres are specialized and process information differently.

Limbic area. The structures at the base of the cerebrum that control emotions.

Long-term potentiation. The increase in synaptic strength and sensitivity that endures as a result of repeated, frequent firings across a synapse between two associated neurons. As of now, it is the accepted mechanism for explaining long-term storage.

Long-term storage. The areas of the cerebrum where memories are stored permanently.

Magnetic resonance imaging (MRI). An instrument that uses radio waves to disturb the alignment of the body's atoms in a magnetic field to produce computer-processed, high-contrast images of internal structures.

Massed practice. The repetition of a skill over short time intervals to gain initial competence.

Mnemonic. A word or phrase used as a device for remembering unrelated information, patterns, or rules.

Motivation. The influence of needs and desires on behavior.

Motor cortex. The narrow band across the top of the brain from ear to ear that controls movement.

Myelin. A fatty substance that surrounds and insulates a neuron's axon.

Neural efficiency. The ability of the brain to use fewer neurons to accomplish a repetitive task.

Neuron. The basic cell making up the brain and nervous system, consisting of a cell body, a long fiber (axon) which transmits impulses, and many shorter fibers (dendrites) which receive them.

Neuroplasticity. The brain's lifelong ability to reorganize neural networks as a result of new experiences.

Neurotransmitter. One of several dozen chemicals stored in axon sacs that transmit impulses from neuron to neuron across the synaptic gap.

Nonassociative learning. A learning whereby the individual responds unconsciously to a stimulus.

Nondeclarative memory. Knowledge of motor and cognitive skills to which we have no conscious access, such as riding a bicycle.

Perceptual representation system. A form of nondeclarative memory in which the structure and form of objects and words that can be prompted by prior experience.

Phonemes. The minimal units of sound in a language that combine to make syllables.

Phonemic awareness. The ability to hear, identify, and manipulate phonemes in spoken syllables and words.

Phonological awareness. In addition to phonemic awareness, it includes the ability to recognize that sentences are comprised of words, words are comprised of syllables, and syllables are comprised of onsets and rimes that can be broken down into phonemes.

Plasticity. The ability of the brain to change as a result of daily learning.

Positron emission tomography (PET) scanner. An instrument that traces the metabolism of radioactively tagged sugar in brain tissue producing a color image of cell activity.

Practice. The repetition of a skill to gain speed and accuracy.

Primacy-recency effect. The phenomenon whereby one tends to remember best that which comes first in a learning episode and second best that which comes last.

Prime-time. The time in a learning episode when information or a skill is more likely to be remembered.

Procedural memory. A form of nondeclarative memory that allows the learning of motor (riding a bicycle) and cognitive (learning to read) skills.

Prosody. The rhythm, cadence, accent patterns, and pitch of a language.

Psychological-cognitive cycle. One of the body's circadian rhythms that determines the degree of focus one has during cognitive processing.

Rate of learning. The amount of time it takes one to learn cognitive information with sufficient confidence that it will be consolidated into long-term memory.

Rate of retrieval. The amount of time it takes one to recall information from long-term memory to working memory.

Rehearsal. The reprocessing of information in working memory.

Retention. The preservation of a learning in long-term storage in such a way that it can be identified and recalled quickly and accurately.

Reticular activating system (RAS). The dense formation of neurons in the brain stem that controls major body functions and maintains the brain's alertness.

Self-concept. Our perception of who we are and how we fit into the world.

Semantic memory. Knowledge of facts and data that may not be related to any event.

Sensory memory. The short-lived (usually in milliseconds) retention of information, such as recalling what someone just said to us, although we were not paying attention to the speaker.

Specialization. The notion that certain brain regions are mainly dedicated to accomplishing specific tasks, such as Broca's area.

Suprachiasmatic nuclei. A tiny cluster of neurons (located just above where the optic nerves cross on their way to the visual cortex) that monitors the intensity of signals along the optic nerve to determine the intensity of external light and start the sleep cycle.

Synapse. The microscopic gap between the axon of one neuron and the dendrite of another.

Thalamus. A part of the limbic system that receives all incoming sensory information, except smell, and shunts it to other areas of the cortex for additional processing.

Transfer. The influence that past learning has on new learning, and the degree to which the new learning will be useful in the learner's future. Positive transfer aids, and negative transfer inhibits, the acquisition of new learning.

Wait-time. The period of teacher silence that follows the posing of a question before the first student is called to respond.

White matter. The support tissue that lies beneath the cerebrum's gray matter (cortex).

Window of opportunity. An important period during which the young brain responds to certain types of input to create or consolidate a neural network.

Working memory. The temporary memory wherein information is processed consciously.

References

Abeles, H. F., & Sanders, E. M. (2005). *Final assessment report: New Jersey Symphony Orchestra's Early Strings Program.* New York: Center for Arts Education Research, Columbia University.

Acebo, C., Wolfson, A., & Carskadon, M. (1997). Relations among self-reported sleep patterns, health, and injuries in adolescents. *Sleep Research, 27,* 149.

Amunts, K., Schlaug, G., Jancke, L., Steinmetz, H., Schleicher, A., Dabringhaus, A., & Zilles, K. (1997). Motor cortex and hand motor skills: Structural compliance in the human brain. *Human Brain Mapping, 5,* 206–215.

Anderson, L. W. (Ed.), Krathwohl, D. R. (Ed.), Airasian, P. W., Cruikshank, K. A., Mayer, R. E., Pintrich, P. R., Raths, J., & Wittrock, M. C. (2001). *A taxonomy for learning, teaching, and assessing: A revision of Bloom's Taxonomy of Educational Objectives* (Complete edition). New York: Longman.

Anvari, S. H., Trainor, L. J., Woodside, J., & Levy, B. A. (2002, October). Relations among musical skills, phonological processing, and early reading ability in preschool children. *Journal of Experimental Child Psychology, 83,* 111–130.

Baddeley, A. (1995). Working memory. In M. S. Gazzaniga (Ed.), *The cognitive neurosciences,* pp. 755–764. Cambridge, MA: MIT Press.

Banich, M. (1997). *Neuropsychology: The neural bases of mental function.* New York: Houghton Mifflin.

Baron-Cohen, S. (2003). *The essential difference: The truth about the male and female brain.* New York: Basic Books.

Barry, N., Taylor, J., & Walls, K. (2002). The role of the fine and performing arts in high school dropout prevention. In R. J. Deasy (Ed.), *Critical links: Learning in the arts and student academic and social development* (pp. 74–75). Washington, DC: Arts Education Partnership.

Bassok, M., & Holyoak, K.J. (1989). Interdomain transfer between isomorphic topics in algebra and physics. *Journal of Experimental Psychology: Learning, Memory and Cognition, 15,* 153–166.

Bateman, B. Warner, J. O., Hutchinson, E., Dean, T., Rowlandson, P., Gant, C., Grundy, J., Fitzgerald, C., & Stevenson, J. (2004). The effects of a double blind, placebo controlled artificial food colorings and benzoate preservative challenge on hyperactivity in a general population sample of preschool children. *Archives of Diseases in Childhood, 89,* 506–511.

Bates, E. (1999, July-August). Language and the infant brain. *Journal of Communication Disorders, 32,* 195–205.

Beatty, J. (2001). *The human brain: Essentials of behavioral neuroscience.* Thousand Oaks, CA: Sage Publications.

Begley, S. (2000, January 1). Rewiring your gray matter. *Newsweek,* 63–65.

Blanchette, I., & Dunbar, K. (2000). How analogies are generated: The roles of structural and superficial similarity. *Memory & Cognition, 28,* 108–124.

Blanchette, I. & Dunbar, K. (2002). Representational change and analogy: How analogical inferences alter target representations. *Journal of Experimental Psychology: Learning, Memory, and Cognition, 28,* 672–685.

Blood, A. J., Zatorre, R. J., Bermudez, P., & Evans, A. C. (1999, April). Emotional responses to pleasant and unpleasant music correlate with activity in paralimbic brain regions. *Nature Neuroscience*, *2*, 382–387.

Bloom, B. S. (Ed.), Engelhart, M. D., Furst, E. J., Hill, W. H., & Krathwohl, D. R. (1956). *Taxonomy of educational objectives: The classification of educational goals. Handbook I: Cognitive domain.* New York: David McKay.

Bloom, B. S. (1976). *Human characteristics and school learning*. New York: McGraw-Hill.

Bor, D., Duncan, J., Wiseman, R. J., & Owen, A. M. (2003, January). Encoding strategies dissociate prefrontal activity from working memory demand. *Neuron, 37,* 361–367.

Bower, J. M., & Parsons, L. M. (2003, August). Rethinking the lesser brain. *Scientific American, 289,* 51–57.

Brannon, E. M. & van der Walle, G. (2001). Ordinal numerical knowledge in young children. *Cognitive Psychology, 43,* 53–81.

Bromley, K., Irwin-DeVitis, L., & Modlo, M. (1995). *Graphic organizers*. New York: Scholastic.

Brooks, J. G., & Brooks, M. G. (1999). *In search of understanding: The case for constructivist classrooms* (2nd ed.) Alexandria, VA: Association for Supervision and Curriculum Development.

Buckner, R. L., Kelley, W. M., & Petersen, S. E. (1999, April). Frontal cortex contributions to human memory formation. *Nature Neuroscience*, *2*, 311–314.

Burton, J. M., Horowitz, R., & Abeles, H. (2000). Learning in and through the arts: The question of transfer. *Studies in Art Education, 41,* 228–257.

Butterworth, B. (1999). *What counts: How every brain is hardwired for math*. New York: Free Press.

Butzlaff, R. (2000, Fall). Can music be used to teach reading? *Journal of Aesthetic Education, 34,* 167–178.

Buzan, T. (1989). *Use both sides of your brain* (3rd ed.). New York: Penguin.

Buzzell, K. (1998). *The children of Cyclops: The influence of television viewing on the developing human brain*. San Francisco: Association of Waldorf Schools of North America.

Cahill, L. (2005, May). His brain, her brain. *Scientific American, 292,* 40–47.

Cahill, L., & McGaugh, J. (1998). Mechanisms of emotional arousal and lasting declarative memory. *Trends in Neuroscience*, *21*, 294–299.

Calvin, W., & Ojemann, G. (1994). *Conversations with Neil's brain: The neural nature of thought and language*. Menlo Park, CA: Addison-Wesley.

Cardoso, S. H. (2000, Fall). Our ancient laughing brain. *Cerebrum, 2,* 15–30.

Carskadon, M. A., Acebo, C., Wolfson, A. R., Tzischinsky, O., & Darley, C. (1997). REM sleep on MSLTS in high school students is related to circadian phase. *Sleep Research*, *26*, 705.

Carter, R. (1998). *Mapping the mind.* Los Angeles: University of California Press.

Carter, T., Hardy, C. A., & Hardy, J. C. (2001, December). Latin vocabulary acquisition: An experiment using information-processing techniques of chunking and imagery. *Journal of Instructional Psychology, 28,* 225–228.

Catterall, J., Chapleau, R., & Iwanga, J. (1999, Fall). Involvement in the arts and human development: Extending an analysis of general associations and introducing the special cases of intense involvement in music and in theater arts. *Monograph Series No. 11*. Washington, DC: Americans for the Arts.

Chapman, C. (1993). *If the shoe fits: Developing the multiple intelligences classroom*. Thousand Oaks, CA: Corwin Press.

Chapman, C., & King, R. (2000). *Test success in the brain compatible classroom*. Tucson, AZ: Zephyr.

Cheour, M., Ceponiene, R., Lehtokoski, A., Luuk, A., Allik, J., Alho, K., & Näätänen, R. (1998, September). Development of language-specific phoneme representations in the infant brain. *Nature Neuroscience*, *1*, 351–353.

Chularut, P., & DeBacker, T. K. (2004, July). The influence of concept mapping on achievement, self-regulation, and self-efficacy in students of English as a second language. *Contemporary Educational Psychology, 29,* 248–263.

Chung, S-C., Tack, G-R., Lee, B., Eom, G-M., Lee, S-Y., & Sohn, J-H. (2004, December). The effect of 30% oxygen on visuospatial performance and brain activation: An fMRI study. *Brain and Cognition, 56,* 279– 285.

Courchesne, E. (1999, March 23). An MRI study of autism: The cerebellum revisited. Letter in *Neurology, 52*, 1106–1107.

Cowan, N. (2001). The Magical Number 4 in Short-term Memory: A Reconsideration of Mental Storage Capacity. *Behavioral and Brain Sciences, 24.* Available online at www.bbsonline.org/documents

Cumming, J., & Hall, C. (2002, February). Deliberate imagery practice: The development of imagery skills in competitive athletes. *Journal of Sports Sciences, 20,* 137–145.

Dale, P. S., Simonoff, E., Bishop, D.V.M., Eley, T. C., Oliver, B., Price, T. S., Purcell, S., Stevenson, J., & Plomin, R. (1998, August). Genetic influence on language delay in two-year-old children. *Nature Neuroscience, 1*, 324–328.

Damasio, A. (1999). *The feeling of what happens: Body and emotion in the making of consciousness*. New York: Harcourt Brace.

Danesi, M. (1990). The contribution of neurolinguistics to second and foreign language theory and practice. *System, 3*, 373–396.

Davis, J. (1997). *Mapping the mind: The secrets of the human brain and how it works*. Secaucus, NJ: Birch Lane Press.

de Fockert, J. W., Rees, G., Frith, C. D., & Lavie, N. (2001). The role of working memory in visual selective attention. *Science, 291,* 1803–1806.

Dehaene, S. (1997). *The number sense: How the mind creates mathematics*. New York: Oxford University Press.

Dehaene, S., Spelke, E., Pinel, P., Stanescu, R., & Tsivkin, S. (1999, May 7). Sources of mathematical thinking: Behavioral and brain-imaging evidence. *Science, 284*, 970–974.

DeHouwer, A. (1999). *Two or more languages in early childhood: Some general points and practical recommendations.* Washington, DC: ERIC Clearinghouse on Languages and Linguistics.

Diamond, J. (1992). *The third chimpanzee: The evolution and future of the human animal*. New York: Harper Perennial.

Diamond, M., & Hopson, J. (1998). *Magic trees of the mind: How to nurture your child's intelligence, creativity, and healthy emotions from birth through adolescence*. New York: Dutton.

Droz, M., & Ellis, L. (1996). *Laughing while learning: Using humor in the classroom*. Longmont, CO: Sopris West.

Duggan, G. B., & Payne, S. J. (2001, December). Interleaving reading and acting while following procedural instructions. *Journal of Experimental Psychology: Applied, 7,* 297–307.

Eisner, E. (2002a, September). What the arts do for the young. *School Arts, 102,* 16–17.

Eisner, E. (2002b). *The arts and the creation of mind.* New Haven, CT: Yale University Press.

Ericsson, K. A. (2003, June). Exceptional memories: Made, not born. *Trends in Cognitive Sciences, 7,* 233–235.

Everhart, D. E., Shucard, J. L., Quatrin, T., & Shucard, D. W. (2001, July). Sex-related differences in event-related potentials, face recognition, and facial affect processing in prepubertal children. *Neuropsychology, 15,* 329–341.

Fagan, J., Prigot, J., Carroll, M., Pioli, L., Stein, A., & Franco, A. (1997, December). Auditory context and memory retrieval in young infants. *Child Development, 68*, 1057–1066.

Fields, R. D. (2005, February). Making memories stick. *Scientific American, 292,* 75–81.

Fiske, E. B. (Ed.). (1999). *Champions of change: The impact of the arts on learning*. Washington, DC: President's Committee on the Arts and the Humanities.

Fleck, D. E., Berch, D. B., Shear, P. K., & Strakowski, S. M. (2001, Spring). Directed forgetting in explicit and implicit memory: The role of encoding and retrieval mechanisms. *The Psychological Record, 51,* 207–221.

Fredrickson, B. L., & Branigan, C. (2005). Positive emotions broaden the scope of attention and thought-action repertoires. *Cognition and Emotion, 19,* 313–332.

Gallup Poll (2004a). *Most teens associate school with boredom, fatigue.* Available online at http://www.gallup.com/poll

Gallup Poll (2004b). *In teens own words: Which teachers motivate you?* Available online at http://www.gallup.com/poll

Gardner, H. (1993). *Frames of mind: The theory of multiple intelligences.* (Rev. Ed.) New York: Basic Books.

Gazzaniga, M. S. (1967, August). The split brain in man. *Scientific American, 207,* 24–29.

Gazzaniga, M. S. (1989). Organization of the human brain. *Science, 245,* 947–952.

Gazzaniga, M. S. (1998a). *The mind's past.* Berkeley: University of California Press.

Gazzaniga, M. S. (1998b, July). The split brain revisited. *Scientific American, 279,* 48–55.

Gazzaniga, M. S., Ivry, R. B., & Mangun, G. R. (2002). *Cognitive neuroscience: The biology of the mind,* (2nd Ed). New York: Norton.

Gobet, F., Lane, P. C. R., Croker, S., Cheng, P., Jones, G., Oliver, I., & Pine, J. M. (2001, June). Chunking mechanisms in human learning. *Trends in Cognitive Sciences, 5,* 236–243.

Goldberg, E. (2001). *The executive brain: Frontal lobes and the civilized mind.* New York: Oxford.

Goleman, D. (1995). *Emotional intelligence: Why it can matter more than I.Q.* New York: Bantam.

Graziano, A. B., Peterson, M., & Shaw, G. L. (1999, March 15). Enhanced learning of proportional math through music training and spatial-temporal training. *Neurological Research, 21,* 139–152.

Gur, R., Turetsky, B., Matsui, M., Yan, M., Bilker, W., Hughett, P., & Gur, R.E. (1999, May 15). Sex differences in brain gray and white matter in healthy young adults: Correlations with cognitive performance. *The Journal of Neuroscience, 19,* 4065–4072.

Gur, R. C., Alsop, D., Glahn, D., Petty, R., Swanson, C. L., Maldjian, J. A., Turetsky, B. I., Detre, J. A., Gee, J., & Gur, R. E. (2000, September). An fMRI study of sex differences in regional activation to a verbal and a spatial task. *Brain and Language, 74,* 157–170.

Guterl, F. (2003, Sept. 8). Overloaded? *Newsweek,* E4–E8.

Haier, R. J., Jung, R. E., Yeo, R. A., Head, K., & Alkire, M. T. (2004, September). Structural brain variation and general intelligence. *NeuroImage, 23,* 425–433.

Hallam, S. (2002). The effects of background music on studying. In R. J. Deasy (Ed.), *Critical links: Learning in the arts and student academic and social development* (pp. 74–75). Washington, DC: Arts Education Partnership.

Hannon, E. E., & Johnson, S. P. (2005, June). Infants use meter to categorize rhythms and melodies: Implications for musical structure learning. *Cognitive Psychology, 50,* 354–377.

Hart, L. (1983). *Human brain and human learning.* New York: Longman.

Harwood, C., Cumming, J., & Hall, C. (2003, September). Imagery use in elite youth sport participants: Reinforcing the applied significance of achievement goal theory. *Research Quarterly for Exercise and Sport, 74,* 292–300.

Hawkins, J. & Blakeslee, S. (2004). *On intelligence.* New York: Times Books.

Hedges, L., & Nowell, A. (1995). Sex differences in mental test scores: Variability and numbers of high scoring individuals. *Science, 269,* 41–45.

Hetland, L. (2000a, Fall). Listening to music enhances spatial-temporal reasoning: Evidence for the "Mozart Effect." *Journal of Aesthetic Education, 34,* 105–148.

Hetland, L. (2000b, Fall). Learning to make music enhance spatial reasoning. *Journal of Aesthetic Education, 34,* 179–238.

High School Survey of Student Engagement Project (HSSSE). (2005). *The 2004 high school student engagement survey.* Bloomington, IN: Indiana University. Available online at http://www.indiana.edu/~nsse/hssse/

Ho, Y-C., Cheung, M-C., & Chan, A. S., (2003, July). Music training improves verbal but not visual memory: Cross-sectional and longitudinal explorations in children. *Neuropsychology, 17,* 439–450.

Hunter, M. (2004). *Mastery teaching.* Thousand Oaks, CA: Corwin Press.

Hyerle, D. (1996). *Visual tools for constructing knowledge.* Alexandria, VA: Association for Supervision and Curriculum Development.

Hyerle, D. (2004). *Student successes with thinking maps: School-based research, results, and models for achievement using visual tools.* Thousand Oaks, CA: Corwin Press.

Iverson, P., Kuhl, P. K., Akahane-Yamada, R., Diesch, E., Tohkura, Y., Kettermann, A., & Siebert, C. (2003, February). A perceptual interference account of acquisition difficulties for non-native phonemes. *Cognition, 87,* B47–B57.

Jausovec, N., & Jausovec, K. (2000, April 3). EEG activity during the performance of complex mental problems. *International Journal of Psychophysiology*, *36*, 73–88.

Johnson, J., & Newport, E. (1991). Critical period effects on universal properties of language: The status of subjacency in the acquisition of a second language. *Cognition*, *39*, 215–258.

Kempermann, G., & Gage, F. (1999, May). New nerve cells for the adult brain. *Scientific American, 280,* 48–53.

Key, N. (1991). *Research methodologies for whole-brained integration at the secondary level.* Report No. SP 037894. Pueblo, CO: U.S. Government Document Service.

Kim, A-H., Vaughn, S., Wanzek, J., & Wei, S. (2004). Graphic organizers and their effects on the reading comprehension of students with LD: A synthesis of research. *Journal of Learning Disabilities, 37,* 105–118.

Kim, K., Relkin, N., Lee, K., & Hirsch, J. (1997). Distinct cortical areas associated with native and second languages. Letter to *Nature*, *388*, 171–174.

Kimura, D. (1992, September). Sex differences in the brain. *Scientific American, 267,* 119– 124.

Kimura, D. (1997). *Sex and cognition.* Cambridge, MA: MIT Press.

Knecht, S., Deppe, M., Drager, B., Bobe, L., Lohmann, H., Ringelstein, E., & Henningsen, H. (2000, January). Language lateralization in healthy right-handers. *Brain*, *123*, 74–81.

Korol, D. L., & Gold, P. E. (1998). Glucose, memory, and aging. *American Journal of Clinical Nutrition*, *67*, 764S–771S.

Kosslyn, S. M., Pascual-Leone, A., Felician, O., Camposano, S., Keenan, J. P., Thompson, W. L., Ganis, G., Sukel, K. E., & Alpert, N. M. (1999, April 2). The role of Area 17 in visual imagery: Convergent evidence from PET and rTMS. *Science*, *284*, 167–170.

Kotulak, R. (1996). *Inside the brain: Revolutionary discoveries of how the mind works.* Kansas City, MO: Andrews McMeel.

Kripke, D. F., Youngstedt, S. D., & Elliot, J. A. (1997). Light brightness effects on melatonin duration. *Sleep Research*, *26*, 726.

Kuhlmann, S., Kirschbaum, C., & Wolf, O. T. (2005, March). Effects of oral cortisol treatment in healthy young women on memory retrieval of negative and neutral words. *Neurobiology of Learning and Memory, 83,* 158–162.

Laviola, G., Adriani, W., Terranova, M. L., & Gerra, G. (1999). Psychobiological risk factors for vulnerability to psychostimulants in human adolescents and animal models. *Neuroscience Biobehavior Review*, *23*(7), 993–1010.

LeBoutillier, N., & Marks, D. F. (2003, February). Mental imagery and creativity: A meta-analytic review study. *British Journal of Psychology, 94,* 29–44.

Leonard, J. (1999, May-June). The sorcerer's apprentice: Unlocking the secrets of the brain's basement. *Harvard Magazine*, 56–62.

Lieberman, B. (2005, June). Study narrows search for brain's memory site. *Brain in the News, 12,* 4.

Loftus, E. (1997, September). Creating false memories. *Scientific American, 277,* 51–55.

Loomans, D., & Kolberg, K. (1993). *The laughing classroom: Everyone's guide to teaching with humor and play*. New York: H. J. Kramer.

Luciana, M., Conklin, H. M., Hooper, C. J., & Yarger, R. S. (2005). The development of nonverbal working memory and executive control processes in adolescents. *Child Development, 76,* 697–712.

Lutchmaya, S., Baron-Cohen, S., & Raggatt, P. (2002). Fetal testosterone and vocabulary size in 18– and 24-month-old infants. *Infant Behavior and Development, 24,* 418–424.

Lynch, G. (2002). Memory enhancement: The search for mechanism-based drugs. *Nature Neuroscience, 5,* 1035–1038.

Maquire, E. A., Frith, C. D., & Morris, R. G. M. (1999, October). The functional neuroanatomy of comprehension and memory: The importance of prior knowledge. *Brain, 122*, 1839–1850.

Mazard, A., Laou, L., Joliot, M., & Mellet, E. (2005, August). Neural impact of the semantic content of visual mental images and visual percepts. *Cognitive Brain Research, 24,* 423–435.

Menon, V., & Levitin, D. J. (2005, October). The rewards of music listening: Response and physiological connectivity of the mesolimbic system. *NeuroImage, 28,* 175–184.

Merzenich, M. M., Jenkins, W. M., Johnston, P., Schreiner, C., Miller, S. L., & Tallal, P. (1996, January 5). Temporal processing deficits of language-learning impaired children ameliorated by training. *Science*, 271.

Mestre, J. (2002). *Transfer of learning: Issues and research agenda.* Arlington, VA: National Science Foundation.

Miller, G. A. (1956). The magical number seven, plus-or-minus two: Some limits on our capacity for processing information. *Psychological Review, 101*, 343–352.

Millichap, J. G., & Yee, M. M. (2003). The diet factor in pediatric and adolescent migraine. *Pediatric Neurology, 28,* 9–15.

Millman, R. P. (2005, June). Excessive sleepiness in adolescents and young adults: Causes, consequences, and treatment strategies. *Pediatrics, 115,* 1774–1786.

Moore, K. D. (2005). *Effective instructional strategies: From theory to practice.* Thousand Oaks, CA: Sage Publications.

Muftuler, L. T., Bodner, M., Shaw, G. L., & Nalcioglu, O. (1999). *fMRI of Mozart effect using auditory stimuli.* Abstract presented at the 7th meeting of the International Society for Magnetic Resonance in Medicine, Philadelphia.

Nakamura, S., Sadato, N., Oohashi, T., Nishina, E., Fuwamoto, Y., & Yonekura, Y. (1999, November 19). Analysis of music-brain interaction with simultaneous measurement of regional cerebral blood flow and electroencephalogram beta rhythm in human subjects. *Neuroscience Letters, 275*, 222–226.

National Center for Education Statistics. (NCES). (2003). *The nation's report card, 2003.* Washington, DC: Author.

National Governors Association (NGA). (2005). *2005 Rate Your Future Survey.* Washington, DC: Author. Available online at http://www.nga.org

National Reading Panel. (NRP). (2000). *Teaching children to read: An evidence-based assessment of the scientific research literature and its implications for reading instruction.* Washington, DC: National Institute of Child Health and Human Development.

Neubauer, A. C., Grabner, R. H., Fink, A., & Neuper, C. (2005). Intelligence and neural efficiency: Further evidence of the influence of task content and sex on the brain-IQ relationship. *Cognitive Brain Research, 25,* 217–225.

Neubauer, A. C., Grabner, R. H., Freudenthaler, H. H., Beckmann, J. F., & Guthke, J. (2004, May). Intelligence and individual differences in becoming neurally efficient. *Acta Psychologica, 116,* 55–74.

Njemanze, P. C. (2005, March). Cerebral lateralization and general intelligence: Gender differences in a transcranial Doppler study. *Brain and Language, 92,* 234–239.

Norton, A., Winner, E., Cronin, K., Overy, K., Lee, D. J., & Schlaug, G. (2005). Are there pre-existing neural, cognitive, or motoric markers for musical ability? *Brain and Cognition*.

Oberauer, K., & Kliegl, R. (2004, August). Simultaneous cognitive operations in working memory after dual-task practice. *Journal of Experimental Psychology: Human Perception and Performance, 30,* 689–707.

Oberman, L. M., Hubbard, E. M., McCleery, J. P., Altschuler, E. L., Ramachandran, V. S., & Pineda, J. A. (2005, July). EEG evidence for mirror neuron dysfunction in autism spectrum disorders. *Cognitive Brain Research, 24,* 190–198.

Ornstein, R., & Thompson, R. (1984). *The amazing brain*. Boston: Houghton Mifflin.

Parrott, C. A. (1986). Visual imagery training: Stimulating utilization of imaginal processes. *Journal of Mental Imagery, 10*, 47–64.

Parsons, L. M., & Osherson, D. (2001, October). New evidence for distinct right and left brain systems for deductive versus probabilistic reasoning. *Cerebral Cortex, 11,* 954–965.

Patterson, M. N. (1997). *Every body can learn*. Tucson, AZ: Zephyr.

Paus, T. (2005). Mapping brain maturation and cognitive development during adolescence. *Trends in Cognitive Sciences, 9,* 60–68.

Penhune, V. B., & Doyon, J. (2005, July). Cerebellum and M1 interaction during early learning of timed motor sequences. *NeuroImage, 26,* 801–812.

Perkins, D., & Salomon, G. (1988, September). Teaching for transfer. *Educational Leadership*, *46*, 22–32.

Perani, D., & Abutalebi, J. (2005, April). The neural basis of first and second language processing. *Current Opinion in Neurobiology, 15,* 202–206.

Petrosini, L., Graziano, A., Mandolesi, L., Neri, P., Molinari, M., & Leggio, M. G. (2003, June). Watch how to do it! New advances in learning by observation. *Brain Research Reviews, 42,* 252–264.

Pinker, S. (1994). *The language instinct: How the mind creates language*. New York: Harper Perennial.

Poe, M. D., Burchinal, M. R., & Roberts, J. E. (2004). Early language and the development of children's reading skills. *Journal of School Psychology, 42,* 315–332.

Press, D. Z., Casement, M. D., Pascual-Leone, A., & Robertson, E. M. (2005). The time course of off-line motor sequence learning. *Cognitive Brain Research, 25,* 375–378.

Rabkin, N., & Redmond, R. (2004). *Putting the arts in the picture: Reforming education in the 21st century.* Chicago: Columbia College.

Raths, J. (2002, Autumn). Improving instruction. *Theory Into Practice, 41,* 233–237.

Rauscher, F. H., & Zupan, M. A. (2000). Classroom keyboard instruction improves kindergarten children's spatial-temporal performance: A field experiment. *Early Childhood Research Quarterly, 15,* 215–228.

Rauscher, F. H., Shaw, G. L., Levine, L. J., Wright, E. L., Dennis, W. R., & Newcomb, R. L. (1997). Music training causes long-term enhancement of preschool children's spatial-temporal reasoning. *Neurological Research*, *19*, 2–8.

Reiss, D., Neiderheiser, J., Hetherington, E. M., & Plomin, R. (2000). *The relationship code: Deciphering genetic and social influences on adolescent development*. Cambridge, MA: Harvard University Press.

Restak, R. M. (2001). *The secret life of the brain.* Washington, DC: Dana Press.

Restak, R. M. (2003). *The new brain: How the modern age is rewiring your mind.* New York: Rodale.

Ringo, J. L., Doty, R. W., Demeter, S., & Simard, P. Y. (1994). Time is of the essence: A conjecture that hemispheric specialization arises from interhemispheric conduction delays. *Journal of the Cerebral Cortex, 4,* 331–343.

Roberts, P., & Kellough, D. (2003). *A guide for developing interdisciplinary thematic units* (3rd Ed.). Englewood Cliffs, NJ: Prentice Hall.

Rodier, P. (2000, February). The early origins of autism. *Scientific American*, *282*, 56–63.

Roediger, H. L., III, & McDermott, K. B. (1995). Creating false memories: Remembering words not presented in lists. *Journal of Experimental Psychology: Learning, Memory, and Cognition*, *21*, 803–814.

Root-Bernstein, R. S. (1997, July 11). Art for science's sake. *Chronicle of Higher Education*, B6.

Rose, S. (1992). *The making of memory*. New York: Doubleday.

Rose, S. (2005). *The future of the brain: The promise and perils of tomorrow's neuroscience.* New York: Oxford University Press.

Rowe, M. B. (1974). Wait-time and rewards as instructional variables: Their influence on language, logic, and fate control. *Journal of Research on Science Teaching*, *2*, 81–94.

Russell, P. (1979). *The brain book*. New York: E. P. Dutton.

Schacter, D. L. (1996). *Searching for memory: The brain, mind, and the past*. New York: Basic Books.

Schacter, D. L. (2001). *The seven sins of memory.* New York: Houghton Mifflin.

Schafer, G. (2005). Infants can learn decontextualized words before their first birthday. *Child Development, 76,* 87–96.

Schank, R. C. (1990). *Tell me a story: Narrative and intelligence.* Evanston, IL: Northwestern University Press.

Schlaug, G., Jancke, L., Huang, Y. X., & Steinmetz, H. (1995). In-vivo evidence of structural brain asymmetry in musicians. *Science*, *267*, 699–701.

Schmidt, S. R. (1995). Effects of humor on sentence memory. *Journal of Experimental Psychology: Learning, Memory and Cognition, 20,* 953–967.

Schmidt, S. R. (2002). The humour effect: Differential processing and privileged retrieval. *Memory, 10,* 127–138.

Schmithhorst, V. J., & Holland, S. K. (2004, January). The effect of musical training on the neural correlates of math processing: A functional magnetic resonance imaging study in humans. *Neuroscience Letters, 354,* 193–196.

Scholey, A. B., Moss, M. C., Neave, N., & Wesnes, K. (1999, November). Cognitive performance, hyperoxia, and heart rate following oxygen administration in healthy young adults. *Physiological Behavior*, *67*, 783–789.

Scott-Simmons, D., Barker, J., & Cherry, N. (2003, May). Integrating research and story writng. *The Reading Teacher, 56,* 742–745.

Shadmehr, R., & Holcomb, H. H. (1997, August 8). Neural correlates of motor memory consolidation. *Science*, *277*, 821–825.

Shallice, T. (1999, July). The origin of confabulations. *Nature Neuroscience*, *2*, 588–590.

Shaywitz, S. E. (2003). *Overcoming dyslexia: A new and complete science-based program for reading problems at any level.* New York: Knopf.

Shaywitz, B. A., Shaywitz, S. E., & Gore, J. (1995). Sex differences in the functional organization of the brain for language. *Nature*, *373*, 607–609.

Shaywitz, S. E., Shaywitz, B. A., Pugh, K. R., Fulbright, R. K., Constable, R. T., Mencl, W. E., Shankweiler, D. P., Liberman, A. M., Skudlarski, P., Fletcher, J. M., Katz, L., Marchione, K. E., Lacadie, C., Gatenby, C., & Gore, J. C. (1998, March 3). Functional disruption in the organization of the brain for reading in dyslexia. *Neurobiology*, *5*, 2636–2641.

Shearer, B. (2004). Multiple intelligences theory after 20 years. *Teachers College Record, 106,* 2–16.

Silverberg, S., & Samuel, A. G. (2004, October). The effect of age of second language acquisition on the representation and processing of second language words. *Journal of Memory and Language, 51,* 381–398.

Smith, E. E., & Jonides, J. (1999, March 12). Storage and executive processes in the frontal lobes. *Science*, *283*, 1657–1661.

Sousa, D. A. (1998a, May). Brain research can help principals reform secondary schools. *NASSP Bulletin*, *82*, 21–28.

Sousa, D. A. (1998b, December 16). Is the fuss about brain research justified? *Education Week*, p. 52.

Sousa, D. A. (2003). *The leadership brain: How to lead today's schools more effectively.* Thousand Oaks, CA: Corwin Press.

Sousa, D. A. (2005). *How the brain learns to read.* Thousand Oaks, CA: Corwin Press.

Sowell, E. R., Thompson, P. M., Holmes, C. J., Jernigan, T. L., & Toga, A. W. (1999). In-vivo evidence for post-adolescent brain maturation in frontal and striatal regions. *Nature: Neuroscience*, *2*, 859–861.

Spencer, S. J., Steele, C. M., & Quinn, D. M. (1999, January). Stereotype threat and women's math performance. *Journal of Experimental Social Psychology*, *35*, 4–28.

Sperry, R. (1966). Brain bisection and consciousness. In Eccles, J. (Ed.), *How the self controls its brain.* New York: Springer-Verlag.

Springer, S. P., & Deutsch, G. (1998). *Left brain/right brain* (5th ed.). New York: W. H. Freeman.

Squire, L. R., & Kandel, E. R. (1999). *Memory: From mind to molecules*. New York: W. H. Freeman.

Stahl, R. J. (1985). *Cognitive information processes and processing within a uniprocess superstructure/microstructure framework: A practical information-based model*. Unpublished manuscript, University of Arizona, Tucson.

Stein, H. (1987, July-August). Visualized notetaking: Left-right brain theory applied in the classroom. *The Social Studies*.

Steinberg, L. (2005). Cognitive and effective development in adolescence. *Trends in Cognitive Sciences, 9,* 69–74.

Sternberg, R. J., Ferrari, M., Clinkenbeard, P. R., & Grigorenko, E. L. (1996). Identification, instruction, and assessment of gifted children: A construct validation of a triarchic model. *Gifted Child Quarterly, 40,* 129–137.

Sternberg, R. J., Grigorenko, E. L., Jarvin, L., Clinkenbeard, P., Ferrari, M., & Torfi, B. (2000, Spring). The effectiveness of triarchic teaching and assessment. *National Research Center on the Gifted and Talented Newsletter,* 3–8.

Tallal, P., Miller, S. L., Bedi, G., Byma, G., Wang, X., Nagarajan, S., Schreiner, C., Jenkins, W. M., & Merzenich, M. M. (1996, January 5). Fast-element enhanced speech improves language comprehension in language-learning impaired children. *Science*, *271*, 81–84.

Terry, W. S. (2005). Serial position effects in recall of television commercials. *Journal of General Psychology, 132,* 151–163.

Thomas, E. (1972, April). The variation of memory with time for information appearing during a lecture. *Studies in Adult Education*, 57–62.

Thomas, L. (1979). *The Medusa and the snail*. New York: Viking Press.

Tuma, R. S. (2005, July-August). An eye on shut-eye. *Brain Work, 15,* p. 6.

United States Department of Education. (USDOE). (2000). *Elementary and secondary survey, 2000.* Washington, DC: Author.

Van Petten, C., & Bloom, P. (1999, February). Speech boundaries, syntax, and the brain. *Nature Neuroscience*, *2*, 103–104.

Vaughn, K. (2000, Fall). Music and mathematics: Modest support for the oft-claimed relationship. *Journal of Aesthetic Education, 34,* 149–166.

Vaughn, K., & Winner, E. (2000, Fall). SAT scores of students who study the arts: What we can and cannot conclude about the association. *Journal of Aesthetic Education, 34,* 77–89.

Wagner, A. D., Schacter, D. L., Rotte, M., Koutstaal, W., Maril, A., Dale, A. M., Rosen, B. R., & Buckner, R. L. (1998, August 21). Building memories: Remembering and forgetting of verbal experiences as predicted by brain activity. *Science*, *281*, 1188–1191.

Walker, M. P., Stickgold, R., Alsop, D., Gaab, N., & Schlaug, G. (2005). Sleep-dependent motor memory plasticity in the human brain. *Neuroscience, 133,* 911–917.

Weinberger, N. M. (2004, November). Music and the brain. *Scientific American, 291,* 89–95.

Weisman, D. H., & Banich, M. T. (2000). The cerebral hemispheres cooperate to perform complex but not simple tasks. *Neuropsychology*, *14*, 41–59.

West, C. K., Farmer, J. A., & Wolff, P. M. (1991). *Instructional design: Implications from cognitive science.* Englewood, Cliffs, NJ: Prentice-Hall.

Wigfield, A., & Eccles, J. S. (2002). Students' motivation during the middle school years. In J. Aronson (Ed.), *Improving academic development: Impact of psychological factors in education.* New York: Academic Press.

Witney, A. G. (2004, November). Internal models for bi-manual tasks. *Human Movement Science, 23,* 747–770.

Wixted, J. T. (2004). The psychology and neuroscience of forgetting. *Annual Review of Psychology, 55,* 235–269.

Wolfson, A., & Carskadon, M. (1998). Sleep schedules and daytime functioning in adolescents. *Child Development, 69*, 875–887.

Wulf, G., Shea, C. H., & Matschiner, S. (1998). Frequent feedback enhances complex motor skill learning. *Journal of Motor Behavior, 30,* 180–192.

Zimmerman, F. J., & Christakis, D. A. (2005, July). Children's television viewing and cognitive outcomes: A longitudinal analysis of national data. *Archives of Pediatrics and Adolescent Medicine, 159,* 619–625.

Resources

Books

Berninger, V., & Richards, T. (2002). *Brain literacy for educators and psychologists.* San Diego, CA: Academic Press.

Calvin, W. (2004). *A brief history of the mind: From apes to intellect and beyond.* New York: Oxford University Press.

Damasio, A. (2003). *Looking for Spinoza: Joy, sorrow and the feeling brain.* New York: Harcourt Brace.

Edelman, G. (2004). *Wider than the sky: The phenomenal gift of consciousness.* New Haven, CT: Yale University Press.

Juslin, P. N., & Sloboda, J. A. (2001). *Music and emotion: Theory and research.* New York: Oxford University Press.

Pinker, S. (2002). *The blank slate: The modern denial of human nature.* New York: Viking.

Ridley, M. (2003). *Nature via nurture: Genes, experience, and what makes us human.* New York: Harper Collins.

Strauch, B. (2003). *The primal teen: What the new discoveries about the teenage brain tell us about our kids.* New York: Doubleday.

Sylwester, R. (2005). *How to explain a brain: An educator's handbook of brain terms and cognitive processes.* Thousand Oaks, CA: Corwin Press.

Internet Sites

Brain Connection

www.brainconnection.com

Brainland: The Neuroscience Information Center

www.brainland.com

Although this site is designed for professionals in neuroscience, educators interested in brain research will find a lot of interesting information.

The Center for Applied Linguistics

www.cal.org

This is a private, non-profit organization that uses the findings of linguistics and related sciences in identifying and addressing language-related problems. CAL carries out a wide range of activities including research, teacher education, analysis and dissemination of information, design and development of instructional materials, technical assistance, and program evaluation.

The Center for Arts Education

www.cae-nyc.org

This Center is committed to restoring, stimulating, and sustaining quality arts education as an essential part of every child's education. It identifies, funds, and supports exemplary partnerships and programs that demonstrate how the arts contribute to learning and student achievement. Although the Center mainly supports New York City's schools, its Web site has useful information about arts programs and resources.

Dana Alliance for Brain Initiatives

www.dana.org

Earobics Literacy Launch

Cognitive Concepts, Inc.
www.earobic.com

A research-based supplemental reading program for students in pre-kindergarten through grade 3. A combination of computer technology, multimedia tools, and print materials support components in phonological awareness, vocabulary, fluency, phonics, and reading comprehension.

Education Resources Information Center (ERIC)

www.eric.ed.gov

Fast ForWord Reading Language Program

Scientific Learning Corporation
www.scientificlearning.com

A scientifically based computer program that is designed for helping beginning readers develop phonemic awareness, letter-sound correspondences, fluent word recognition, vocabulary, and an appreciation of literature. Programs for older struggling readers are also available.

Inspiration Software, Inc.

http://inspiration.com

This company produces software that helps students construct all types of visual organizers for improving comprehension and building thinking skills. *Kidspiration* is designed for grades K through 5, and *Inspiration* is for grade 6 and higher. Demonstration versions can be downloaded from the site.

National Institutes of Health
www.nih.gov

National Network for Early Language Learning (NNELL)
www.nnell.org

This is an organization for educators involved in teaching foreign languages to children. The organization facilitates cooperation among organizations directly concerned with early language learning; facilitates communication among teachers, teacher educators, parents, program administrators, and policymakers; and disseminates information and guidelines to assist in developing programs of excellence.

Neuroscience for Kids
http://faculty.washington.edu/chudler/neurok.html

The Society for Neuroscience
www.sfn.org

Educators will find useful information in *Brain Briefings* and *Brain Backgrounders.*

Thematic Units Sites:
Lesson Plans for K-12 Teachers: http://library.csus.edu/guides/rogenmoserd/educ/lesson.htm
A to Z Teacher Stuff/Themes: http://atozteacherstuff.com/Themes/
CA Dept. of Education/Recommended Literature: http://www.cde.ca.gov/ci/rl/ll/
Lessonplanz.com Thematic Units: http://lessonplanz.com/Lesson_Plans/Thematic_Units/
Teacher Guide.com Thematic Units: http://www.theteachersguide.com/Thematicunits.html

U.S. Department of Education
www.ed.gov

Whole Brain Atlas
www.med.harvard.edu/AANLIB/home.html

Hundreds of different types of brain scans.

Index

Page numbers in **boldface** are **Practitioner's Corners.**

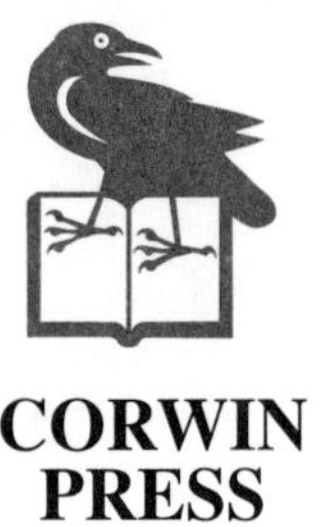

The Corwin Press logo—a raven striding across an open book—represents the union of courage and learning. Corwin Press is committed to improving education for all learners by publishing books and other professional development resources for those serving the field of PreK–12 education. By providing practical, hands-on materials, Corwin Press continues to carry out the promise of its motto: **"Helping Educators Do Their Work Better."**